WN 100

Normal Variants and Pitfalls in Imaging

JAMES B. VOGLER, III, M.D.
Chief of Skeletal Radiology
Department of Radiology
David Grant U.S. Air Force Medical Center
Travis Air Force Base, California

CLYDE A. HELMS, M.D.
Associate Professor of Radiology
University of California Medical Center
School of Medicine
San Francisco, California

PETER W. CALLEN, M.D.
Associate Professor of Radiology,
Obstetrics and Gynecology
University of California Medical Center
School of Medicine
San Francisco, California

1986

W. B. SAUNDERS COMPANY
Philadelphia - London - Toronto - Mexico City
Rio de Janeiro - Sydney - Tokyo - Hong Kong

W. B. Saunders Company: West Washington Square
                          Philadelphia, PA   19105

Library of Congress Cataloging in Publication Data

Vogler, James B., III

Normal variants and pitfalls in imaging.

1. Diagnostic imaging.   I. Helms, Clyde A.
II. Callen, Peter W.   III. Title. [DNLM: 1. Nuclear
Magnetic Resonance—diagnostic use. 2. Nuclear Medicine.
3. Technology, Radiologic. 4. Tomography, X-Ray Computed.
5. Ultrasonic Diagnosis. WN 160 V883]

RC78.7.D53V64 1986   616.07'57   85–18304

ISBN 0–7216–1457–4

Disclaimer

The opinions expressed herein are those of the authors and do not necessarily reflect the official policy of the U.S. Department of Defense or the U.S. Air Force.

Editor: Dana Dreibelbis
Designer: Terri Siegel
Production Manager: Bill Preston
Manuscript Editor: Kate Mason
Illustration Coordinator: Walt Verbitski
Page Layout Artist: Patti Maddaloni

Normal Variants and Pitfalls in Imaging   ISBN   0–7216–1457–4

Last digit is the print number: 9   8   7   6   5   4   3   2   1

To James B. Vogler, Jr. and Sarah C. Vogler—
there are those you can never repay

—JBV

To Tracy Gene Helms
1955–1985
my brother and close friend

—CAH

To Brooke and Melanie

—PWC

Contributors

WILLIAM E. BRANT, M.D.
Chief of Ultrasound and Computed Tomography, Department of Radiology, and Chief of Diagnostic Radiology, David Grant U.S. Air Force Medical Center, Travis Air Force Base, California.

PETER W. CALLEN, M.D.
Associate Professor of Radiology, Obstetrics and Gynecology, Department of Radiology, University of California School of Medicine, San Francisco, California.

FREDERIC A. CONTE, M.D.
Fellow, Nuclear Medicine Service/SGHQRI, Wilford Hall U.S. Air Force Medical Center, Lackland Air Force Base, Texas.

CHARLES M. GLASIER, M.D.
Assistant Professor of Radiology and Pediatrics and Pediatric Radiologist, Arkansas Children's Hospital and University of Arkansas for Medical Sciences, Little Rock, Arkansas.

ALBERT S. HALE, M.D.
Chairman, Department of Radiology, Wilford Hall U.S. Air Force Medical Center/SGHQR, Lackland Air Force Base, Texas.

CLYDE A. HELMS, M.D.
Associate Professor of Radiology, Department of Radiology, University of California School of Medicine, San Francisco, California.

HEDVIG HRICAK, M.D.
Associate Professor of Radiology and Neurology, Department of Radiology, University of California School of Medicine, San Francisco, California.

DONALD E. JACKSON, M.D.
Assistant Chief of Nuclear Medicine Section, Department of Radiology, David Grant U.S. Air Force Medical Center, Travis Air Force Base, California.

R. BROOKE JEFFREY, JR., M.D.
Associate Professor of Radiology, University of California, San Francisco, School of Medicine, San Francisco, California.

WILLIAM M. KELLY, M.D.
Assistant Clinical Professor of Neuroradiology, University of California, San Francisco; Chief of Neuroradiology, David Grant U.S. Air Force Medical Center, Travis Air Force Base, California.

DAVID L. LAMASTERS, M.D.
Chief of Diagnostic and Interventional Neuroradiology, Wilford Hall U.S. Air Force Medical Center, Lackland Air Force Base, Texas.

BARRY S. MAHONY, M.D.
Assistant Professor, Department of Radiology, and Attending Radiologist, Duke University Medical Center, Durham, North Carolina.

JAMES R. McCONNELL, M.D.
Assistant Professor of Radiology and Pediatrics and Pediatric Radiologist, Arkansas Children's Hospital and University of Arkansas for Medical Sciences, Little Rock, Arkansas.

JOSEPH A. ORZEL, M.D.
Assistant Chief, Nuclear Medicine Service/SGHQRI, Wilford Hall U.S. Air Force Medical Center, Lackland Air Force Base, Texas.

CHARLES E. PETERSON, M.D.
Clinical Assistant Professor, Wright State University School of Medicine, Dayton; Chairman, Nuclear Medicine, U.S. Air Force Medical Center, Wright-Patterson Air Force Base, Ohio.

MICHAEL L. RICHARDSON, M.D.
Assistant Professor of Radiology, Department of Radiology, University of Washington, Seattle; Director of Skeletal Radiology, Harborview Medical Center, Seattle, Washington.

HANS RINGERTZ, M.D.
Professor of Diagnostic Radiology, Karolinska Institute, Stockholm; Chairman of Diagnostic Radiology, Huddinge University Hospital, Stockholm, Sweden.

ARTHUR T. ROSENFIELD, M.D.
Professor of Diagnostic Radiology, Yale University School of Medicine; Head, Section of Computed Tomography, Yale–New Haven Hospital, New Haven, Connecticut.

EDWARD A. SICKLES, M.D.
Associate Professor of Radiology, University of California School of Medicine, San Francisco; Chief, Breast Imaging Section, University of California Medical Center, San Francisco, California.

JAMES B. VOGLER, III, M.D.

Chief of Skeletal Radiology, Department of Radiology, David Grant U.S. Air Force Medical Center, Travis Air Force Base, California.

SUSAN D. WALL, M.D.

Assistant Professor of Radiology, University of California School of Medicine, San Francisco, California.

W. RICHARD WEBB, M.D.

Associate Professor of Radiology, University of California School of Medicine, San Francisco, California.

FREDERICK L. WEILAND, M.D.

Chief and Program Director, Nuclear Medicine Service/ SGHQRI, Wilford Hall U.S. Air Force Medical Center, Lackland Air Force Base, Texas.

ROBERT K. ZEMAN, M.D.

Associate Professor of Radiology, Georgetown University School of Medicine; Chief of Abdominal Imaging Division and Computerized Tomography Laboratory, Georgetown University Hospital, Washington, D.C.

Preface

Knowledge advances by steps, and not by leaps.
—THOMAS BABINGTON MACAULAY, 1828

Long before the advent of radiology, variations in normal human anatomy had been recognized by physicians and anatomists. The importance of these normal variants has been reinforced throughout the history of medicine by the publication of numerous articles describing some of them in detail. Knowledge of many of the variants, however, was passed on only by the teachings of more experienced physicians to younger apprentices. Because of the commonplace nature of some of the variants, documentation was not always felt to be necessary. As the field of medicine expanded, the need to document many of these normal variations increased. It no longer seemed possible to pass on the rapidly expanding fund of knowledge by direct teaching. Without documentation, many individuals entering the practice of medicine were left to agonize over whether these variants were, in fact, normal or pathologic. Much effort was duplicated in researching these entities, often with little success.

The radiograph is but an image of anatomy; thus, the above scenario has been repeated innumerable times since the advent of the specialty of radiology. Many individuals in the field of radiology have recognized the need to document variations in normal anatomy so that others might benefit from their experience. Attempts to catalogue these variants have been ongoing for years. These efforts began with *Pediatric X-Ray Diagnosis* by Dr. John Caffey and *Borderlands of the Normal and Early Pathologic in Skeletal Roentgenology* by Dr. Alban Kohler and continued with the works of Dr. Theodore E. Keats, including *An Atlas of Normal Roentgen Variants That May Simulate Disease*. To these individuals, we owe a debt of gratitude. The practice of radiology has benefited by their efforts.

The specialty of radiology has dramatically expanded with the addition of several different imaging modalities over a relatively short period of time. With all the changes that have occurred, and the different ways in which the anatomy of the human body can now be imaged, there still remains the task of differentiating the normal from the abnormal and the pathologic from the non-pathologic. A normal variation remains just that, whether it is visualized on standard radiographs or on computed tomography scans. Yet, just as normal anatomy is seen in a different perspective with the newer modalities, so are normal anatomic variations. Thus, the need arises, as in the past, to document the appearance of these variations so that others who may encounter them will not have to "reinvent the wheel."

Normal variants represent only a portion of the problem encountered in the use of imaging modalities other than conventional radiography. The sophisticated imaging modalities of today bring with them sophisticated problems. It is no longer enough to recognize the normal variations in anatomy that may mimic pathology; one must now also be able to recognize technologic artifacts, many of which may also simulate pathology, produced by these sophisticated machines. These artifacts are the pitfalls of modern imaging.

The normal variants and pitfalls illustrated in this text are grouped primarily by imaging modality. In each major section dealing with a specific modality, each respective chapter, where applicable, deals with a specific organ system or anatomic region. Running heads throughout the book direct the reader to more specific anatomic sites within the chapters. Separation of each imaging modality allows the reader quick access to the specific imaging question at hand; inherent in this format, however, is the repetition of certain variants and pitfalls within each major section and between the different imaging modalities.

Scattered throughout the text are examples of pathologic processes; there are several reasons for their inclusion. Since many of the normal variants and pitfalls mimic pathologic processes, some of these pathologic entities are included for the purpose of comparison. Additionally, some of the pitfalls relate to compromised interpretation of pathologic processes, owing to technical artifacts; in these instances, examples of pathology have also been included.

Because of the nature of many of the examples, pathologic proof was not consistently available. In most instances, it was difficult to justify subjecting a patient to biopsy of what almost certainly represents a benign process. Thus, we were left to prove the nature of many entities as best we could, realizing that, in the future, some of the explanations offered may not prove to be correct.

When possible, references are included to indicate the source where an illustrated entity was described or documented. Many of the variants and pitfalls lack documentation, resulting, in part, from the relatively recent introduction and short use of some imaging modalities. In certain instances, the illustrated entities simply may have not yet been documented in the literature. Similarly, no established explantations exist as to why some of the technical artifacts are seen while others remain only partially explained. With time and increased understanding of the technology, the explanations may become apparent. At present, however, this uncertainty remains a stimulus to investigation for some and a source of frustration for others. With the publication of this text, it is hoped that false-positive diagnoses will decrease and diagnostic accuracy will improve, to the benefit of both patient and physician.

JAMES B. VOGLER, III
CLYDE A. HELMS
PETER W. CALLEN

Acknowledgments

An undertaking of this size rarely results from the efforts of only a few individuals. We wish to thank the many people without whose efforts this project would never have been possible. To the contributing authors, we are indeed grateful. It seems that the busiest people somehow always find the time to take on one more important project. Additionally, we are grateful to these individuals for recognizing the need for a text such as this and for approaching their contributions in a professional manner. Several of the illustrations used by the contributors and ourselves were reprinted from other works; we are indebted to the many authors and publishers who graciously allowed us to reproduce their figures.

Special acknowledgment is due Dr. Theodore E. Keats, who many years ago, without his knowing it, provided the inspiration and foundation for this work through his book *An Atlas of Normal Roentgen Variants That May Simulate Disease*. The recognized excellence of that text was the stimulus to provide a similar service in the newer imaging modalities of radiology.

The secretarial and administrative assistance necessary to a project such as this is indeed substantial. Sheer numbers prohibit recognizing each of these individuals; however, to all of those who provided such assistance to us and to the contributors, we offer our deep appreciation.

Finally, we would like to express our sincere thanks to the many individuals at the W. B. Saunders Company who believed in this project from its inception and who then helped us along the way. Specifically, we would like to thank Dana Dreibelbis, executive editor, for methodically directing the editorial staff and for coordinating each step of this massive undertaking; Janice McCusker, editorial assistant, for untiring support; Kate Mason, copy editor, for meticulous and invaluable manuscript editing; Bill Preston, production manager, for skillful scheduling of book production; Terri Siegel, designer, for innovative internal and book cover design; and Walt Verbitski, illustration coordinator, for accomplishing the difficult task of coordinating and processing the thousands of illustrations appearing in this book.

JAMES B. VOGLER, III
CLYDE A. HELMS
PETER W. CALLENS

Contents

III
NUCLEAR MEDICINE

I

COMPUTED TOMOGRAPHY (CT)

Physics and Artifacts

WILLIAM E. BRANT, M.D.

Figure 1–1. VOLUME AVERAGING. Each CT image is a two-dimensional representation of a three-dimensional slice of patient tissue produced by averaging the x-ray attenuation of small volumes of patient tissue. Each two-dimensional picture element (pixel) represents a three-dimensional volume of patient tissue (voxel). A CT number representing the calculated volume average attenuation of each voxel is assigned to each pixel. The CT number is characteristic of the tissue in each voxel only if the voxel is homogeneous. When objects of widely different x-ray attenuation occupy the same volume element of patient tissue, the calculated attenuation value (CT number) is proportional to their average value and is characteristic of neither. Volume average effect is present in every CT image and must always be considered in image interpretation.

Figure 1–1A. A low-density area *(arrows)* in the left lobe of the liver simulates a mass lesion. The pixels in this low-density area represent a volume average of fat surrounding the heart and liver parenchyma. No mass lesion is present. In the slice just above the one shown, pericardial fat was present in the same area as the lesion. Careful analysis of sequential slices near suspected lesions will usually reveal the source of the volume average artifact.

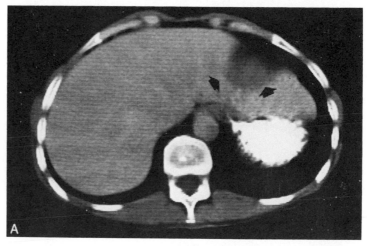

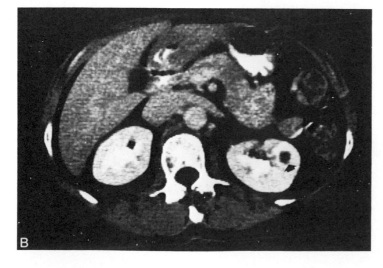

Figure 1–1B. A low-density lesion *(arrow)* is demonstrated in the left kidney. Because the size of the lesion is approximately equal to the thickness of the image slice (10 mm), volume average effect will be significant. Although this lesion was confirmed by ultrasound to be a simple renal cyst, its average CT number was +27 HU, well above the range usually accepted as cystic fluid. This elevation of average CT number is due to the presence of high-density contrast–enhanced renal parenchyma within the same voxels shared by the cyst. Volume average effect can be minimized by using thin slices and small pixel sizes (targeted or "zoom" reconstructed images).

Ref.: Goodenough D, Weaver K, Davis D, LaFalce S. Volume averaging limitations of computed tomography. AJR 1982; 138:313–316.

Figure 1–2. BLOOMING—POINT SPREAD EFFECT. Manipulation of the window width and window level controls can have a significant influence on measurements of size of structures in the CT image.

    Studies by Baxter and Sorenson indicate that size measurements are most accurate when the window level is centered midway between the background density and the object density. Small spherical objects must be centered within the CT slice, and the slice thickness must be less than the diameter of the sphere. If these conditions are met, the size measurements are accurate to approximately 1 mm.

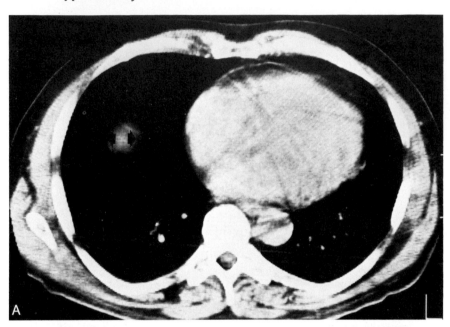

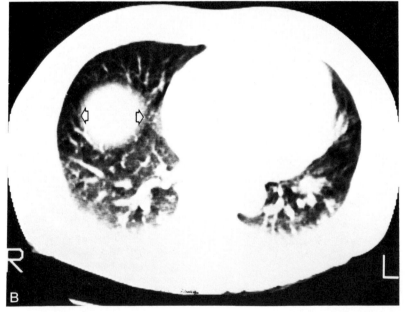

Figure 1–2A and B. In *A,* the diameter of the dome of the right hemidiaphragm measures 24 mm *(arrows)* at a window width of 250 HU and window level of +30 HU. The same slice at window width 1000 HU and window level −500 HU is shown in *B.* The diameter of the dome of the right hemidiaphragm now measures 43 mm *(arrows).* This variation in measurement is related to two factors. The first is volume averaging. The diaphragm and underlying dome of the liver arc through the 10-mm slice thickness occupy a different percentage volume of adjacent voxels. Second, only a portion of a wide range of CT numbers is represented in the viewed image at any particular setting of window width and window level. The tissues of interest may exceed this range and may not be visualized. This results in object boundaries that appear to shift position at different viewing settings.

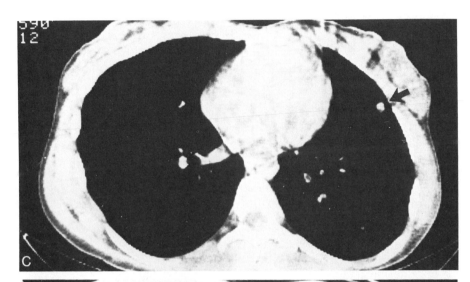

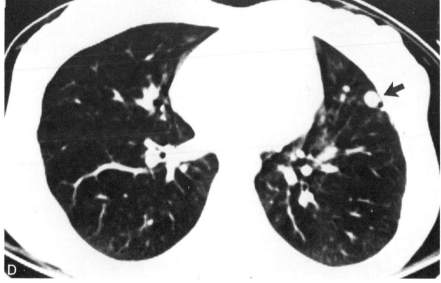

Figure 1–2C and D. The clinical significance of the measurement error demonstrated in A and B is apparent in C and D. The left lung nodule *(arrow)* measures 8 mm at "soft tissue" settings (window width 250 HU, window level +35 HU) in C and measures 13 mm at "lung" window settings (window width 1000 HU, window level −500 HU) in D. Change in size is an important parameter in assessment of benignancy versus malignancy on serial examinations and in following response to therapy; therefore, measurement of size must be made as accurately and reproducibly as possible.

Ref.: Baxter BS, Sorenson JA. Factors affecting the measurement of size and CT number in computed tomography. Invest Radiol 1981; 16:337–341.

Figure 1–3. ***NOISE.*** Noise appears visually as a mottled pattern of gray, white, and black dots superimposed on the anatomic information of the image. A primary determinant of noise in the CT image is the number of x-ray photons used to calculate the attenuation value of each pixel forming the CT image. Noise is inversely proportional to the number of photons per pixel. Factors that affect the number of photons per pixel include milliamperage setting, scan time (number and duration of views), pixel size, and slice thickness.

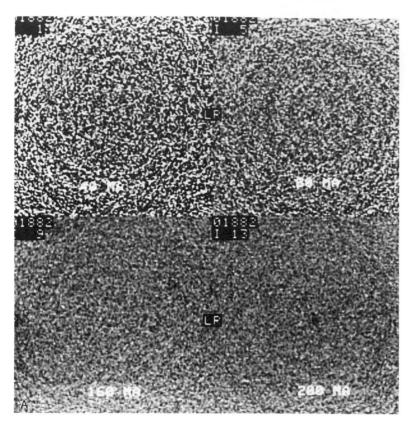

Figure 1–3A. A composite of four images taken on a homogeneous phantom at four different milliamperage settings is shown. All other scan technique factors were unchanged. The image on the *upper left* (No. 1) was obtained at 40 mA, the image on the *upper right* (No. 2) at 80 mA; the image on the *lower left* (No. 9) was obtained at 160 mA, and that on the *lower right* (No. 13) at 200 mA. The mottled pattern of noise is seen to decrease progressively with the increased numbers of photons per image provided by increasing the milliamperage.

Figure 1–3B. Four images from a lumbar spine CT are shown. The increased mottling due to noise seen in image 4 *(lower right)* compared to the other three images is due to decreasing the milliamperage setting from 600 to 320 mA. Technicians may do this to decrease interscan delay time due to tube cooling.

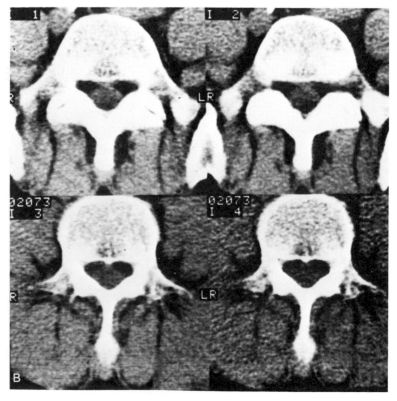

Figure 1–3C. Images 9, 10, and 11 in this lumbar spine CT were obtained with a 10-mm slice thickness. Image 12 *(lower right)* shows a marked increase in noise due to changing the slice thickness from 10 mm to 5 mm. The thecal sac is not adequately demonstrated to make a diagnosis. Decreasing the slice thickness often requires an increase in milliamperage setting to maintain diagnostic quality of the image.

Noise and patient dose are inversely related. A certain level of noise must be accepted to limit patient dose but excessive noise may make the image diagnostically uninterpretable.

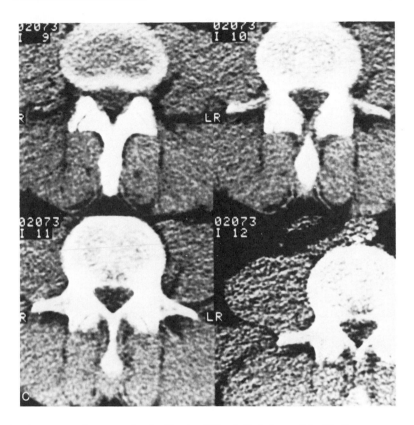

Ref.: Hanson KM. Noise and contrast discrimination in computed tomography. In: Newton TH, ed. Radiology of the Skull and Brain, Vol. 5: Technical Aspects of Computed Tomography. St. Louis: C. V. Mosby, 1980; pp 3941–3955.

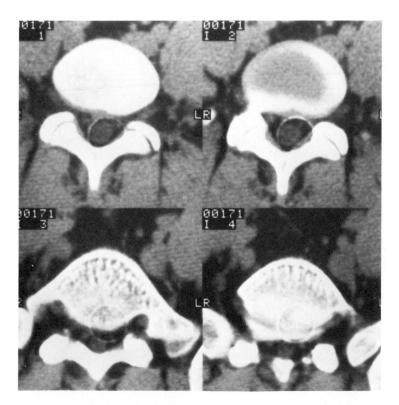

Figure 1–4. RING ARTIFACT. A high-density artifactual ring is demonstrated on multiple images of a dedicated scan of the lumbar spine. CT scanners with rotating detectors are prone to ring artifacts when detectors are out of calibration. Each detector is responsible for a ring of data as the gantry rotates. The calibration error is therefore projected in the data ring of the faulty detector. The presence of the artifact is confirmed by identifying it on multiple scans and in different patients scanned on the same day.

Ref.: Joseph PM. Artifacts in computed tomography. In: Newton TH, ed. Radiology of the Skull and Brain, Vol. 5: Technical Aspects of Computed Tomography. St. Louis: C. V. Mosby, 1980; pp 3956–3992.

Figure 1–5. RING ARTIFACT SIMULATING ASCITES.

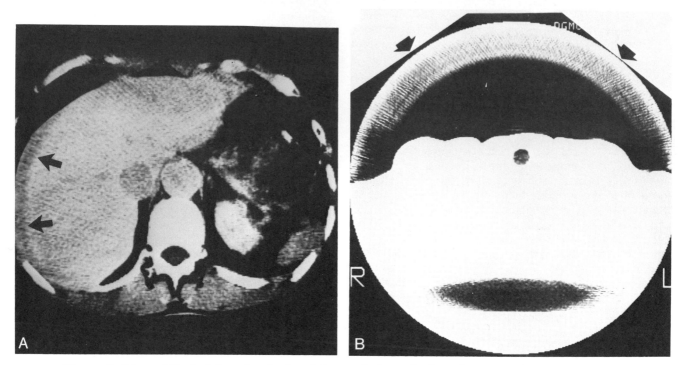

Figure 1–5A and B. *A,* A low-density band *(arrows)* along the lateral margin of the liver has the appearance of ascites. However, this low-density band is a ring artifact due to faulty x-ray detector calibration in the CT scanner. *B,* The presence of a ring artifact is confirmed. This scan at a different level in the same patient examined at low window settings demonstrates the ring artifact *(arrows)* projected in air.

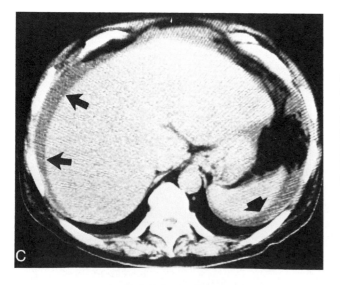

Figure 1–5C. A case of true ascites is shown. Fluid density is seen along the margin of the spleen *(arrowhead)* as well as along the margin of the liver *(arrows).* Since this band of lucency is not in the same data ring, it represents a true finding and not an artifact. On scans lower in the abdomen, fluid could also be seen outlining bowel and mesentery. This would not be found with ring artifacts.

Ref.: Jolles H, Coulam CM. CT of ascites: Differential diagnosis. AJR 1980; 135:315–322.

Figure 1–6. BEAM HARDENING ARTIFACT. As the polychromatic x-ray beam generated by CT scanners passes through patient tissue, low-energy photons are attenuated to a greater extent than are high-energy photons. The mean energy of the beam is progressively increased. Attenuation is less at the end of an x-ray beam than at its beginning. This phenomenon is called beam hardening. Most CT reconstruction algorithms assume that any change in beam intensity is due to a change in tissue attenuation and thus make errors in areas of beam hardening. Intense beam hardening errors are demonstrated visually as areas or streaks of low density extending from structures of high x-ray attenuation.

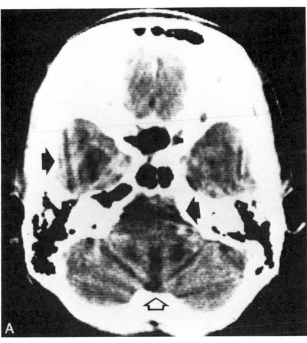

Figure 1–6A. A scan through the skull base demonstrates beam hardening artifact from the petrous bones, causing low density in the brain stem and streaks through the temporal lobes *(solid arrowheads)*. Additional lucent streaks extend through the posterior fossa due to beam hardening caused by the internal occipital protuberance *(open arrowhead)*.

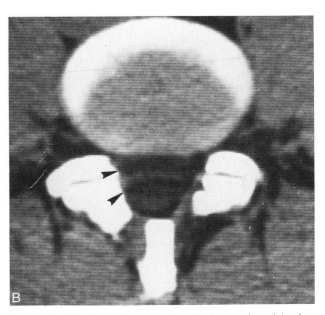

Figure 1–6B. Low-density streaks *(arrowheads)*, due to beam hardening by the facet joints, obscure the thecal sac in this lumbar spine scan.

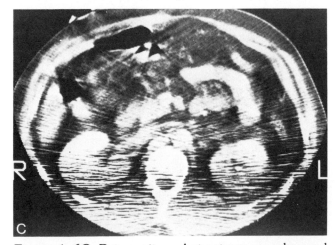

Figure 1–6C. Retroperitoneal structures are obscured by the beam hardening effects of the patient's arms being left at his sides during this abdominal scan. Dense structures outside the field of view may cause prominent artifacts.

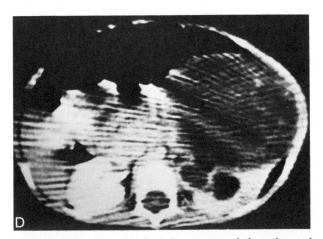

Figure 1–6D. The child's left arm was left at his side during immobilization for this abdominal CT scan. Prominent beam hardening effect from the arm obscures the internal septations important in the diagnosis of this multilocular cystic nephroma.

Ref.: Young SW, Muller HH, Marshall WH. Computed tomography: Beam hardening and environmental density artifact. Radiology 1983; 148:279–283.

Figure 1–7. STREAK ARTIFACT. Streaks in the CT image reflect errors in radiation detection along a projected beam. High-density sharp-edged objects, particularly vascular clips and dental fillings, are prone to produce streak artifacts. The source of the artifact is usually obvious when the entire slice is viewed.

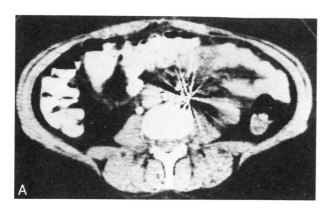

Figure 1–7A. Several metallic clips adjacent to the aorta cause prominent streak artifacts in this CT scan of the lower abdomen.

Figure 1–7B. When only a portion of the slice is viewed, as in this targeted image reconstruction of the lumbar spine, recognition of the source of the artifact may be more difficult. The streaks in this case project from a clip just outside the reconstructed image.

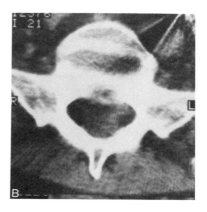

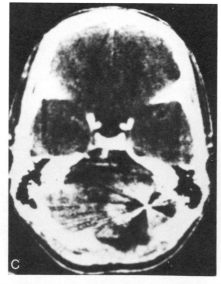

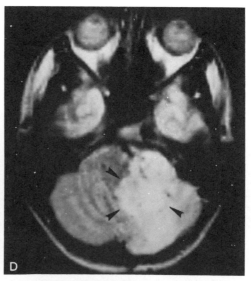

Figure 1–7C and D. Alternate imaging modalities may be necessary to make a diagnosis when excessive clip artifact is present. In *C,* a surgical clip in the posterior fossa obscures evidence of recurrence of a cerebellar astrocytoma. In the magnetic resonance image from the same patient shown in *D,* the tumor is clearly demonstrated *(arrowheads)* with no streak artifacts present. The surgical clip was not ferromagnetic.

Changes in the CT reconstruction algorithms offer promise of minimizing streak artifact from high-density objects. (Courtesy of Dr. Michael N. Brant-Zawadzki and Dr. William M. Kelly.)

Ref.: Morin RL, Raeside DE. A pattern recognition method for the removal of streaking artifact in computed tomography. Radiology 1981; 141:229–233.

Figure 1–8. STREAK ARTIFACT—RENAL STRIATIONS.

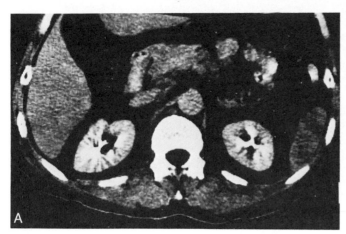

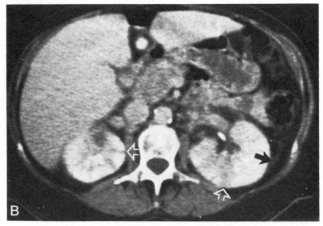

Figure 1–8A. Beam hardening and streak artifacts cause lucent and dense bands in the renal parenchyma on this CT scan of the kidneys. The streaks obscure renal parenchymal detail and simulate the striations due to edema seen in renal inflammatory disease. High-density contrast medium concentrated in the calyces is the source of the prominent streak artifact. Note that the striations radiate from the renal collecting structures and that they consist of both dense and lucent bands. There are no other signs of renal inflammation.

Figure 1–8B. A CT scan of bilateral acute pyelonephritis demonstrates linear lucencies *(open arrowheads)* in the renal parenchyma. Note that the lucencies do not extend from the renal collecting structures. Thickened renal fascia *(closed arrow)* provides additional evidence of inflammation.

Ref.: Morehouse HT, Weiner SN, Hoffman JC. Imaging in inflammatory disease of the kidney. AJR 1984; 143:135–141.

Figure 1–9. MOTION ARTIFACT. Errors in image reconstruction are produced when structures move to different positions during image acquisition. Motion is demonstrated in the image as prominent streaks from high- to low-density interfaces or as a blurred or duplicated image.

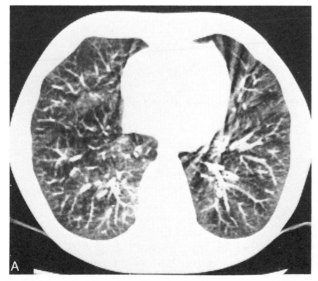

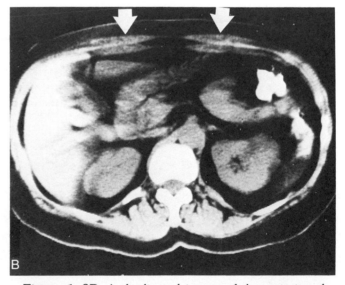

Figure 1–9A. Streak artifact in the lung is seen adjacent to the beating heart on this CT scan of the chest. The continuous movement of the heart is a common source of motion artifact in chest CT.

Figure 1–9B. A duplicated image of the anterior abdominal wall *(arrows)* is shown on this abdominal CT scan. Breathing during scan acquisition is the source of this artifact. Physiologic motion artifact due to cardiac motion, vessel pulsation, and peristalsis can be minimized by fast scan times. Voluntary motion in the uncooperative patient can be minimized by immobilization and sedation.

Ref.: Joseph PM. Artifacts in computed tomography. In: Newton TH, ed. Radiology of the Skull and Brain, Vol. 5: Technical Aspects of Computed Tomography. St. Louis: C. V. Mosby, 1980; 3956–3992.

Figure 1–10. "FAT MAN" ARTIFACT. "Fat man," or truncated view, artifacts in CT attenuation values occur whenever the patient is too large for the maximum field of view of the CT scanner or when any part of the patient extends outside the field of view. X-ray beams intended for reference detectors are attenuated by patient tissue rather than air. Reference detectors used to measure variations in x-ray tube output present faulty data that causes errors in CT attenuation value calculations. Visual disturbance in the image is usually not severe. The artifact should be suspected whenever the whole patient cross section is not included in the image and a halo is noted at the periphery of the image.

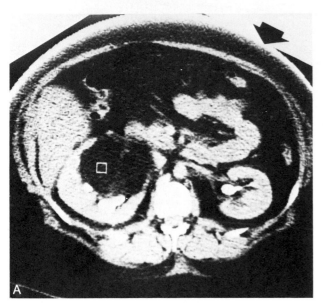

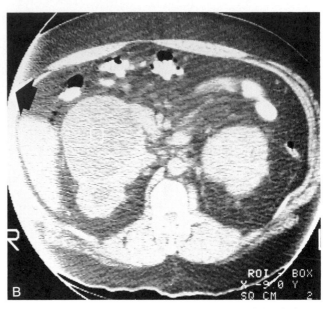

Figure 1–10A. The renal peripelvic cyst *(white open box)* in this abdominal CT scan has a mean attenuation value of −169 HU; subcutaneous fat has a mean attenuation value of −213 HU. The cystic nature of the peripelvic mass was confirmed by ultrasound. Note the halo *(arrow)* at the periphery of the reconstructed image.

Figure 1–10B. A cystic adenocarcinoma of the kidney *(white open box)* has a mean attenuation value of −43 HU suggesting a fat-containing lesion. Percutaneous aspiration cytology yielded the correct diagnosis. Note again the halo *(arrow)* at the periphery of the image.

Ref.: Lehr JL. Truncated-view artifacts: Clinical importance on CT. AJR 1983; 141:183–191.

Figure 1–11. VISUAL ILLUSION ERRORS—BACKGROUND CONTRAST EFFECT. Visual assessment of the density of an object in a CT image is dependent in part on the background surrounding the object of interest. Objects of equal x-ray attenuation displayed on the CT image as the same shade of gray may be visually assessed as being of different visual density if the background in which they are displayed is of different density. This phenomenon is illustrated in

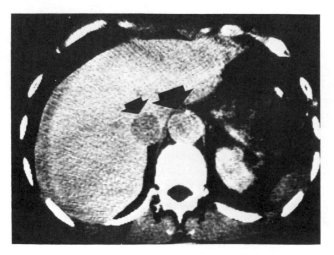

this computed tomogram of the abdomen. Both the inferior vena cava *(small arrow)* and the aorta *(large arrow)* have measured mean attenuation values of 52 HU. However, the high-density background of contrast-enhanced liver parenchyma makes the inferior vena cava appear more lucent, whereas a background of fat makes the aorta appear more dense.

This visual illusion is related to the Mach effect and results from lateral inhibitory impulses in the retina of the eye. This phenomenon is explained in detail in the article by Daffner (see below). Range of interest or identification mode may be used to clarify these visual illusion errors in interpretation.

Ref.: Daffner RH. Visual illusions in computed tomography: Phenomena related to Mach effect. AJR 1980; 134:261–264.

2

Head

DAVID L. LAMASTERS, M.D.

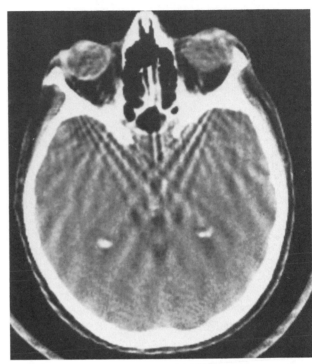

Figure 2–1. MOTION ARTIFACT. Axial CT section centered at the level of the orbits demonstrates the typical linear streak artifacts caused by patient motion. The symmetric pattern is caused by rotational motion about a central axis; that is, moving the head from side to side.

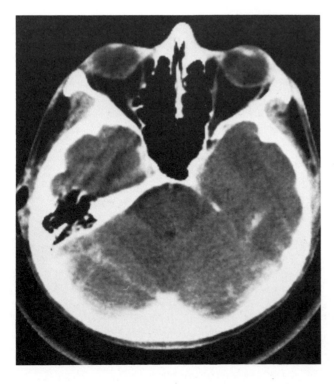

Figure 2–2. BRACHYCEPHALY. Axial CT scan through the orbits and posterior fossa in this patient demonstrates a diminished anteroposterior dimension to the calvarial vault. The brain is normal. Craniostenoses generally do not produce abnormalities of the brain with the exception of kleeblattschlädel (closure of all the cranial sutures). The cranial abnormality in this case is due to symmetric early closure of the coronal sutures.

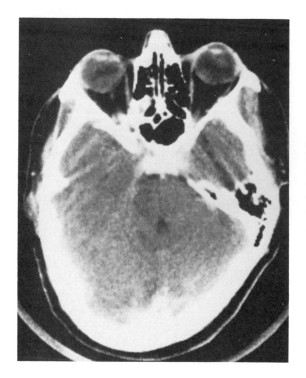

Figure 2–3. PLAGIOCEPHALY. Axial CT scan through the temporal lobes and posterior fossa shows flattening of the left occiput. The volume of the left hemisphere is diminished, but the underlying brain parenchyma is normal. This is typical of unilateral early closure of the lambdoid suture. Intellect is usually normal; this finding is often incidentally encountered during evaluation for an unrelated clinical problem.

Figure 2–4. CRANIOPLASTY PROSTHESIS.

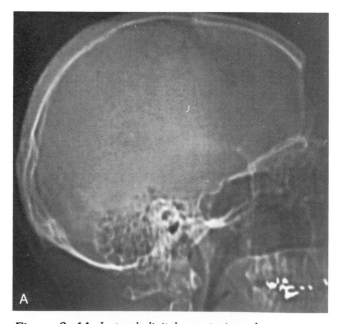

Figure 2–4A. Lateral digital scout view demonstrates a bifrontal craniotomy. The prosthesis is difficult to discern.

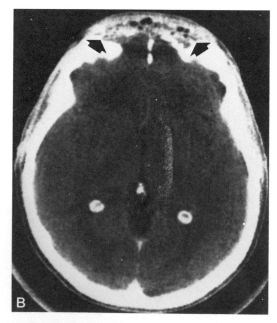

Figure 2–4B. Axial CT scan at the level of the third ventricle demonstrates the nature of the prosthesis *(arrows)*, which in this instance is made of Silastic. Neither an inner nor an outer table is present. The normal hyperdense diploë of the calvarium is replaced by the prosthesis with amorphous granular material of mixed attenuation that is partially air-containing.

Figure 2–5. HYPEROSTOSIS FRONTALIS INTERNA.
Two images through the upper calvarium demonstrate thickening and irregularity of the inner table of the skull in the frontal region (arrowheads). This is most marked on the more cephalad images. This finding is typically noted in women in the middle to older age groups. Hyperostosis from meningiomas may be confused with hyperostosis frontalis interna, although symmetry would argue against this as a possible diagnosis. Another entity that may produce somewhat similar irregular bone is Paget's disease due to the hyperostotic reaction typically seen in this disorder.

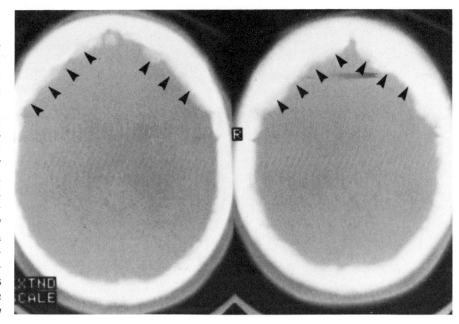

Ref.: Dilhmann W. Computerized tomography in typical hyperostosis cranii (THC). Eur J Radiol 1981; 1:2–8.

Figure 2–6. MARKED HYPEROSTOSIS FRONTALIS INTERNA.

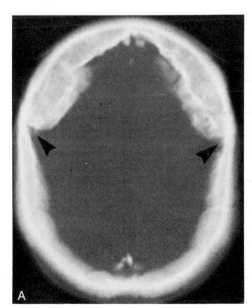

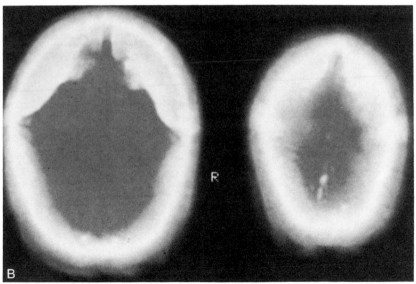

Figure 2–6A. In this case of an 89-year-old woman, the changes typically seen in hyperostosis frontalis interna are markedly exaggerated. Such findings are more typical in the older age groups. Note that the notch (arrowheads) behind the hyperostotic bone in the frontal region is a defect normally seen for the coronal suture.

Figure 2–6B. On axial CT scans obtained through the vertex, the effect is even more pronounced because a greater cross-sectional area of the hyperostotic bone is encountered. As with A, considerations in the differential diagnosis include meningioma and Paget's disease as well as fibrous dysplasia and other primary bony anomalies such as cranial metaphyseal dysplasia, von Buchem's disease, and osteopetrosis.

Ref.: von Babo H. Hyperostosis of the skull. Plain film and microradiography. Radiologe 1981; 21:12–18.

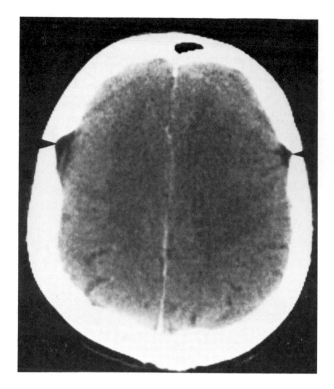

Figure 2–7. INNER TABLE SCALLOPING FROM THE CORONAL SUTURE. Axial scans through the cerebral hemispheres and upper aspect of the calvarium demonstrate two areas of inner table scalloping *(arrowheads)*. These represent the position of the coronal suture on axial CT scans. This should not be mistaken for a pathologic variant, as it corresponds to the normal location of the coronal sutures.

Figure 2–8. SCALLOPING OF THE INNER TABLE. Axial CT section through the posterior fossa shows an area of scalloping involving the inner table of the occipital bone on the left *(arrowheads)*. Mild undulation of the calvarial surface is quite common; however, when it is seen to this degree, the differential diagnosis should include adjacent subarachnoid cyst, leptomeningeal cyst (when the region of scalloping extends through the outer table as well), prominent dural sinus, and erosion from a cortical vein in a patient with an arteriovenous malformation or cranial lacunae. In this instance, because there is no adjacent abnormality within the calvarium, this represents a benign variant.

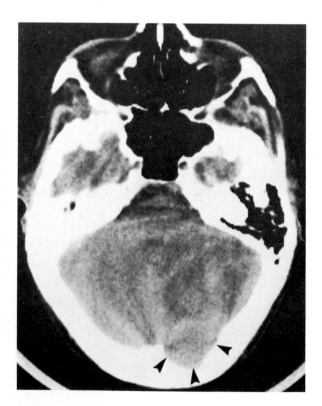

Ref.: Ethier R, Scowalt N: Thickness and texture. In: Newton TH, Potts DG, eds. Radiology of the Skull and Brain: The Skull, Vol. 1, Part 1, St. Louis: C. V. Mosby, 1971; pp 154–215.

Figure 2–9. ASYMMETRIC PNEUMATIZATION OF THE SPHENOID SINUS.

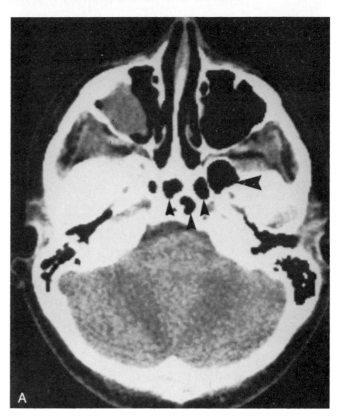

Figure 2–9A. A large air-filled loculus *(large arrowhead)* is present to the left of the sphenoid body. It is separated from the three centrally located sphenoid sinus loculi *(small arrowheads)*. Note also the right maxillary retention cyst.

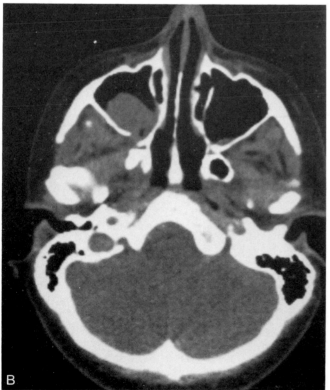

Figure 2–9B. The lateral sphenoid sinus pneumatization extends inferiorly to the level of the pterygoid plates on the left. Lateral pneumatization of the sphenoid sinus is not uncommon. Communication with other sinus loculi is by means of small ostia. While extensive lateral sphenoid pneumatization is usually symmetric, unequal aeration can cause confusion on sinus films, due to the differential density seen through the maxillary sinuses. This problem is easily rectified with CT.

Figure 2–10. EXTENSIVE MASTOID PNEUMATIZATION.

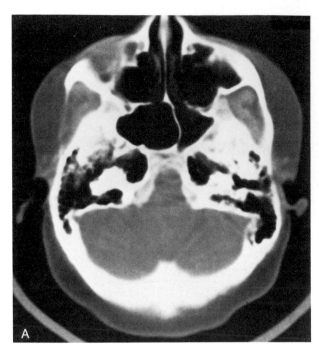

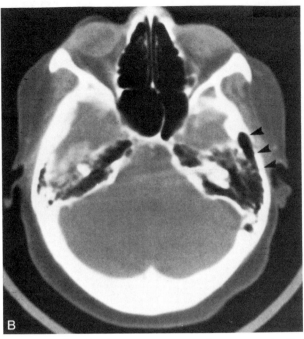

Figure 2–10A. The high-resolution bone windows demonstrate extensive mastoid pneumatization. Whereas pneumatization laterally in the region of the mastoid tip and even of the temporal squamosa is frequently encountered, extensive medial pneumatization extending into the petrous tip adjacent to the sphenoid is not commonly found. Although pneumatization in this case is extensive, note that the mastoids are undiseased, in that the individual air cells may be appreciated with wide window settings and there is no evidence of tissue density within the mastoids to suggest the possibility of cholesteatoma formation or chronic mastoid infection.

Figure 2–10B. In the same case as A, pneumatization has extended into the temporal squamosa proper *(arrowheads).* Again, extensive pneumatization involving the petrous apex as well as the mastoid complex is seen.

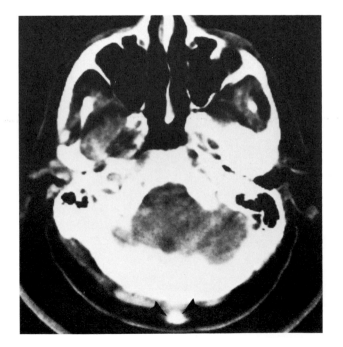

Figure 2–11. EXTERNAL OCCIPITAL PROTUBER-ANCE. The axial CT scan obtained through the posterior fossa and maxillary sinuses demonstrates a solitary calcification *(arrowheads)* in the soft tissues posterior to the occipital bone. This is another effect of partial volume averaging, in that on the next cephalad CT section, the external occipital protuberance is encountered. Although this is a normal variant, in patients with acromegaly, marked enlargement of the external occipital protuberance can be found on axial CT sections, as well as other secondary signs such as thickening of the soft tissues, enlargement of the sella turcica, and prominence of the frontal sinuses.

Figure 2–12. DURAL CALCIFICATION.

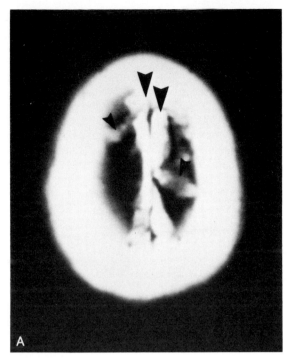

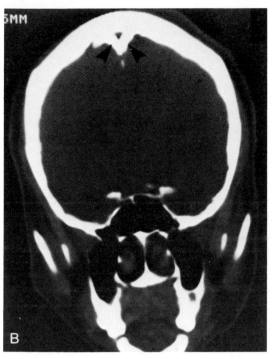

Figure 2–12A. In this axial CT image taken through the vertex of the calvarium, extensive calcification is seen along the sulci *(small arrowheads)* and in a paramedian position adjacent to the superior sagittal sinus *(large arrowheads)*.

Figure 2–12B. The findings in *A* are seen in this coronal scan. The calcification *(arrowheads)* parallels the dura that forms the superior sagittal sinus. The small triangle in the midline represents the blood pool capacity of the superior sagittal sinus.

Figure 2–13. EXTENSIVE FALX CALCIFICATION.
The anterior portion of the falx cerebri is heavily calcified. Note that the contour of the calcification is irregular on the left margin but smooth on the right. The posterior portion of the falx is uncalcified and is visualized because of the dense fibrous nature of the falx and secondarily because of intravenous contrast enhancement.

Ref.: Zimmerman RD, Yurberg E, Russell EJ, Leeds NE. Falx and interhemispheric fissure on axial CT: I. normal anatomy. AJR 1982; 138:899–904.

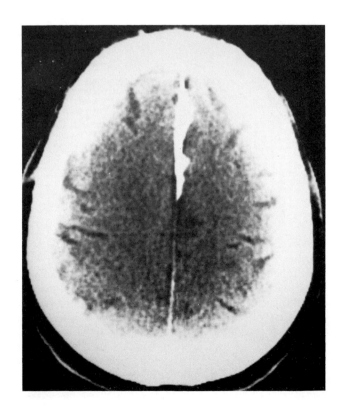

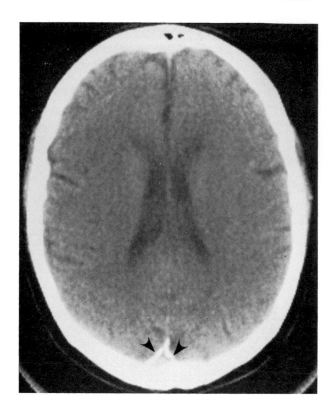

Figure 2–14. CALCIFICATION IN THE LEAVES OF THE SUPERIOR SAGITTAL SINUS. This non-contrast scan demonstrates a triangularly configured area of hyperdensity *(arrowheads)* in the region of the descending portion of the superior sagittal sinus, prior to its junction with the torcular. Like physiologic dural calcifications elsewhere, sinus calcifications tend to be linear in appearance and are usually short in length and small in overall area. Confusion can occur if a non-contrast scan is mistaken for one with intravenous enhancement, as this appearance on the latter is suggestive of superior sagittal sinus thrombosis with the central low density representing clot.

Ref.: Patronas NJ, Duda EE, Mirfakraee, M. Superior sagittal sinus thrombosis diagnosed by computed tomography. Surg Neurol 1981; 15:11–15.

Figure 2–15. DENSE FALX CALCIFICATION.

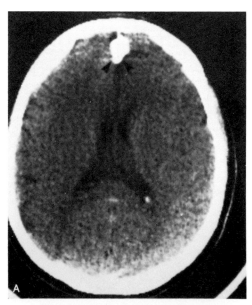

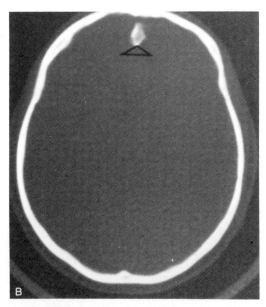

Figure 2–15A. A high-density calcified midline mass *(arrowheads)* is noted in the region of the anterior portion of the falx cerebri. This example of exuberant but idiopathic calcification of the falx is more clump-like than is usually seen. Normally, falx calcification is linear and present in the anterior third of the falx. Other causes for falx calcification include calcified meningioma, chronic calcified falcine subdural hematoma, and extensive calcification of all dural surfaces in basal cell nevus syndrome (Gorlin's syndrome).

Figure 2–15B. In this scan, taken at wide window settings to emphasize bone detail, the densely calcified nature of this variant is better appreciated *(open arrowhead).*

Figure 2–16. **TENTORIAL CALCIFICATION.** As with other dural surfaces, the tentorium may also calcify. This is much less common than calcifications of the falx, petroclinoid ligaments, and other dural surfaces.

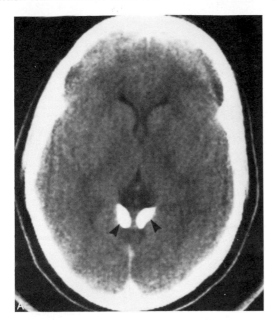 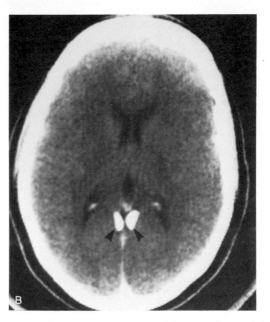

Figure 2–16A. The dense calcification of the tentorial edge *(arrowheads)* is easily apparent situated posterior to the superior cerebellar cistern.

Figure 2–16B. The two tentorial lesions *(arrowheads)* are almost fused.

Figure 2–17. **PARTIAL VOLUME AVERAGING EFFECT—FRONTAL SINUS, ORBITAL ROOF.**

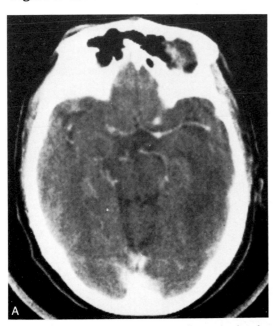 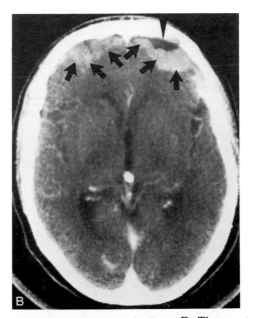

Figure 2–17. A, Axial CT section through the frontal sinuses shows extensive pneumatization. *B,* The next most cephalad section demonstrates a left frontal lucency *(arrowhead)* and bifrontal densities *(multiple arrows)* suggesting possible frontal calcified lesions. Because of the prominent frontal sinus in this patient, the left sinus loculus is "partially seen" on the higher CT section, as are the anterior portions of the orbital roofs. Partial volume averaging effects are most common (and also most confusing) when the structure in question is inclined at a slight angle to the CT plane of section, or lies in a small percentage of the collimated slice.

   Problems regarding partial volume averaging effects usually can be resolved by analyzing the anatomic structures immediately sub- and supra-adjacent to the image in question. Pertinent negative information includes lack of mass effect (i.e., cisternal, sulcal, and ventricular compression and vascular displacement), lack of focal cerebral edema, and most important, lack of appropriate pathologic explanation.

Figure 2–18. DOMINANT ANTERIOR CEREBRAL ARTERY.

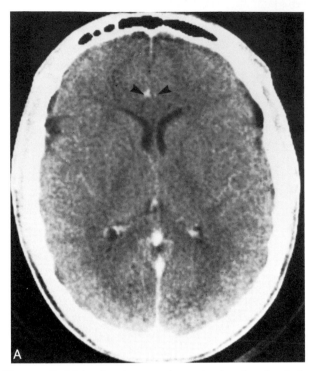

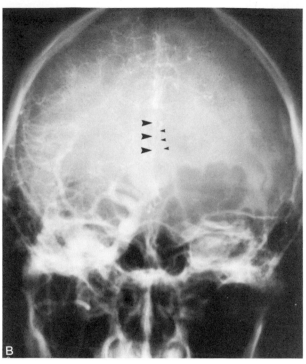

Figure 2–18A. Axial scan through the level of the frontal horns of the lateral ventricles demonstrates asymmetry of the anterior cerebral arteries *(arrowheads)* with the right being larger than the left.

Figure 2–18B. Cerebral angiography confirms the finding seen in A *(large arrowheads,* right anterior cerebral artery; *small arrowheads,* left anterior cerebral artery).

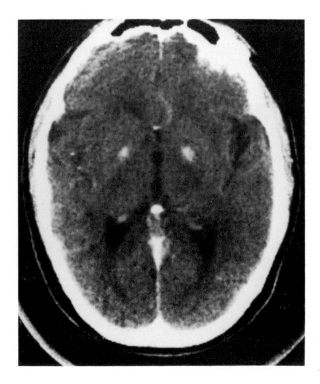

Figure 2–19. CALCIFICATIONS OF THE BASAL GANGLIA. In this axial CT image taken through the diencephalon there are two high-density foci situated within the globus pallidus and putamen. This appearance is quite typical of basal ganglia calcification, which occurs in roughly 1 per cent of the patient population studied. Usually this is an incidental finding; however, it may be associated with hypoparathyroidism, hyperphosphatemia, pseudohypoparathyroidism, pseudopseudohypoparathyroidism, and a variety of less common syndromes including Wilson's disease, Fahr's disease, and Cockayne's syndrome. Basal ganglia calcification also occurs in a variety of hypercalcemic states.

Ref.: Sachs C, Ericson K, Erasmie U, Bergström M. Incidence of basal ganglia calcifications on computed tomography. J Comput Assist Tomogr 1979; 3:339–344.

Figure 2–20. EXTENSIVE CALCIFICATION OF THE BASAL GANGLIA. Extensive calcification of the globus pallidus, putamen, caudate nucleus and thalamic pulvinar (idiopathic).

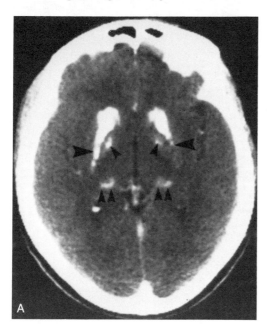

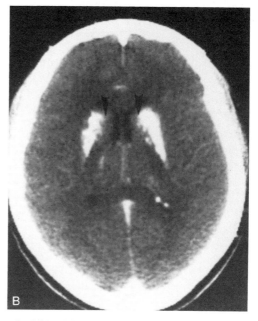

Figure 2–20A. Axial CT section through the third ventricle shows heavy, dense, symmetric calcification of the pulvinar *(double small arrowheads)*, globus pallidus *(single small arrowheads)* and putamen *(large arrowheads)*.

Figure 2–20B. Above, at the level of the frontal horns of the lateral ventricles, the calcification extends medially to involve the heads of the caudate nuclei *(arrowheads)*.

This degree of nuclear calcification in the diencephalon is unusual. There was, however, no clinical history of toxic substance or radiation exposure. A metabolic work-up initiated by this finding was unremarkable. The CT scan was initially ordered to evaluate atypical migraine.

Differential diagnostic considerations in this case would include endocrinopathies of the thyroid and parathyroid glands, heavy metal poisoning (lead, antimony and bismuth), anoxia (especially that due to exposure to carbon monoxide), Wilson's disease, ferrocalcinosis, and a variety of rare syndromes including Cockayne's.

Figure 2–21. PROMINENT VEIN OF GALEN (CONTRAST-ENHANCED SCAN). This axial CT section taken at the level of the third ventricle shows a soft-tissue density mass *(lower paired small arrowheads)* in the superior aspect of the quadrigeminal plate cistern. Its density approximates that of surrounding vascular structures. (*Upper paired small arrowheads,* internal cerebral veins; *large arrowheads,* basal veins of Rosenthal.)

The soft-tissue mass is large, but otherwise its appearance is normal for the vein of Galen.

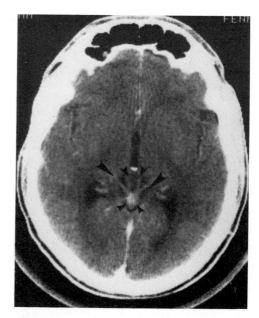

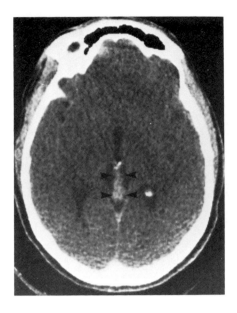

Figure 2–22. PROMINENT VEIN OF GALEN. Axial scan obtained through the posterior third ventricle and atria of the lateral ventricles with intravenous contrast enhancement demonstrates a tubular midline enhancing structure *(arrowheads)* just posterior to the pineal calcification and situated within the superior cerebellar cistern. This is the normal anatomic location of the vein of Galen prior to its junction with the sinus rectus. In this patient, the vein of Galen appears prominent but is still within normal limits. Enlargement of the vein of Galen can be pathologically related to arteriovenous malformations (such as the vein of Galen ''aneurysm'') and hypervascular tumors with increased blood flow that drain centrally or from bases of the dural sinuses.

Figure 2–23. LIPOMA OF THE QUADRIGEMINAL PLATE CISTERN. The axial CT section through the tentorial hiatus demonstrates a lucency *(open white arrow)* bounded by the collicular plate (anterior) and the leaves of the tentorium (posterolateral). This collection is of lower density than the cerebrospinal fluid within the atrium of the left lateral ventricle *(arrowhead)*. No distortion of, or mass effect on, the mesencephalon is noticeable.

Supratentorial lipomas of the central nervous system are congenital or hamartomatous tumors. In a functional sense their discovery in the adult is usually incidental, as the patient's clinical symptoms are most often unrelated to the location of the lipoma. Other sites include the corpus callosum and tuber cinereum.

Ref.: Kazner E, Stockdorph O, Wende S, Grumme T. Intracranial lipoma. Diagnostic and therapeutic considerations. J Neurosurg 1980; 52:234–245.

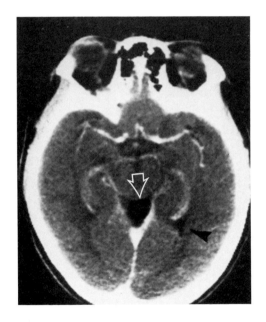

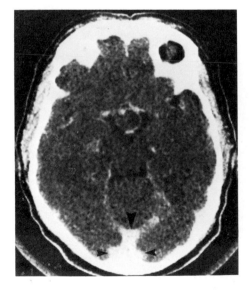

Figure 2–24. PROMINENT TORCULAR HEROPHILI AND STRAIGHT SINUS. In this axial CT scan obtained through the parasellar region, mesencephalon, superior cerebellar vermis, and occipital lobes, a prominent enhancing structure is seen posterior in the midline. Its most anterior aspect *(large arrowhead)* represents the termination of the straight sinus, or sinus rectus. The posterior extent is the torcular Herophili *(small arrowheads)*, which is large in this patient.

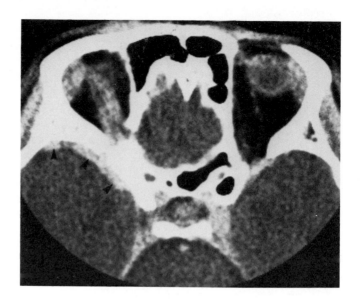

Figure 2–25. SPHENOPARIETAL SINUS. This axial CT section coned down to the orbital region demonstrates an enhancing tubular structure *(arrowheads)* paralleling the greater wing of the sphenoid. On other axial cuts, this is contiguous medially with the cavernous sinus. This sinus drains blood from the sylvian fissure through the superficial middle cerebral vein.

Ref.: Galligioni F, Bernardi R, Pellone M, Iraei G. The superficial sylvian vein in normal and pathlogic cerebral angiography. AJR 1969, 107:565–579.

Figure 2–26. BASILAR ARTERY ECTASIA.

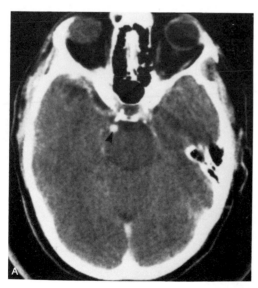

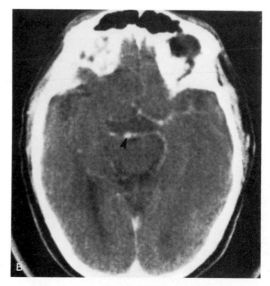

Figure 2–26A. Axial CT image obtained at the level of the pons shows a round enhancing object *(arrowhead)* situated in the basal cistern.

Figure 2–26B. On the next higher CT section, the basilar artery has migrated *(arrowhead)* toward the midline. Ectasia of the basilar artery is common, particularly in the elderly. For this reason it is a poor marker of the midline.

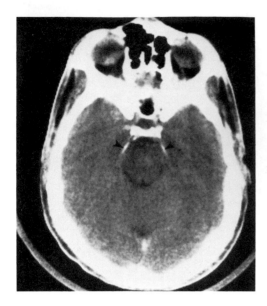

Figure 2–27. PETROCLINOID LIGAMENT CALCIFICATION. Axial CT section taken through the sella turcica and brain stem shows two calcified linear structures *(arrowheads)* extending posterolaterally from the posterior clinoid processes. These are the petroclinoid ligaments, which in the adult are often calcified. They course inferiorly from dorsum to petrous apex and may be seen on contiguous axial CT sections. While symmetry is the rule, unilateral calcification of a petroclinoid ligament can be confused with atherosclerotic vascular calcification of the superior cerebellar or posterior cerebral vessels. The latter can be differentiated by their circumferential course around the brain stem.

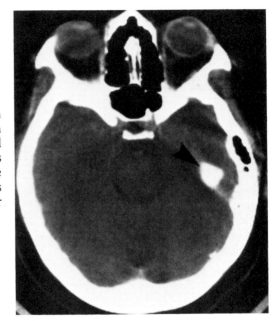

Figure 2–28. ARCUATE EMINENCE. In this axial CT section taken through the region of the brain stem, orbits, and temporal lobes, a high-attenuation structure *(arrowhead)* is noted centered in the lateral aspect of the left temporal lobe just medial to the uncus. This represents partial volume averaging of the arcuate eminence of the petrous bone, which houses the superior semicircular canal. This should not be mistaken for hyperostosis from a meningioma or for an intrinsic calcified temporal lobe mass.

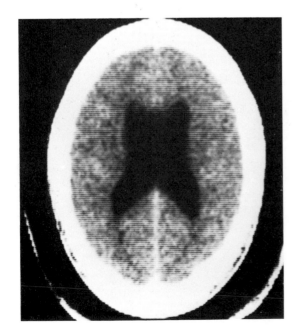

Figure 2–29. ABSENCE OF THE SEPTUM PELLUCIDUM. This axial CT scan obtained through the bodies of the lateral ventricles demonstrates conjoined lateral ventricles without a midline septum pellucidum. Absence of the septum pellucidum may occur as a single event or may be associated with a range of midline defects that include septo-optic dysplasia of deMorsier, the holoprosencephalies (lobar, semilobar and alobar) and severe hydrocephaly.

Refs.: (1) Byrd SE, Harwood-Nash DC, Fitz CR, Rogovitz DM. Computed tomography evaluation of holoprosencephaly in infants and children. Comput Assist Tomogr 1977; 1:456–463. (2) O'Dwyer JA, Newton TH, Hoyt WF. Radiologic features of septo-optic dysplasia: deMorsier syndrome. Am J Neurorad 1980; 1:443–447.

Figure 2–30. CAVUM SEPTI PELLUCIDI AND CAVUM VERGAE (CHILD). The cavum septi pellucidi and cavum vergae are developmental abnormalities related to nonfusion of the two leaves of the septum pellucidum. These are commonly found in the neonatal state but usually fuse by the age of two months. The cavum septi pellucidi should be distinguished from a cyst of the cavum septi pellucidi, which by definition would cause obstructive hydrocephalus. The posterior extension of the cavum septi pellucidi is the cavum vergae. This is the remnant of the cyst posterior to the foramen of Monro.

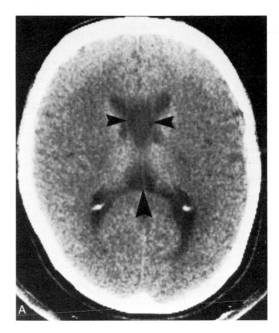

Figure 2–30A. Axial CT scan taken at the level of the frontal horns of the lateral ventricles demonstrates a cerebrospinal fluid collection positioned between the frontal horns of the lateral ventricles. The two leaves of the septum pellucidum can be seen splayed by the midline collection *(small arrowheads).* The rostral cerebrospinal fluid collection is the cavum septi pellucidi. More posteriorly a triangular cerebrospinal fluid collection anterior to the atrial region represents the cavum vergae *(large arrowhead).*

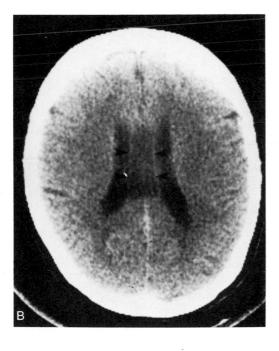

Figure 2–30B. More cephalad at the level of the body of the lateral ventricles, the leaves of the septum pellucidum can again be seen splayed by the cerebrospinal fluid collection *(arrowheads).*

Refs.: (1) Shaw CM, Alvord EC Jr. Cavum septi pellucidi et vergae: their normal and pathologic states. Brain 1969; 92:213–224. (2) Healy JF, Wickbom GI, Janon E. Computed tomographic illustration of cavum vergae. CT 1981; 5:336–339.

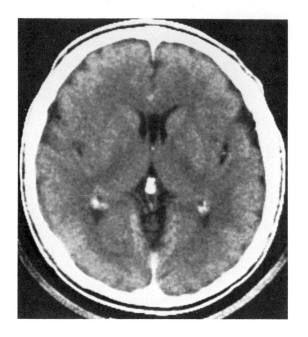

Figure 2–31. CAVUM SEPTI PELLUCIDI (ADULT). Axial scans obtained through the brain at the level of the frontal horns demonstrate a cerebrospinal fluid density separating the frontal horns. This terminates at the level of the foramen of Monro. It does not extend posteriorly along the bodies of the lateral ventricles. These findings are diagnostic of a cavum septi pellucidi. An extension of midline cerebrospinal fluid density beyond the level of the foramen of Monro is by definition a cavum vergae.

Figure 2–32. DENSELY CALCIFIED CHOROID OF THE THIRD VENTRICLE. In this axial CT section, the choroid plexus *(arrowheads)* of the third ventricle is seen. The CT section was taken at the level of the frontal horns of the lateral ventricles and the body of the third ventricle. Dense calcification of the third ventricular choroid is less commonly seen than calcification in the glomus of the lateral ventricles or the lateral tuft of choroid in the fourth ventricle.

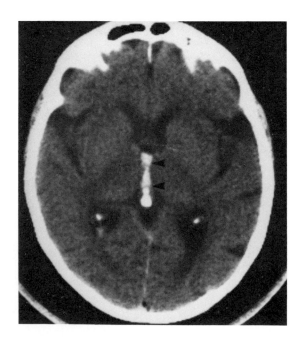

Figure 2–33. **EXTENSIVE CALCIFICATION OF THE CHOROID PLEXUS.** Calcification is seen on high-resolution computed tomography approximately 9 to 15 times more frequently than on plain skull radiography. Although this degree of calcification is normal, calcification in the temporal horns has been noted in association with neurofibromatosis. Extensive glomus calcification has been associated with choroid plexus papillomas. Physiologic calcification of the choroid is an incidental finding in approximately half the computed tomograms obtained in the adult population. It increases in relative frequency as the patient's age increases, with an incidence approaching 86 per cent in the eighth decade of life.

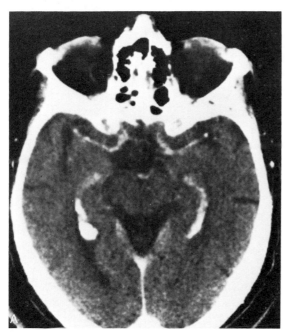

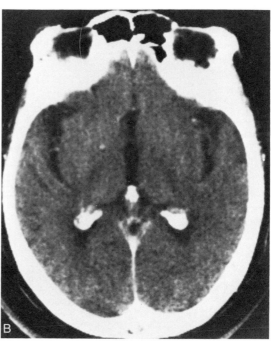

Figure 2–33A. Axial CT section through the temporal horns and atria of the lateral ventricle demonstrates extensive calcification within the glomus and calcification extending into the temporal horn proper. This effectively outlines the entire length of the temporal horn.

Figure 2–33B. A CT section taken at the level of the glomus of the choroid plexus again demonstrates heavy clump-like calcification bilaterally. Incidentally noted is cortical atrophy with enlargement of the sylvian fissures and third ventricle.

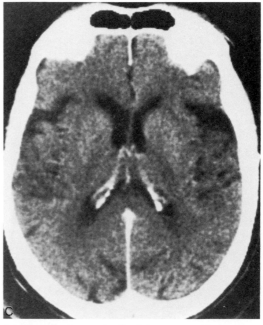

Figure 2–33C. Image taken at the level of frontal horns and bodies of lateral ventricles demonstrates calcification extending into the bodies proper as far forward as the foramen of Monro.

Refs.: (1) Modic MT, Weinstein MA, Rothner DA, et al. Calcification of the choroid plexus visualized by computed tomography. Radiology 1980; 135:369–372. (2) Norman D, Diamond C, Boyd D. Relative detectability of intracranial calcifications on computed tomography and skull radiography. J Comput Assist Tomogr 1978; 2:61–64.

Figure 2–34. PROMINENT CHOROID PLEXUS ENHANCEMENT IN THE LATERAL VENTRICLES.

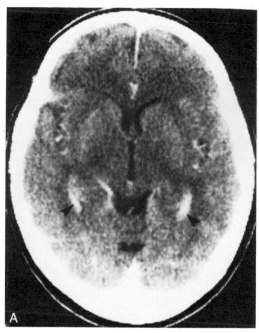

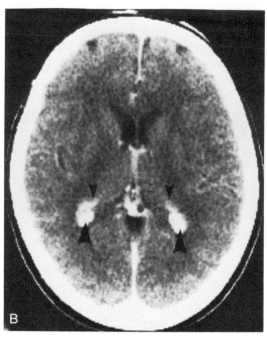

Figure 2–34A. Axial CT section taken at the level of the frontal horns demonstrates enhancement bilaterally *(arrowheads)* posterior to the sylvian fissures.

Figure 2–34B. Enhancement is also noted in the region of the glomus of the choroid plexus. The posterior aspect of the glomus in this instance is calcified *(large arrowheads)*. The more anterior aspect of the choroid plexus is enhanced but shows no calcification *(small arrowheads)*.

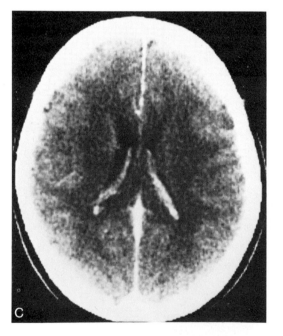

Figure 2–34C. At the level of the body of the lateral ventricles enhancement can be seen in the choroid extending from glomus posteriorly to the foramen of Monro anteriorly. While a small amount of enhancement is generally seen in the choroid plexus, significant enhancement such as this may suggest other diagnoses. Marked uptake of contrast material by the choroid plexus is found in cases of intraventricular infection (ependymitis), intraventricular seeding of tumor (especially medulloblastoma and ependymoma) and in post-hemorrhagic states.

Refs.: (1) Warmser GP, Shashan A. Ventriculitis complicating gram negative meningitis in an adult. Mt Sinai J Med (NY) 1980; 47:575–578. (2) Sullivan WT, Dorwart RH. Leakage of iodinated contrast media into the cerebral ventricles in an adult with ependymitis. Am J Neurorad 1983; 4:1251–1253.

Figure 2–35. ASYMMETRIC CHOROID PLEXUS OF THE TEMPORAL HORN.

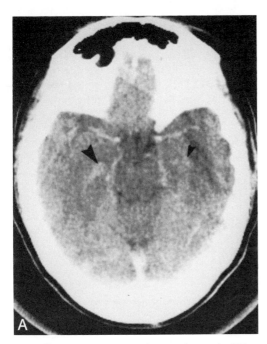

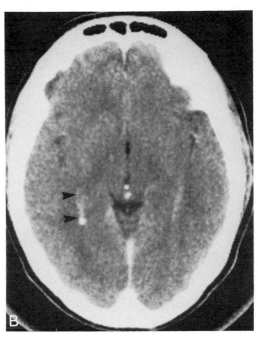

Figure 2–35A. Contrast-enhanced axial CT section obtained at the level of the temporal lobe, mesencephalon, and tentorial incisura demonstrates a small, comma-shaped hyperdense nodule *(large arrowhead)* just behind the uncus of the mesial temporal lobe. A smaller, less obvious nodule is present opposite *(small arrowhead).*

Figure 2–35B. One section higher, these nodules are contiguous with two hyperdense linear streaks of choroid in the posterior aspect of the temporal horn *(arrowheads).*

Figure 2–35C. At the level of the frontal horns the choroid of the temporal horns merges with that of the atria. Note that noncalcified but hyperdense choroid *(open arrowhead)* lies anterior to the calcified glomus.

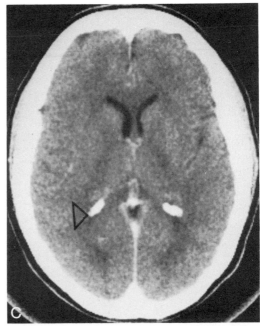

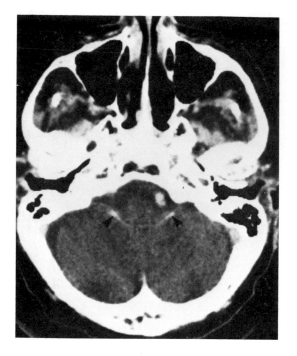

Figure 2–36. CHOROID PLEXUS OF THE FOURTH VEN-TRICLE. High-density linear structure noted just posteriorly to the medulla *(arrowheads)* extends laterally to the cerebellopontine angle. Although partially calcified, the high-density structure also demonstrates contrast enhancement. This represents choroid plexus within the lateral recesses of the fourth ventricle passing laterally to the foramen of Luschka. The choroid plexus of the fourth ventricle when identified serves as a useful anatomic landmark. Not infrequently a tuft of choroid outside the fourth ventricle extends into the cerebellopontine angle; it should not be mistaken for a mass lesion.

Ref.: Hayman LA, Evans RA, Hinck VC. Choroid plexus of the fourth ventricle: Useful CT landmark. AJR 1979; 133:285–288.

Figure 2–37. VERMIAN PSEUDOTUMOR. An axial CT scan obtained with intravenous contrast medium through the posterior fossa at the level of the body of the fourth ventricle demonstrates an elliptical region of hyperdensity *(arrowheads)* in the inferior vermis. There is no mass effect on the fourth ventricle; also, no edema is seen laterally in the cerebellar hemispheres. This is characteristic of pseudotumor of the inferior vermis, originally described by Kramer.

Differential diagnostic possibilities include midline noncystic cerebellar hemangioblastoma, an infiltrating vermian glioma, and an aneurysm of the posterior medullary segment of the posteroinferior cerebellar artery.

Ref.: Kramer RA. Vermian pseudotumor. A potential pitfall of CT brainscanning with contrast enhancement. Neuroradiology 1979; 13:229–230.

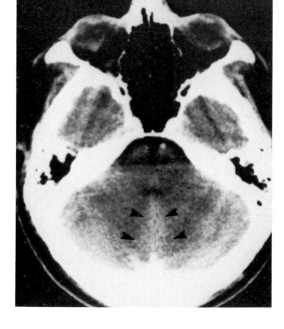

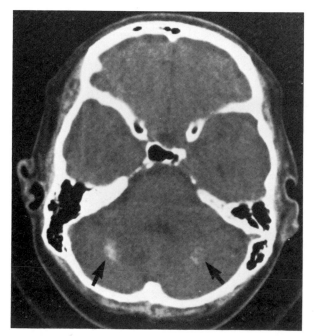

Figure 2–38. DENTATE NUCLEUS CALCIFICATION. Axial scan obtained through the posterior fossa demonstrates two areas of high density *(arrows)* in each cerebellar hemisphere lateral to the middle cerebellar peduncle. This is the anatomic location of the dentate nuclei of the cerebellum. This finding may be seen in ferrocalcinosis, hypercalcemic states, and Cockayne's syndrome; however, most frequently it is idiopathic and should be considered a normal variant. Its frequency relative to calcification of basal ganglia is significantly less.

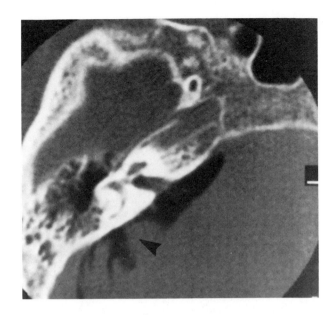

Figure 2–39. THE CEREBELLAR FLOCCULUS. On this air-enhanced CT angle study, the cerebellar flocculus *(arrowhead)* is well outlined with gas in the cerebellopontine angle cistern. In the past the flocculus has been mistaken for a cerebellopontine angle tumor. This structure is part of the flocculonodular lobe of the cerebellar vermis. On routine axial scans with intravenous contrast medium, this may appear as a slightly higher density than the adjacent cerebellum.

Ref.: Daniels DL, Haughton VM, Williams AL, Berns TF. Flocculus in computed tomography. AJNR 1981; 2:227–229.

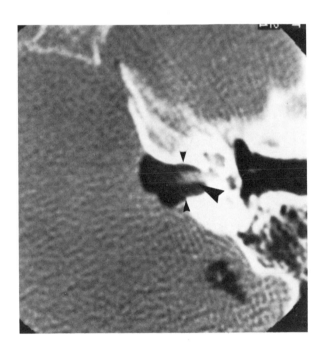

Figure 2–40. PATULOUS INTERNAL AUDITORY CANAL. In this patient receiving a work-up for sensorineural hearing loss, the plain films showed a discrepancy of 2 mm between the right and left sides of the vertical measurement of the internal auditory canal. The axial CT image in the lateral decubitus position (left side up) obtained as part of the air-enhanced CP angle CT evaluation shows a patulous canal that is widened also in the anterior to posterior dimension *(small arrowheads)*. The seventh and eighth cranial nerves are visualized as a small soft-tissue mass *(large arrowhead)* at the most lateral aspect of the internal auditory canal. These paired structures should not be mistaken for an acoustic tumor. A patulous internal auditory canal is also seen pathologically even without an acoustic tumor in neurofibromatosis, due to the dural ectasia.

Ref.: Holt JF. Neuhauser lecture: Neurofibromatosis in children. AJR 1978; 130:615–640.

Figure 2–41. JUGULAR TUBERCLE. Axial CT image through the posterior fossa demonstrates a high-density structure protruding into the left cerebellopontine angle cistern *(arrowhead)*. No comparable finding is seen on the contralateral side. This is the jugular tubercle. This has been mistaken in the past for a variety of lesions including aneurysms or meningioma. The jugular tubercle is the most medial boundary of the jugular fossa. It lies directly above the occipital condyle. Anatomically, it is part of the clivus. While visualization of one side without the other is most frequently a function of poor patient positioning, the jugular tubercles may normally be asymmetric, as in this case.

Refs.: (1) Osborn AG, Brinton WR, Smith WH. Radiology of the jugular tubercles. AJR 1978; 131:1037–1040. (2) Williams IL, Haughton VM. Jugular foramen: Anatomic and computed tomographic study. Am J Neurorad 1983; 4:1227–1232.

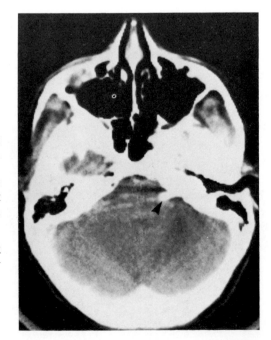

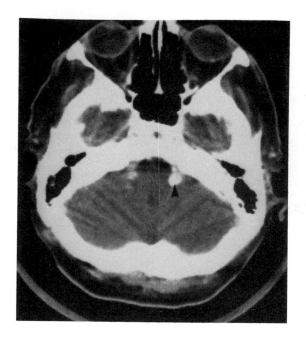

Figure 2–42. JUGULAR TUBERCLES. A single left-sided calcified density *(arrowhead)* is noted adjacent to the medial tip of the petrous bone. This is the jugular tubercle, which lies above the hypoglossal canal and occipital condyle. In the 0-degree, or anthropologic, plane this is not usually apparent as a distinct entity; however, when the scan plane is +15 degrees or greater, the jugular tubercle can be seen as an isolated piece of bone. This has been mistaken in the past for an aneurysm of the vertebral artery. Its true nature can be revealed by obtaining thinner section CT above and below the plane and noting its continuity with the medial aspect of the temporal bone.

Ref.: Osborn AG, Brinton WR, Smith WH. Radiology of the jugular tubercles. AJR 1978; 131:1037.

Figure 2–43. MEGA CISTERNA MAGNA. In these axial images obtained through the posterior fossa, a large, low-density midline structure is apparent. It is of cerebrospinal fluid density. This is an enlarged, or mega, cisterna magna. It can be differentiated from a subarachnoid cyst, which would have similar CT characteristics but would be expected to demonstrate some effacement of cerebellar sulci and no displacement and obliteration of the fourth ventricle. An enlarged cisterna magna may be associated with some degree of hypoplasia of the inferior vermis. Usually there is no neurologic deficit.

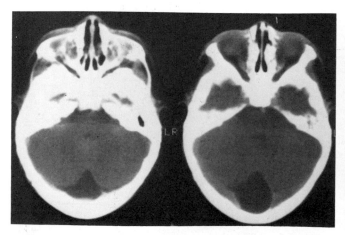
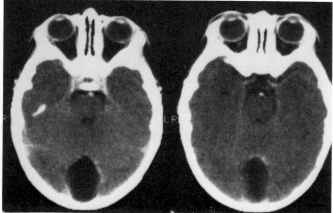

Refs.: (1) Archer CR, Darwish H, Smith K Jr. Enlarged cisterna magna and posterior fossa cyst simulating Dandy-Walker syndrome on computed tomography. Radiology 1978; 127:681–686. (2) Adams R., Greenberg JO. The mega cisterna magna. J Neurosurg 1978; 48:190–192.

Figure 2–44. MEGA CISTERNA MAGNA.

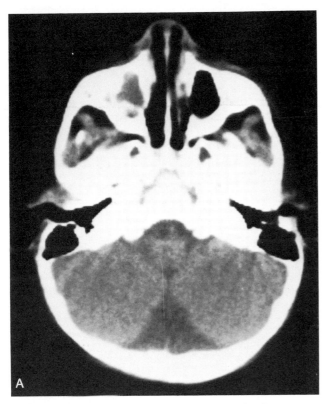

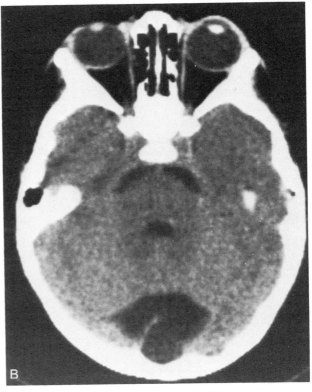

Figure 2–44A. Axial CT scan through the lower posterior fossa shows a cerebrospinal fluid density collection posterior to the medulla and medial to the cerebellar hemispheres. This collection is in communication with the cerebrospinal fluid spaces anterior to the medulla by means of vallecular and intramedullary cisterns. This represents an anatomic variant known as the mega cisterna magna, which is a simple enlargement of the cisterna magna unrelated to neurologic deficit.

Figure 2–44B. On more cephalad CT scans, the mega cisterna magna is seen to wrap around the inferior vermis and communicate directly with the superior cerebellar cistern.

Refs.: (1) Just NWM, Goldenberg M. Computed tomography of the enlarged cisterna magna. Radiology 1979; 1131:385–391. (2) Adam R, Greenberg JO. The mega cisterna magna. J Neurosurg 1978; 48:190–192.

Figure 2–45. PROMINENT TRANSVERSE SINUSES. Axial CT sections through the posterior fossa demonstrate the tubular enhancing transverse sinuses (arrowheads) that terminate near the edge of the tentorium. The sinuses are particularly prominent in this individual and are roughly the same size. Normally the sinus is closely applied to the occipital bone and sits in its own groove. In this case, however, the sinus appears to be surrounded by cerebrospinal fluid, as the patient has cerebellar atrophy.

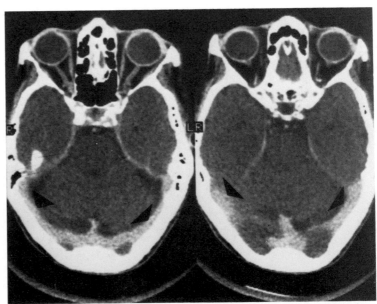

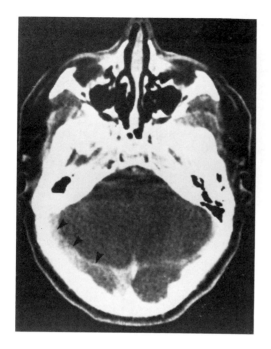

Figure 2–46. **PROMINENT TRANSVERSE SINUS.** In this instance, an axial CT section through the posterior fossa demonstrates a prominent enhancing structure posterior to the right cerebellar hemisphere. This represents a prominent transverse sinus *(arrowheads)*. Note that the contralateral transverse sinus is significantly smaller. In angiographic studies the right transverse sinus is normally larger than the left, being a direct continuation of the superior sagittal sinus in approximately 20 per cent of patients.

Ref.: Browning H. The confluence of the dural venous sinuses. Am J Anat 1959; 93:307–329.

Figure 2–47. **PROMINENT VERTEBRAL ARTERY.** Axial CT section through the foramen magnum demonstrates a high-density object *(arrowhead)* adjacent to the left lateral aspect of the medulla and anterior to the cerebellar tonsil. This is a large left vertebral artery. No right vertebral artery is identified. The left vertebral artery is larger than the right in 42 per cent of cases. One vertebral artery, most commonly the right, may be hypoplastic. This degree of asymmetry may be pathologic when associated with arteriovenous malformations or other high-flow states of the posterior fossa.

Ref.: Krayenbuhl H, Yasargil MG: Erkrankungen im Gebiet der Arteria Vertebralis, und Arteria Basialis. Stuttgart: Thieme, 1959.

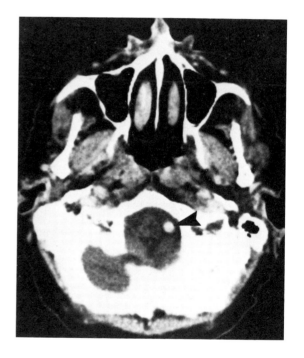

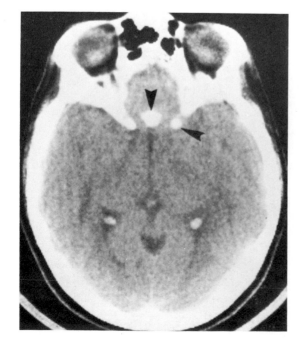

Figure 2–48. **PROMINENT PLANUM SPHENOIDALE.** The planum sphenoidale *(arrowhead, top)* is seen in this 0-degree axial CT section as an isolated bony protuberance, due to the partial volume averaging effect. This effect also causes the left anterior clinoid process *(arrowhead, below, right)* to appear separate from the lesser sphenoid wing. Diagnostic errors and unnecessary additional work-up can be avoided by examining the CT section above and below the region in question and noting adjacent anatomic structures, or by correlating the CT section in question with the digital scout radiograph.

An en plaque subfrontal meningioma causing hyperostosis may simulate a prominent planum; however, with the former, some degree of contrast enhancement is usually detectable. Spheno-ethmoidal mucoceles and mucopyoceles will expand the planum upward, but in these instances a lower CT section will reveal expanded sinus chambers with thin cortical margins.

Figure 2–49. SELLAR SPINE.

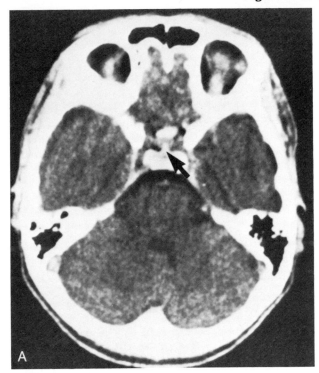

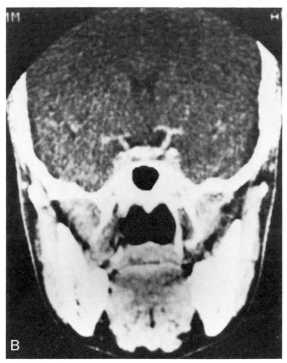

Figure 2–49A. Axial scan through the sella demonstrates a bony protuberance *(arrow)* extending anteriorly from the dorsum sella. This extends directly into the gland proper.

Figure 2–49B. Coronal view obtained through the floor of the sella demonstrates the internal carotid branching into the anterior and middle cerebral arteries and also shows a calcific high-density, midline focus. This is characteristic of a bony anomaly, which is a normal variant, known as the sellar spine. This anomaly is most likely a congenital defect in the formation and subsequent incomplete regression of the most cephalad notochord segment.

Refs.: (1) Lang J. Structure and postnatal organization of heretofore uninvestigated and infrequent associations in the sella turcica region. Acta Anat 1977; 99:121–139. (2) LaMasters DL., Boggan JE, Wilson CB. Computerized tomography of the sellar spine. J Neurosurg 1982; 57:407–409.

Figure 2–50. CAVERNOUS SINUS FAT. Axial scan of the parasellar region demonstrates low density *(arrowheads)* within the cavernous sinus proper. This material measures approximately −60 CT units, which approximates the value for adipose tissue. Although fat within the cavernous sinus has not to our knowledge been reported, its extension from the orbit would be relatively easy to explain because there is communication through the superior orbital fissure for the nerves of ocular motion as well as the superior ophthalmic vein. The latter structure directly communicates with the cavernous sinus as a pathway for venous drainage of the orbit and frontal region. While the cranial nerves within the cavernous sinus may be seen, their uniform density is not as low as in this example.

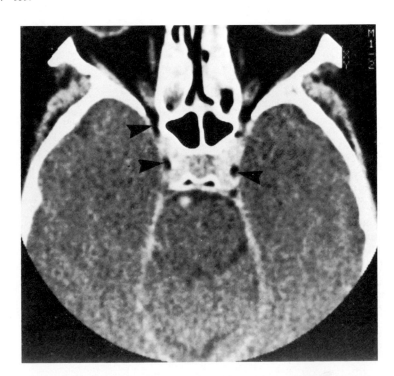

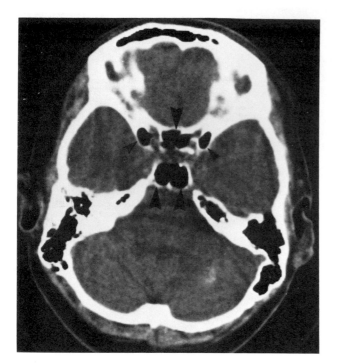

Figure 2–51. EXTENSIVE PNEUMATIZATION OF THE CLINOIDS. Axial scan obtained through the orbital roofs, parasellar region, and petrous bones demonstrates extensive pneumatization of both anterior clinoid processes *(small arrowheads),* the tuberculum *(single large arrowhead),* and the entire dorsum sella *(paired large arrowheads).* This is a relatively frequent finding on axial CT, and these gas collections should not be confused with free air within the cranial vault.

Figure 2–52. THINNING OF THE ORBITAL ROOFS. The coronal views of this patient show two regions of discontinuity *(arrowheads)* in the orbital roofs. This effect is caused by partial volume averaging of the very thinnest portion of the orbital plate of the frontal bone. This should not be mistaken for erosive phenomena from an adjacent tumor.

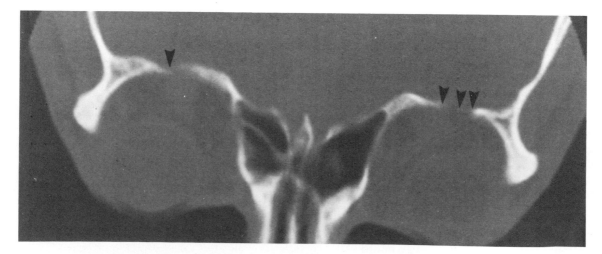

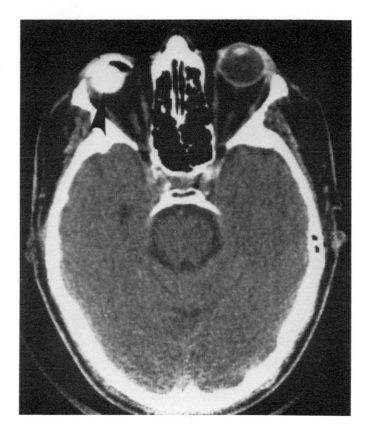

Figure 2–53. PROSTHETIC GLOBE. This axial CT scan obtained at the level of the sella turcica and orbits demonstrates a hyperdense right globe *(arrowhead)*, partially separated from the eyelid medially by a gas collection. This is the typical configuration of a globe prosthesis implanted following enucleation. Globe prostheses usually consist of two components, an anterior cornea/iris/sclera replacement which matches the contralateral visible autologous eye, and an intraorbital sphere designed to fill the enucleated orbital volume.

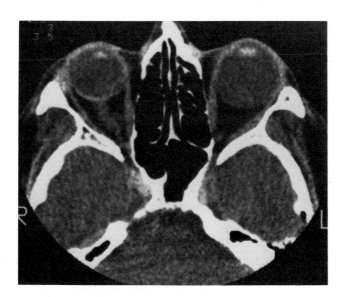

Figure 2–54. MYOPIA. Contrast-enhanced axial CT scan through the orbit shows disparity in the size of the two globes; the right is normal and the left is enlarged. Note that the enlargement is predominantly in the posterior chamber. This finding is frequently noted in myopia. Note also that there is thinning of the posterior scleral border compared with the normal right side.

Ref.: Moseley IF, Sanders MD. Computerized Tomography in Neuro-Ophthalmology. Philadelphia: W. B. Saunders Co., 1982; p 244.

Figure 2–55. BANDING OF THE GLOBE FOR RETINAL DETACHMENT. While not a normal variant, visualization of the band used in this particular surgical procedure is not an infrequent incidental finding on CT scans of the brain.

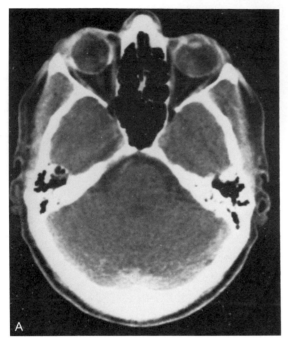

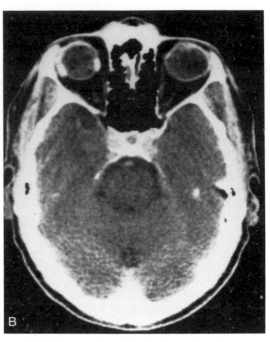

Figure 2–55A. Two high-density structures are seen in the posterior third of the right globe. This is a retinal band used to compress the globe to reduce a retinal detachment.

Figure 2–55B. At a level just above the lens, a more cephalad portion of the band is visible.

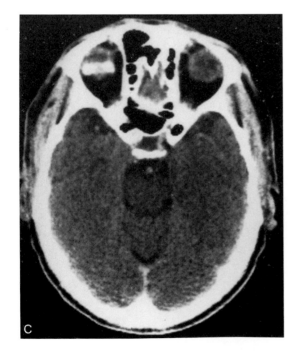

Figure 2–55C. The top portion of the band, a rectangular area of high density, is now appreciated. This band encircles the entire globe and is seen on multiple CT sections.

Ref.: Bensen WE. Retinal Detachment. Hagerstown, MD: Harper & Row, 1980; pp 101–138.

Figure 2–56. ASYMMETRY OF THE SUPERIOR ORBITAL FISSURES. Asymmetry of the superior orbital fissures can be a normal variant; however, when a significant portion of the greater wing of the sphenoid bone is absent, the diagnosis of neurofibromatosis with sphenoid dysplasia must be considered. In neurofibromatosis, however, there is usually herniation of the temporal lobe through the sphenoid defect into the orbit. Clinically this produces proptosis and exophthalmos. These findings are not present in examples below, and the widening of the fissure is considered to be secondary to an anatomic variant.

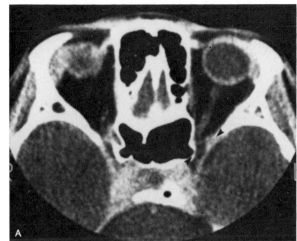

Figure 2–56A. In this axial CT section through the orbits, there is asymmetry of the superior orbital fissures, with the left superior orbital fissure being widened compared with the right.

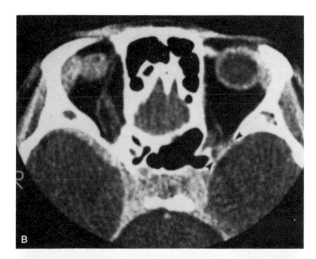

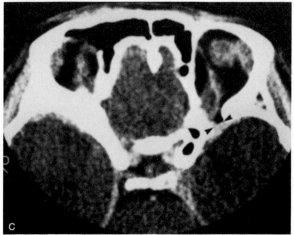

Figure 2–56B and C. This finding persists on contiguous cephalad axial images.

Ref.: Holt JF. Neurofibromatosis in children. AJR 1978; 130:615–640.

CHAPTER 3

Spine

CLYDE A. HELMS, M.D.
JAMES B. VOGLER, III, M.D.

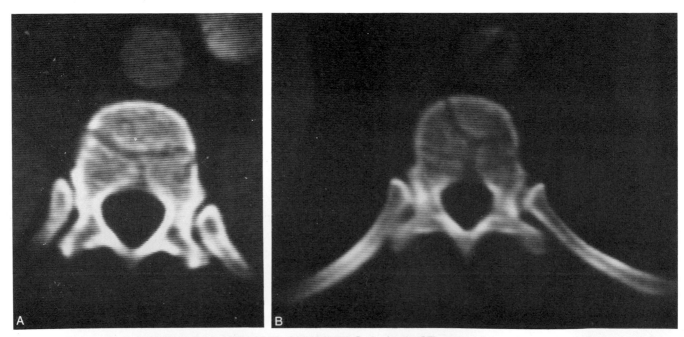

Figure 3–1. INCOMPLETE SCANNING PROTOCOL. This particular scanning protocol, with scans parallel to the disc and several scans above and below the disc, leaves gaps in the scanning sequence in the central canal *(arrows)*, which are areas where free fragments or spinal stenosis could be missed.

Figure 3–2. VERTEBRAL VENOUS CHANNELS. In both CT scans, linear lucencies are seen in the mid-portion of the vertebral body extending into the basivertebral plexus. These are characteristic for vertebral venous channels and should not be confused with fractures. They can be differentiated by their location exclusive to the mid-vertebral body slice.

Refs.: (1) Haughton VM, Syvertsen A, Williams AL. Soft-tissue anatomy within the spinal canal as seen on CT. Radiology 1980; 134:649–655. (2) Dorwart RH, Sauerland EK, Haughton VM, et al. In: Newton TH, Potts DG, eds. CT of the Spine and Spinal Cord. San Anselmo, CA: Clavadel Press, 1983; p 94.

Figure 3–3. VERTEBRAL BODY VENOUS CHANNELS AND FRACTURE.

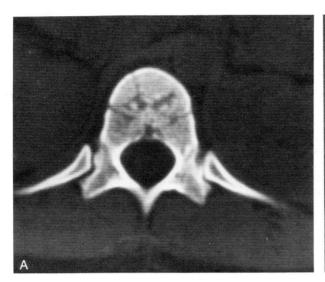
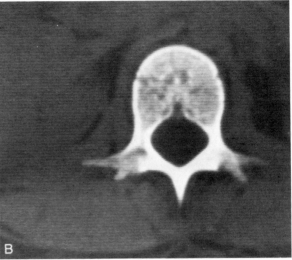

Figure 3–3A and B. Vertebral body veins draining into the basivertebral plexus are seen in the mid-vertebral body slices of thoracic vertebrae at two levels in this patient.

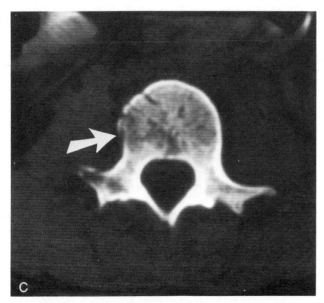
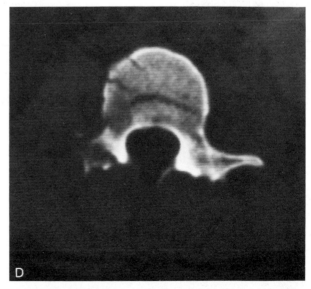

Figure 3–3C. A fracture can be seen through the mid-vertebral body with a step-off of the cortex laterally *(arrow)*.

Figure 3–3D. Multiple linear structures can be differentiated from venous channels by their location (removed from the mid-vertebral body level) and their lack of communication with the basivertebral plexus.

Figure 3–4. BASIVERTEBRAL PLEXUS.

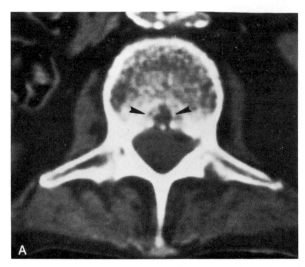

Figure 3–4A. The basivertebral plexus is found in the mid-vertebral body level posteriorly and usually presents as a distinct lucency *(arrowheads)*.

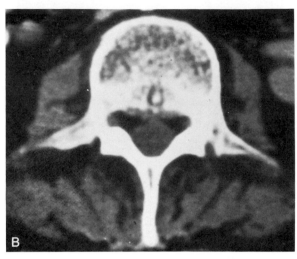

Figure 3–4B. A small amount of calcification can be seen within the plexus.

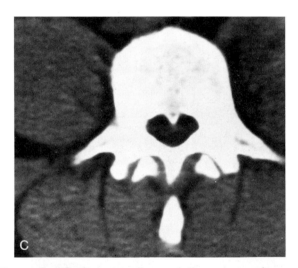

Figure 3–4C. Occasionally a calcific spur can be seen protruding from the basivertebral plexus.

Refs.: (1) Haughton VM, Syvertsen A, Williams AL. Soft-tissue anatomy within the spinal canal as seen on CT. Radiology 1980; 134:649–655. (2) Dorwart RH, Sauerland EK, Haughton VM, et al. Normal lumbrosacral spine. In: Newton TH, Potts, DG, eds. CT of the Spine and Spinal Cord. San Anselmo, CA: Clavadel Press, 1983; p 94.

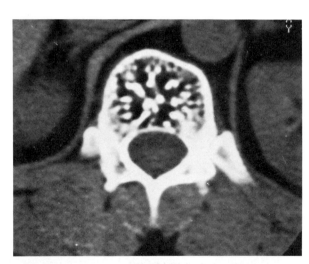

Figure 3–5. HEMANGIOMA. A vertebral body hemangioma has a characteristic CT appearance with hypertrophied individual trabecular struts giving a wild-looking pattern such as this.

Ref.: Helms CA, Vogler JB, Genant HK. Characteristic CT manifestations of uncommon spinal disorders. Orthop Clin North Am 1985; 16:445–459.

Figure 3–6. FOCAL HEMANGIOMA.

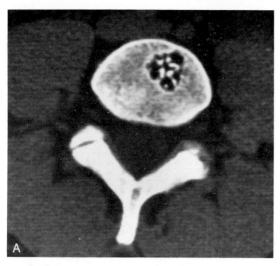

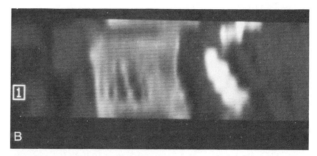

Figure 3–6A. A focal area of hypertrophied trabecular struts, characteristic of a hemangioma, is seen in this vertebral body.

Figure 3–6B. A sagittal reformation through this lesion shows a "corduroy striped" appearance that is characteristic of hemangioma.

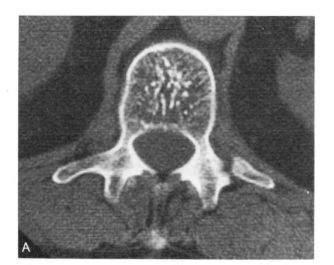

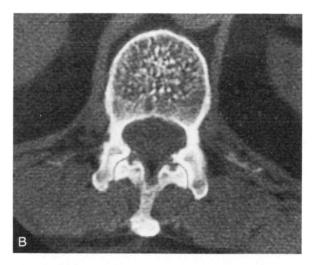

Figure 3–7. OSTEOPOROSIS SIMULATING HEMANGIOMA. Osteoporosis can sometimes be associated with apparent hypertrophy of the trabeculae and thus mimic hemangiomas, as in these scans from the same patient. Osteoporosis will generally have this appearance at multiple levels, whereas hemangiomas most commonly will involve only a single level. It can on occasion be difficult to differentiate these two entities.

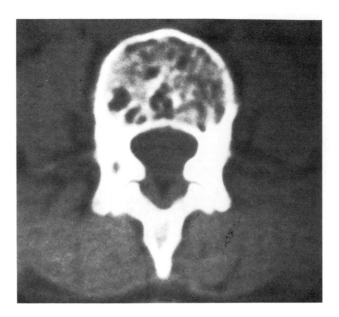

Figure 3–8. MULTIPLE MYELOMA. Multiple irregular lucencies are seen throughout the vertebral body in this patient with known multiple myeloma. The plain films in this patient showed only mild osteopenia. The pattern shown here is characteristic for early multiple myeloma and should not be confused with osteoporosis in which the lucencies generally appear more regular and have trabeculae within (compare Figure 3–7B).

Ref.: Helms CA, Genant HK. CT in the early detection of skeletal involvement with multiple myeloma. JAMA 1982; 248:2886–2887.

Figure 3–9. MULTIPLE MYELOMA. This is multiple myeloma in a more chronic form than that shown in Figure 3–8. The trabecular struts have undergone compensatory hypertrophy giving it a sclerotic appearance on CT. The plain film in this case showed only striking osteopenia.

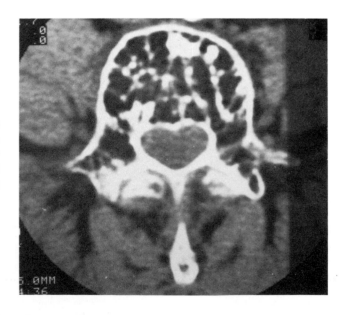

Ref.: Helms CA, Vogler JB, Genant HK. Characteristic CT manifestations of uncommon spinal disorders. Orthop Clin North Am 1985; 16:445–459.

Figure 3–10. PAGET'S DISEASE.

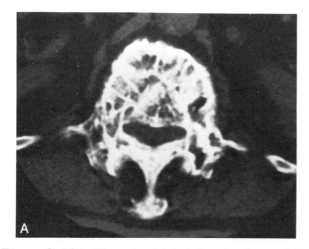

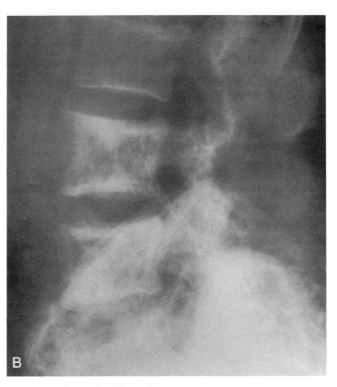

Figure 3–10A. The mixed lytic/sclerotic phase of Paget's disease can mimic multiple myeloma (as seen in Figure 3–9) or even hemangioma. Encroachment on the central canal by bony overgrowth, however, helps make the diagnosis of Paget's disease.

Figure 3–10B. Plain films in this case demonstrate sclerotic, overgrown vertebrae. For the diagnosis of myeloma to be considered, the appearance would have to be osteopenic.

Ref.: Helms CA, Vogler JB, Genant HK. Characteristic CT manifestations of uncommon spinal disorders. Orthop Clin North Am 1985; 16:445–459.

Figure 3–11. PAGET'S DISEASE. Diffuse sclerosis involving the vertebral body and the posterior elements with encroachment on the central canal is characteristic of Paget's disease. Degenerative disease of the facets can occasionally have a similar appearance.

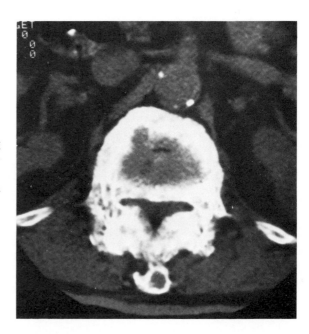

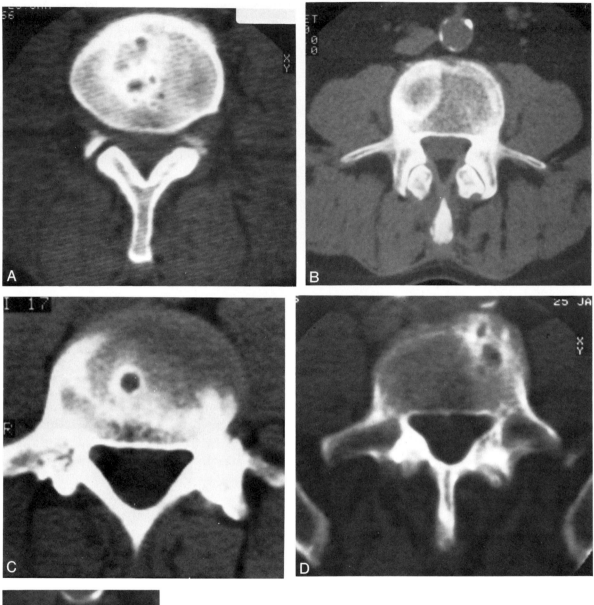

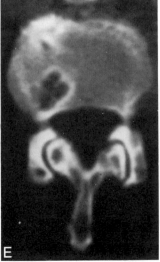

Figure 3–12. SCHMORL'S NODES. Multiple examples of Schmorl's nodes are shown *(A–E)*. On CT, Schmorl's nodes are characterized by a sclerotic periphery with various degrees of lucency within. They are typically located adjacent to the disc space. These characteristics help differentiate Schmorl's nodes from other processes such as metastatic disease. Rarely, a metastatic focus can have a similar appearance.

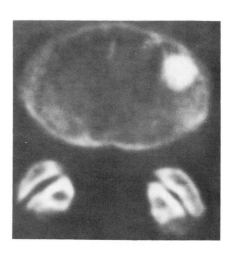

Figure 3–13. METASTATIC DISEASE. A prostate metastasis in this ventral body appears as a blastic focus with a lucent periphery. Note the difference between this and the Schmorl's node, which has a lucent centrum and a sclerotic periphery (compare Figure 3–12).

Figure 3–14. SCHMORL'S NODES AND METASTATIC DISEASE.

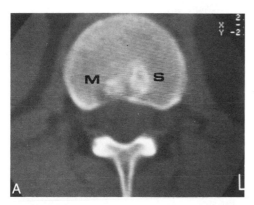

Figure 3–14A. CT scan shows two sclerotic processes, both of which originally were diagnosed as Schmorl's nodes. The lesion with the lucent periphery represents a metastatic focus (M); the lesion with the sclerotic periphery and lucent centrum is a Schmorl's node (S).

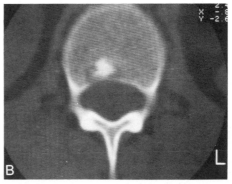

Figure 3–14B. In a CT section adjacent to A, the lesion with the lucent periphery is seen best.

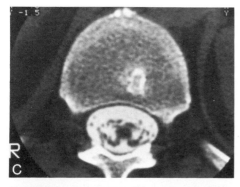

Figure 3–14C. In a metrizamide-enhanced repeat scan performed three months later, the lesion with the sclerotic periphery (labeled S in A) is unchanged.

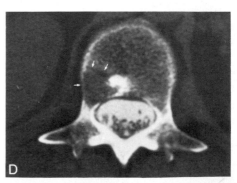

Figure 3–14D. Another section of the repeat scan shows that the lesion with the lucent periphery has progressed to destroy more of the vertebral body (*arrows*).

Figure 3–15. PSEUDODISC SECONDARY TO PARTIAL VOLUME AVERAGING.

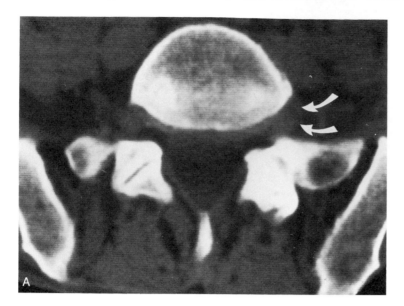

Figure 3–15A. An apparent lateral disc *(arrows)* is noted on the left side.

Figure 3–15B. The next most caudal scan shows that the left pedicle is in this region, raising the question of partial volume averaging of this structure.

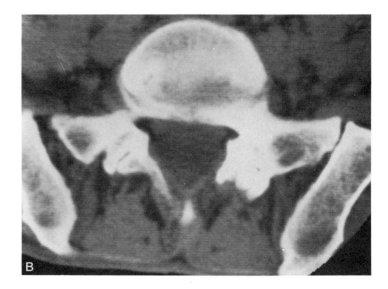

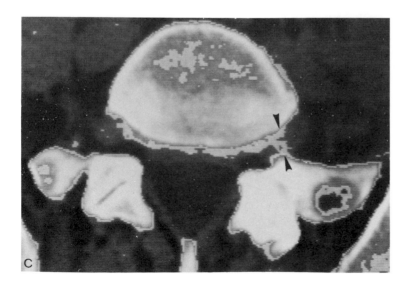

Figure 3–15C. In reviewing the first slice *(A)* with the blink mode, part of the increased density *(arrowheads)* is shown to be columnar in shape and increased in density over the remainder of the mass. This is partial volume averaging of the pedicle and accounts for a portion of the mass, with the nerve root or dorsal root ganglion making up the remainder. A small amount of the disc material can be seen blinking as it extends beyond the posterior margin of the endplate. This is the same density as the partially volume averaged pedicle.

Figure 3–16. INTERFACET ARTIFACT.

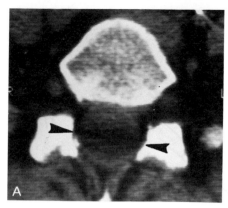

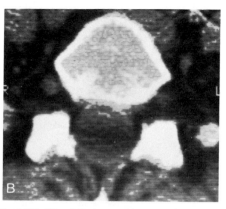

Figure 3–16A. An interfacet artifact *(arrowheads)* is seen crossing the thecal sac. This gives the anterior portion of the thecal sac a relative increase in density over the posterior portion, mimicking a large disc protrusion.

Figure 3–16B. The blink mode is used to visualize disc material. The anterior portion of the thecal sac is shown not to be highlighted at disc densities.

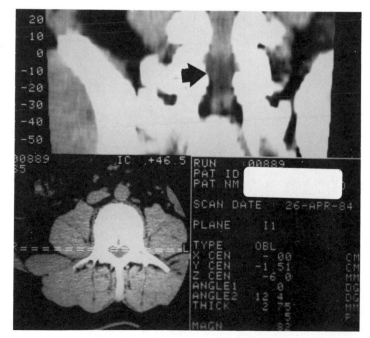

Figure 3–17. FACET ARTIFACT. A coronal reformation through the lumbar spine shows an area of decreased attenuation *(arrow)* which is the result of a facet artifact. These can occur in both axial or reformatted images and should be considered whenever an area of low attenuation is seen that cannot be easily explained.

Figure 3–18. PSEUDO–LATERAL DISCS SECONDARY TO SCOLIOSIS. Contiguous axial scans in this patient with marked scoliosis demonstrate pseudo–lateral disc herniations *(arrow and arrowheads)* that are due to the oblique angulation of the disc in relation to the axial scan.

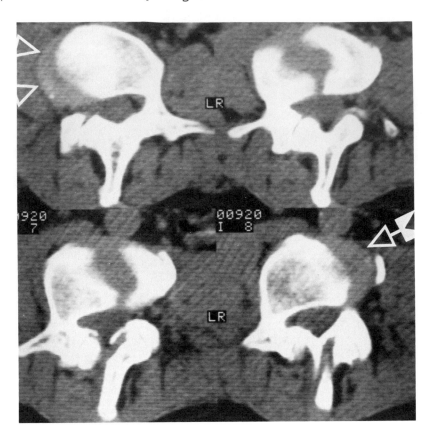

Figure 3–19. PSEUDODISC AT L5–S1.

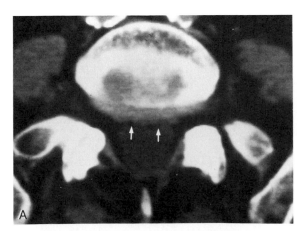

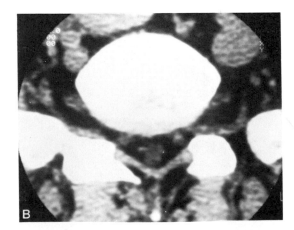

Figure 3–19A. The disc at L5–S1 normally has a convex posterior configuration, which together with a marked lordosis can make this appear to be a broad-based disc protrusion. Note the preserved epidural fat *(arrows)* between the thecal sac and the disc in this normal example.

Figure 3–19B. This is another example of the convex appearance of the L5–S1 disc.

Figure 3–20. OSTEOPHYTOSIS. Osteophytes can be anterior or posterior. Differentiation of an osteophyte from a calcified disc protrusion cannot be reliably made on CT.

Figure 3–20A. This CT scan shows anterior osteophyte formation.

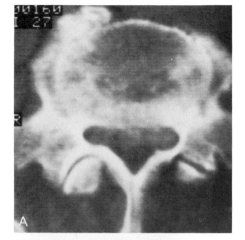

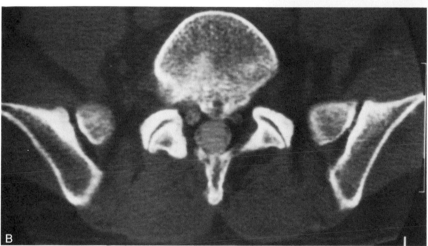

Figure 3–20B. Osteophyte formation is located posteriorly in this CT scan.

Figure 3–21. BODY OF SACRUM SIMULATING DISC PROTRUSION.

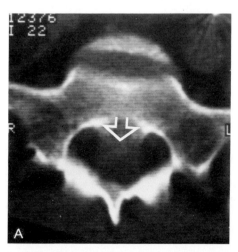

Figure 3–21A. An apparent osteophyte or disc protrusion into the central canal is noted *(arrow)*.

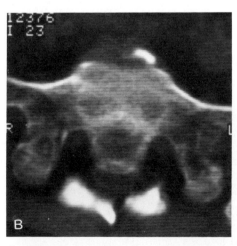

Figure 3–21B. The caudal slice adjacent to A shows this to represent partial volume averaging of the normal body of the sacrum, which often has this appearance.

Figure 3–22. CALCIFIED INTERVERTEBRAL DISC.

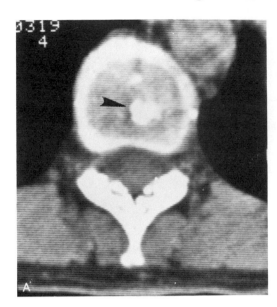

Figure 3–22A. Blastic-appearing lesions *(arrowhead)* are identified in a lower thoracic vertebra.

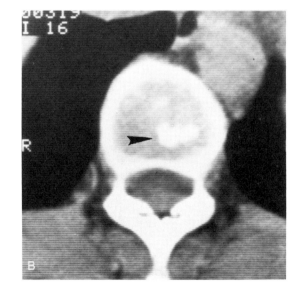

Figure 3–22B. Blastic-appearing lesions *(arrowheads)* are also demonstrated at a level adjacent to *A.*

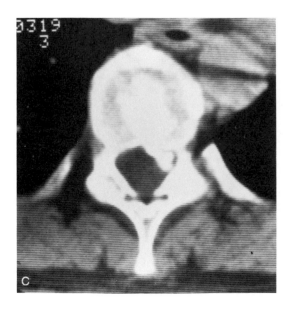

Figure 3–22C. A contiguous slice confirms that the "lesion" seen in *A* and *B* actually represents portions of a calcified disc that have extended into the vertebral body (calcified Schmorl's node). Note also that the calcified disc has herniated into the central canal.

Figure 3–23. COMPRESSION FRACTURE. A compression fracture may have a bizarre appearance and mimic infection or a metastatic destructive process. In this example, the paravertebral masses were believed to be hematomas. This patient was biopsied and found to have no infection or tumor.

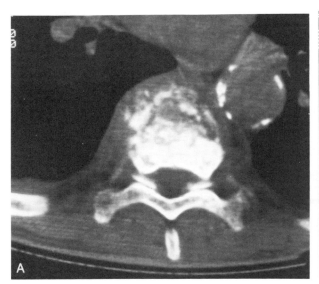
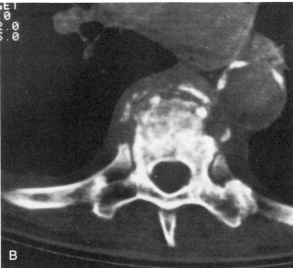

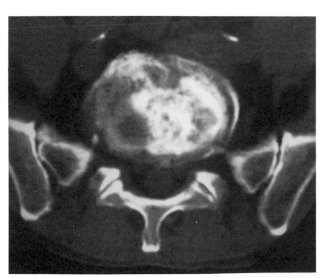

Figure 3–24. DEGENERATIVE DISC DISEASE. Severe degenerative disc disease can sometimes mimic infection or metastatic disease, as in this example of severe degenerative changes involving the inferior endplate of L5. The absence of destructive foci in the vertebral body, the lack of cortical breakthrough, and normal paravertebral soft tissues help to exclude more aggressive processes.

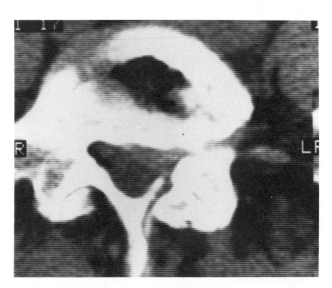

Figure 3–25. VACUUM DISC. A vacuum disc is commonly seen in degenerative disc disease and should not be interpreted as gas secondary to an infection.

Ref.: Larde D, Mathieu D, Frija J. Spinal vacuum phenomenon: CT diagnosis and significance. J Comput Assist Tomogr 1982; 6:671–676.

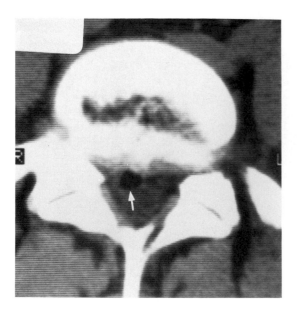

Figure 3–26. GAS IN THE CENTRAL CANAL. In this axial scan in a patient with a vacuum disc phenomenon, gas is seen in the central canal *(arrow)*, which in this example was secondary to a defect in the anulus fibrosus that allowed gas to leak into the central canal. This does not necessarily indicate a herniated nucleus pulposus.

Figure 3–27. INTERVERTEBRAL VACUUM CLEFT.

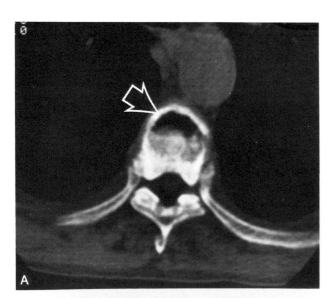

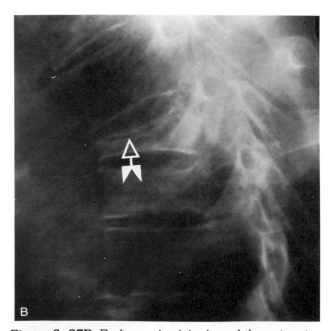

Figure 3–27A. A subchondral gas density *(arrow)* on CT can mimic a vacuum disc; however, if it can be localized to the vertebral body, it is said to be pathognomonic for aseptic necrosis.

Figure 3–27B. Radiograph of the lateral thoracic spine in this patient shows a collapsed vertebral body with a subchondral lucency *(arrow)*. This plain film appearance has been termed an intervertebral vacuum cleft and is said to be a reliable indicator of aseptic necrosis. When it is present, metastatic disease can be excluded as the cause of the collapse.

Ref.: Maldague BE, Noel HM, Malghem JJ. The intervertebral vacuum cleft: A sign of ischemic vertebral collapse. Radiology 1978; 129:23–29.

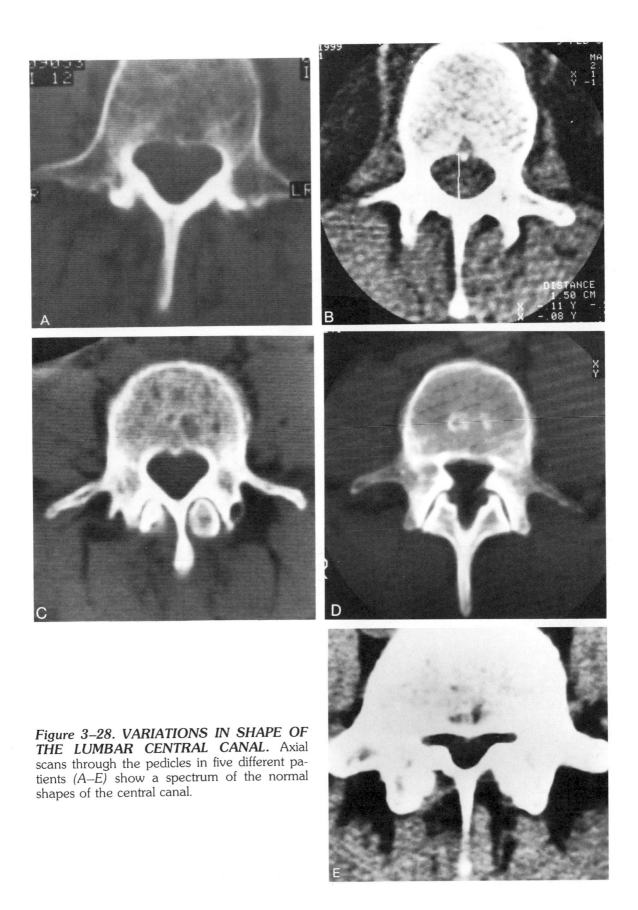

Figure 3–28. VARIATIONS IN SHAPE OF THE LUMBAR CENTRAL CANAL. Axial scans through the pedicles in five different patients *(A–E)* show a spectrum of the normal shapes of the central canal.

Figure 3–29. EFFECT OF WINDOW SETTING ON CENTRAL CANAL SIZE.

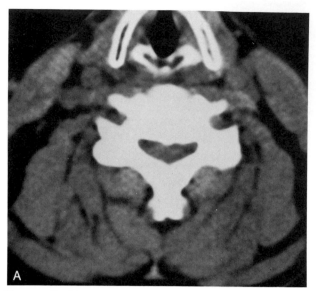

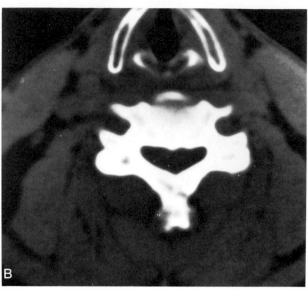

Figure 3–29A. An axial scan of the cervical spine shows apparent central canal stenosis when viewed at soft-tissue windows.

Figure 3–29B. When viewed at bone window settings, the central canal appears within normal limits (compare with A).

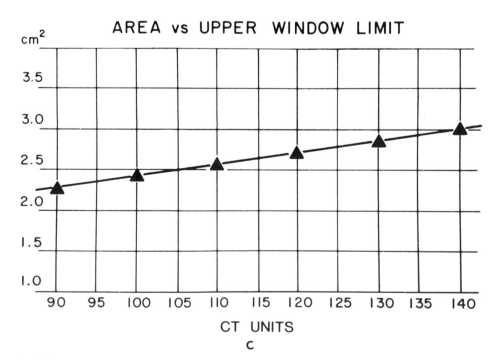

Figure 3–29C. This graph illustrates the effect of the window setting on the apparent area of the spinal canal.

Ref.: Ullrich CG, Binet EF, Sanecki MG, Kieffer SA. Quantitative assessment of the lumbar spinal canal by CT. Radiology 1980; 134:137–143. Figure 3–29C reprinted with permission.

Figure 3–30. UNRELIABILITY OF MEASUREMENTS IN DIAGNOSING SPINAL STENOSIS.

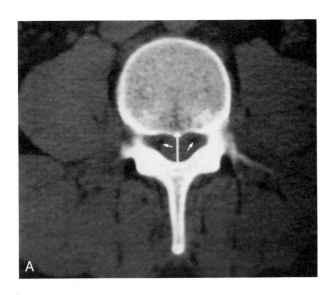

Figure 3–30A. Axial scan through the lumbar spine with cursor measurements shows the anteroposterior diameter of the central canal to be 11.4 mm. Even though this measurement is below the lower limit of normal (12 mm), this patient had no evidence clinically of spinal stenosis. Patients with small-diameter central canals do not necessarily have clinical spinal stenosis if their thecal sacs are proportionally small. Note the spherical shape of the thecal sac and the presence of epidural fat *(arrows)*.

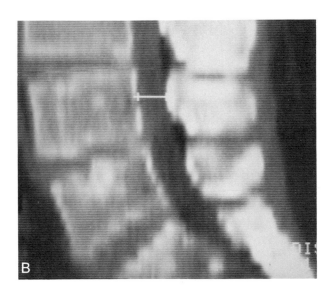

Figure 3–30B. A sagittal reformation of the lumbar spine (same patient as in A) with a cursor measurement of the central canal again shows an 11.2-mm diameter. Note the absence of bony impingement on the thecal sac.

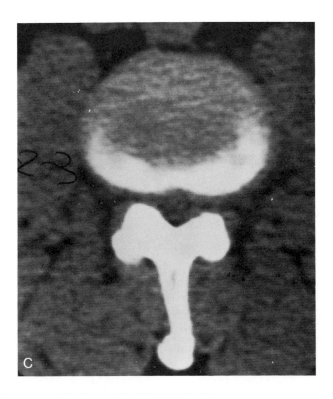

Figure 3–30C. Note that in this patient with spinal stenosis, the thecal sac appears to be compressed in an anteroposterior direction and the epidural fat is obliterated in comparison with the axial scan of the patient shown in A.

Ref. Helms CA, Vogler JB. CT of spinal stenoses and arthroses. Clin Rheum Dis 1983; 9:417–441.

Figure 3–31. **UNRELIABILITY OF CENTRAL CANAL MEASUREMENTS IN DIAGNOSING SPINAL STENOSIS.**

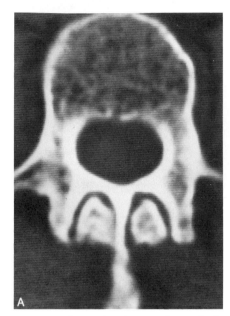

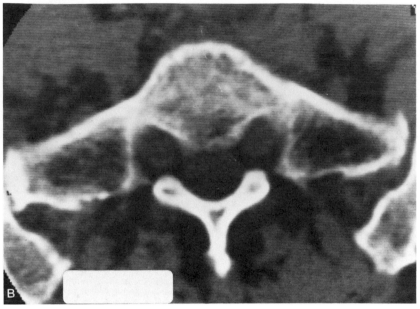

Figure 3–31A. Axial scan through the lumbar spine in this patient with normal measurements of the bony central canal and classic symptoms of spinal stenosis shows obliteration of the epidural fat at this level.

Figure 3–31B. Axial scan through the S1 level shows disproportion between the size of the central canal and that of the neural elements. The nerve roots and the thecal sac are much larger than are normally seen at this level. Subsequent surgical decompression laminectomy relieved this patient's symptoms of spinal stenosis. This is an example of normal bony measurements with disproportionate enlargement of the thecal sac and nerve roots, resulting in clinical spinal stenosis.

Figure 3–32. **ANTERIOR INTERNAL EPIDURAL VEINS.**

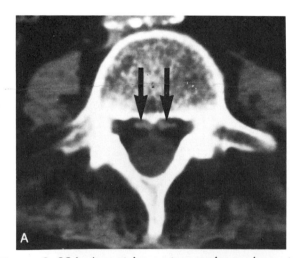

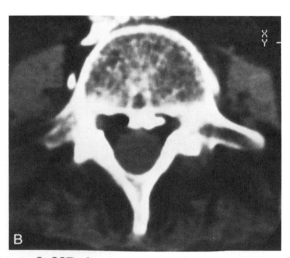

Figure 3–32A. An axial scan in a cadaver shows two soft-tissue densities anterior to the thecal sac *(arrows)* that are characteristic for the anterior internal epidural veins. They are typically isodense or near-isodense to the neural elements and therefore should be differentiated from a free disc fragment, which would be increased in density. The veins are usually most prominent adjacent to the basivertebral plexus in the mid-vertebral body area.

Figure 3–32B. In the same cadaver specimen, the veins were injected with contrast material, confirming the vascular nature of these densities. (Courtesy of Dr. Robert Dorwart.)

Ref.: Dorwart RH, Sauerland EK, Haughton VM, et al. Normal lumbosacral spine. In: Newton TH, Potts DG, eds. CT of the Spine and Spinal Cord. San Anselmo, CA: Clavadel Press, 1983; p 94.

Figure 3–33. VARIATION IN NERVE ROOT SHEATH SIZE.

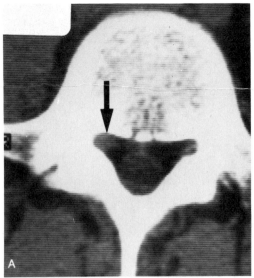

Figure 3–33A. Considerable variation in the size of the nerve root sheaths can be seen in normal and pathologic conditions. In this asymptomatic patient the right nerve root *(arrow)* is considerably larger than the left, and this is considered a normal variant.

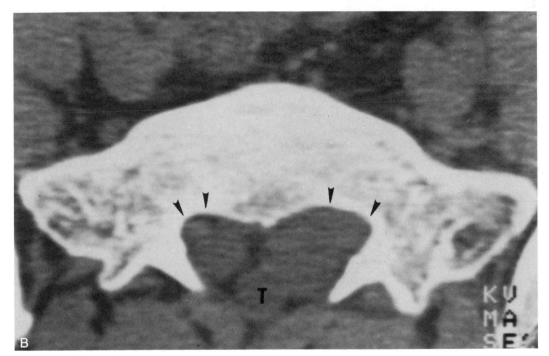

Figure 3–33B. In this patient with spina bifida, gross enlargement of the nerve root sheaths is seen bilaterally with some erosion of the lateral recesses *(arrowheads)*. Cystic dilatations of the nerve root sheaths are known as Tarlov cysts. These should be isodense to the thecal sac (T) and thereby differentiated from free disc fragments. Conjoined nerve roots may be confused with Tarlov cysts. Both conjoined nerve roots and Tarlov cysts are thought to be asymptomatic.

Figure 3–34. POSTOPERATIVE FIBROSIS.

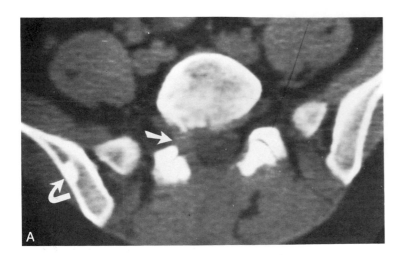

Figure 3–34A. Postoperative fibrosis usually is seen on CT as a soft-tissue mass with a density greater than that of the thecal sac, as seen on the right side *(straight arrow)*. Incidentally noted is a bone island in the right iliac wing *(curved arrow)*.

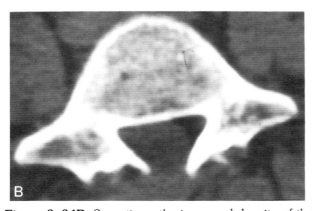

Figure 3–34B. Sometimes the increased density of the postoperative fibrosis can be difficult to appreciate, as seen here.

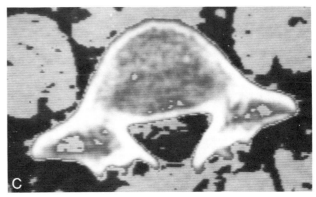

Figure 3–34C. In cases such as *B*, the blink mode can be useful in separating the fibrosis from the thecal sac, as in this example. Since disc fragments would also be expected to be increased in density over the thecal sac and could have similar configurations as these examples, it may be extremely difficult to differentiate disc fragments from fibrosis.

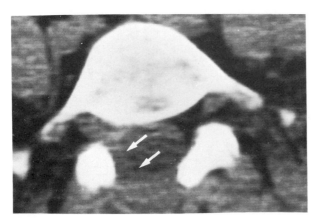

Figure 3–35. POSTOPERATIVE FIBROSIS. Obliteration of epidural fat often occurs secondary to postoperative fibrosis. Characteristically, as in this example, the fibrosis *(arrows)* is increased in density in comparison with the thecal sac and has been reported to be generally decreased in density in comparison with disc fragments; however, this can be difficult to appreciate.

Ref.: Teplick JG, Haskin ME. CT of the postoperative lumbar spine. Radiol Clin North Am 21:395, 1983.

Figure 3–36. CONJOINED NERVE ROOTS.

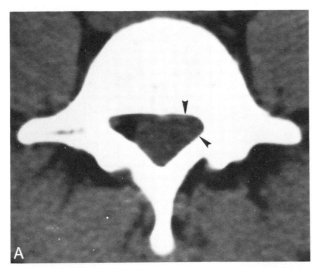

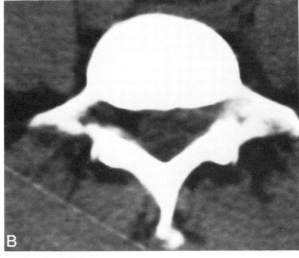

Figure 3–36A. An asymmetric soft-tissue density is seen in the left lateral recess *(arrowheads)*. It appears isodense to the thecal sac.

Figure 3–36B. A contiguous caudal slice shows the soft-tissue density on the left side persisting.

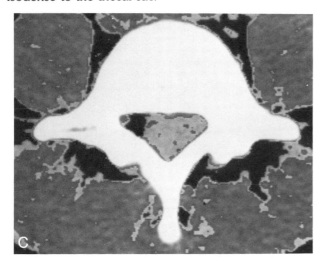

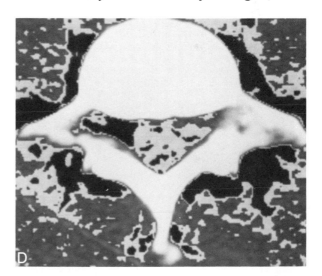

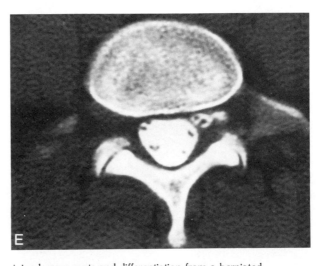

Figure 3–36C, D, and E. *C and D,* The blink mode demonstrates that the soft-tissue density in the left lateral recess is isodense to the thecal sac and nerve roots. This will differentiate a conjoined nerve root, as in these examples, from a free disc fragment. The asymmetric shape of the lateral recesses is also helpful in making this differentiation. Because of the decreased amount of cerebrospinal fluid in the nerve root sheaths, the conjoined nerve root may appear slightly increased in density in comparison with the thecal sac but is never high enough in density to mimic disc fragments. *E,* A metrizamide CT scan in this patient confirms the double rootlet or conjoined nerve root on the left side.

From: Helms CA, Dorwart R, Gray MB. The CT appearance of conjoined nerve roots and differentiation from a herniated nucleus pulposus. Radiology 1982; 144:803–807. Reproduced with permission.

Figure 3–37. CONJOINED NERVE ROOT.

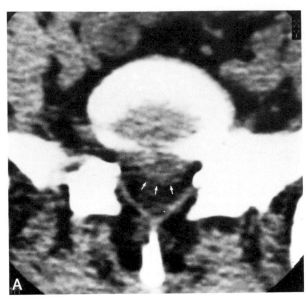

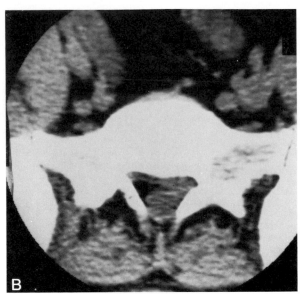

Figure 3–37A. An axial scan through the L5–S1 level shows a large focal disc herniation *(arrows).* Note the increase in density of the disc material in comparison with the thecal sac.

Figure 3–37B. A section caudal to the L5–S1 disc shows soft-tissue density in the left lateral recess that was felt to be consistent with a free disc fragment.

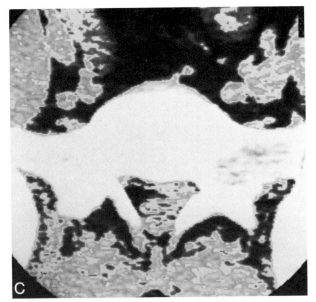

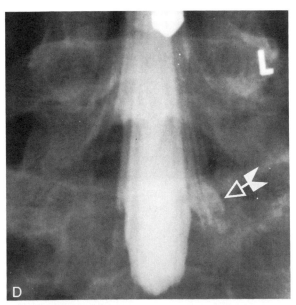

Figure 3–37C. The blink mode shows this soft-tissue density to be isodense to the thecal sac, making the diagnosis of a conjoined nerve root more likely. A disc fragment would have increased soft-tissue density in comparison with the thecal sac. Note also the asymmetry of the left lateral recess in comparison to the right.

Figure 3–37D. A myelogram in this case shows the conjoined nerve root at L5–S1 on the left side *(arrow).* The disc herniation is not seen on the anteroposterior view but was confirmed at surgery.

Figure 3–38. CONJOINED NERVE ROOT.

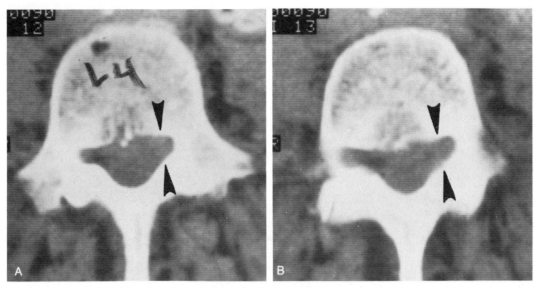

Figure 3–38A and B. Contiguous axial scans through the L4 vertebral body and superior portion of the L4–5 intervertebral disc demonstrate asymmetry of the soft tissues and bony margins of the lateral recesses. Epidural fat is absent in the left lateral recess due to the presence of a conjoined nerve root. Enlargement of the bony margins *(arrowheads)* of the left lateral recess is an ancillary finding seen in association with conjoined nerve roots.

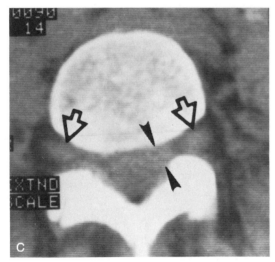

Figure 3–38C. Dorsal root ganglia *(open arrows)* are identified in the neuroforamina. Note the mild asymmetry of the thecal sac on the left *(arrowheads)*, as a result of the conjoined nerve root.

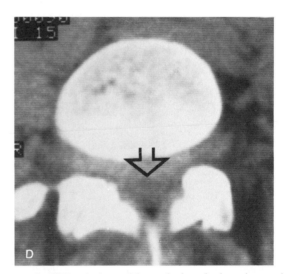

Figure 3–38D. A broad-based disc bulge *(arrow)* is evident at the superior portion of the intervertebral disc. In cases such as this, the soft-tissue asymmetry of the recesses seen in *A* and *B* has sometimes been mistaken for extruded disc fragments. The bony asymmetry of the lateral recesses then becomes a key finding to identify the conjoined nerve root as the etiology of the soft-tissue asymmetry.

Ref.: Hoddick WK, Helms CA. Bony spinal canal changes that differentiate conjoined nerve roots from herniated nucleus pulposus. Radiology 1985; 154:119–120.

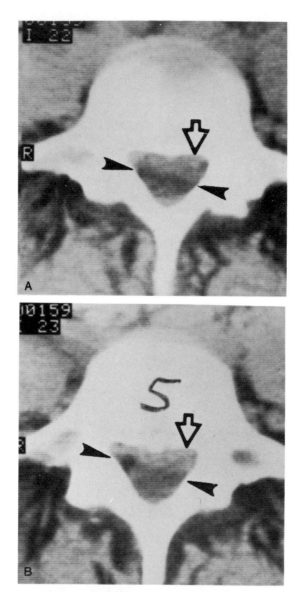

Figure 3–39. CONJOINED NERVE ROOT AND INTERFACET ARTIFACT. On contiguous axial CT scans in this patient with a conjoined nerve root *(open arrow)*, an interfacet artifact *(arrowheads)* has made the conjoined nerve root in these scans appear relatively increased in density, thereby mimicking a free disc fragment. The bony asymmetry of the left lateral recess compared to the right (a secondary sign of conjoined nerve roots) will help to differentiate this from a free disc fragment. Evaluation of CT attenuation numbers or blink mode would show the conjoined nerve root to be considerably decreased in density compared to disc tissue.

Figure 3–40. CONJOINED NERVE ROOT AND INTERFACET ARTIFACT.

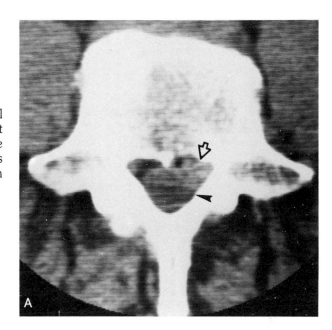

Figure 3–40A. An axial scan through the L5 vertebral body shows a soft-tissue density *(open arrow)* in the left lateral recess that appears increased in density over the thecal sac. A facet artifact *(arrowhead)*, also noted, is causing the thecal sac to be artificially decreased in density.

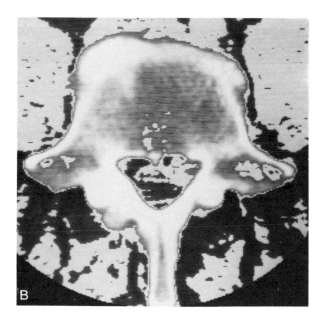

Figure 3–40B. When the blink mode is applied to the scan in *A* and set at usual thecal sac levels (60 HU), the soft-tissue mass is highlighted, indicating that it has similar density.

Figure 3–40C. The thecal sac becomes highlighted when the blink mode level is set at negative values—near those of epidural fat. This case illustrates how a facet artifact can artifically lower the density of one structure (the thecal sac), making an isodense structure (a conjoined root in this case) resemble a free disc fragment.

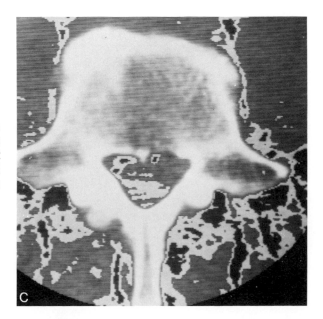

Figure 3–41. INTRASPINAL SYNOVIAL CYSTS.

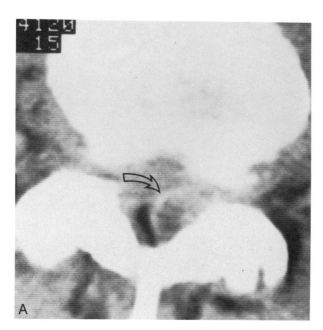

Figure 3–41A. This axial scan demonstrates a spherical soft-tissue density with a sharp rim *(arrow)* arising adjacent to a degenerated facet joint. This appearance is characteristic for an intraspinal synovial cyst. Most investigators believe that these are asymptomatic in nature and often spontaneously decompress. The characteristic location and appearance should be diagnostic. They are always located adjacent to the facet joints and are considered by some to be analogous to synovial ganglion cysts seen in other joints.

Figure 3–41B. Bone window scans of two sections at the same level as *A* again demonstrate the synovial cyst *(arrows)* but show more clearly the degenerative changes in the facet joints with which these cysts are often associated.

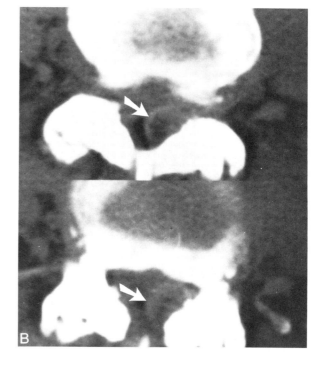

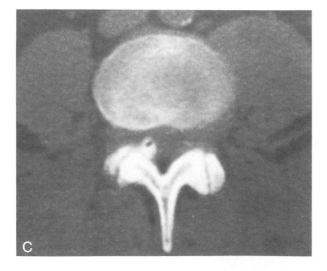

Figure 3–41C. In a different patient, a facet arthrogram with subsequent CT scan has been performed. In this case the synovial cyst has filled with contrast material, confirming the intra-articular association.

Ref.: Hemminghytt S, Daniels DL, Williams AL, Haughton VM. Intraspinal synovial cysts: Natural history and diagnosis by CT. Radiology 1982; 145:375, 1982.

Figure 3–42. CALCIFICATION OF THE POSTERIOR LONGITUDINAL LIGAMENT.

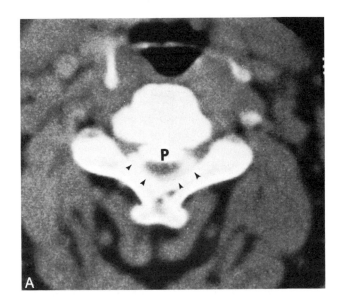

Figure 3–42A. This metrizamide CT scan through the cervical spine shows calcification of the posterior longitudinal ligament (P), causing encroachment on the spinal cord. The remainder of the cord is outlined with metrizamide *(arrowheads)*. Calcification of the posterior longitudinal ligament is reported to occur in up to 25 per cent of patients with diffuse idiopathic skeletal hyperostosis (DISH).

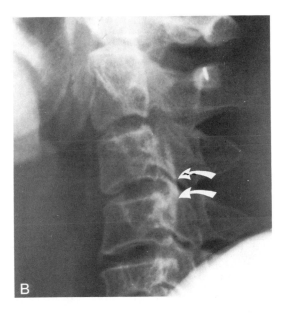

Figure 3–42B. A lateral plain film in this case shows calcification of the posterior longitudinal ligament *(arrows)* at the C3-4 vertebral body level. Often the calcification is not seen on plain films but is clearly visible in CT.

Figure 3–42C. A lateral radiograph of the thoracic spine shows exuberant anterior osteophytosis *(arrows)* without significant disc-space narrowing—typical findings of DISH.

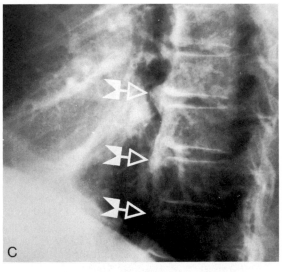

From: Helms CA, Vogler JB. Spinal stenosis and degenerative lesions. In: Newton TH, Potts, DG, eds. CT of the Spine and Spinal Cord. San Anselmo, CA: Clavadel Press, 1983; p 257. Reproduced with permission.

Ref.: Resnick D, Guerra J, Robinson CA, Vint VC. Association of diffuse idiopathic skeletal hyperostosis (DISH) and calcification and ossification of the posterior longitudinal ligament. AJR 1978; 131:1049–1053.

Figure 3–43. **CALCIFICATION OF THE POSTERIOR LONGITUDINAL LIGAMENT.**

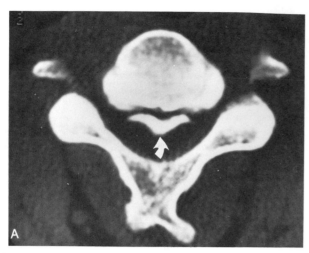

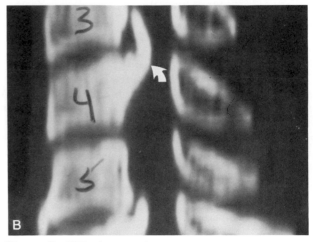

Figure 3–43A. Axial scan of the cervical spine shows calcification of the posterior longitudinal ligament *(arrow)*, which appears separated from the vertebral body on this section.

Figure 3–43B. A sagittal reformation through the cervical spine shows bulky calcification *(arrow)* posterior to C3-4. As in *A,* this finding should not be mistaken for a free disc fragment or osteophyte, especially when it is seen extending over one or more vertebral body levels.

Figure 3–44. **ASCENDING LUMBAR VEINS.**

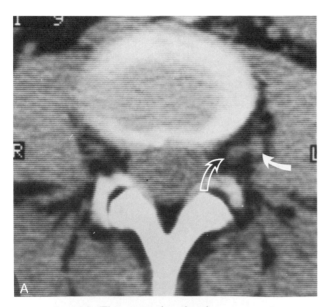

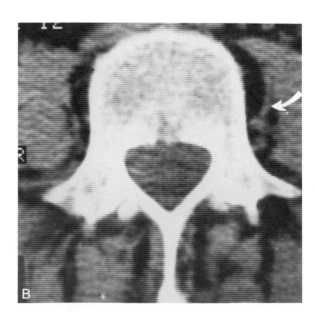

Figure 3–44A. The ascending lumbar veins often have a variable course. In some patients, the veins *(solid arrow)* may lie adjacent to the dorsal root ganglia *(open arrow).* These should not be confused with lesions arising from or near the dorsal root ganglia.

Figure 3–44B. A more caudal scan demonstrates branching of the venous structure *(arrow)* to allow this differentiation.

Refs.: (1) Dorwart RH, DeGroot J, Sauerland EK, et al. Computed tomography of the lumbosacral spine: Normal anatomy, anatomic variants, and pathologic anatomy. Radiographics 1982; 2:459–499. (2) Dorwart RH, Sauerland EK, Haughton VM, et al. Normal lumbosacral spine. *In:* Newton TH, Potts DG, eds. CT of the Spine and Spinal Cord. San Anselmo, CA: Clavadel Press, 1983; p 94.

Figure 3–45. ENLARGED TRANSVERSE FORAMEN.
This metrizamide-enhanced axial CT section through C7 demonstrates a large left transverse foramen. The transverse foramen in this instance is almost twice that of the opposite side. At C7 there is considerable variability in the size and number of transverse foramina. Transverse foramina may be single, duplex or triplex. When more than one foramen are present on the same side, usually the vertebral artery passes through the larger of the two and paravertebral veins pass through the other. Enlargement as in this case is normally not pathologic; however, when expansion of this foramen is present, the possibility of a spinal arteriovenous malformation fed by the vertebral artery must be considered. (Case courtesy of David LaMasters, M.D.)

Ref.: Taitz C, Nathan H, Arensburg B. Anatomical observations of the foramina transversaria. J Neurol Neurosurg Psychiatry 1978; 41:170–176.

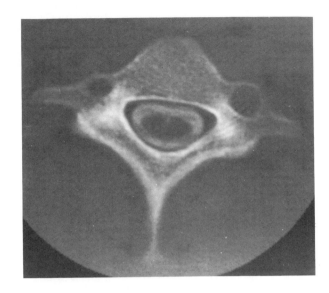

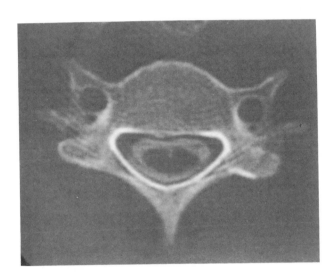

Figure 3–46. DUPLICATED TRANSVERSE FORAMINA. This axial metrizamide-enhanced CT section through C6 demonstrates duplicated transverse foramina bilaterally. The smaller, more posterior foramen normally conducts the paravertebral veins, whereas the larger, anterior foramen conducts the vertebral artery. This is a very common anomaly within the cervical spine. (Case courtesy of David LaMasters, M.D.)

Ref.: Taitz C, Nathan H, Arensburg D. Anatomical observations of the foramina transversaria. J. Neurol Neurosurg Psychiatry 1978; 41:170–176.

Figure 3–47. BIFID SPINOUS PROCESS OF C2. The axial CT image obtained through the C2 vertebral body (axis) demonstrates a widely bifid spinous process. The posterior arch is fused at the inner laminar line; however, the spinous process continues posteriorly as two separate bony elements. C2 is the most common cervical vertebra to have a duplicated spinous process. (Case courtesy of David LaMasters, M.D.)

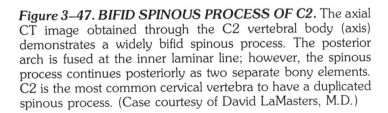

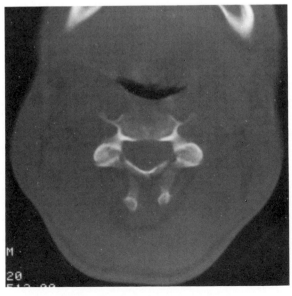

Figure 3–48. MOTION ARTIFACT.

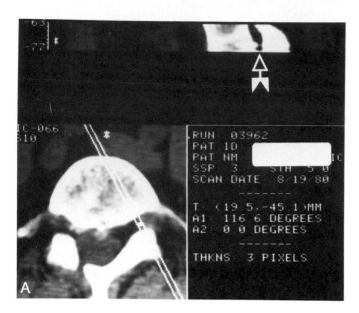

Figure 3–48A. An oblique reformation through the left neural foramen shows an apparent spur intruding into the neural foramen *(arrow)*; this spur, in fact, represents a misregistration artifact caused by motion. When reformations are performed, it is imperative that motion artifacts be recognized.

Figure 3–48B. A reformatted image through the right neural foramen shows encroachment on the neural foramen secondary to an osteophyte or calcified disc protrusion. Compare this with *A* to appreciate how difficult it may be to recognize motion artifacts. True bony pathology should also be present on the axial scans.

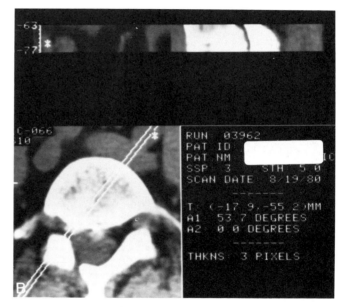

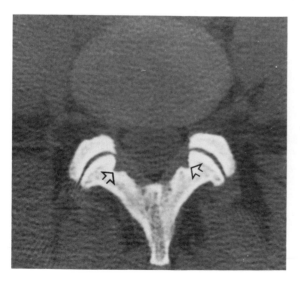

Figure 3–49. IRREGULARITIES OF THE LAMINAE. Irregular bony indentations *(arrows)* in the laminae are often seen near the facet, as in this example. It is believed that these represent the normal insertion sites of the joint capsule.

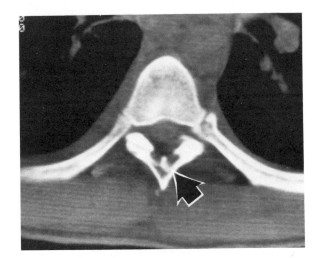

Figure 3–50. IRREGULARITY OF THE LAMINAE. Irregularity of the laminae *(arrow)* is often seen in the thoracic spine. It is thought that this represents the junction point of the laminae with the spinous process.

Figure 3–51. INTERLAMINAR SPACE. The interlaminar space can mimic a post-laminectomy defect, as in these examples.

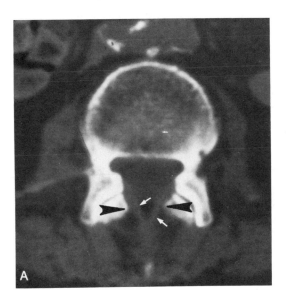

Figure 3–51A. On this axial scan, the interlaminar space *(arrowheads)* appears very prominent. Features that aid in differentiating this from a laminotomy defect include presence of the ligamentum flavum *(arrows)* and symmetric-appearing soft tissues.

Figure 3–51B. Occasionally, in postoperative examples, the ligamentum flavum can appear intact, as in this case. Therefore, there is no substitute for clinical history.

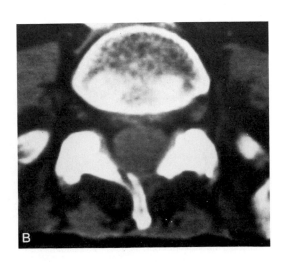

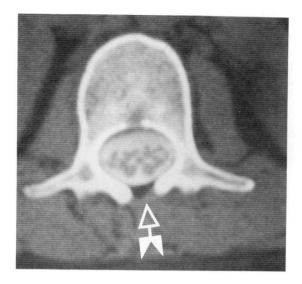

Figure 3–52. SPINA BIFIDA OCCULTA. In contrast to the interlaminar defect that is seen at the level of the facets, this laminar defect *(arrow)* is seen in the mid-body and represents a spina bifida occulta. The CT metrizamide shows that this defect is not associated with a meningocele.

Figure 3–53. DEVELOPMENTAL ANOMALIES OF C1.

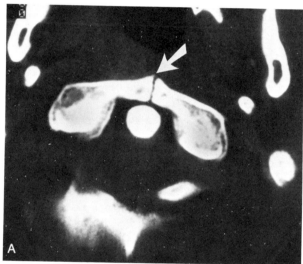

Figure 3–53A. A linear lucency *(arrow)* is seen through the anterior arch of C1. This is a fusion defect and should not be confused with a fracture.

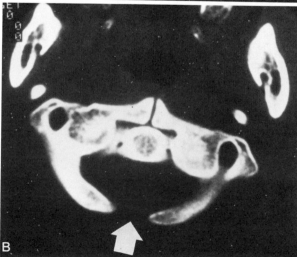

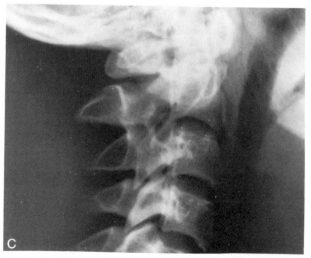

Figure 3–53B. In the same patient, in addition to the fusion defect anteriorly, note the hypoplastic arch posteriorly *(arrow)*. These developmental defects often occur at multiple sites, although they can be present in an isolated fashion.

Figure 3–53C. On a lateral plain film of the cervical spine in this patient, the hypoplastic posterior arch of C1 is difficult to visualize. Defects of this nature are often difficult to see on plain films and may be first appreciated on CT.

Figure 3–54. PSEUDARTHROSIS OF THE TRANSVERSE PROCESS OF L5 WITH THE SACRUM.

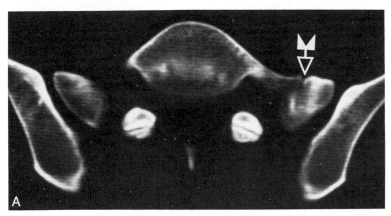

Figure 3–54A. Pseudarthrosis *(arrow)* of the transverse process of L5 with the sacrum is a common normal variant. Although frequently asymptomatic, it can be a source of pain.

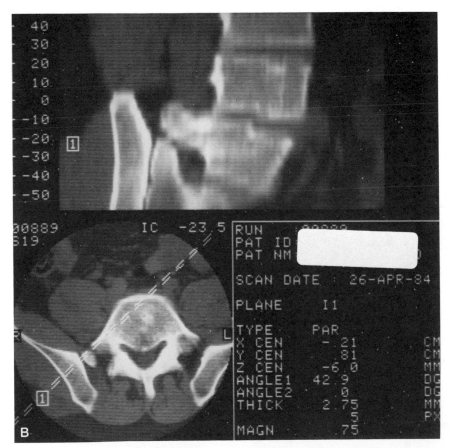

Figure 3–54B. Pseudarthrosis should be recognized on CT quite easily in axial scans such as *A*, but occasionally reformations, such as this example, show it somewhat more clearly.

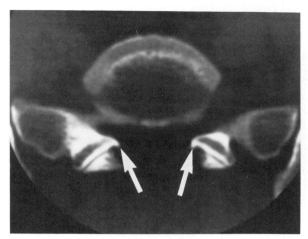

***Figure 3–55. LAMINAE SIMULATING OSTEO-
PHYTES.*** Partial volume averaging of the laminae
(arrows) at the junction of the laminae with the facets
can simulate osteophytes. The absence of other degenerative changes in the facet joints, in addition to a
normal appearance of the facets on contiguous slices,
favors partial volume averaging.

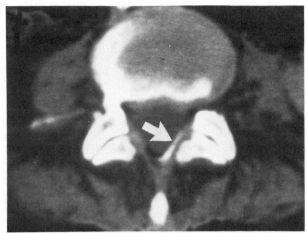

***Figure 3–56. LAMINAE SIMULATING CALCIFI-
CATION OF THE LIGAMENTUM FLAVUM.*** Scans
through the margins of the laminae can mimic calcification of the ligamentum flavum *(arrow)*, due to partial
volume averaging of the laminae. The adjacent CT
scan would show the laminae conforming to the configuration of the "calcification."

Figure 3–57. SPUR OF THE PARS INTERARTICULARIS.

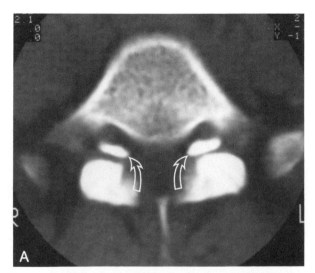

Figure 3–57A. An axial scan shows symmetric bony
protuberances *(arrows)* in the region of the neural
foramen.

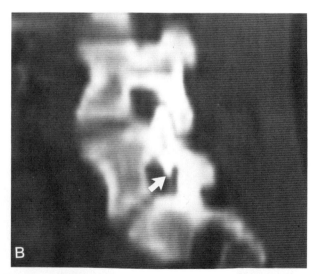

Figure 3–57B. A sagittal reformation of the right side
shows a bony protuberance *(arrow)* extending inferiorly
from the pars into the neural foramen. This is a normal
variant that is seen occasionally and that has never
been reported to be symptomatic.

Ref.: Grogan JP, Hemminghytt S, Williams AL, et al. Spondylolysis studied with computed tomography. Radiology 1982;
145:737–742.

Figure 3–58. BONY SPUR OF THE PEDICLE.

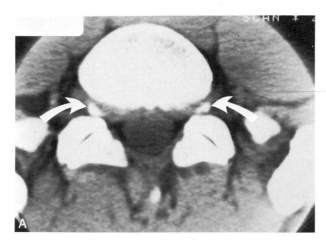

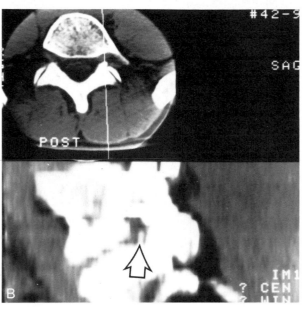

Figure 3–58A. As in Figure 3–57, symmetric bony spurs *(arrows)* are seen extending into the neural foramen on the axial scan.

Figure 3–58B. On the sagittally reformatted image, the spur *(arrow)* extends cephalad from the pedicle into the neural foramen. (Case courtesy of St. Mary's Hospital, Dept. of Radiology, San Francisco, Cal.)

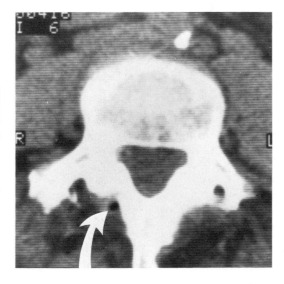

Figure 3–59. GAS ADJACENT TO FACETS. Gas *(arrow)* can often be seen adjacent to facet joints, as in this example. It is said to have been extruded from vacuum facet joints and is considered to represent nitrogen in a synovial cyst. The facet joints often demonstrate degenerative change.

Ref.: Schulz EE, West WL, Hinshaw DB, et al. Gas in a lumbar extradural juxta-articular cyst: Sign of synovial origin. AJR 1984; 143:875–876.

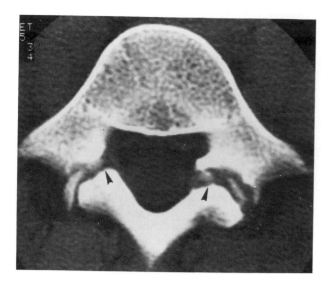

Figure 3–60. SPONDYLOLYSIS. On an axial CT scan spondylolysis is seen as an additional linear lucency *(arrowheads)* in the lamina that can mimic facet joints. When facets are present on the same section, as in this example, a so-called double facet sign will be noted. If the scan plane does not include the facet joints, spondylolysis can mimic the facets and thereby be missed. The lamina should be a solid ring at the level of the basivertebral plexus (mid-vertebral body level). When the lamina is not intact at the basivertebral plexus, the presence of spondylolysis should be considered.

Ref.: Grogan JP, Hemminghytt S, Williams AL, et al. Spondylolysis studied with computed tomography. Radiology 1982; 145:737–742.

Figure 3–61. SPONDYLOLYSIS WITH SPONDYLO-LISTHESIS AND A PSEUDODISC. This patient has spondylolysis with a spondylolisthesis of L5 on S1. The L5 vertebral body is anterior to S1, and the S1 endplate, which is partially visualized just anterior to the central canal, mimics a calcified disc fragment. The fusiform shape of the central canal and the thecal sac are both secondary signs of a spondylolisthesis.

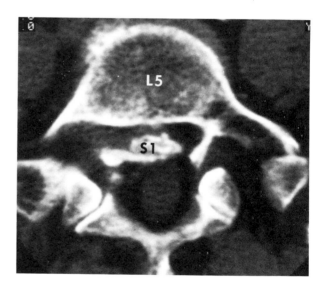

Ref.: Grogan JP, Hemminghytt S, Williams AL, et al. Spondylolysis studied with computed tomography. Radiology 1982; 145:737–742.

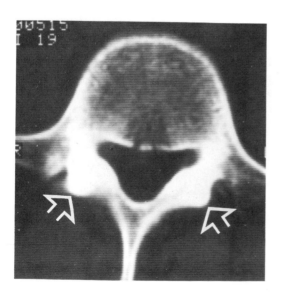

Figure 3–62. BONY TUBERCLE ON THE LAMINA. Most laminae have a bony protuberance or tubercle *(arrows)* that can mimic healing through an area of spondylolysis. This should not be mistaken for callus formation.

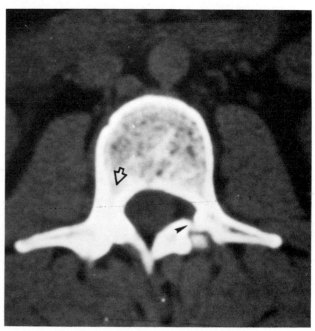

Figure 3–63. UNILATERAL ARCH HYPERTROPHY. A congenital, or even acquired, defect in the pedicle or lamina *(arrowhead),* as in this example, can result in compensatory hypertrophy through the contralateral pedicle *(open arrow),* causing unilateral arch hypertrophy. When this degree of hypertrophy is present, the contralateral defect should be considered chronic and not an acute fracture. The hypertrophied side can present on plain films as a dense pedicle and mimic metastatic disease.

Ref.: Maldague BE, Malghem JJ. Unilateral arch hypertrophy with spinous process tilt: A sign of arch deficiency. Radiology 1976; 121:567–574.

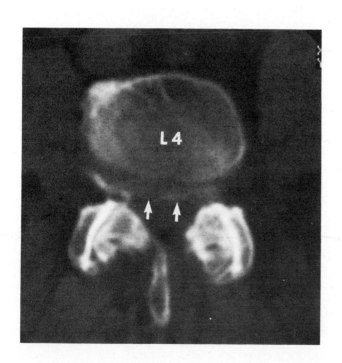

Figure 3–64. DEGENERATIVE SPONDYLOLISTHE-SIS. The L4 vertebral body is anterior to the L5 vertebral body *(arrows),* indicating spondylolisthesis; however, no pars defect could be found. The reason for the slippage is seen in the facet joints in this patient. The facets are severely degenerated and slightly subluxed, with the superior articular facets slightly offset from the inferior facets. This has been termed degenerative spondylolisthesis.

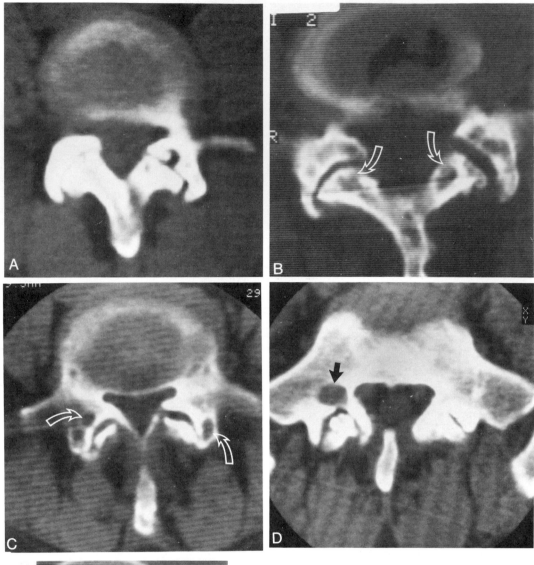

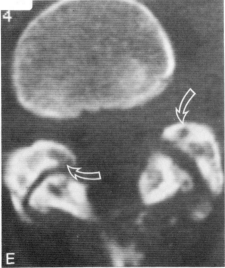

Figure 3–65. DEGENERATIVE DISEASE OF THE ARTICULAR FACETS. Degenerative disease of the articular facets can have all of the findings of degenerative disease in any synovial joint (joint space narrowing, sclerosis, osteophytosis, subchondral cysts); however, hypertrophy of the facets is a common prominent finding. Some degree of hypertrophy is present in all of these examples as is joint-space narrowing or irregularity and sclerosis with osteophytosis. Note that examples *B–E* also demonstrate prominent geodes *(arrows)*, or subchondral cysts. The geodes in *B, C, D,* and *E* were believed by some examiners to possibly represent metastatic disease; however, their subchondral location adjacent to degenerated facet joints makes them characteristic for subchondral cysts.

Figure 3–66. LUCENCY IN THE VERTEBRAL BODY.

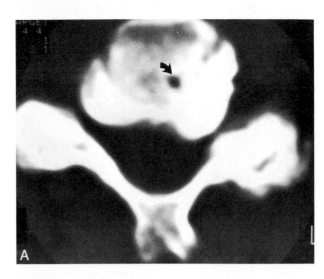

Figure 3–66A. An axial scan through the cervical spine in this patient with advanced degenerative disease of the facets and the uncovertebral joints demonstrates a subchondral cyst, or geode *(arrow)*, in the vertebral body adjacent to the uncovertebral joint. The presence of severe degenerative disease in the adjacent joints enables one to distinguish this low density defect from a more aggressive process.

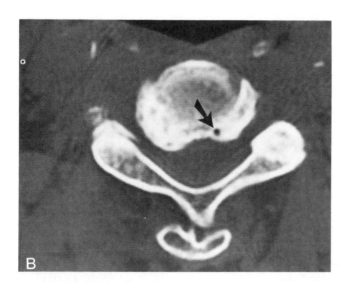

Figure 3–66B. A similar process with a small geode *(arrow)*.

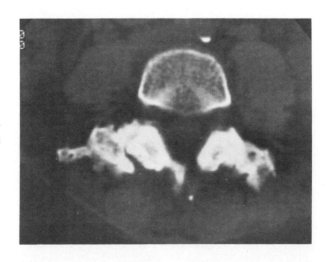

Figure 3–67. DEGENERATIVE FACET DISEASE. Extreme hypertrophy of the facets simulating posterior fusion masses is seen in this patient with degenerative facet disease.

Figure 3–68. POSTSURGICAL CHANGES. Postsurgical changes in the lumbar spine can have many appearances, as in these examples.

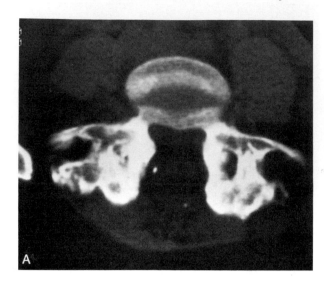

Figure 3–68A. Large laminectomy defect with bilateral fusion grafts in place.

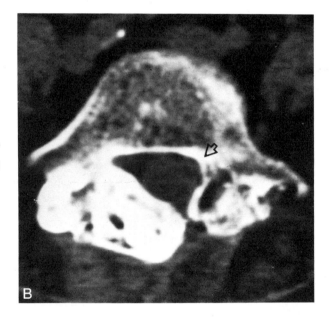

Figure 3–68B. A process similar to *A* is seen in this CT scan, with partial obliteration of the left lateral recess *(arrow)* due to ingrowth of the fusion graft.

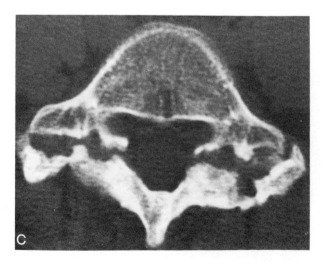

Figure 3–68C. Grafting around a spondylolysis defect with possible pseudarthrosis is demonstrated. Reformations are often necessary to evaluate the integrity of postoperative fusion grafts.

Ref.: Teplick JG, Haskin ME. CT of the postoperative lumbar spine. Radiol Clin North Am 1983; 21:395.

CHAPTER 4

Chest

W. RICHARD WEBB, M.D.

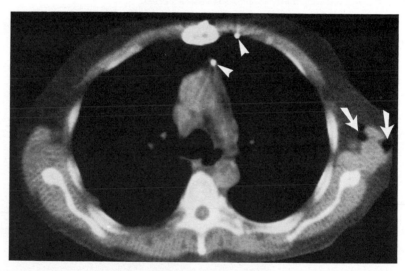

Figure 4–1. MEDIASTINAL CLIPS AND STERNAL WIRE SUTURES. Metal clips and sutures *(arrowheads)*, which might simulate calcification, are visible in this patient following cardiac surgery. At wider window widths, the metallic structures should appear denser than calcification. Also note subcutaneous emphysema *(arrows)*.

Figure 4–2. RADIOPAQUE CATHETER.

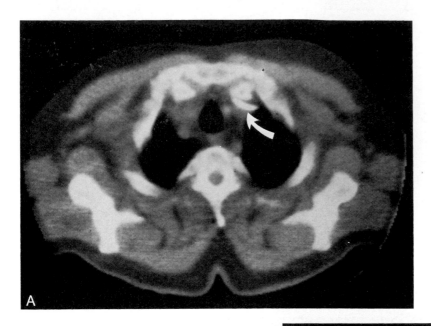

Figure 4–2A. A radiopaque central venous catheter *(arrow)* is visible in the left brachiocephalic vein, posterior to the left clavicular head.

Figure 4–2B. At a lower level, the catheter *(arrow)* with associated artifacts is positioned in the superior vena cava.

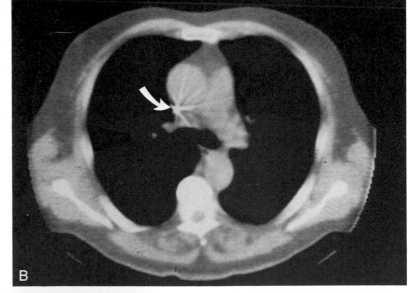

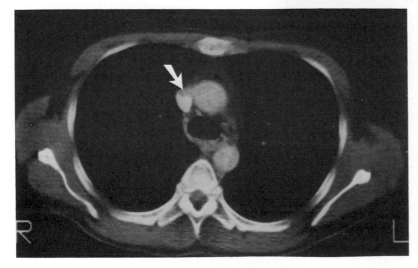

Figure 4–3. FLOW DEFECT. With bolus injection of contrast into a single arm vein, streaming of opacified blood in the superior vena cava can mimic an intraluminal thrombus *(arrow)*. (See also Figures 4–11 and 4–19.)

Ref.: Godwin JD, Webb WR. Contrast-related flow phenomena mimicking pathology on thoracic computed tomography. J Comput Assist Tomogr 1982; 6:460–464.

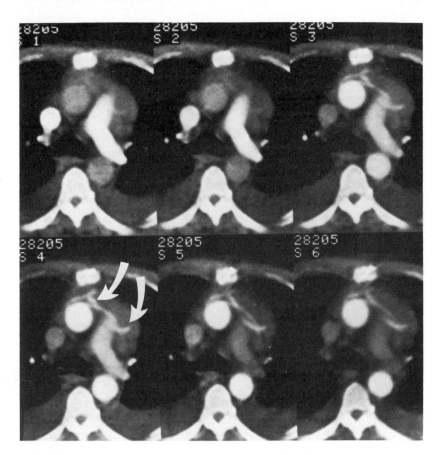

Figure 4–4. CORONARY ARTERY BYPASS GRAFTS. Coronary artery bypass grafts *(arrows)* are visible on sequential images (1–6) following the bolus injection of contrast. They opacify at the same time as the aorta. Wire sternal sutures also are visible.

Ref.: Godwin JD, Califf RM, Korobkin M, et al.: Clinical value of coronary bypass graft evaluation with CT. AJR 140:649–655, April 1983.

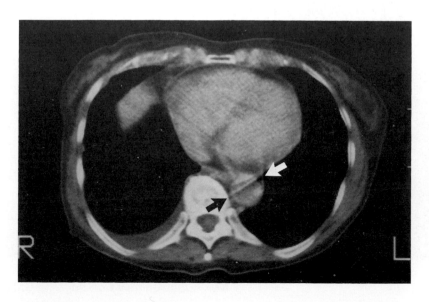

Figure 4–5. STREAK ARTIFACT. A streak artifact paralleling left heart border *(arrows)* mimics a descending aortic dissection. However, note that it extends past the edge of the aorta *(black arrow)*.

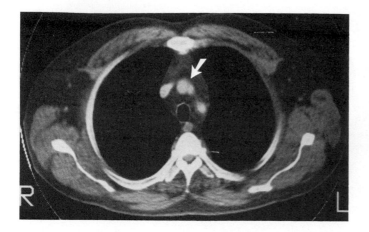

Figure 4–6. MEDIASTINAL LIPOMATOSIS. Fat accumulated in the mediastinum of this patient results in mediastinal widening. The benign nature of this is easily determined at CT. Also note the common origin *(arrow)* of the innominate and right carotid arteries.

Ref.: Baron RL, Levitt RG, Sagel SS, Stanley RJ. Computed tomography in the evaluation of mediastinal widening. Radiology 1981; 138:107–113.

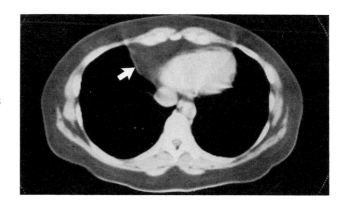

Figure 4–7. EPICARDIAC FAT PAD. A large fat pad is visible in the right cardiophrenic angle *(arrow)*.

Figure 4–8. NORMAL THYMUS GLAND. The normal thymus gland *(arrows, A–E)* is somewhat variable in size. It generally appears bilobed or arrowhead-shaped on CT. It is most prominent in children, adolescents, and young adults.

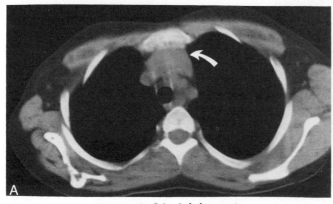

Figure 4–8A. Adolescent.

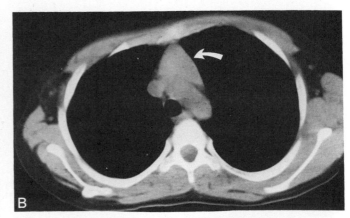

Figure 4–8B. Adolescent.

Illustration continued on opposite page

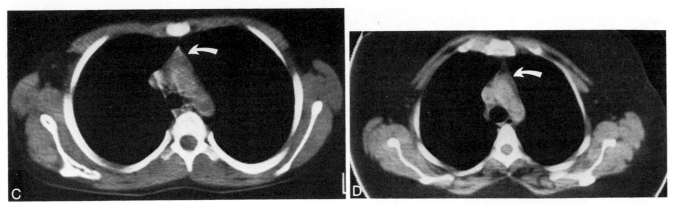

Figure 4–8C. Young Adult.   **Figure 4–8D.** Adult.

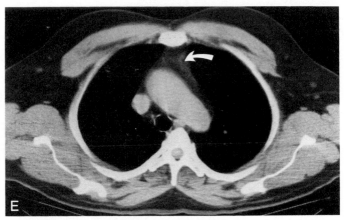

Figure 4–8E. Adult.

Refs.: (1) Baron RL, Lee JKT, Sagel SS, Peterson RR. Computed tomography of the normal thymus. Radiology 1982; 142:121–125. (2) Moore AV, Korobkin M, Olanow W, et al. Age-related changes in the thymus gland: CT–pathologic correlation. AJR 1983; 141:241–246.

Figure 4–9. MEDIASTINAL THYROID GLAND.
The lower poles of the thyroid gland *(arrows)* in this normal patient extend into the mediastinum, closely related to the trachea.

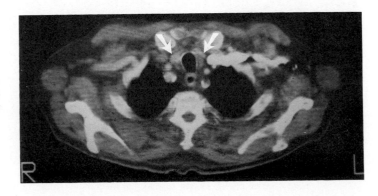

Figure 4–10. NORMAL MEDIASTINAL LYMPH NODES.

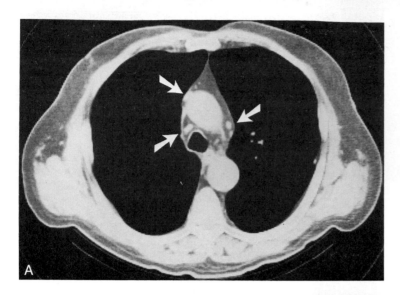

Figure 4–10A. Normal mediastinal lymph nodes *(arrows)* are visible in the prevascular space, pretracheal space, and aorticopulmonary window.

Figure 4–10B. Normal nodes *(solid arrow)* can be seen in the pretracheal space at a slightly lower level. Volume averaging of the left pulmonary artery simulates a mass in the aorticopulmonary window *(open arrow)*. Calcified pleural plaques resulting from asbestos exposure can also be seen.

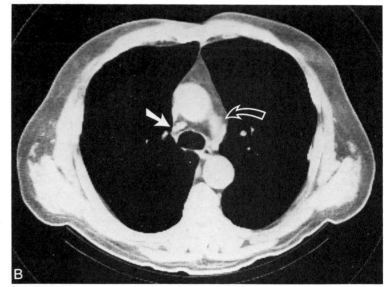

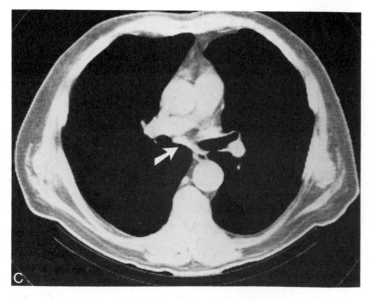

Figure 4–10C. Normal nodes in the subcarinal space can be larger than those seen in other areas. Note also the normal concave azygoesophageal recess *(arrow)*.

Ref.: Genereux GP, Howie JL. Normal mediastinal lymph node size and number: CT and anatomic study. AJR 1984; 142:1095–1100.

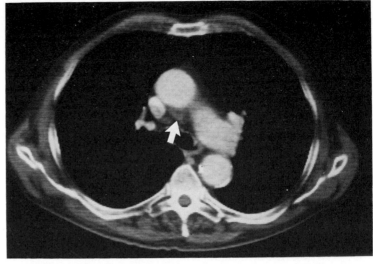

Figure 4–11. SUPERIOR PERICARDIAL RECESS. In 50 per cent of normal individuals, an extension of the pericardial sac *(arrow)* posterior to the aorta can mimic a lymph node; in 18 per cent, the extension is large enough to be of concern. Also note a normal-sized lymph node and a flow defect in the superior vena cava.

Ref.: Aronberg DJ, Glazer HS, Peterson RR, et al. Ascending aortic appendage: A pitfall of mediastinal CT. Radiology 1983; 149(P):170.

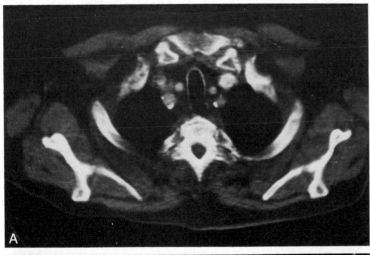

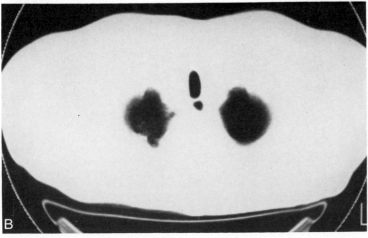

Figure 4–12. SABER-SHEATH TRACHEA. These two images (*A* and *B*) made at different window settings demonstrate a saber-sheath trachea. Side-to-side narrowing of the trachea below the thoracic inlet, usually occurring in patients with obstructive pulmonary disease, has been termed saber-sheath trachea. It can mimic compression by a mass or tracheal stenosis. Not uncommonly, the coronal diameter of the trachea is less than half of the sagittal diameter. Also note the air-filled esophagus behind the trachea.

Ref.: Gamsu G, Webb WR. Computed tomography of the trachea: Normal and abnormal. AJR 1982; 139:321–326.

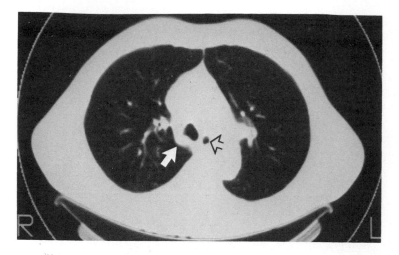

Figure 4–13. TRACHEAL IRREGULARITY. Near the tracheal carina, the trachea can be irregular in shape or triangular. In this patient, the azygos vein *(solid arrow)* behind the trachea simulates a mass compressing the tracheal lumen. Note the air-filled esophagus *(open arrowhead)*.

Ref.: Gamsu G, Webb WR. Computed tomography of the trachea: Normal and abnormal. AJR 1982; 139:321–326.

Figure 4–14. WINDOW LEVEL. In the same patient and at the same level as in Figure 4–13, viewing the scan at a mediastinal rather than lung window setting markedly alters the apparent diameter of the trachea and esophagus.

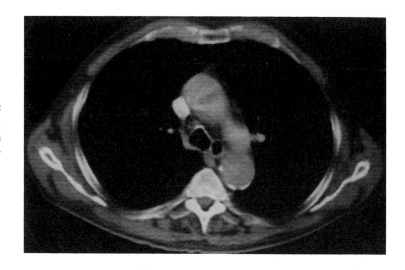

Figure 4–15. ESOPHAGUS MIMICKING BRONCHUS.

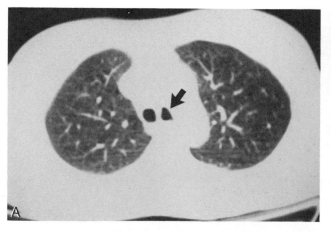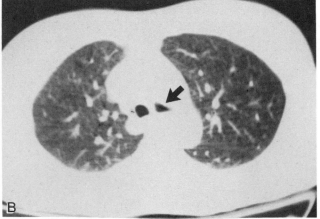

Figure 4–15A and B. At two levels, the air-filled esophagus *(arrows)* mimics an abnormally narrowed left main bronchus.

Illustration continued on opposite page

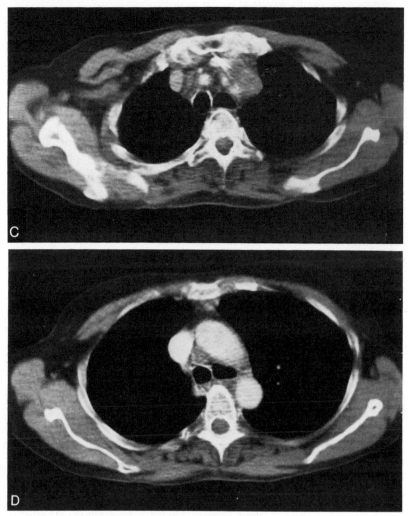

Figure 4–15C and D. At mediastinal window settings, the trachea *(right)* shows calcification of cartilages whereas the esophagus *(left)* does not.

Figure 4–16. ESOPHAGEAL AIR-FLUID LEVEL. Air and fluid in the esophagus are not uncommonly visible on CT of the mediastinum and their presence does not imply obstruction or abnormal motility. They are found most commonly just below the aortic arch, as in this patient *(arrow)*. Also note an azygos lobe and fissure (see Figure 4–61).

Ref.: Halber MD, Daffner RH, Thompson WM: CT of the esophagus: I. Normal appearance. AJR 1979; 133:1047–1050.

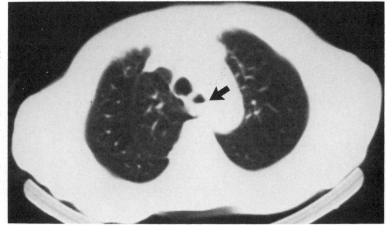

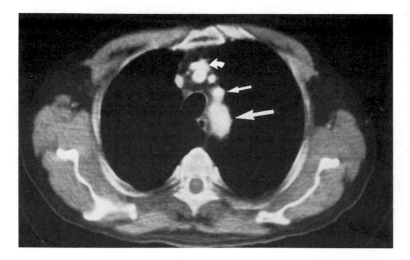

Figure 4–17. AORTIC ARCH POSTERIOR TO THE LEFT SUBCLAVIAN ARTERY. Although the left subclavian artery usually arises from the most superior aspect of the aorta, the aortic arch can occasionally be seen as a separate structure *(large arrow)* behind the subclavian artery *(small straight arrow)*. The left brachiocephalic vein *(curved arrow)* can be seen crossing the mediastinum anterior to the innominate artery.

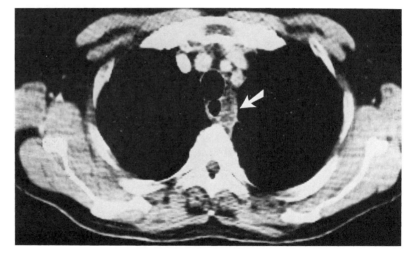

Figure 4–18. VOLUME AVERAGING OF AORTIC ARCH SIMULATING MEDIAS-TINAL MASS. A contrast-enhanced CT scan shows opacified vessels anterior and lateral to the trachea. Volume averaging of the top of the aortic arch *(arrow)* posterior to the left subclavian artery and lateral to the air-filled esophagus mimics a soft-tissue density mass.

Figure 4–19. AORTIC ARCH CALCIFICATION—FLOW DEFECTS.

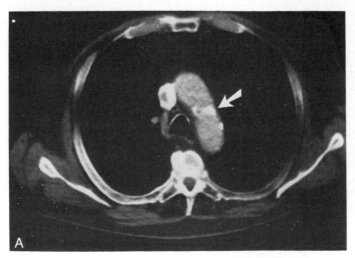

Figure 4–19A. Calcification is present at the under-surface of the aortic arch *(arrow).*

Illustration continued on opposite page

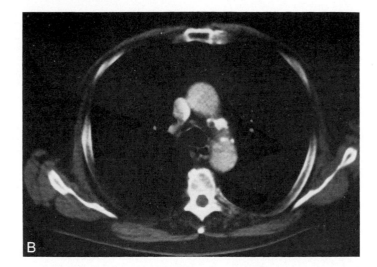

Figure 4–19B. The calcification seen in *A* mimics calcified nodes or a mass at a lower level in the aortic pulmonary window. Also note flow defects in the superior vena cava at both levels.

Figure 4–20. HIGH MAIN PULMONARY ARTERY.

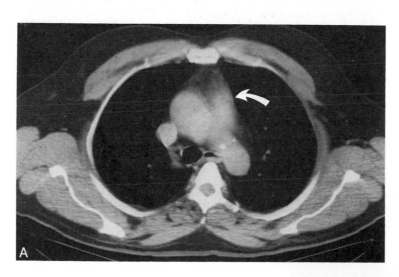

Figure 4–20A. In some patients, the main pulmonary artery *(arrow)* is high, being visible anterior to the aortic arch, thus mimicking a mass lesion.

Figure 4–20B. At lower levels, however, it is evident that this represents the artery. Note also a tortuous azygos arch.

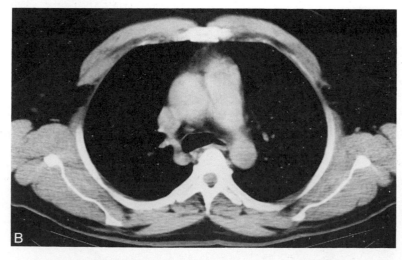

Ref.: Mencini RA, Proto AV. The high left and main pulmonary arteries: A CT pitfall. J Comput Assist Tomogr 1982; 6:452–459.

Figure 4–21. AORTICOPULMONARY WINDOW.

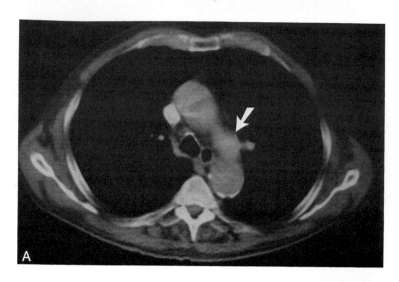

Figure 4–21A. Volume averaging of the undersurface of the aortic arch (see Figures 4–10B and 4–19) or the superior main or left pulmonary artery can mimic a mass *(arrow)* in the aorticopulmonary window.

Figure 4–21B. Continuity of the "mass" *(asterisk)* with the pulmonary artery, which is visible at the level below A, enables the correct diagnosis to be made.

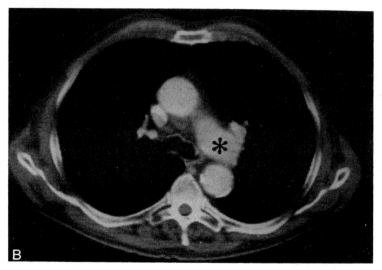

Figure 4–22. PROMINENT LEFT ATRIAL APPENDAGE.

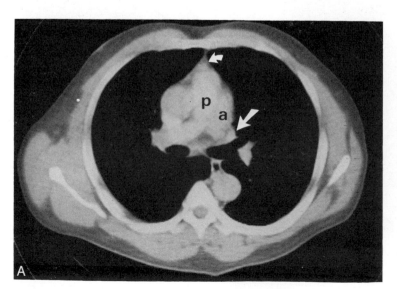

Figure 4–22A. The superior left atrial appendage (a) extends anterior to the left superior pulmonary vein *(straight arrow)* lateral to the main pulmonary artery (p) and can mimic a mediastinal mass. Also note normal thymic tissue *(curved arrow)* anterior to the great vessels.

Illustration continued on opposite page

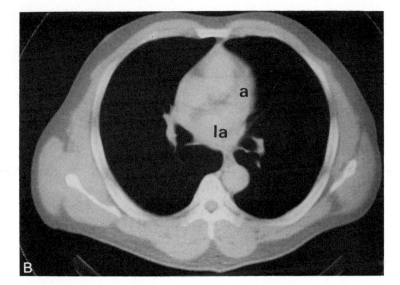

Figure 4–22B. At a lower level, the atrial appendage (a) is seen to be contiguous with the left atrium (la).

Ref.: Guthaner DF, Wexler L, Harell G. CT demonstration of cardiac structures. AJR 1979; 133:75–81.

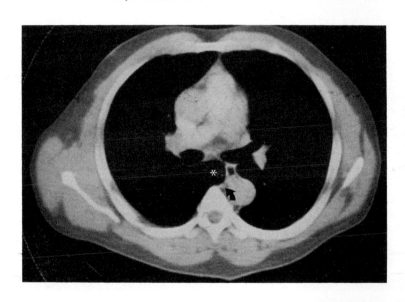

Figure 4–23. DEEP AZYGOESOPHAGEAL RECESS. In a normal subject, the azygoesophageal recess *(asterisk)* can extend across the midline and contact the left main bronchus and the right esophageal wall. The azygos vein is posterior *(arrow)*.

Figure 4–24. CONVEX AZYGOESOPHAGEAL RECESS—ESOPHAGUS. The normal esophagus *(arrow)* can produce a convexity of the azygoesophageal recess. This is seen most frequently in children or young adults.

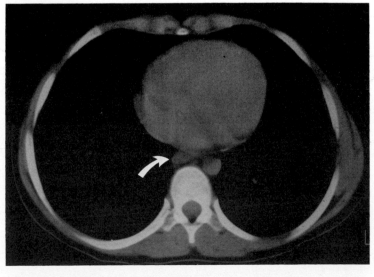

Ref.: Onitsuka H, Kuhns LR. Dextroconvexity of the mediastinum in the azygoesophageal recess. A normal CT variant in young adults. Radiology 1980; 135:126.

Figure 4–25. CONVEX AZYGOESOPHAGEAL RECESS—AZYGOS VEIN.

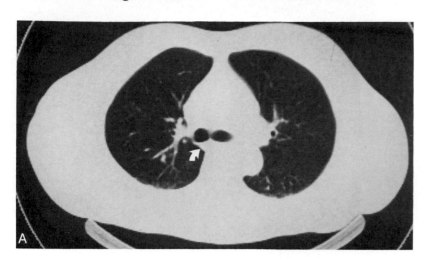

Figure 4–25A. At a lung window setting, a small convexity *(arrow)* is visible in the azygoesophageal recess.

Figure 4–25B. The same convexity *(arrow)* can be seen at a level adjacent to A (lung window setting).

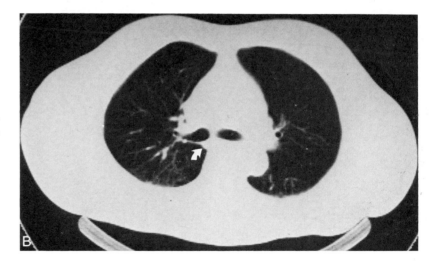

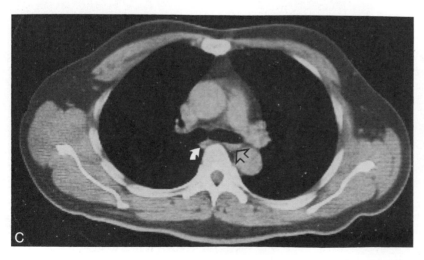

Figure 4–25C. At a mediastinal window setting, this is seen to be the azygos vein *(curved arrow).* The esophagus *(open arrow)* is to the left of the vertebral body.

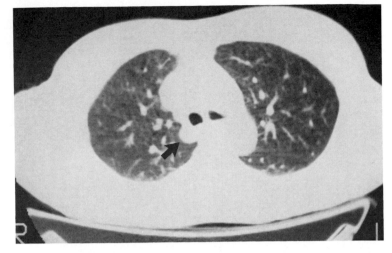

Figure 4–26. TORTUOUS AZYGOS ARCH.
A somewhat dilated tortuous posterior portion of the azygos arch *(arrow)* can simulate a lung or mediastinal mass.

Ref.: Rockoff SD, Druy EM. Tortuous azygos arch simulating a pulmonary lesion. AJR 1982; 138:577–579.

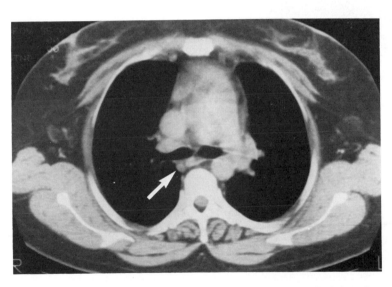

Figure 4–27. AZYGOS VEIN. In 9 per cent of subjects the azygos vein *(arrow)* can be seen behind the right main or upper lobe bronchus, simulating a mediastinal lymph node *(see also Figure 4–20)*. The esophagus is just medial to the vein.

Ref.: Landay MJ. Azygos vein abutting the posterior wall of the right main and upper lobe bronchi: A normal CT variant. AJR 1983; 140:461–462.

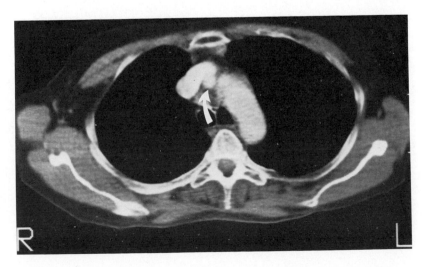

Figure 4–28. INNOMINATE ARTERY MIMICKING NODE. The origin of the innominate artery *(arrow)* can appear to be separate from the aorta, thus mimicking a mediastinal lymph node. Following the course of the vessel, however, will allow the correct diagnosis to be made.

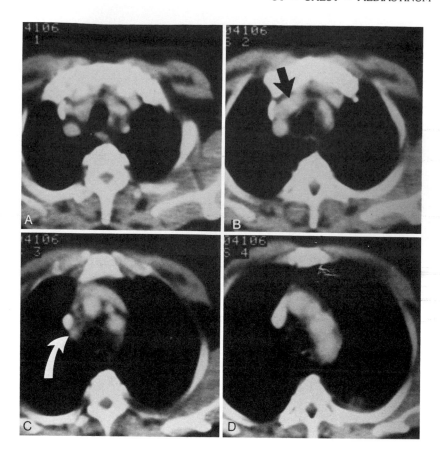

Figure 4–29. TORTUOUS INNOMI-NATE ARTERY. Because the innominate artery is tortuous, the right subclavian artery *(arrow, C)* is visible below the level of the horizontally oriented innominate artery *(arrow, B)*, thus mimicking a lymph node. This appearance is not uncommon in patients with a tortuous artery. Note contrast agent in the right subclavian vein and superior vena cava.

Figure 4–30. ANOMALOUS RIGHT SUBCLAVIAN ARTERY. This is a common anomaly, occurring in approximately 1 of 200 patients.

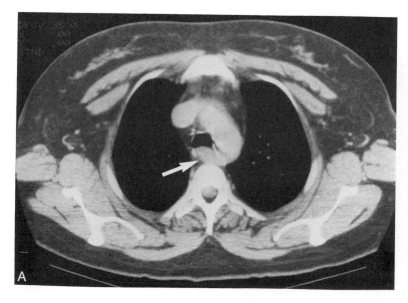

Figure 4–30A. The anomalous artery arises from the posterior aortic arch *(arrow).*

Illustration continued on opposite page

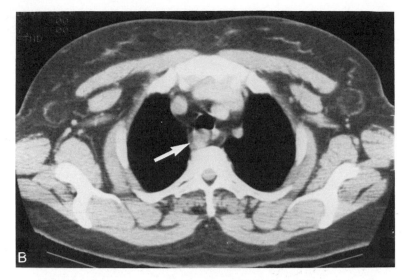

Figure 4–30B. The anomalous artery *(arrow)* then passes behind the esophagus; in this location it can mimic a mediastinal mass. Without contrast medium, it may be difficult to separate these two structures.

Ref.: Webb WR, Gamsu G, Speckman JM, et al. CT demonstration of mediastinal aortic arch anomalies. J Comput Assist Tomogr 1982; 6:445–451.

Figure 4–31. ANOMALOUS RIGHT SUBCLAVIAN ARTERY.

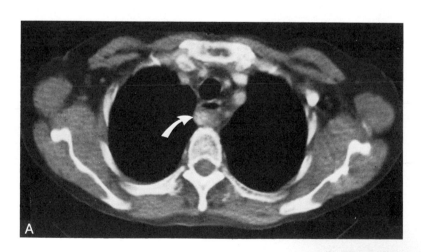

Figure 4–31A. The anomalous artery *(arrow)* is visible behind the esophagus.

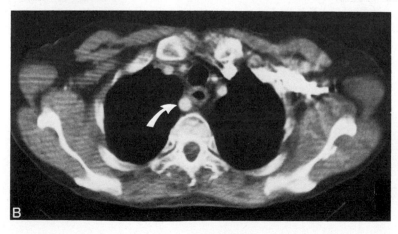

Figure 4–31B. At a higher level, the artery *(arrow)* can be seen to the right of the esophagus.

Figure 4–32. RIGHT AORTIC ARCH WITH ANOMALOUS LEFT SUBCLAVIAN ARTERY.
This anomaly, which occurs in 1 in 1000 people, is much the same as anomalous right subclavian artery with left aortic arch.

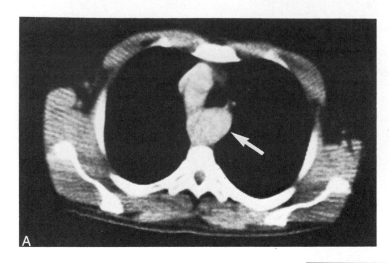

Figure 4–32A. The anomalous artery arises behind the esophagus, often from an aortic diverticulum *(arrow)*.

Figure 4–32B. At higher levels, the anomalous artery *(arrow)* is posterior in the mediastinum.

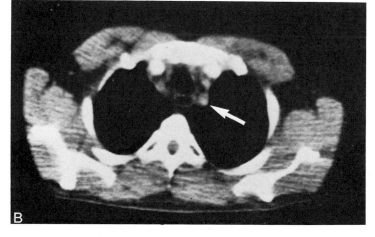

Figure 4–33. DOUBLE AORTIC ARCH.

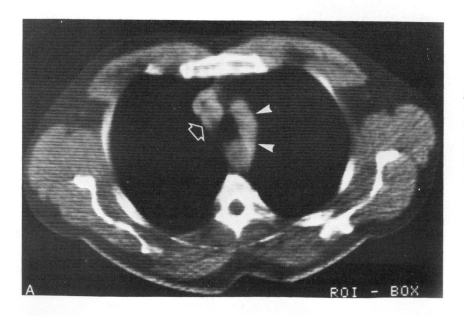

Figure 4–33A. A small left aortic arch *(arrowheads)* is visible with the descending aorta being posterior to the trachea. The right ascending aorta *(open arrow)* simulates a mass lesion posterior to the superior vena cava.

Illustration continued on opposite page

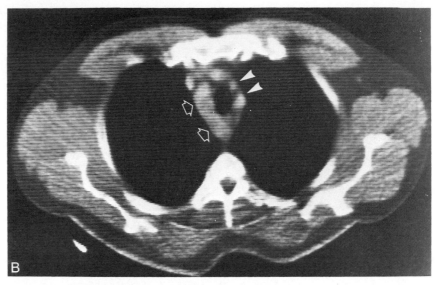

Figure 4–33B. At a higher level, the right aortic arch *(open arrows)* passes to the right of the trachea to join the descending aorta. The left subclavian and carotid arteries *(arrowheads)* arise from the left arch. At an even higher level, the right subclavian and carotid arteries would be seen as separate branches of the right arch.

From: Webb WR, Gamsu G, Speckman JM, et al. CT demonstration of mediastinal aortic arch anomalies. J Comput Assist Tomogr 1982; 6:445–451. Reproduced with permission.

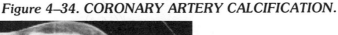

Figure 4–34. CORONARY ARTERY CALCIFICATION.

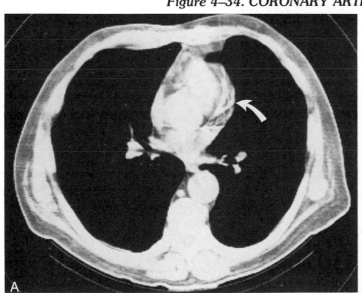

Figure 4–34A. Calcification of the left coronary artery *(arrow)* is demonstrated.

Figure 4–34B. In this image, calcification of the right coronary artery *(arrow)* is seen.

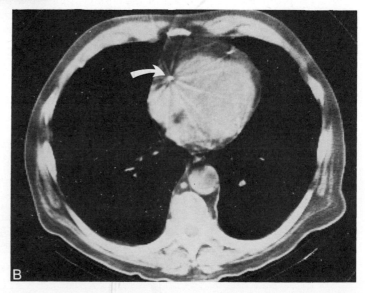

Figure 4–35. BRACHIOCEPHALIC VEIN ANTERIOR TO AORTA. The left brachiocephalic vein usually crosses the mediastinum anterior to the left carotid and right brachiocephalic arteries (see Figures 4–17 and 4–36).

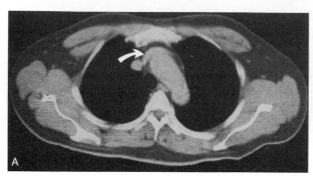

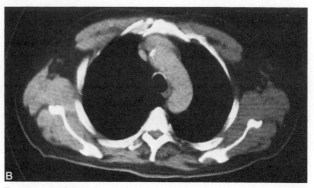

Figure 4–35A. In occasional cases, the vein *(arrow)* crosses anterior to the aortic arch, mimicking a mediastinal mass. Also, the fat plane separating the brachiocephalic vein and anterior aortic wall can simulate the intimal flap of dissecting aortic aneurysm.

Figure 4–35B. In this case, the anterior aortic wall is identified by calcification, and the vein appears even more masslike.

Ref.: Taber P, Chang LWM, Campion GM. The left brachiocephalic vein simulating aortic dissection on computed tomography. J Comput Assist Tomogr 1979; 3:360.

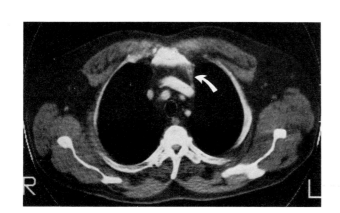

Figure 4–36. INTERNAL MAMMARY VEIN. The right or left internal mammary vein *(arrow)* is sometimes visible, extending anteriorly from the brachiocephalic vein. This should not be confused with pleural thickening.

Figure 4–37. AZYGOS AND HEMIAZYGOS CONTINUATION OF THE INFERIOR VENA CAVA. The azygos arch *(arrow)* is dilated in scan A. At a lower level *(B)*, the azygos vein *(arrow)* is prominent at the level of the heart. In C, the azygos vein communicates with the hemiazygos vein *(arrow)* behind the aorta. In a retrocrural location *(D)*, note the dilated hemiazygos vein *(arrow)*. Wire sternal sutures and mediastinal clips are also present.

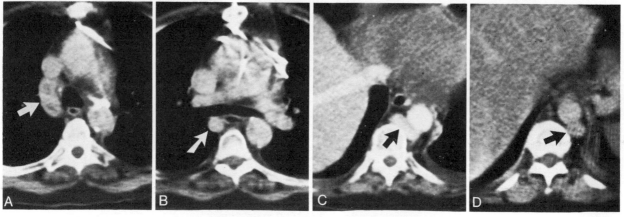

From: Webb WR, Gamsu G, Speckman JR, et al. Computed tomographic demonstration of mediastinal venous anomalies. AJR 1982; 139:157–161. Reproduced with permission.

Figure 4–38. PERSISTENT LEFT SUPERIOR VENA CAVA. Sequential scans at contiguous levels (top left to bottom right) shows a right superior vena cava *(open arrows)* and a persistent left superior vena cava *(solid arrows)* descending along the left mediastinum, anterior to the left hilum. It is densely opacified. This anomaly occurs in 0.3 per cent of the population.

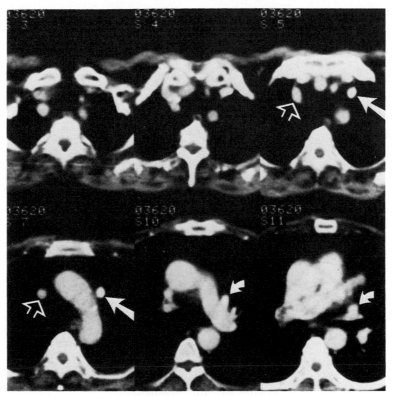

From: Webb WR, Gamsu G, Speckman JM, et al. Computed tomographic demonstration of mediastinal venous anomalies. AJR 1982; 139:157–161. Reproduced with permission.

Figure 4–39. ANOMALOUS LEFT BRACHIOCEPHALIC VEIN. Contiguous scans (A–C) in this patient demonstrate the left brachiocephalic vein *(arrow)* descending along the left mediastinum, as in the case of a persistent left superior vena cava (see Figure 4–38), before entering the aorticopulmonary window, crossing the midline, and joining with the right superior vena cava.

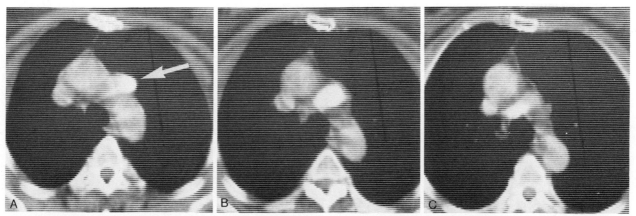

From: Webb WR, Gamsu G, Speckman JM, et al. Computed tomographic demonstration of mediastinal venious anomalies. AJR 1982; 139:157–161. Reproduced with permission.

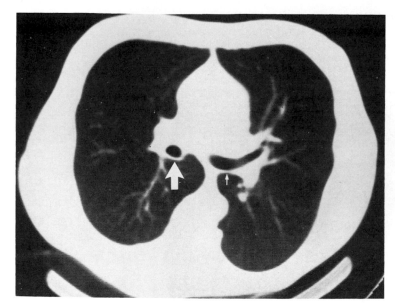

Figure 4–40. NORMAL POSTERIOR BRON-CHIAL WALLS. The posterior wall of the right bronchus intermedius *(large arrow)* is always visible in normal subjects and measures a few millimeters in thickness. The posterior bronchial wall on the left *(small arrow)* is typically visible only at the level of the left upper lobe bronchus.

Ref.: Webb WR, Glazer G, Gamsu G. Computed tomography of the normal pulmonary hilum. J Comput Assist Tomogr 1981; 5:476–484.

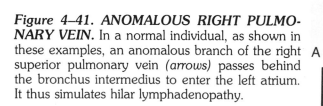

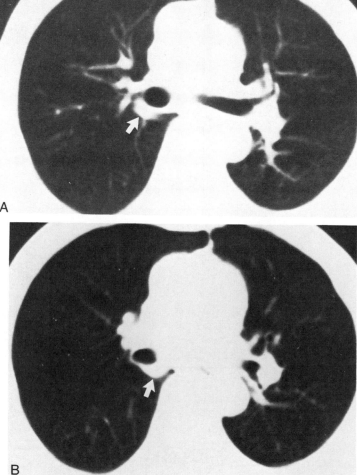

Figure 4–41. ANOMALOUS RIGHT PULMO-NARY VEIN. In a normal individual, as shown in these examples, an anomalous branch of the right superior pulmonary vein *(arrows)* passes behind the bronchus intermedius to enter the left atrium. It thus simulates hilar lymphadenopathy.

A

B

From: Webb WR, Hirji M, Gamsu G. Posterior wall of the bronchus intermedius: Radiographic–CT correlation. AJR 1984; 141:907–911. Reproduced with permission.

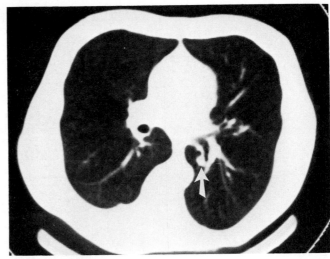

Figure 4–42. LEFT PULMONARY VEIN. In some normal subjects, a branch of the left pulmonary vein *(arrow)* passes medial to the superior segment bronchus and behind the main bronchus. As in Figure 4–41, this can simulate a lymph node.

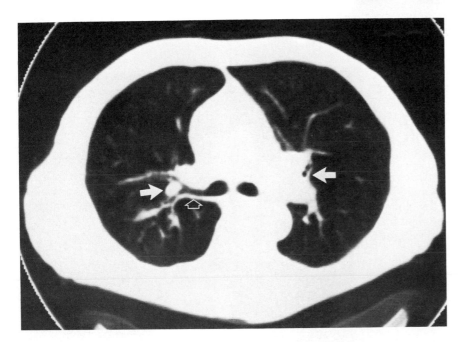

Figure 4–43. NORMAL UPPER HILA. Within the right hilum, a vein branch *(arrow)* lies between the anterior and posterior segmental bronchi of the right upper lobe. The posterior wall of the right upper lobe bronchus is sharply outlined by lung, but the azygos vein *(open arrow)* can obscure it (see Figure 4–27). On the left, in most patients, lung contacts the lateral bronchial wall *(arrow).*

Ref.: Webb WR, Glazer G, Gamsu G. Computed tomography of the normal pulmonary hilum. J Comput Assist Tomogr 1981; 5:476–484.

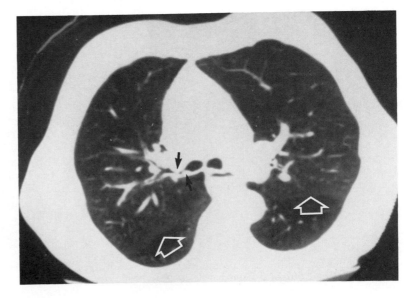

Figure 4–44. BRONCHIAL MUCUS. Collections of mucus *(solid arrows)* within the trachea or bronchi can simulate the appearance of an endobranchial lesion. However, they will disappear with coughing. Compare the appearance of the right upper lobe bronchus in this case with that seen in Figure 4–43. Note that the major fissures *(open arrows)* are visible as vague bands of density (see also Figure 4–56B).

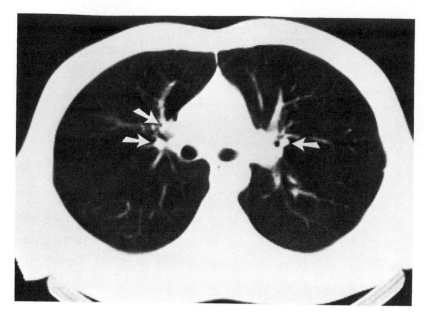

Figure 4–45. HILAR VEINS. Right hilar vein branches *(arrows)* result in a variable appearance of the anterior right hilum, simulating adenopathy. On the left, a vein branch *(arrow)* lying lateral to the bronchus (see Figure 4–43) simulates a lymph node. This vein is visible in less than half of the patient population.

Figure 4–46. NORMAL RIGHT HILAR FAT. A collection of fat, sometimes containing normal-sized nodes *(arrows)* is commonly visible in the anterior right hilum, lateral to the bifurcation of the right main pulmonary artery. This should not be misinterpreted as a mass.

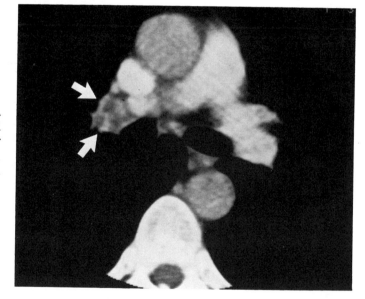

Figure 4–47. LEFT UPPER LOBE ARTERY SIMULATING MASS.

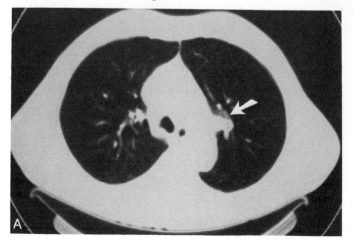

Figure 4–47A. The rather variable branching pattern of the left main pulmonary artery *(arrow)* into left upper lobe arterial branches can sometimes simulate a hilar or mediastinal mass.

Illustration continued on opposite page

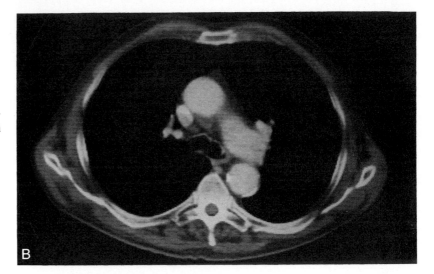

Figure 4–47B. Continuity with the pulmonary artery at lower levels is helpful in reaching the correct diagnosis.

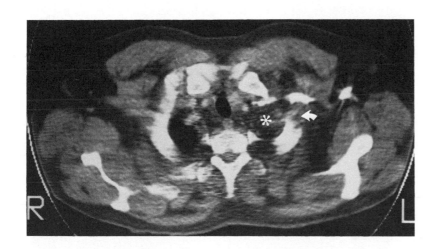

Figure 4–48. APICAL ASYMMETRY SIMULATING MASS. Slight malpositioning of the patient can result in asymmetry of aerated lung at the apex, simulating an apical mass *(asterisk)*. Also note that partial visualization of the left first rib simulates destruction *(arrow)*.

Figure 4–49. BULLAE. Bullae, although not normal, are not uncommonly visible on CT and should not be mistaken for pneumothorax or lung destruction as a result of an acute disease process.

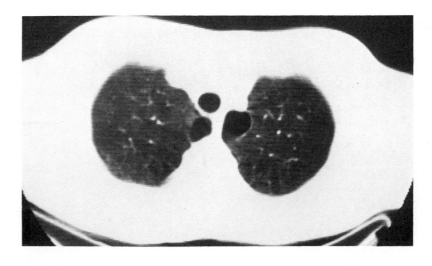

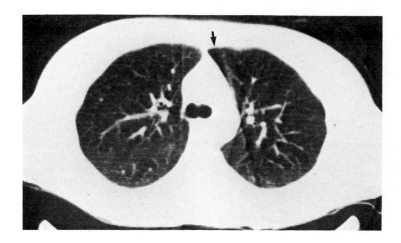

Figure 4–50. STREAK ARTIFACTS. Streak artifacts can result in areas of apparent lucency *(arrow)* as well as density. These should not be mistaken for pathology such as a pneumomediastinum or pneumothorax.

Figure 4–51. FIRST RIB AS NODULE.

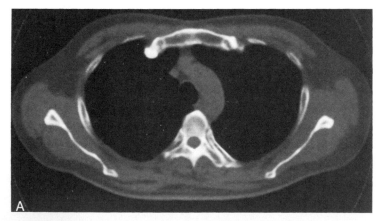

Figure 4–51A. A densely calcified osteophyte is arising from the inferior right first rib.

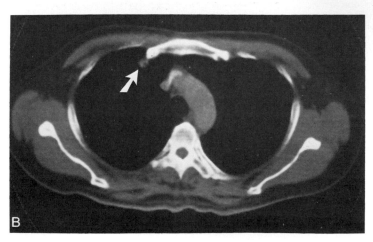

Figure 4–51B. At a slightly lower level, volume averaging with lung makes the first rib appear to be an uncalcified lung nodule *(arrow)*.

Illustration continued on opposite page

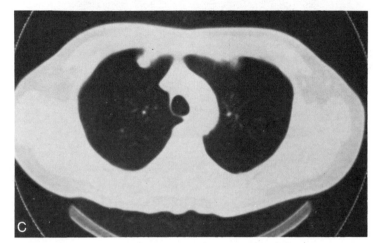

Figure 4–51C. At lung window settings the first rib again appears nodular.

Ref.: Paling MR, Dwyer A. The first rib as a cause of a "pulmonary nodule" on chest computed tomography. J Comput Assist Tomogr 1980; 4:847–848.

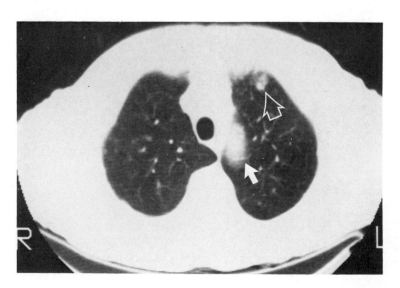

Figure 4–52. PSEUDONODULES. In this subject, both the undersurface of the first rib *(open arrow)* and volume averaging of the top of the aortic arch *(solid arrow)* mimic lung nodules.

Figure 4–53. HEALED RIB FRACTURE MIMICKING LUNG NODULE.

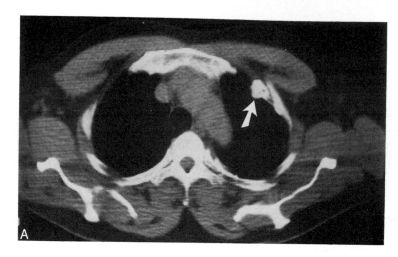

Figure 4–53A. Callus *(arrow)* is demonstrated in a patient with a healed rib fracture.

Figure 4–53B. At lung window settings, the callus seen in *A* can be mistaken for a peripheral lung nodule.

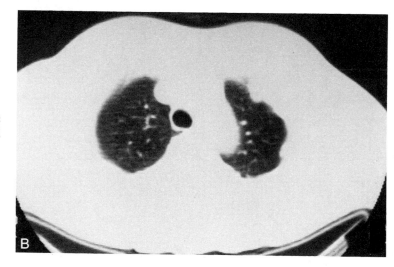

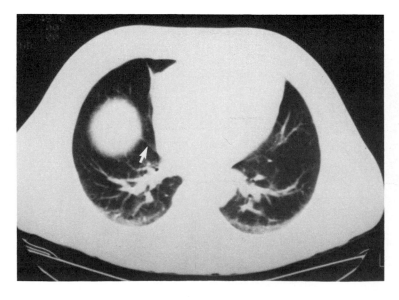

Figure 4–54. NORMAL POSTERIOR LUNG DENSITY. In supine patients a band of increased density is often visible paralleling the posterior chest wall. It probably reflects collapsed and relatively airless lung. Note also the right inferior pulmonary ligament *(arrow)* (see Figures 4–61 and 4–62).

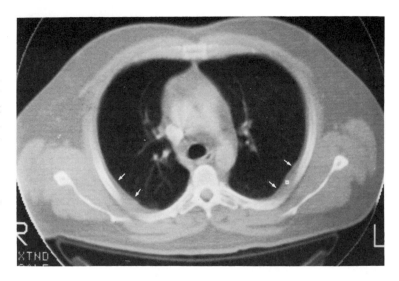

Figure 4–55. EXTRAPLEURAL FAT MIMICKING PLEURAL THICKENING OR FLUID. In this obese patient, extrapleural fat *(arrows)* separates lung and rib. It mimicks fluid but does not occupy the most dependent (posterior) portions of the chest.

Ref.: Sargent EN, Boswell WD Jr, Ralls PW, Markovitz A. Subpleural fat pads in patients exposed to asbestos: Distinction from non-calcified pleural plaques. Radiology 1984; 152:273–277.

Figure 4–56. MAJOR FISSURE.

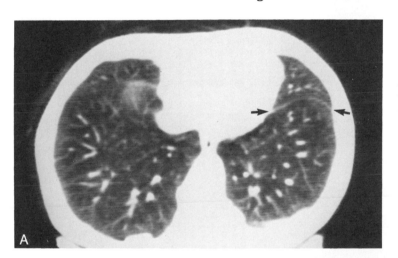

Figure 4–56A. The major fissure is sometimes visible as a thin white line. Typically, this occurs if it is oriented perpendicular to the plane of scan. In this patient, the left major fissure is clearly visible *(arrows)*. A portion of the right major fissure is also seen. Also note peripheral pleural plaques as a result of asbestos exposure.

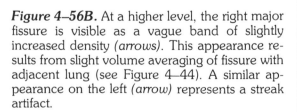

Figure 4–56B. At a higher level, the right major fissure is visible as a vague band of slightly increased density *(arrows)*. This appearance results from slight volume averaging of fissure with adjacent lung (see Figure 4–44). A similar appearance on the left *(arrow)* represents a streak artifact.

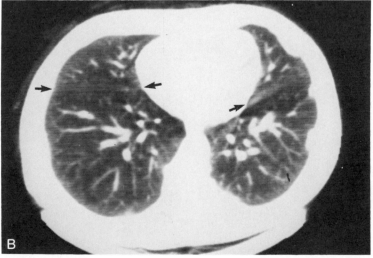

Ref.: Proto AV, Ball JB Jr. Computed tomography of the major and minor fissures. AJR 1983; 140:439–448.

Figure 4–57. MAJOR AND MINOR FISSURES.

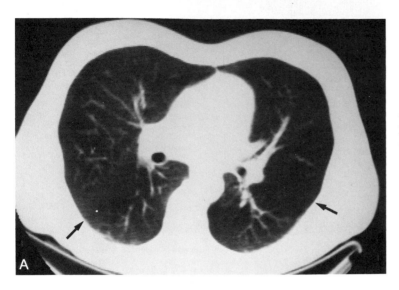

Figure 4–57A. The position of each major fissure *(arrows)* is recognizable primarily by an avascular band of lung representing the peripheral pulmonary parenchyma of the upper and lower lobes on both sides of the fissure.

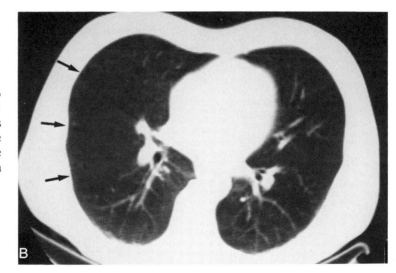

Figure 4–57B. At a lower level and anterior to the major fissure, a large avascular area *(arrows)* represents the plane of the minor fissure. This should not be misinterpreted as abnormal. The minor fissure is almost never seen as a white line. Anterior and medial to this avascular area is the upper lobe.

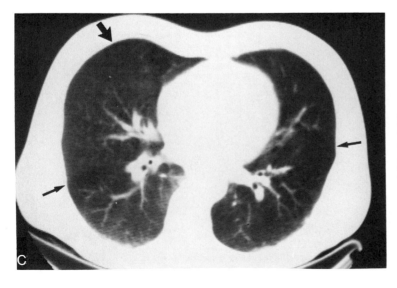

Figure 4–57C. At the level of the right middle lobe, lucent bands representing major fissures *(small arrows)* and the anterior minor fissure *(large arrow)* are visible. On the right, the middle lobe lies between major and minor fissures.

Ref.: Proto AV, Ball JB Jr. Computed tomography of the major and minor fissures. AJR 1983; 140:439–448.

Figure 4–58. MAJOR AND MINOR FIS-SURES. Radiolucent bands mark the positions of the major fissures on both sides *(small arrows).* On the right, vessels anterior to the major fissure are within the right middle lobe; note the position of the middle lobe bronchus (b). Anterior to the middle lobe vessels, an avascular area represents the minor fissure *(large arrow),* descending toward the diaphragm as it extends anteriorly. Anterior and medial to the plane of the minor fissure is the upper lobe.

Ref.: Proto AV, Ball JB Jr. Computed tomography of the major and minor fissures. AJR 1983; 140:439–448.

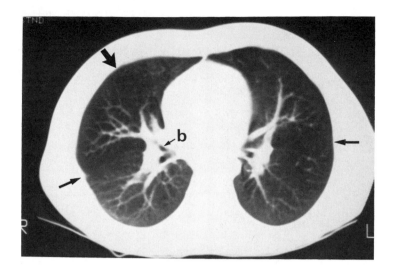

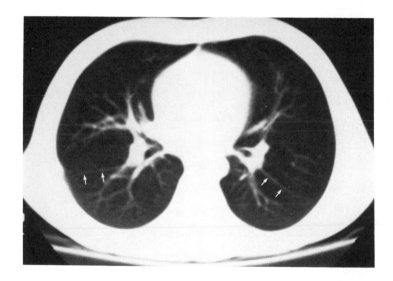

Figure 4–59. VESSELS SIMULATING FIS-SURES. In the patient shown in Figure 4–58, but scanned on another occasion, small vessels on both sides *(arrows)* simulate the major fissures. However, the true locations of the fissures are more anterior.

Figure 4–60. FISSURE SIMULATING LUNG NODULE. Slight thickening of the left major fissure *(large arrow)* simulates a lung nodule. The position of the medial fissure is clearly seen *(small arrow).*

Ref.: Webb WR, Cooper C, Gamsu G. Interlobar pleural plaque mimicking a lung nodule in a patient with asbestos exposure. J Comp Assist Tomogr 1983; 7:135–136.

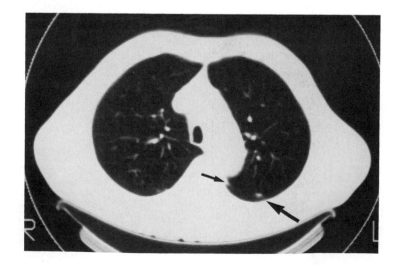

Figure 4–61. AZYGOS LOBE.

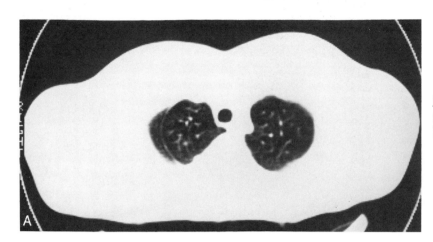

Figure 4–61A. Near the lung apex, the azygos fissure is typically visible as a white line convex laterally.

Figure 4–61B. Several centimeters lower, the azygos arch, originating anteriorly at the level of the left brachiocephalic vein, passes through the lung.

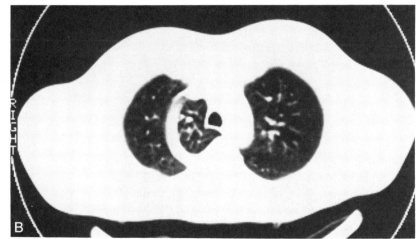

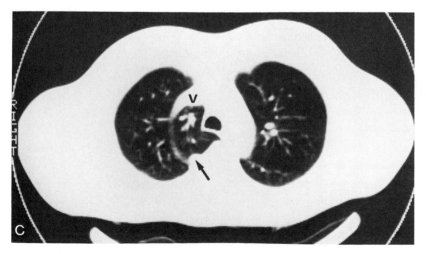

Figure 4–61C. Slightly lower, the azygos arch is only partially seen. The superior vena cava (V) anteriorly and the azygos vein *(arrow)* posteriorly are more prominent than usual. The vena cava can mimic a mass, and the posterior azygos vein can mimic a lung nodule.

Ref.: Speckman J, Gamsu G, Webb WR. Alterations in CT mediastinal anatomy produced by an azygos lobe. AJR 1981; 137:47–50.

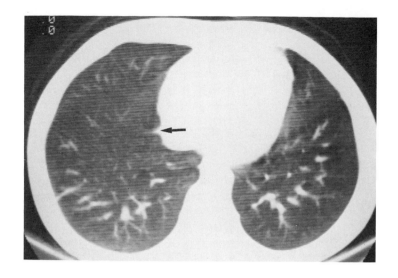

Figure 4–62. RIGHT INFERIOR PULMO-NARY LIGAMENT. The right inferior pulmonary ligament *(arrow)* is visible extending a short distance into the right lung, near the surface of the right hemidiaphragm. It commonly arises near the inferior vena cava. The major fissure is more anterior.

Ref.: Godwin JD, Vock P, Osborne DR. CT of the pulmonary ligament. AJR 1983; 141:231–236.

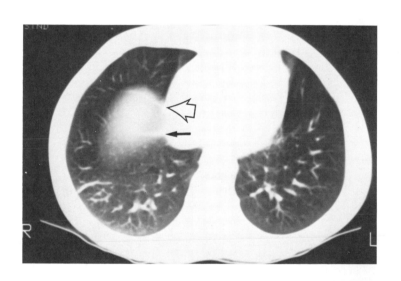

Figure 4–63. RIGHT INFERIOR PULMO-NARY LIGAMENT. The right inferior pulmonary ligament *(solid arrow)* and major fissure *(open arrow)* are visible at the surface of the right hemidiaphragm.

Figure 4–64. LEFT INFERIOR PULMONARY LIGAMENT. The left inferior pulmonary ligament *(arrows)* is visible extending into the lung from below, along the surface of the diaphragm. Fat extending into the left major fissure *(asterisk)* is visible anteriorly (see Figure 4–66).

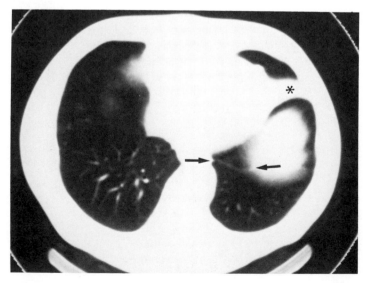

Ref.: Rost RC Jr, Proto AV. Inferior pulmonary ligament: Computed tomographic appearance. Radiology 1983; 148:479–483.

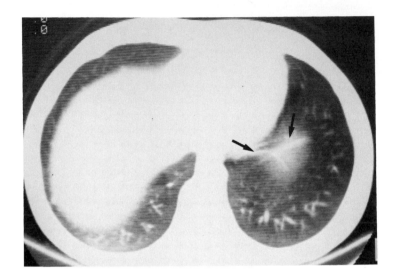

Figure 4–65. LEFT INFERIOR PULMONARY LIGAMENT. Near the surface of the left hemi-diaphragm, the left inferior pulmonary ligament is visible as a branching, linear structure *(arrows)*. The appearance and location are characteristic and allow differentiation from pathologic processes.

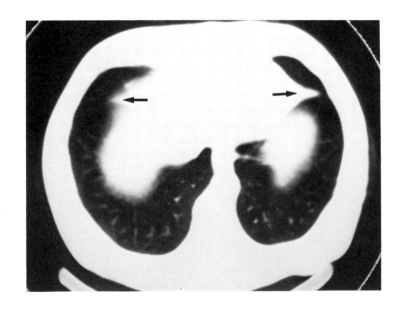

Figure 4–66. FAT EXTENDING INTO FISSURES. Collections of fat *(arrows)*, either from the mediastinum or the surface of the diaphragm, can extend into the fissures, simulating pleural fluid or thickening. Also note the left inferior pulmonary ligament.

Abdomen and Pelvis

SUSAN D. WALL, M.D.
R. BROOKE JEFFREY, M.D.

Figure 5–1. NORMAL ABDOMEN. A CT scan of the mid-abdomen with a single calcification in the pancreas and spleen is displayed. Note the splenic vein *(curved white arrow)* posterior to the pancreas, with a normal interposed fat plane, which should not be mistaken for a dilated pancreatic duct. The splenic artery *(open white arrow)*, also seen on this image, is posterior to the vein and is seen to extend directly into the splenic hilum. The right and left adrenal glands *(straight white arrows)* are demonstrated. Note the thin caudate lobe of the liver anterior to the inferior vena cava (I) and posterior to the portal vein (P). The right and left crura *(black arrow)* of the diaphragm are seen anterior to the aorta.

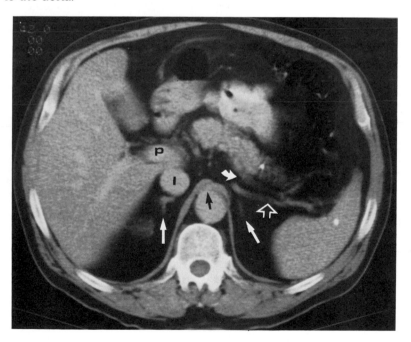

Figure 5–2. FLATTENED INFERIOR VENA CAVA.

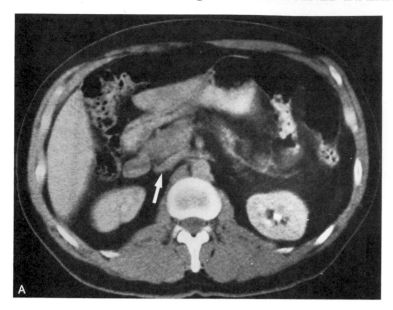

Figure 5–2A. Flattening of the usually round inferior vena cava is normal at the level of entrance of the left renal vein *(arrow)*. The left renal vein is seen crossing anterior to the aorta and posterior to the superior mesenteric artery.

Figure 5–2B. In a second patient, normal flattening of the inferior vena cava *(curved arrow)* is seen at the entrance of the left renal vein *(straight arrow)* in this non-enhanced scan.

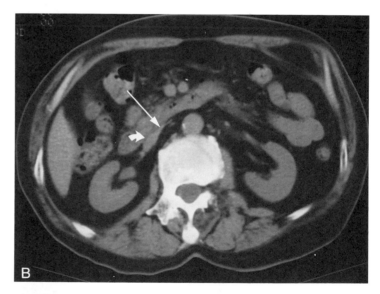

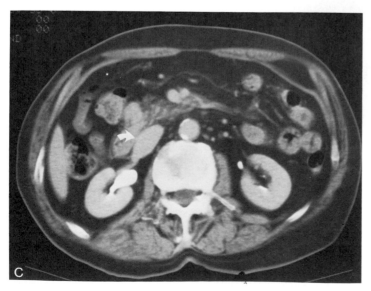

Figure 5–2C. This scan, at the same level as *B,* shows a more dilated inferior vena cava *(curved arrow)* after intravenous contrast enhancement. Note enhancement of the right and left kidneys and excretion of the opacified urine, confirming intravenous contrast administration. (See also Chapter 6, Figure 6–34, for variations of the inferior vena cava.)

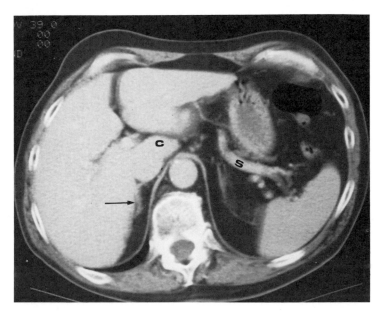

Figure 5–3. SPLENIC VEIN. A large extent of the splenic vein (S) is apparent in this scan. In this subject, most of the splenic vein is seen cephalad to the pancreas rather than directly posterior—a normal variant. Note the normal right adrenal gland *(black arrow)* and the caudate lobe (C) of the liver.

Figure 5–4. NORMAL RENAL VESSELS.

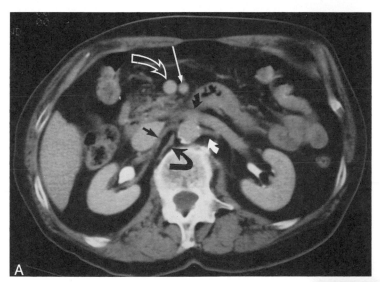

Figure 5–4A. The left renal vein *(small curved black arrow)* is seen to course anterior to the aorta and posterior to the superior mesenteric artery *(straight white arrow)*. The right diaphragmatic crus *(large curved black arrow)*, left renal artery *(small curved white arrow)*, and right renal artery *(small straight black arrow)* can also be seen. The left renal vein is double the size of the left renal artery. This proportion is normal and should not be misinterpreted as obstruction with subsequent dilatation of the left renal vein. The superior mesenteric vein *(large open white arrow)* is well delineated in this intravenous contrast-enhanced image.

Figure 5–4B. The entrance of the left renal vein *(straight black arrow)* into the inferior vena cava (I) is noted, along with partial volume averaging of the take-off of the superior mesenteric artery *(small curved white arrow)*. As in A, the superior mesenteric vein *(large open white arrow)* is well delineated. The uncinate process of the pancreas is seen posterior to the superior mesenteric vein. Note the moderate fatty involution of the pancreatic head, a normal finding in this 54-year-old patient. (See also Chapter 6, Figure 6–2.)

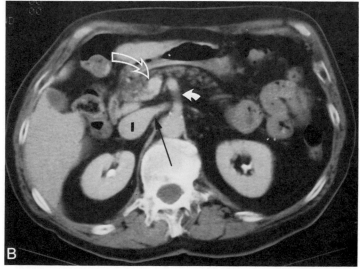

Figure 5–5. **REPLACED RIGHT HEPATIC ARTERY.**

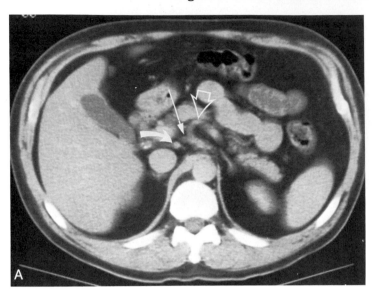

Figure 5–5A. A replaced right hepatic artery *(solid curved white arrow)* is demonstrated, heading cephalad toward the liver. The normal hepatic artery is usually seen anterior to the portal vein; however, a replaced right hepatic artery, arising from the superior mesenteric artery or directly from the aorta, will be seen between the portal vein and the inferior vena cava, as in this case. The splenic artery *(open arrow)* and the main hepatic artery *(straight arrow)* can also be seen.

Figure 5–5B. The replaced right hepatic artery *(solid curved arrow)* is demonstrated, as is the celiac axis *(open curved arrow)* .

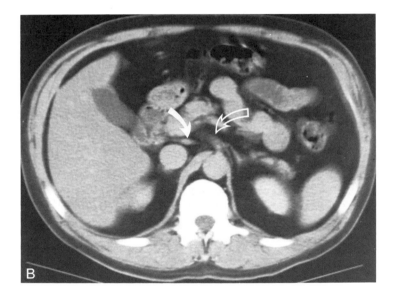

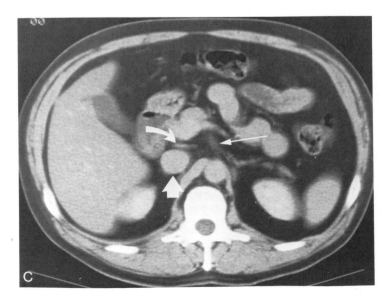

Figure 5–5C. In this image the replaced right hepatic artery *(curved arrow)*, which is horizontal to the plane of the imaging axis shown in *B,* is seen anterior to the inferior vena cava *(straight short arrow)*. The superior mesenteric artery also can be seen *(straight long arrow)*.

Figure 5–6. LEFT INFERIOR VENA CAVA. The levels shown in *A–D* progress from caudal to cephalad; the aorta is indicated by the *curved black arrow*. Bilateral polycystic kidneys are demonstrated in all images.

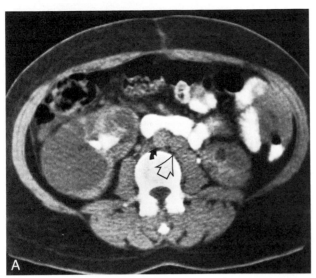

Figure 5–6A. At a level below the left renal hilum, a left inferior cava *(open arrow)* can be seen. Note the opacified transverse duodenum anterior to the aorta and inferior vena cava.

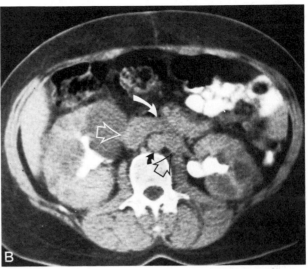

Figure 5–6B. At a slightly more cephalad level, the left renal vein enters the left inferior vena cava. This is the only level at which both the left *(open black arrow)* and the right *(open white arrow)* inferior venae cavae are seen. The crossover to the right inferior vena cava can also be seen *(curved white arrow)* overlying the pancreatic head.

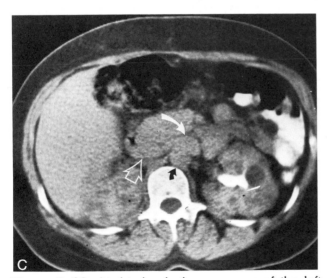

Figure 5–6C. At this level, the crossover of the left inferior vena cava *(curved white arrow)* to the right inferior vena cava *(open white arrow)* can be identified.

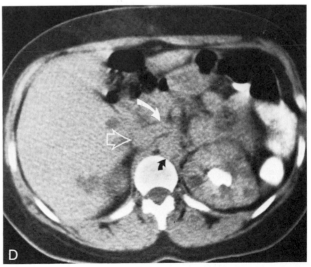

Figure 5–6D. At a slightly more cephalad level, the crossing-over left inferior vena cava *(curved white arrow)* can be seen entering the right inferior vena cava *(open white arrow)*. (See also Chapter 6, Figure 6–34.)

Ref.: Mayo J, Gray R, St. Louis E. Review: Anomalies of the inferior vena cava. AJR 1983; 140:339–345.

Figure 5–7. DUPLICATED INFERIOR VENA CAVA. A duplicated inferior vena cava *(black arrows)* and a right-sided inferior vena cava *(curved arrows)* are seen at all three levels *(A, B, C).*

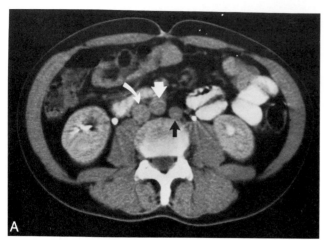

Figure 5–7A. At this level the aorta *(wide arrow)* is demonstrated.

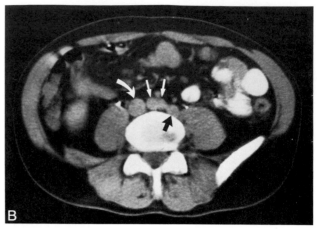

Figure 5–7B. The aorta is seen at the level of its bifurcation in this scan *(straight arrows).*

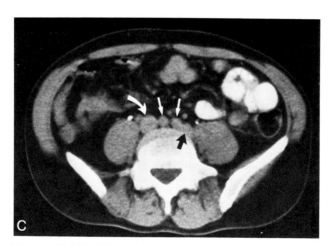

Figure 5–7C. This image, which is 1 cm caudal to *B,* demonstrates the right and left iliac arteries *(straight arrows).*

Ref.: Faer MJ, Lynch RD, Evans HO, Chin FK. Inferior vena cava duplication. Demonstration by computed tomography. Radiology 1979; 130:707–709.

Figure 5–8. DUPLICATED INFERIOR VENA CAVA. In all views *(A–D)* the aorta is demonstrated *(curved arrow)*.

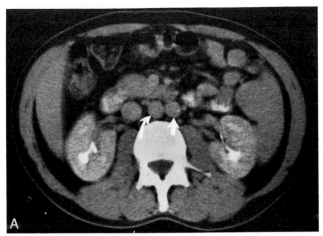

Figure 5–8A. A duplicated inferior vena cava *(straight arrow)* is seen at the level of the renal hila.

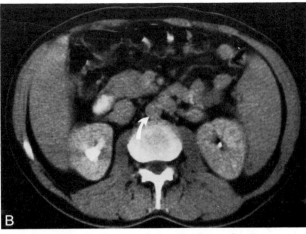

Figure 5–8B. At this level the duplicated inferior vena cava begins to move anterior to the aorta.

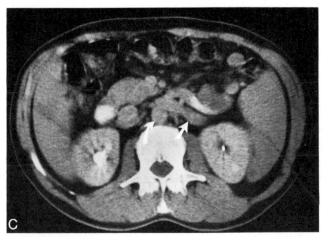

Figure 5–8C. The duplicated inferior vena cava can be seen to cross horizontally toward the right-sided inferior vena cava at the level of the entrance of the left renal vein *(straight arrow)*.

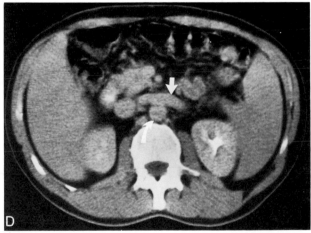

Figure 5–8D. This level, which is 1 cm cephalad to *C*, further demonstrates the course of the duplicated inferior vena cava *(straight arrow)* as it crosses over the aorta *(curved arrow)* to the right-sided inferior vena cava.

Ref.: Royal SA, Callen PW. CT evaluation of anomalies of the inferior vena cava and left renal vein. AJR 1979; 132:759–763.

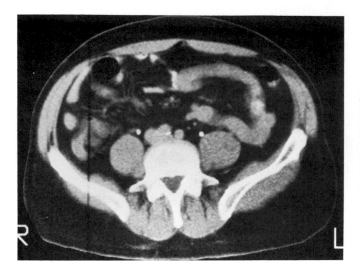

Figure 5–9. NORMAL MESENTERY. The curvilinear lines of the blood vessels and connective tissue of the normal mesentery are well demonstrated in this subject. Note the slight asymmetry of the right and left iliac arteries, psoas muscles, and iliac wings, which is due to positioning and should not be misinterpreted as abnormal.

Figure 5–10. ASYMMETRIC PSOAS MUSCLES. Anterior lobulation of the right psoas muscle *(arrow)* is demonstrated in a young patient; this is a normal variant. Note the normal right ureter, which is situated somewhat lateral to the psoas muscle compared with the left ureter. Both are in a normal position. (See also Chapter 6, Figure 6–27, for variations in the psoas muscles.)

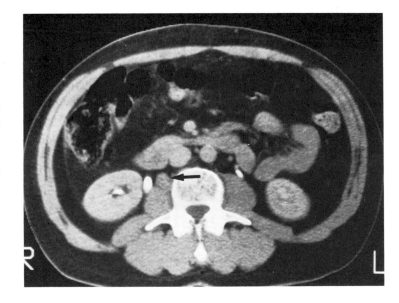

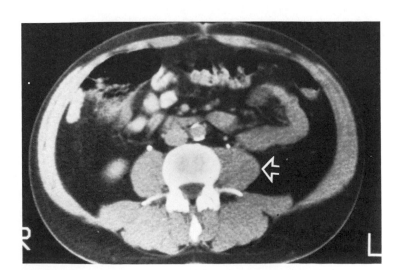

Figure 5–11. ASYMMETRIC PSOAS MUSCLES. This image demonstrates fullness of the left psoas muscle *(arrowhead)* compared with the right; this is a normal variant.

Figure 5–12. ASYMMETRIC PSOAS MUSCLES. Progressive asymmetric atrophy of the psoas muscles is seen in this left-handed/left-legged elderly patient, with greater preservation of the left-sided muscle mass *(straight arrow in B)* than of the right *(curved arrow in B)*. Note that in *B* there is partial volume averaging of the right iliac crest because of asymmetric positioning of the patient within the gantry (more obvious in *C*).

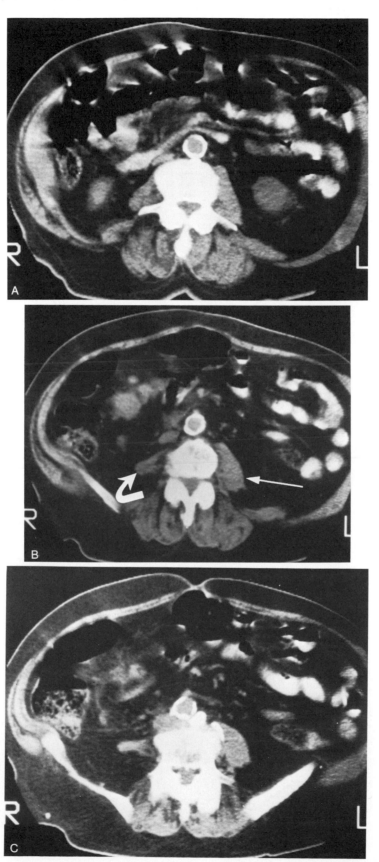

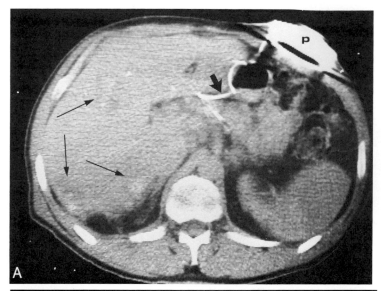

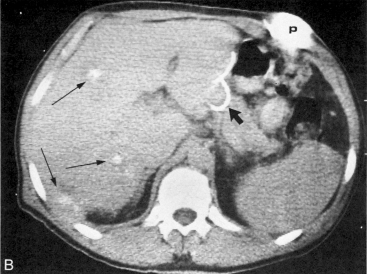

Figure 5–13. HEPATIC ARTERY INFUSION PUMP. In two adjacent sections *(A and B)*, a high-density, curvilinear catheter *(short arrows)* has been positioned into the hepatic artery for selective chemotherapeutic infusion in this patient with metastatic colon cancer *(long arrows)*. The high-density infusion pump (p) has been placed in the left anterior abdominal wall.

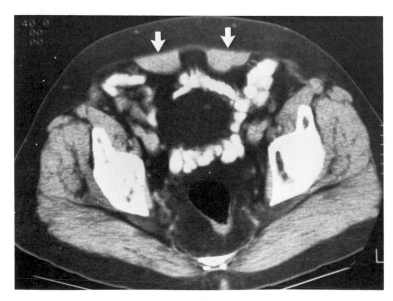

Figure 5–14. RECTUS ABDOMINUS. A midline separation of the right and left rectus abdominus muscles *(arrows)* is demonstrated. Fat is present between the two muscles (a normal variant).

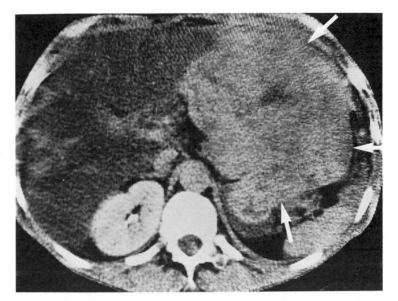

Figure 5-15. INTRA-ABDOMINAL HEMA-TOMA. A huge lesser sac hematoma *(arrows)* from hemorrhagic pancreatitis mimics a solid mass. Note the diffuse hypodensity of the liver, which is due to fatty infiltration.

Figure 5-16. INTRAUTERINE PREGNANCY SIMULATING A TUMOR. This normal intra-uterine pregnancy simulates a large calcium-producing or bone-forming tumor. In these scans the placenta cannot be differentiated from the amniotic fluid because of similar CT attenuation numbers.

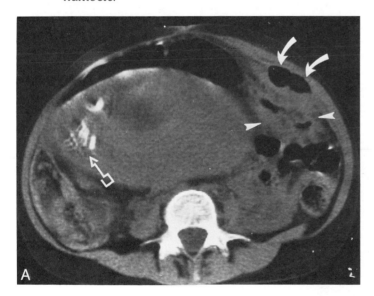

Figure 5-16A. Note the ribs and spine *(open boxed arrow)* of the fetus. Also demonstrated are a thick-ened bowel wall *(arrowheads)* and an associated extraluminal abscess with a gas collection involving the left anterior abdominal wall *(curved arrows);* these are manifestations of Crohn's disease and the reason for this limited CT examination.

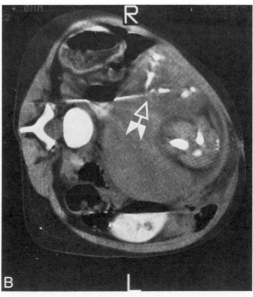

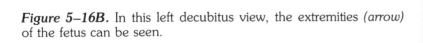

Figure 5-16B. In this left decubitus view, the extremities *(arrow)* of the fetus can be seen.

Figure 5–17. INFERIOR VENA CAVA UMBRELLA.

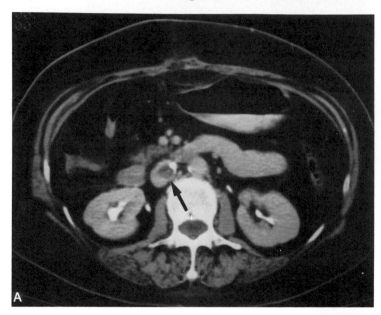

Figure 5–17A. A low-density clot *(arrow)* is present in the inferior vena cava. It is just caudal the umbrella seen in *B* and *C*.

Figure 5–17B. An umbrella *(arrow)* can be seen within the inferior vena cava.

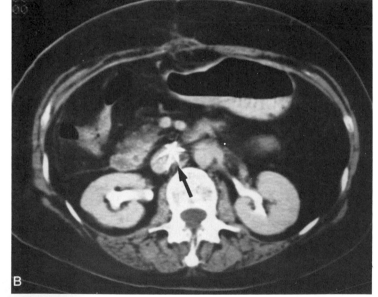

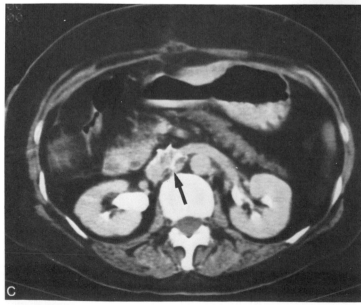

Figure 5–17C. At a level adjacent to *B*, the umbrella *(arrow)* is still visible.

Illustration continued on opposite page

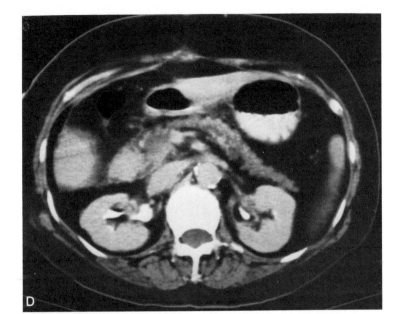

Figure 5–17D. At this level, just cephalad to the umbrella, entrance of the left renal vein into a normal inferior vena cava is demonstrated.

Ref.: Glazer GM, Callen, PW, Parker JJ. CT diagnosis of tumor thrombus in the inferior vena cava: Avoiding the false-positive diagnosis. AJR 1981; 137:1265–1267.

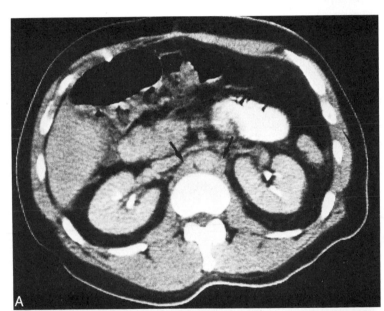

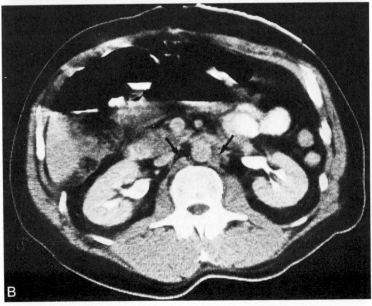

Figure 5–18. PSEUDOADENOPATHY. In these contiguous scans (*A* and *B*) termination of the crura of the diaphragm simulates retroperitoneal adenopathy *(arrows).* (See also Chapter 6, Figure 6–27C for an example of diaphragmatic crus.)

Ref.: Rosen A, Auk YH, Rubenstein WA, et al. CT appearance of diaphragmatic pseudotumor. J Comput Assist Tomogr 1983; 7:995–999.

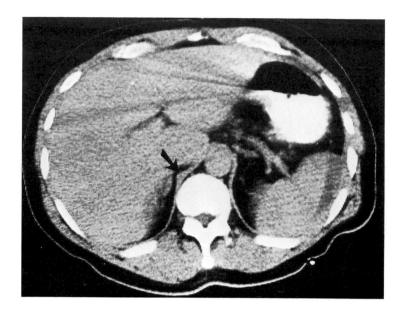

Figure 5–19. NORMAL DIAPHRAGMATIC CRUS. Right crural pseudotumor *(arrow)*, due to the normal nodularity of muscle fibers of the diaphragmatic crus.

Ref.: Callen PW, Korobkin M, Isherwood I. Computed tomographic evaluation of the retrocrural prevertebral space. AJR 1977; 129:907–910.

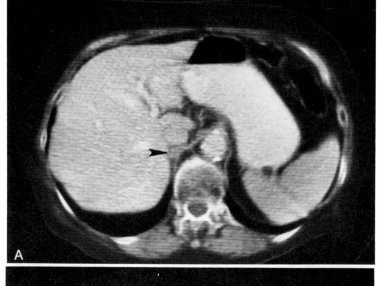

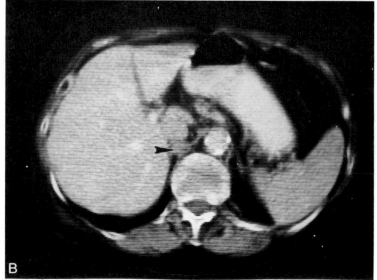

Figure 5–20 PSEUDO–ADRENAL MASS. The knobby right diaphragmatic crus *(arrowhead)* in A and B simulates an adrenal mass.

Illustration continued on opposite page

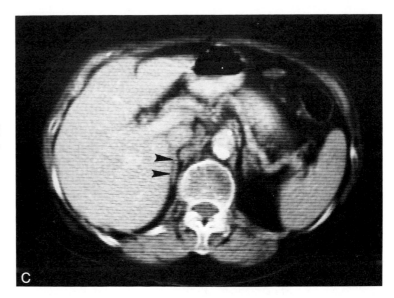

Figure 5–20C. A normal right adrenal gland *(arrowheads)* is demonstrated. (See also Chapter 6, Figure 6–29.)

Ref.: Callen PW, Korobkin M, Isherwood I. Computed tomographic evaluation of the diaphragmatic crura. Radiology 1978; 126:413–416.

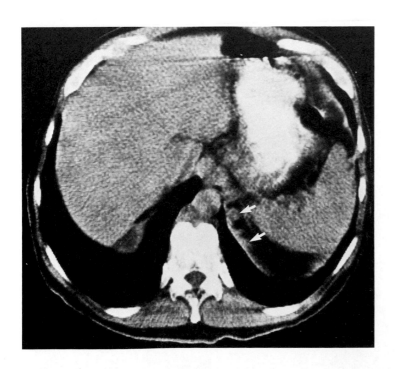

Figure 5–21. DIAPHRAGMATIC PSEUDO-TUMOR. Normal muscle insertions *(arrows)* of the diaphragm can simulate diaphragmatic tumor nodules.

Ref.: Rosen A, Auk YH, Rubenstein WA, et al. CT appearance of diaphragmatic pseudotumor. J Comput Assist Tomogr 1983; 7:995–999.

Figure 5–22. **INTERRUPTED DIAPHRAGM.**

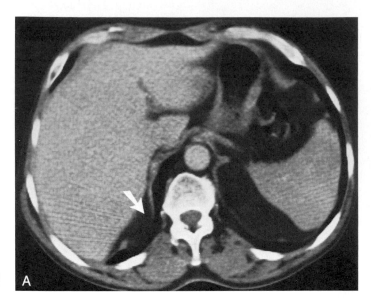

Figure 5–22A. An interrupted right hemidiaphragm *(arrow)* is visible where the high-density curvilinear diaphragmatic muscle bordering the subdiaphragmatic fat is seen to be incomplete; this is a normal variant.

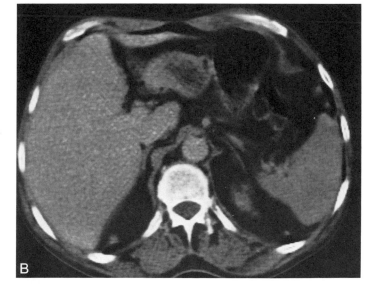

Figure 5–22B. A contiguous caudal section again demonstrates the interruption.

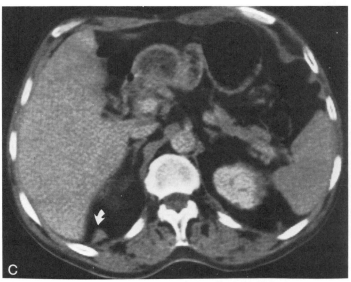

Figure 5–22C. Note the slightly bulbous diaphragmatic muscular insertion *(arrow)* of the posterior aspect of the diaphragm.

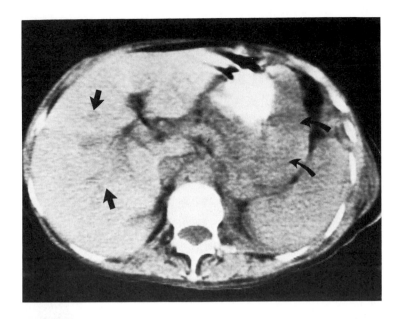

Figure 5–23. PSEUDO–HEPATIC LESIONS. Unopacified hepatic and portal venous structures in this non-contrast scan mimic low-density hepatic lesions *(straight arrows)*. Note the thickened gastric wall in this patient with lymphoma *(curved arrows)*.

Ref.: Kressel HY, Korobkin M, Goldberg HI, et al. The portal venous tree simulating dilated biliary ducts on computed tomography of the liver. J Comput Assist Tomogr 1977; 1:169–175.

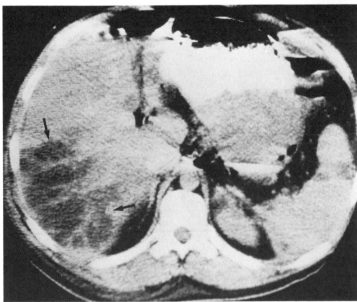

Figure 5–24. FOCAL FATTY INFILTRATION OF THE LIVER. This scan demonstrates fatty infiltration *(arrows)* simulating a low-density mass within the liver. Note the lack of vascular displacement.

Ref.: Scott WW, Sanders RC, Siegelman SS. Irregular fatty infiltration of the liver: Diagnostic dilemmas. AJR 1980; 135:67–71.

Figure 5–25. FOCAL FATTY INFILTRATION OF THE LIVER. Generalized decreased density of the liver compared with the spleen is demonstrated with focal areas *(arrows)* of greater fat accumulation. Note the linear, geographic appearance of areas of focal fatty infiltration.

Ref.: Scott WW, Sanders RC, Siegelman SS. Irregular fatty infiltration of the liver: Diagnostic dilemmas. AJR 1980; 135:67–71.

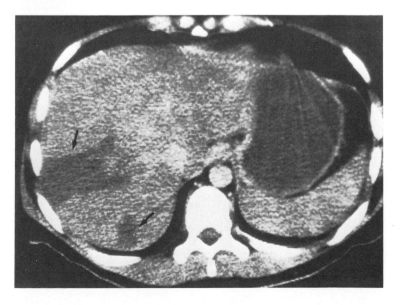

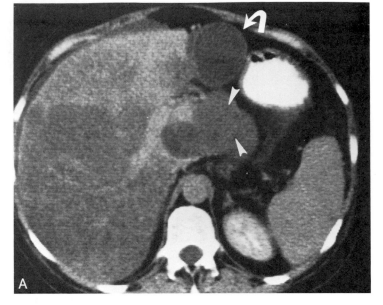

Figure 5–26 FATTY INFILTRATION OF THE LIVER. A, In this patient with alcoholic cirrhosis, a hepatic mass is simulated *(arrowheads)* by the enlarged lobulated caudate lobe that is homogeneously reduced in density by diffuse fatty infiltration. The high attenuation of the enhanced hepatic vessels simulates the border of a mass. Note the gallbladder *(curved arrow)*, which should not be mistaken for a low-density lesion.

In *B*, an image contiguous to *A*, note the more heterogeneous fatty infiltration elsewhere in the liver and the confirmation of the "pseudomass" as the caudate lobe.

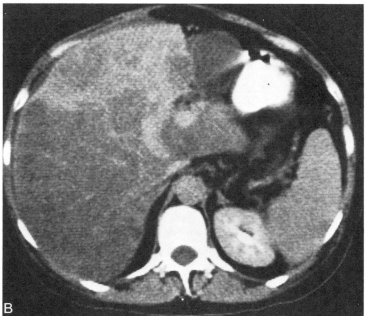

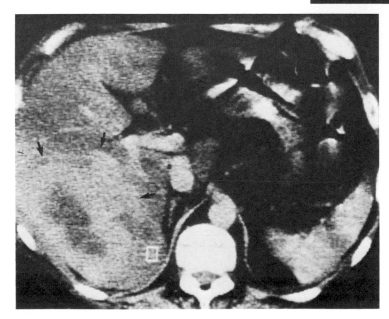

Figure 5–27. FATTY INFILTRATION OF THE LIVER. Hepatic metastasis *(arrows)* is suggested by a high-density lesion in a liver with fatty infiltration *(cursor)*.

Ref.: Lewis E, Bernardino ME, Barnes PA, et al. The fatty liver: Pitfall in the CT and angiographic evaluation of metastatic disease. J Comput Assist Tomogr 1983; 7:235–241.

Figure 5–28. SMALL MEDIAL SEGMENT OF THE LEFT LOBE OF THE LIVER

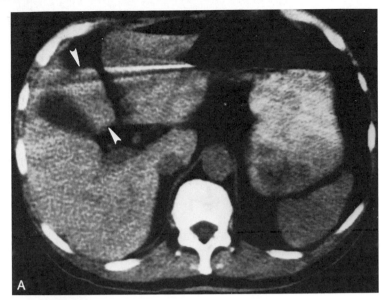

Figure 5–28A. The medial segment of the left lobe of the liver can sometimes be relatively small *(arrowheads)*.

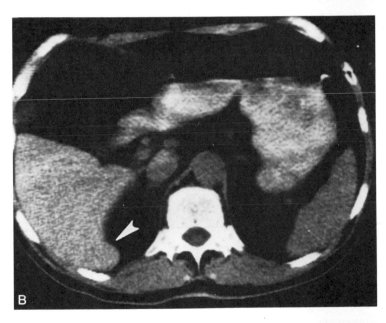

Figure 5–28B. This section is 1 cm caudal to the image in *A* and demonstrates only the right lobe. Note the lobulation of the posterior segment *(arrowhead)* of the right lobe, a normal variant.

Figure 5–29. REGENERATING NODULE. A regenerating nodule in a patient with cirrhosis appears as an isodense lobulated mass *(arrows)*.

Ref.: Laing FC, Jeffrey RB, Federle MP, et al. Non-invasive imaging of unusual regenerating nodules in the cirrhotic liver. Gastrointest Radiol 1984; 7:235–249.

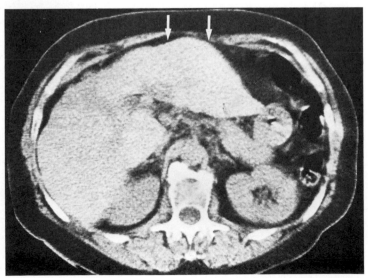

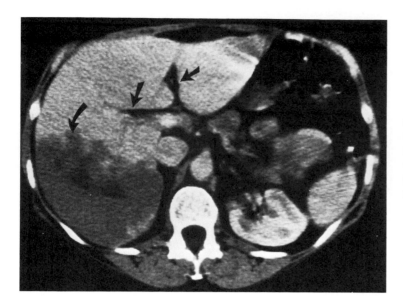

Figure 5–30. FAT WITHIN THE HEPATIC FISSURES. Fat within the hepatic fissures *(straight arrows)* mimics dilated intrahepatic bile ducts. Note the low-density cavernous hemangioma in the posterior segment of the right lobe *(curved arrow)*.

Figure 5–31. HEPATIC LACERATION.

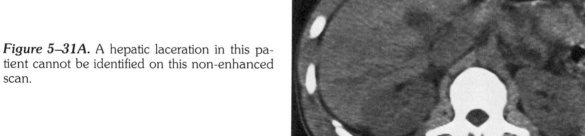

Figure 5–31A. A hepatic laceration in this patient cannot be identified on this non-enhanced scan.

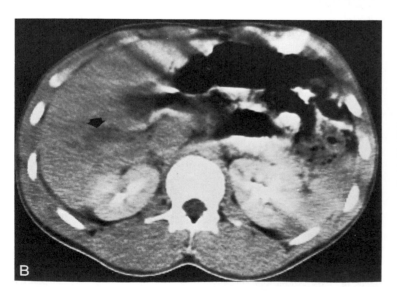

Figure 5–31B. After intravenous contrast enhancement of the normal hepatic parenchyma, a hypodense linear laceration *(arrow)* is demonstrated in the right lobe of the liver on this scan (same level as *A*).

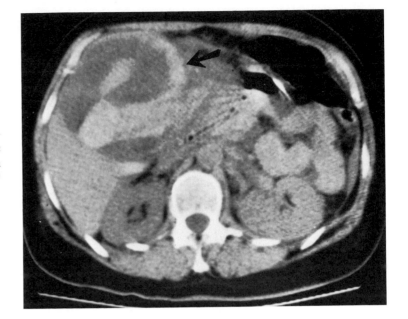

Figure 5–32. HEPATIC HEMORRHAGE. Recent intrahepatic hemorrhage of a hypodense hepatic adenoma gives the appearance of a stretched segment of opacified bowel *(arrow)* because of high attenuation of the fresh blood.

Figure 5–33. STREAK ARTIFACTS.

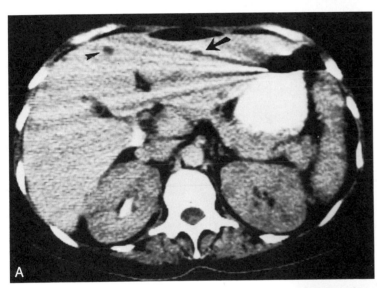

Figure 5–33A. Streak artifacts from the air and Gastrografin interface nearly obscure the "microabscesses" *(arrow)* in the lateral and medial segments of the left lobe of the liver in this patient with disseminated candidiasis. Farther from the streak artifacts, other abscess deposits are more readily seen, such as in the medial segment of the left lobe *(arrowhead).*

Figure 5–33B. In another scan in the same patient in A, abscess deposits are demonstrated in the posterior segment of the right lobe *(arrows).*

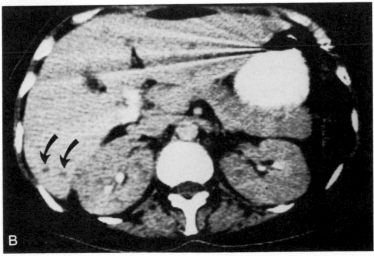

Figure 5–34. STREAK ARTIFACTS. Streak artifacts *(curved arrows)* from the interface of air and high-concentration Gastrografin nearly obscure low-density hepatic lacerations *(arrowheads).*

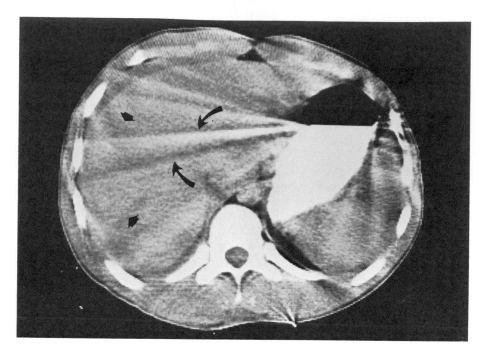

Ref.: Moon KL, Federle MP. Computed tomography in hepatic trauma. AJR 1983; 141:309–324.

Figure 5–35. CLIP ARTIFACTS. High-density streak artifacts from metallic surgical clips impede visualization of a low-density intrahepatic abscess *(arrow).*

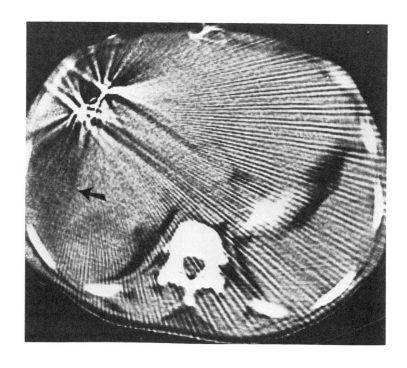

Figure 5–36. LOBULATION OF THE LIVER. Lobulation *(arrow)* of the posterior segment of the right lobe of the liver should not be mistaken for a mass or a fracture.

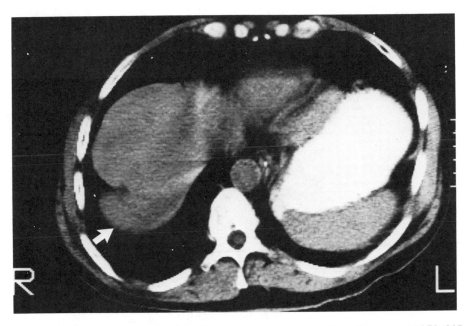

Ref.: Kollins SA. Computed tomography of the liver, spleen and pancreas. Semin Roentgenol 1978; 227–234.

Figure 5–37. BILIARY STENTS. High-density biliary stents are demonstrated in various anatomic locations shown in *A–E,* as well as in a scout view *(F).*

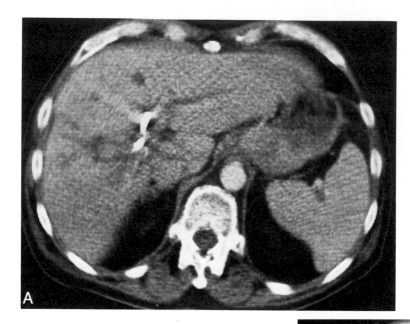

Figure 5–37A. Right and left bile ducts.

Figure 5–37B. Common hepatic duct.

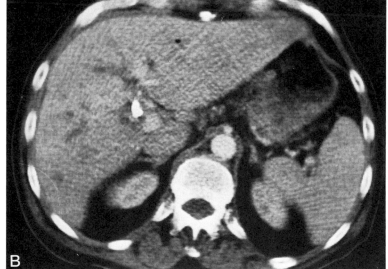

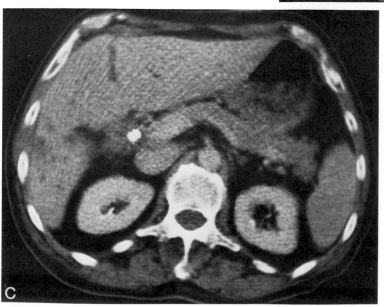

Figure 5–37C. Common bile duct.

Illustration continued on opposite page

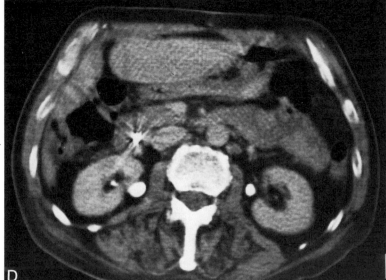

Figure 5–37D. Second portion of the duodenum.

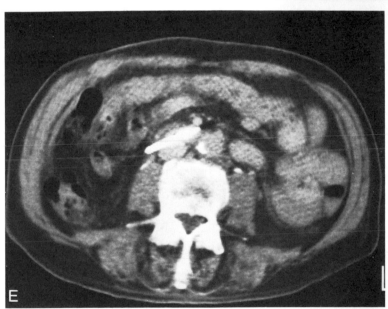

Figure 5–37E. Transverse portion of the duodenum.

Figure 5–37F. Abdominal scout view showing the biliary stent.

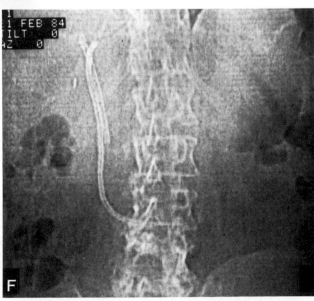

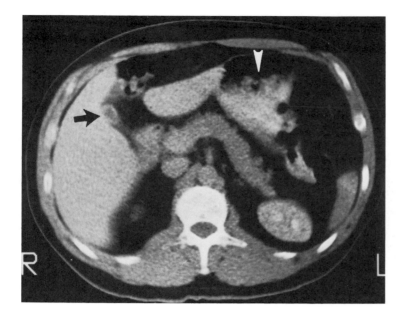

Figure 5–38. NORMAL GALLBLADDER. The small size of the gallbladder *(black arrow)* seen in this patient is due to postprandial contraction. Note the gastric food contents *(white arrowhead)*, which are mixed with oral Gastrografin. It should not be mistaken for the small, shrunken gallbladder of chronic cholecystitis.

Figure 5–39. PSEUDOGALLSTONES.

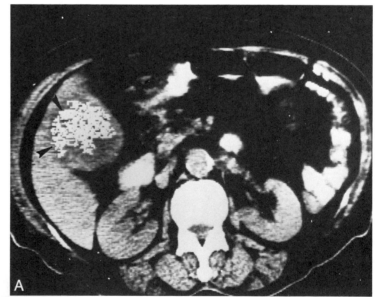

Figure 5–39A. Gallstones *(arrowheads)* are simulated by the use of the blink mode.

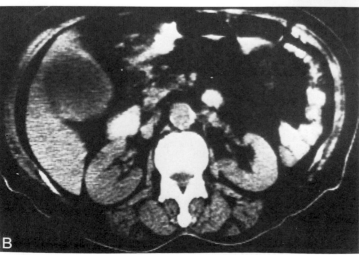

Figure 5–39B. The same image as *A*, without the blink mode, shows no gallstones but some layering of lower-density bile corresponding to the area highlighted by the blink mode.

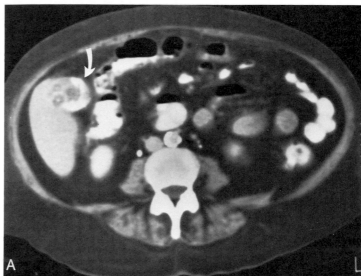

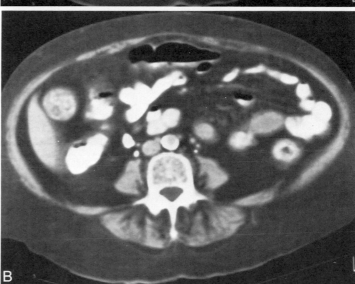

Figure 5–40. PORCELAIN GALLBLADDER.
A calcified gallbladder wall *(arrow, A)* and cholelithiasis are noted.

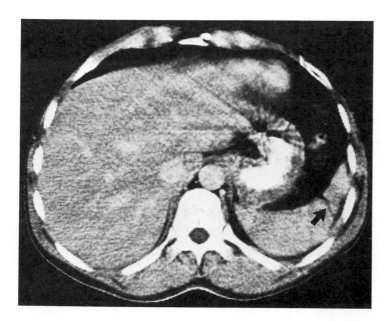

*Figure 5–41. PSEUDO–SPLENIC LACERA-
TION.* A congenital cleft of the spleen *(arrow)*
mimics a splenic laceration in this patient who had
sustained blunt abdominal trauma.

Ref.: Jeffrey RB, Laing FC, Federle MP, et al. Computed
    tomography of splenic trauma. Radiology 1981;
    141:729–732.

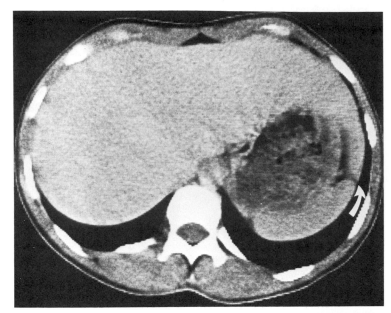

Figure 5–42. PSEUDO–SPLENIC LACERATION. The lateral segment of the left lobe of the liver extends across the midline, and posteriorly it is seen to abut the spleen, simulating a splenic laceration *(arrow)* (see reference, Figure 5–36).

Figure 5–43. SPLENIC CALCIFICATION. This image demonstrates a calcified spleen *(arrow)* from autoinfarction in patient with sickle cell disease.

Ref.: Magid D, Fishman EK, Siegelman SS. Computed tomography of the spleen and liver in sickle cell disease. AJR 1984; 143:245–249.

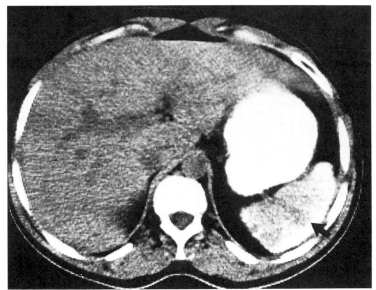

Figure 5–44. TRILOBED SPLEEN.

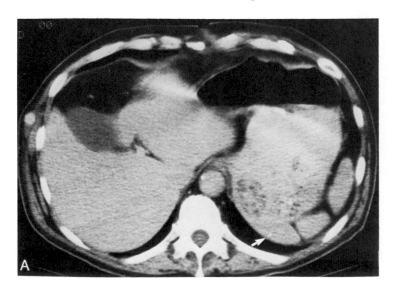

Figure 5–44A. This image shows fat planes interposed between the three lobes of a trilobed spleen, a normal variant. A single calcification *(arrow)* is seen in the most medial lobe.

Illustration continued on opposite page

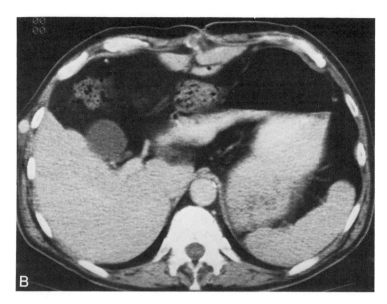

Figure 5–44B. This more caudal image demonstrates the body of the spleen, which is not segmented.

Ref.: Piekarski J, Federle MP, Moss AA, London SS. Computed tomography of the spleen. Radiology 1980; 135:683–689.

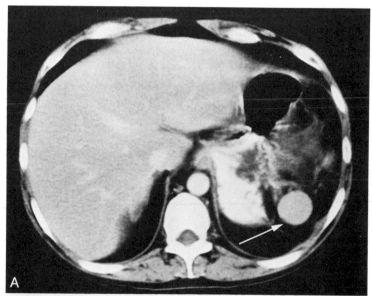

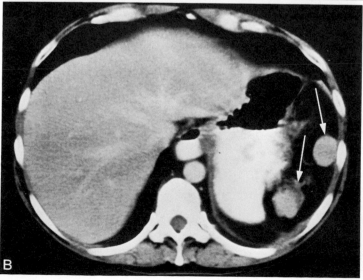

Figure 5–45. ACCESSORY SPLEEN. Accessory splenic tissue *(arrows)* has hypertrophied in the two-year interval since this patient underwent splenectomy because of traumatic laceration. (See also Chapter 6, Figure 6–16.)

Refs.: (1) Beahrs JR, Stephens DH. Enlarged accessory spleens: CT appearance in postsplenectomy patients. AJR 1980; 135:483–486. (2) Glazer GM, Axel L, Goldberg HI, Moss AA. Dynamic CT of the normal spleen. AJR 1981; 137:343–346.

Figure 5–46. PSEUDO–PANCREATIC MASS. A pancreatic mass can be simulated by unopacified small bowel loops.

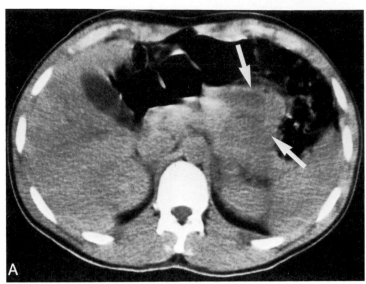

Figure 5–46A. The ill-defined soft-tissue density *(arrows)* in the area of the body of the pancreas could be misinterpreted as a pancreatic mass.

Figure 5–46B. Delayed scans following further administration of oral contrast identified the "mass" as unopacified bowel.

Ref.: Churchill RJ, Reynes CJ, Love L, et al. Pancreatic pseudotumors: Computed tomography. Gastrointest Radiol 1978; 3:251–256.

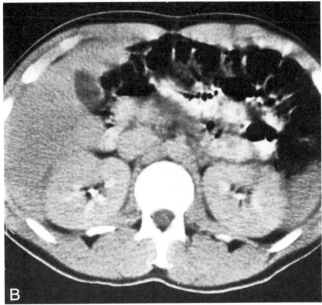

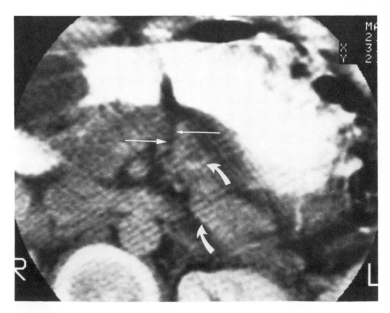

Figure 5–47. PSEUDO–PANCREATIC FRAC-TURE. A pancreatic fracture is simulated by the closeness of unopacified bowel loops. The vertically oriented low density *(straight arrows)* adjacent to the head of the pancreas simulates a pancreatic fracture in a patient who had sustained blunt abdominal trauma. Close scrutiny reveals a very small amount of high-density oral contrast material *(curved arrows)* in adjacent small bowel loops that are mimicking the tail of the pancreas.

Ref.: Jeffrey RB, Federle MP, Crass RA: CT of pancreatic trauma. Radiology 1983; 147:491–494.

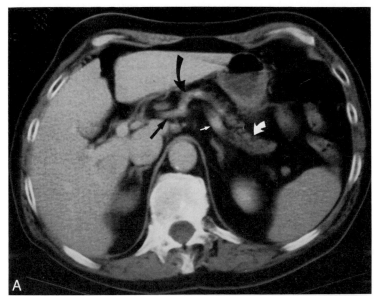

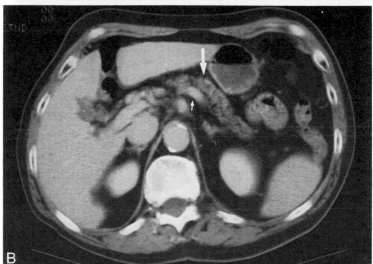

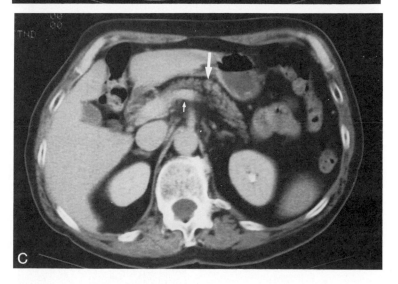

Figure 5–48. AGED PANCREAS. A normal, fatty pancreas is seen in these scans of a 67-year-old patient. The tail *(curved white arrow in A)* and body *(large straight white arrow in B and C)* of the pancreas are seen to have some fatty involution; the pancreas is normal in size, contour, and appearance for the patient's age. The splenic vein *(small straight white arrow in A, B, and C)* is seen to abut the pancreas posteriorly with a slender, fatty plane interposed. The celiac axis and two of its branches, the splenic artery *(curved black arrow in A)* and the hepatic artery *(straight black arrow in A),* are well delineated. Note the normal right and left adrenal glands.

Ref.: Patel S, Bellon EM, Haaga J, Park CH. Fat replacement of the exocrine pancreas. AJR 1980; 135:843–845.

Figure 5–49. PSEUDO–GASTRIC MASS. A pseudo–gastric mass caused by the normal esophagogastric junction *(white arrow)* is seen at the level of the ligamentum venosum *(white arrowhead)*. Area of a hepatocellular carcinoma is also demonstrated *(cursor)*. Note the low-density subcapsular hemorrhage *(black arrows)*.

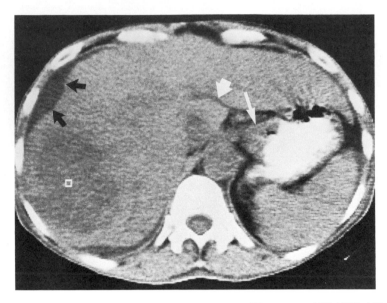

Refs.: (1) Kaye MD, Young SW, Hayward R. Gastric pseudotumor on CT scanning. AJR 1980; 135:190–192. (2) Balfe DM, Mauro MA, Koehler RE, et al. Gastrohepatic ligament: Normal and pathologic CT anatomy. Radiology 1984; 150:485–490.

Figure 5–50. PSEUDO–GASTRIC MASS. This is an example of a pseudotumor of the esophagogastric junction *(black arrow)*. A subphrenic abscess is demonstrated *(curved white arrow)*.

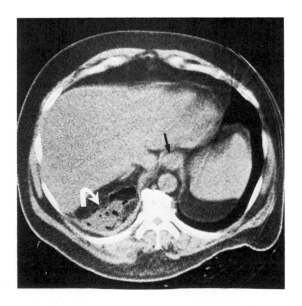

Ref.: Marks WM, Callen PW, Moss AA. Gastroesophageal region: Source of confusion on CT. AJR 1981; 136:359–362.

Figure 5–51. NISSEN FUNDOPLICATION. Normal CT findings following a transabdominal fundoplication (Nissen procedure) are demonstrated in *A–F.* An antireflux operation for hiatal hernia, the Nissen procedure involves wrapping part of the fundus completely around the lower 4 to 6 cm of the esophagus and suturing it in place so that the gastroesophageal sphincter passes through a short tunnel of stomach. Postoperative CT findings simulate thickening of the posterior gastric wall *(arrows, A and B),* a discrete mass *(arrow, C),* and an abscess with gas *(arrows, D–F).*

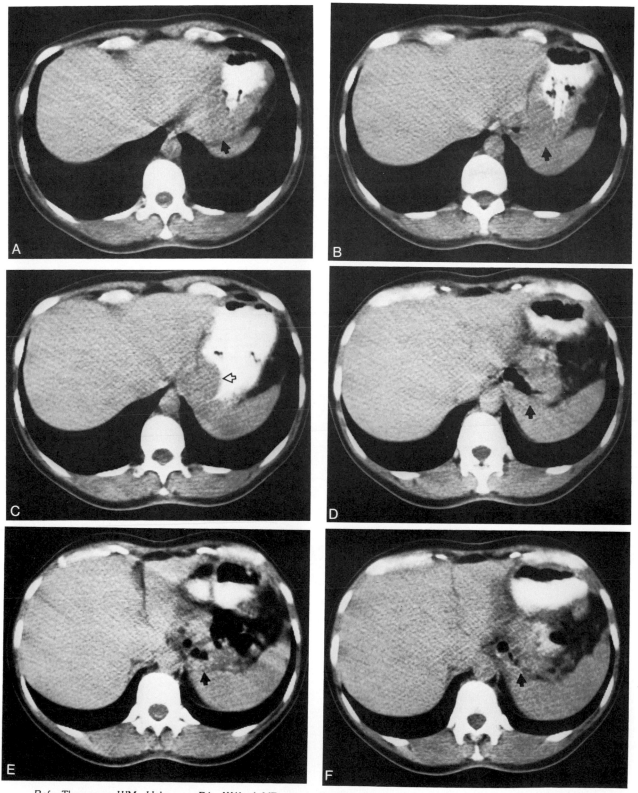

Ref.: Thompson WM, Halvorsen RA, Wilford ME, et al. Computed tomography of the gastroesophageal junction. Radiographics 1982; 2:179–193.

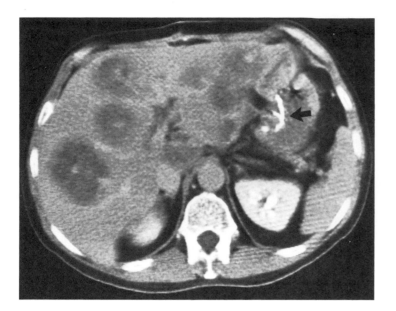

Figure 5–52. SURGICAL STAPLES. High-density surgical staples *(arrow)* are visible along the site of a gastric resection in a patient with recurrent gastric carcinoma and hepatic metastases. Note the low-density metastatic lesions in the liver (with central focus of high attenuation).

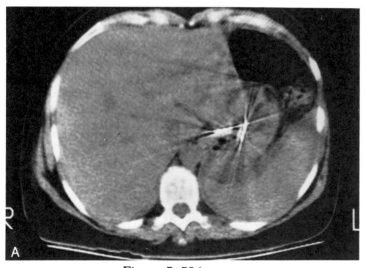

Figure 5–53A

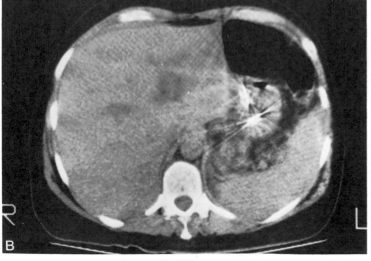

Figure 5–53B

Figure 5–53. PSEUDOCLIPS. The surgical clip–type artifacts demonstrated in *A–E* suggest a history of prior surgery. The high-density structures seen overlying the gastroesophageal junction *(A)* and the stomach *(B, 1 cm caudal)* can be identified as a nasogastric tube filled with a high concentration of oral contrast material, when the more cephalad images *(C–E)* are examined. These images demonstrate the same pseudoclip artifact caused by the nasogastric tube in the esophagus. Note the most cephalad abdominal slice *(E)*, which demonstrates normal breast tissue *(arrowheads)* in the chest wall.

Illustration continued on opposite page

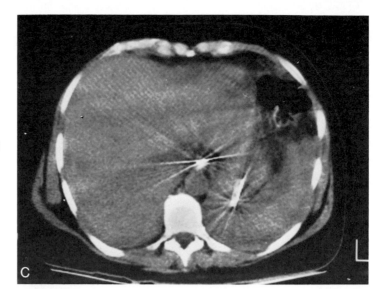

Figure 5–53C

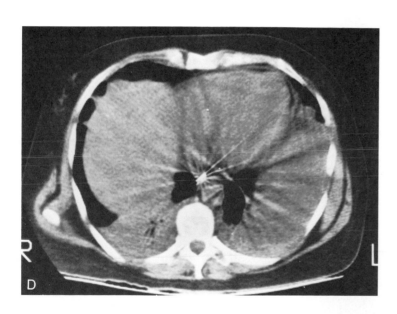

Figure 5–53D

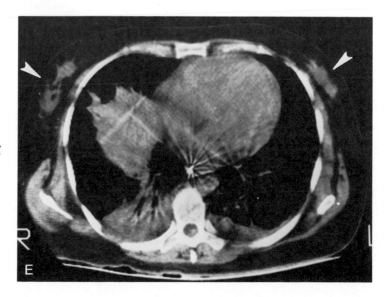

Figure 5–53E

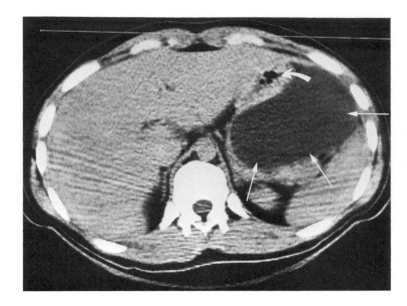

Figure 5–54. PANCREATIC PSEUDOCYST. Large lesser sac pancreatic pseudocyst *(straight arrows)* mimics a dilated, fluid-filled stomach. Note the collapsed stomach *(curved arrow)* anterior to the pseudocyst.

Figure 5–55. HIATAL HERNIA. Varying appearances of a hiatal hernia are shown on axial scans *(A–C)* through the upper abdomen.

Figure 5–55A. Hiatal hernia *(arrowheads)* might be mistaken for a thickened esophageal wall in this scan.

Illustration continued on opposite page

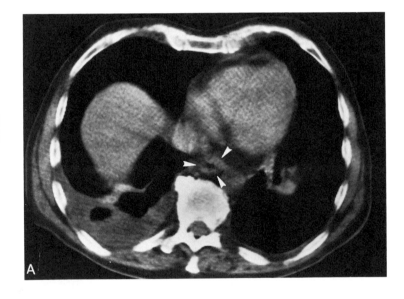

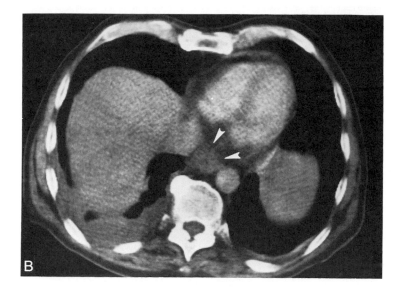

Figure 5–55B. Hiatal hernia mimics an esophageal mass *(arrowheads).*

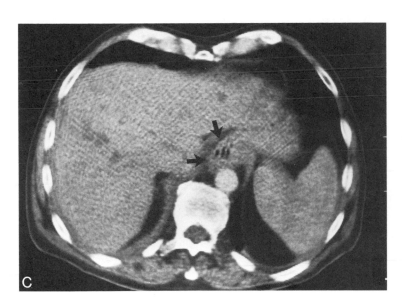

Figure 5–55C. Hiatal hernia simulates a gascontaining abscess *(arrows)* at the gastroesophageal junction.

Refs.: (1) Pupols A, Ruzicka FF. Hiatal hernia causing a cardiac pseudomass on computed tomography. JCAT 1984; 8:699–700. (2) Govoni AF, Whalen JP, Kazam E. Hiatal hernia: A relook. Radiographics 1983; 3:612–644.

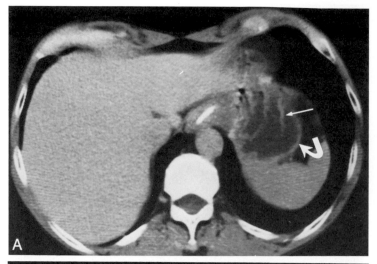

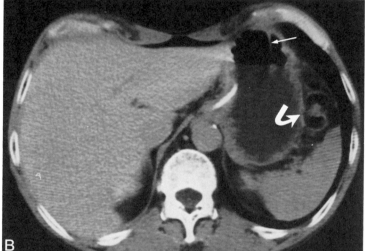

Figure 5–56. NORMAL GASTRIC FOLDS.
Normal gastric folds *(straight arrows, A–C)* are clearly visualized in the unopacified gastric fluid and air contained within the stomach; the gastric wall *(curved arrows, A–C)* can also be identified, due to an extrinsic fat plane and adjacent air-filled colon. Gastric air-fluid level is demonstrated *(B, C)*. Note the high-density nasogastric tube in each image.

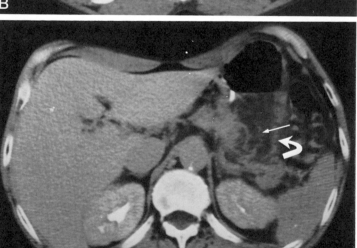

Ref.: Balfe DM, Koehler RE, Karstaedt N, et al. Computed tomography of gastric neoplasms. Radiology 1981; 140:431–436.

Figure 5–57. NASOGASTRIC TUBE. Nasogastric tubes may assume many different configurations on CT.

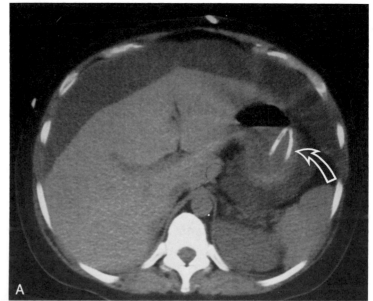

Figure 5–57A. In this patient with extensive ascites, a nasogastric tube *(arrow)* is turned back on itself within the stomach.

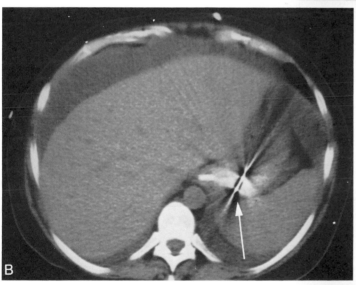

Figure 5–57B. In this more cephalad image, the mercury tip *(urrow)* of the nasogastric tube is demonstrated. Note the streak artifact caused by the mercury. A small amount of oral contrast material is present in the posterior fundus of the stomach.

Figure 5–58. CHILAIDITI'S SYNDROME. Two gas collections *(arrows)* anterior to the lateral segment of the left lobe of the liver were confirmed to be within bowel on adjacent images and should not be mistaken for an abscess collection or for extraluminal gas.

Ref.: Newmark H, Bierros R, Silberman EL, et al. A pitfall in the diagnosis of a subphrenic abscess seen on computed tomography. Comput Tomogr 1980; 40:155–157.

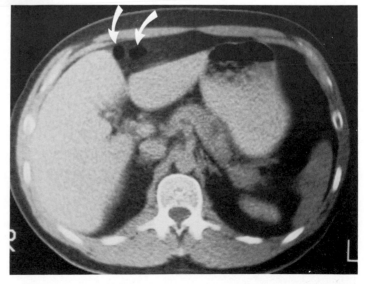

Figure 5–59. **PSEUDOABSCESS.**

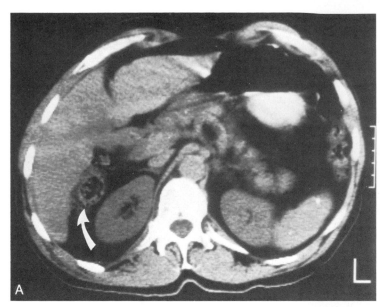

Figure 5–59A. An encapsulated, irregular gas collection *(arrow)* is demonstrated in the hepatorenal fossa in a patient who was thought to have an intra-abdominal abscess.

Figure 5–59B. This image, 1 cm caudal to *A,* identifies the "abscess" as bowel. Note the high-density intraluminal oral-contrast material; also note the pseudo-thickened wall of the contracted gallbladder *(arrow).*

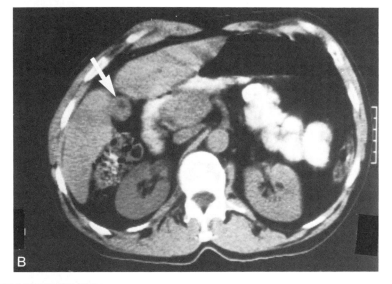

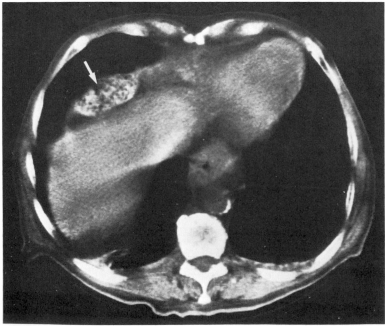

Figure 5–60. **OPACIFIED BOWEL.** Gastrografin within the superior aspect of the hepatic flexure *(arrow)* mimics a calcified liver mass.

Figure 5–61. PSEUDOBOWEL.

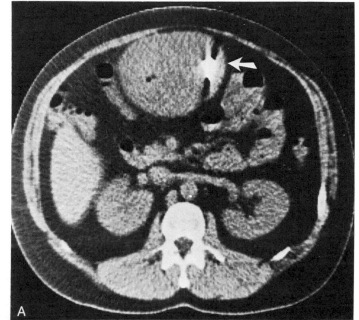

Figure 5–61A. This image demonstrates an abscess from a retained surgical sponge. The sponge has a high-density component *(arrow)* and should not be mistaken for contrast material within bowel.

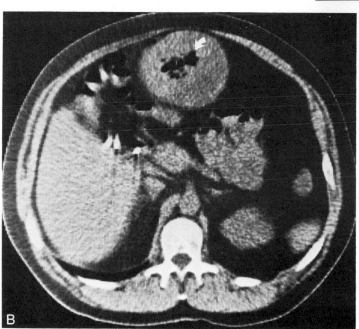

Figure 5–61B. A more cephalad image demonstrates the gas collection *(arrow)* of this abscess.

Ref.: Jeffrey RB, Goodman PC, Federle MP. CT of the lesser peritoneal sac. Radiology 1981; 141:117–122.

Figure 5–62. ILEOCECAL VALVE. The opacified terminal ileum *(straight arrow)* and cecum *(open arrow)* outline a fatty ileocecal valve.

Ref.: Cohen WN, Seidelmann FE, Bryan PJ. Computed tomography of localized adipose deposits presenting as tumor masses. AJR 1977; 128:1007–1011.

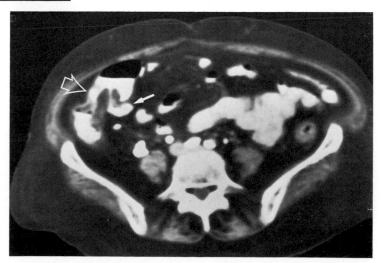

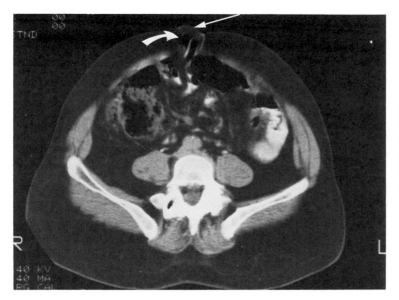

Figure 5–63. UMBILICAL HERNIA. An umbilical hernia is seen in the midline abdomen, where air-filled bowel *(curved arrow)* is seen to extend into the subcutaneous tissue with a slight bulge in the anterior abdominal wall *(straight arrow).*

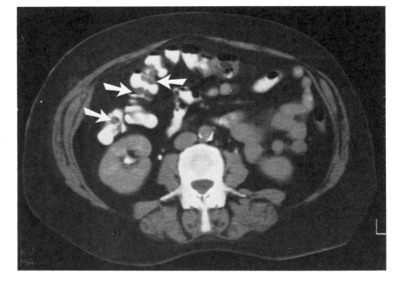

Figure 5–64. NORMAL COLON. Normal haustral markings *(arrows)* are demonstrated in this nondistended, partially opacified bowel.

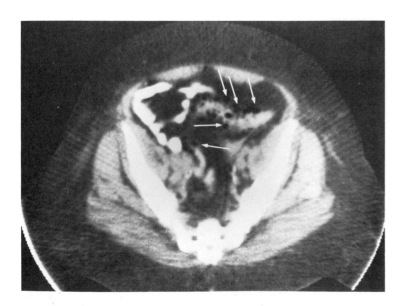

Figure 5–65. SIGMOID DIVERTICULOSIS. Multiple air-filled diverticula *(arrows)* are seen along the opacified sigmoid colon.

Figure 5–66. COLOSTOMY. The radiographic appearance of a normal well-healed colostomy (*white arrow, A, B,* and *C*) is presented in these three contiguous 1-cm images. *B* is at the level of the aortic bifurcation *(black arrows, B).*

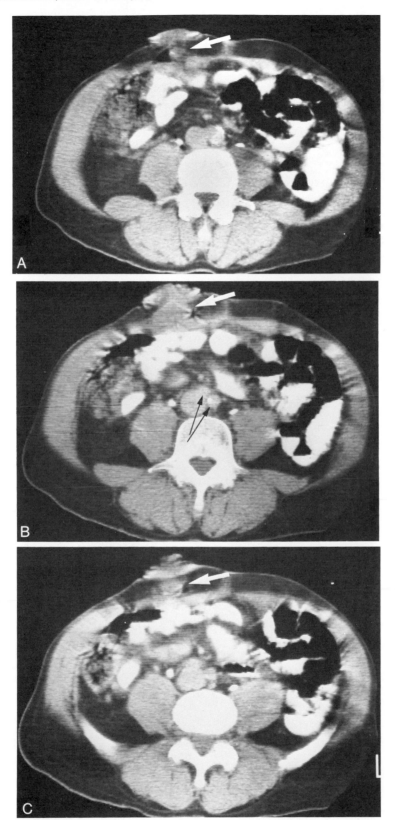

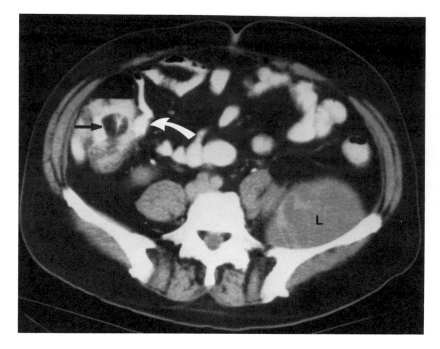

Figure 5–67. ILEOCECAL VALVE.
This image demonstrates a fatty ileocecal valve *(black arrow)*. Note the opacified terminal ileum *(white arrow)*. A leiomyosarcoma (L) is present in the left retroperitoneum.

Ref.: Scanlon MH, Blumberg ML, Ostrum BJ. Computed tomographic recognition of gastrointestinal pathology. Radiographics 1983; 3:201–227.

Figure 5–68. PSEUDOABSCESS.

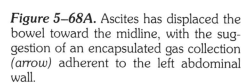

Figure 5–68A. Ascites has displaced the bowel toward the midline, with the suggestion of an encapsulated gas collection *(arrow)* adherent to the left abdominal wall.

Illustration continued on opposite page

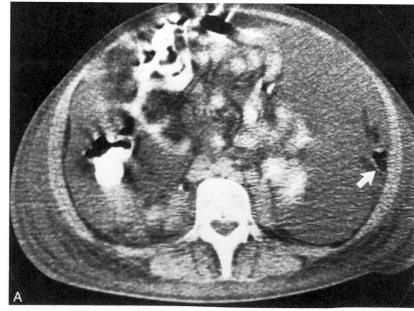

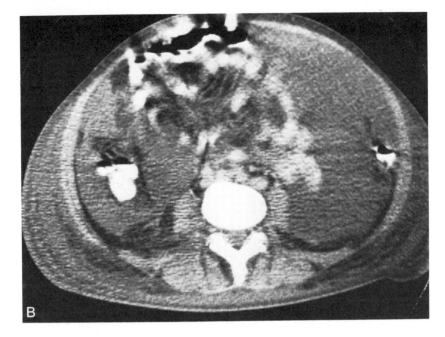

Figure 5–68B. An image 1 cm caudal to A shows this to be air and oral contrast material within a segment of bowel. More caudal images further confirmed this to be the descending colon.

Ref.: Marks WM, Goldberg HI, Moss AA, et al. Intestinal pseudotumors: A problem in abdominal computed tomography solved by directed techniques. Gastrointest Radiol 1980; 5:155–160.

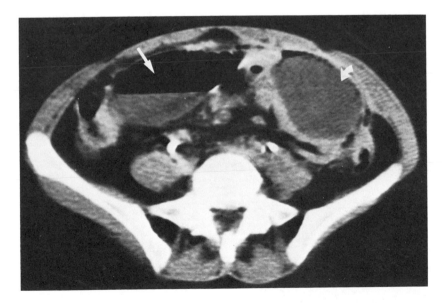

Figure 5–69. BOWEL VERSUS ABSCESS. An air-fluid level *(straight arrow)* in a segment of bowel loop mimics an abscess. A true abscess *(curved arrow)* is seen in the left pelvis and is demonstrated as a low-density collection that has an air-fluid level with a very small amount of air.

Figure 5–70. RETAINED SURGICAL SPONGE.

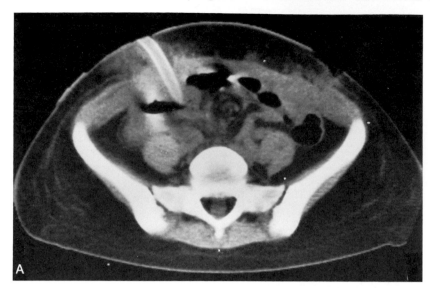

Figure 5–70A. This image demonstrates a percutaneous drainage tube placed at surgery four days prior to this CT study done for a postoperative "abscess search."

Figure 5–70B. Note the unusual appearance of the distal portion of the drainage tube, with an irregular high-density structure surrounding the tube.

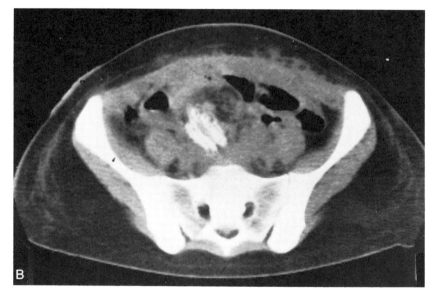

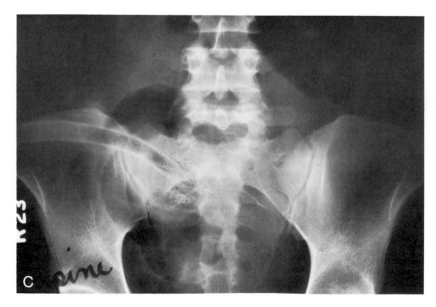

Figure 5–70C. A plain film of the abdomen showed that the structure was a retained surgical sponge. This was confirmed at surgery.

Illustration continued on opposite page

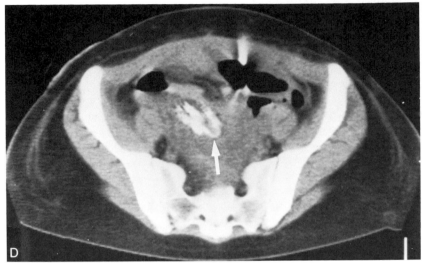

Figure 5–70D. This image shows the most distal tip of the tube *(arrow)*. Note the dissimilarity in the appearance of the tip and that of the surrounding sponge.

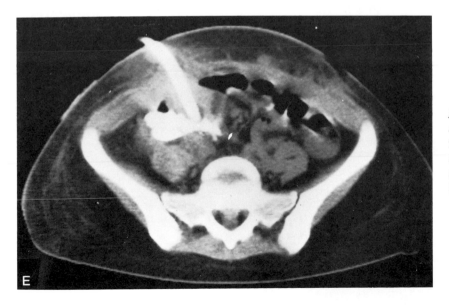

Figure 5–70E. This scan was made after iodinated contrast material was introduced into the drainage tube; it is seen to fill the abscess cavity and to abut a segment of opacified bowel (*see* Figure 5–76).

Figure 5–71. PSEUDOENTERIC FISTULA. These are scans of the same patient shown in Figure 5–70.

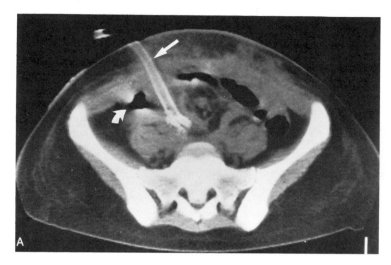

Figure 5–71A. This scan demonstrates a fluid-filled drainage tube *(straight arrow)* with slight opacification of adjacent bowel segments *(curved arrow)* by orally ingested contrast material. The high-density material abutting the tip of the drainage tube represents a retained surgical sponge (see Figure 5–70).

Figure 5–71B. This image is at the same level as A but was taken after contrast material was introduced into the drainage tube and abscess cavity. The increased opacification of the adjacent segment of bowel is due to the passage of time and to the distal propulsion of the orally ingested Gastrografin and should not be mistaken for communication with the abscess cavity.

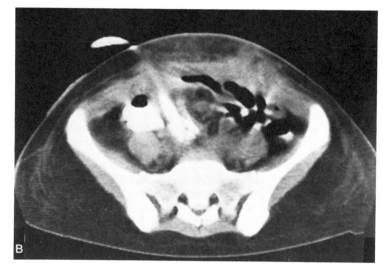

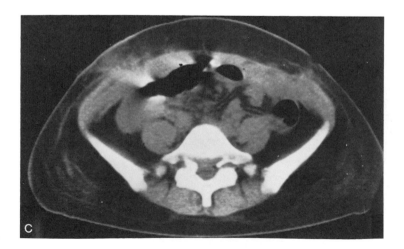

Figure 5–71C. This image, 1 cm cephalad to A, was obtained at the same time as A. Note the minimal opacification of bowel at this time.

Illustration continued on opposite page

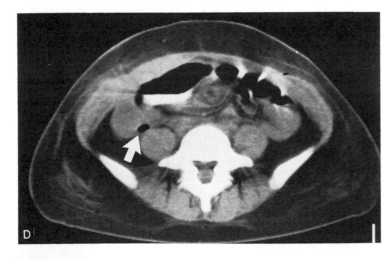

Figure 5–71D. This image was taken at the same level as *C*. The scan was obtained at the same time as *B* and confirms the more distal propulsion of the Gastrografin. The gas bubble *(arrow)* shown here was proved by contiguous images to be within the bowel and did not represent an abscess.

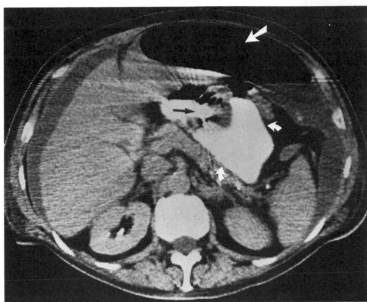

Figure 5–72. GASTRIC PERFORATION. A gastric ulcer has perforated into the lesser sac in this patient, resulting in extravasation of oral contrast material *(curved white arrows)*. The lesser sac is filled with contrast material and mimics an opacified bowel loop. Streaks from a nasogastric tube can be seen in the stomach *(black arrow)*. Note also the large hydropneumoperitoneum *(straight white arrow)* simulating an air-filled, dilated segment of colon.

Figure 5–73. SURGICAL STAPLES. Surgical staples are visible *(curved white arrow)* along the margin of a small bowel resection for Crohn's disease. They should not be mistaken for collecting of oral contrast material, even though there are no streak artifacts associated with them. Note the adjacent low-density postoperative abscess *(straight white arrows)*. Normal ileostomy findings are indicated *(large white arrow)*.

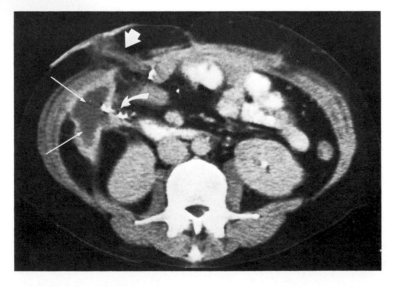

Figure 5–74. **FOLEY CATHETER FILLED WITH OPACIFIED URINE.** The destructive bony lesions *(A, B, C)* are metastatic deposits from prostatic carcinoma.

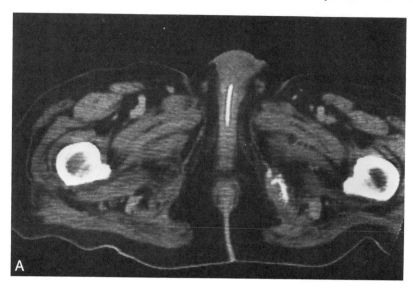

Figure 5–74A. The catheter is demonstrated in the penile urethra.

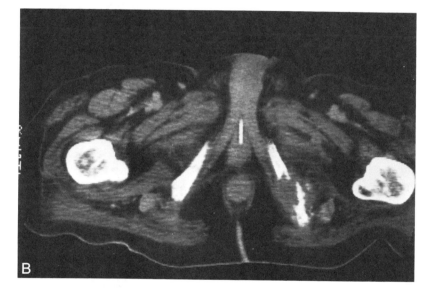

Figure 5–74B. A slightly more cephalad scan shows the catheter in the bulbar portion of the urethra.

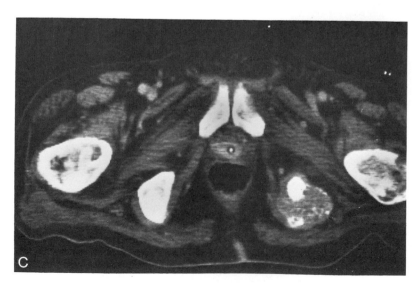

Figure 5–74C. In this image the catheter can be seen in the prostatic urethra.

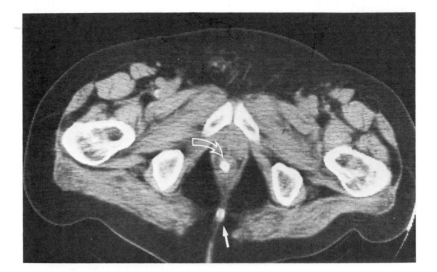

Figure 5–75. RECTAL TUBE. Central high-density structure *(curved arrow)* is a rectal tube filled with dilute Hypaque. The midline, posterior high-density structure *(straight arrow)* is the sacral tip.

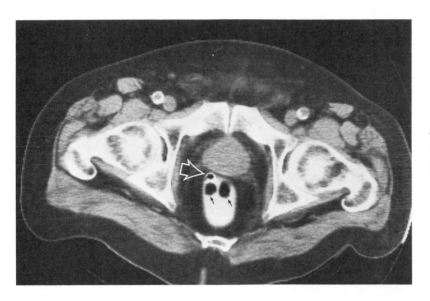

Figure 5–76. RECTAL TUBE. Scan demonstrates an air-filled rectal tube *(open arrows)* among the Hypaque and feces *(black arrows)* filling the rectum.

Figure 5–77. PSEUDOPERFORATION. Partial volume averaging of the curved rectosigmoid colon causes the rectal tube *(arrow)* to appear extraluminal.

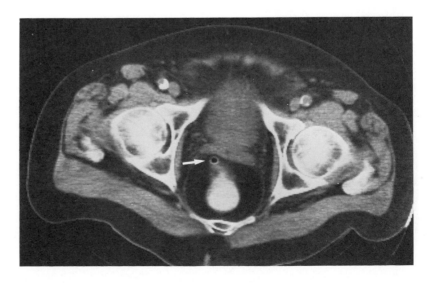

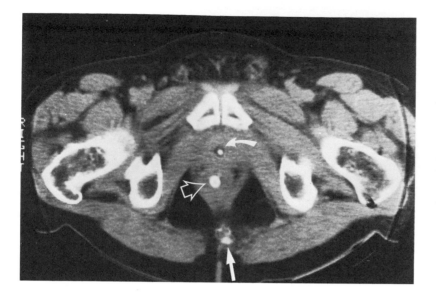

Figure 5–78. NORMAL PELVIS WITH TUBES. Midline high-density structures behind the symphysis pubis represent *(anterior to posterior)* a urine-opacified Foley catheter *(solid curved arrow)* in the prostatic urethra, a Hypaque-filled rectal tube *(open arrow)*, and the tip of the sacrum *(straight arrow)*.

Figure 5–79. PSEUDO–FOLEY CATHETER. The calcification seen in the prostate in both *A* and *B* should not be mistaken for a displaced urine-opacified Foley catheter. Note that the prostate is enlarged. This is not due to adenocarcinoma but to benign prostatic hypertrophy (with calcification). (See also Chapter 6, Figure 6–38.)

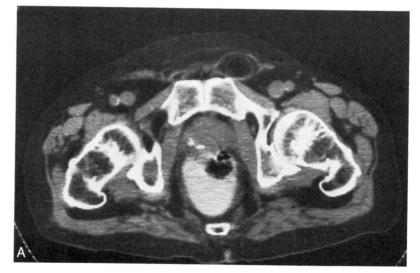

Figure 5–79A. Irregular, non–centrally positioned calcification is demonstrated.

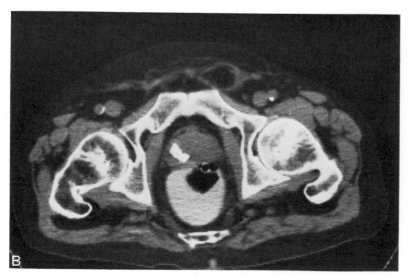

Figure 5–79B. In an image that is 1 cm more caudal than *A*, the calcification is more prominent.

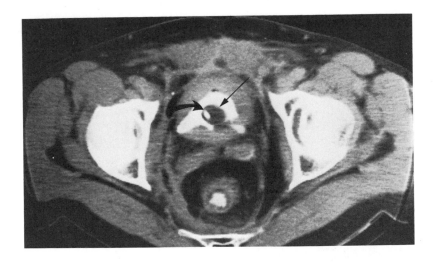

Figure 5–80. **PSEUDO–BLADDER MASS.** Unusual appearance of the urinary bladder is demonstrated in this patient who had hemorrhagic cystitis secondary to Cytoxan chemotherapy. The urine-opacified bladder is poorly distended, and there is thickening of the wall. The central low density *(straight arrow)* is not a mass within the bladder; it is the water-filled balloon of the Foley catheter, with opacified urine within the catheter lumen *(curved arrow).* (See also Chapter 6, Figure 6–36.)

Figure 5–81. **PSEUDO–ENTEROVESICAL FISTULA.** The water-filled balloon of this Foley catheter should not be mistaken for a lesion within the urine-opacified bladder. Note the opacified urine within the catheter lumen *(black arrow)* in both *A* and *B*. Irregularity of the posterior bladder wall was caused by a transitional cell carcinoma.

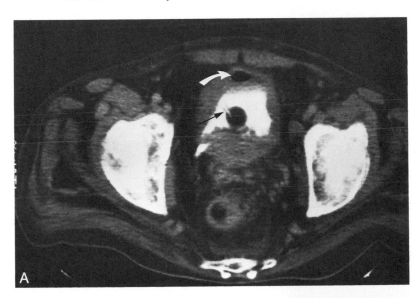

Figure 5–81A. Air *(curved white arrow)* within the bladder, introduced via the catheterization, should not be interpreted as evidence of an enterovesical fistula.

Figure 5–81B. The typical appearance of a Foley catheter is again shown. Note that it appears to be lower in density than the adjacent mass.

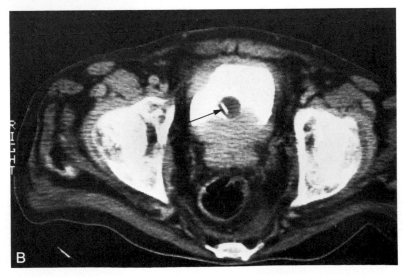

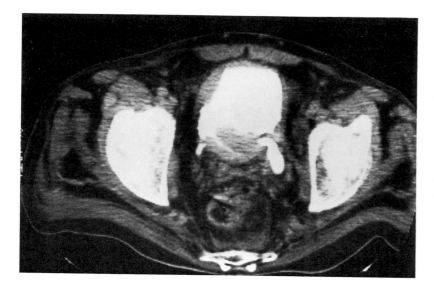

Figure 5–82. PSEUDOEXTRAVASA-TION. Pseudoextravasation of opacified urine is demonstrated in this image of the same patient seen in Figure 5–67. Tumor infiltration of the posterior bladder wall causes partial obstruction of the ureters, which is more evident on the left than the right. (See also Chapter 6, pp. 208–210.)

Figure 5–83. BRICKER CONDUIT. A Bricker conduit and ileostomy are demonstrated in a patient who had undergone a cystectomy for a transitional cell carcinoma. The right ureter *(straight arrow, A, B, and C)* and left ureter *(curved arrow, A and B)* are seen to lead into the opacified segment of ileum *(open arrow, A–D)* before it exits the right anterior abdominal wall at the site of the ileostomy *(solid arrow in C).*

Illustration continued on opposite page

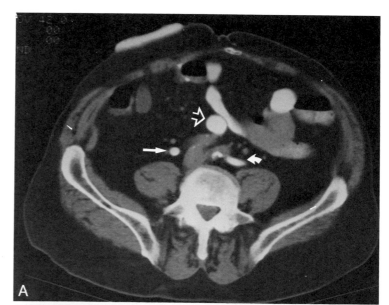

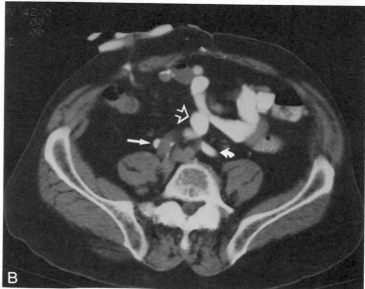

Figure 5–83 A and B

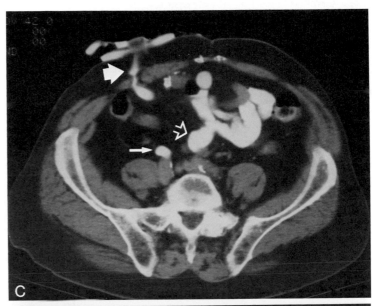

Figure 5–83 C and D

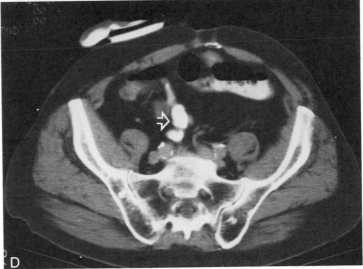

Figure 5–84. PROSTATE.

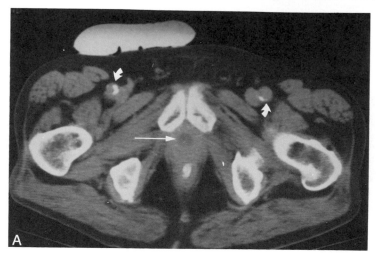

Figure 5–84A. An image of the pelvis demonstrates a post–prostatic urethrotomy defect as a round, hypodense area *(straight arrow)* within the prostate. Note also the calcification of the femoral arteries *(curved arrows)*, clearly seen on this wider window image (500 HU). (See also Chapter 6, Figure 6–38.)

Figure 5–84B. In this narrower window image (250 HU), note the enhanced tissue contrast and increased visibility of the urethrotomy defect *(arrow)*.

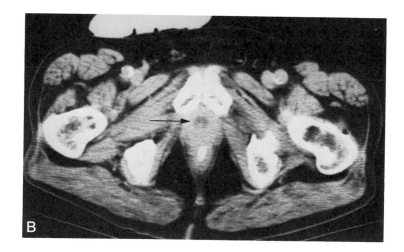

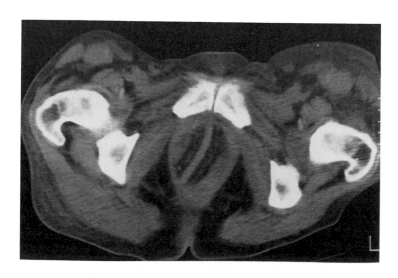

Figure 5–85. NEOVAGINA. A neovagina is demonstrated in this patient who had undergone pelvic exenteration for an extensive malignancy and subsequently underwent reconstructive surgery.

Figure 5–86. URETEROSTOMY.

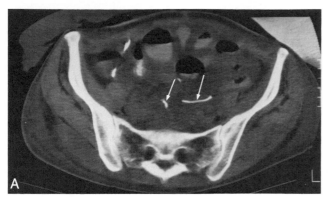

Figure 5–86A. Ureterostomy stents are demonstrated in the left and right ureters *(arrows)*.

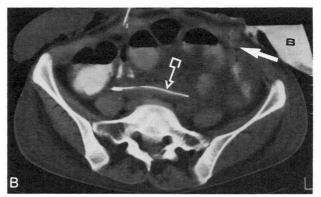

Figure 5–86B. The left stent extends across the midline *(boxed open arrow)*. Note the colostomy *(closed arrow)* and the opacified ostomy bag (B).

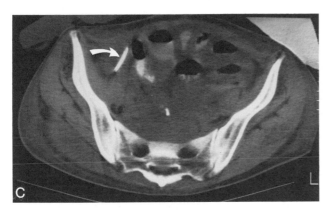

Figure 5–86C. The left stent approaches *(arrow)* the right anterior abdominal wall in this image.

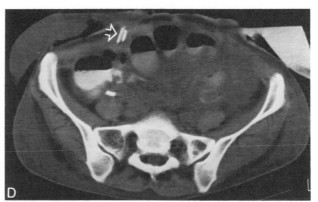

Figure 5–86D. In this scan, the left stent *(arrow)* passes through the anterior right abdominal wall.

Genitourinary System and Retroperitoneum

ROBERT K. ZEMAN, M.D.
ARTHUR T. ROSENFIELD, M.D.

Figure 6–1. ORGAN MOTION SECONDARY TO RESPIRATION. Three sequential scans through the abdomen after the injection of intravenous contrast medium are presented in a patient with chronic lymphatic leukemia who has had a splenectomy and who is known to have ascites and left perinephric fluid.

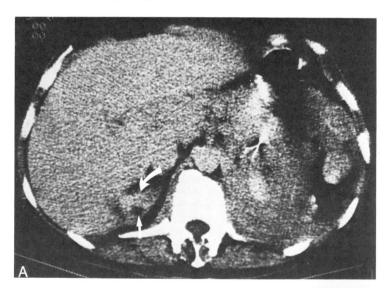

Figure 6–1A. On the initial scan there is an apparent right adrenal mass *(curved arrow)* with a low density center *(straight arrow).*

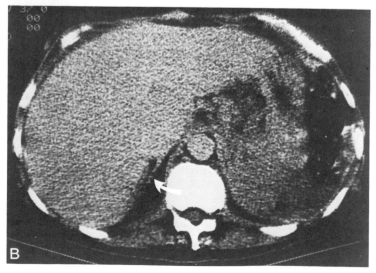

Figure 6–1B. This scan, obtained 1 cm below A, shows a normal right adrenal *(curved arrow).*

Illustration continued on opposite page

Figure 6–1C. The final scan, obtained 2 cm below A, shows a cyst in an otherwise normal right kidney. However, A and C are at virtually identical levels. The impression of a right suprarenal mass was created by respiratory motion. Failure to obtain scans with the same degree of inspiration or expiration is a potential pitfall in all abdominal CT imaging.

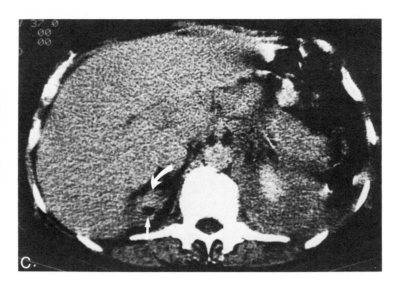

Figure 6–2. NORMAL RENAL VEIN/RENAL SINUS LIPOMATOSIS/RENAL CYST.

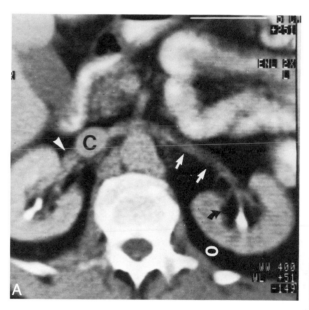

Figure 6–2A. Scan through the mid-abdomen following intravenous injection of urographic contrast medium clearly demonstrates the right renal vein *(arrowhead)* and left renal vein *(white arrows)* converging on the inferior vena cava (C). Although the renal veins often lie at different levels, they may occasionally be seen on a single section. Also note the abundant renal sinus lipomatosis on the left *(curved black arrow)*. The infundibula are being draped by tissue of characteristic fat density; compare with retroperitoneum *(circle)*.

Figure 6–2B. Scan in another patient demonstrates slight narrowing of the left renal vein *(arrowhead)* as it "squeezes" between the aorta (A) and the mesenteric vessels (artery, *straight arrow;* vein, *curved arrow*). This is a common variant. Incidentally noted is a large renal cyst (C), characterized by homogeneous water density, smooth margins, well-defined "claws," and a barely perceptible thin wall. (See also Chapter 5, Figure 5–4, for examples of normal renal vessels.)

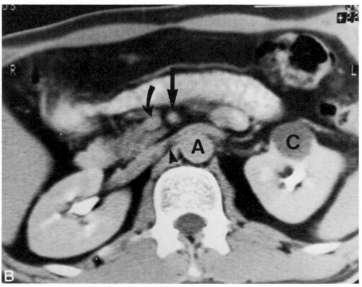

Ref.: Buschi AJ, Harrison RB, Brenbridge AG, et al. Distended left renal vein: CT/sonographic normal variant. AJR 1980; 135:339–342.

Figure 6–3. NORMAL RENAL ARTERY AND VEIN/SEPTUM OF BERTIN.

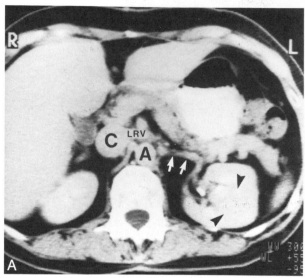

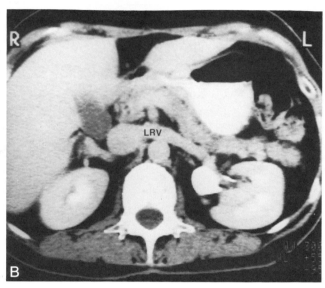

Figure 6–3A. The left renal artery *(arrows)* is unusually well seen in this patient. It is uncommon to see both the proximal and distal arteries on a single section. The left renal vein (LRV), inferior vena cava (C), and aorta (A) are also identified. Incidentally noted is a left septum of Bertin *(arrowheads)*. This should not be mistaken for a renal mass (see Figure 6–12).

Figure 6–3B. The left renal vein (LRV) is more clearly seen on this slightly more caudad section.

Figure 6–4. CIRCUMAORTIC RENAL VEIN. The presence of a circumaortic renal vein has been reported in 7 per cent of autopsy specimens. It is slightly more common than a single isolated retroaortic renal vein. During early embryonic life, the subcardinal and supracardinal veins are connected via a renovascular collar. The dorsal (retroaortic) component usually atrophies, but if it fails to do so, the circumaortic renal venous drainage persists into adult life. It is an important anomaly to recognize, as the anomalous veins may be injured in many types of abdominal surgery including aortic bypass, nephrectomy, shunt creation for relief of portal hypertension, and caval interruption procedures.

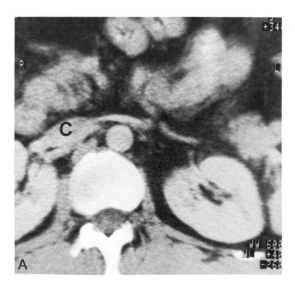

Figure 6–4A. Computed tomography during infusion of intravenous contrast medium demonstrates the left renal vein *(arrow)* in its usual position, passing in front of the aorta to enter the inferior vena cava (C).

Illustration continued on opposite page

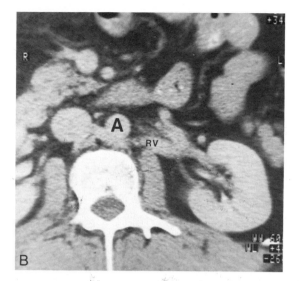

Figure 6–4B. In this scan 1 cm lower than *A,* a second left renal vein (RV) is seen passing behind the aorta (A).

Refs.: (1) Reed MD, Friedman AC, Nealey P. Anomalies of the left renal vein: Analysis of 433 CT scans. J Comput Assist Tomogr 1982; 6:1124–26. (2) Parikh SJ, Peters JC, Kihm RH. The anomalous left renal vein: CT appearance and clinical implications. CT 1981; 5:529–533.

Figure 6–5. PELVIC KIDNEY. CT scan following oral and intravenous administration of contrast medium demonstrates a transversely oriented kidney (K) just below the level of the iliac crests. The right kidney was present in its normal position on other sections. Ectopic kidneys should be distinguished from the ptotic kidney. The former has never been located in its proper anatomic position, has a short (or long) ureter, and has a vascular supply arising from nearby vessels. The arterial supply of a pelvic kidney is from the distal aorta or iliac arteries. These anomalies are important to recognize because of their predisposition to hydronephrosis and calculi formation. (Case courtesy of Peter Choyke, M.D., Washington, D.C.)

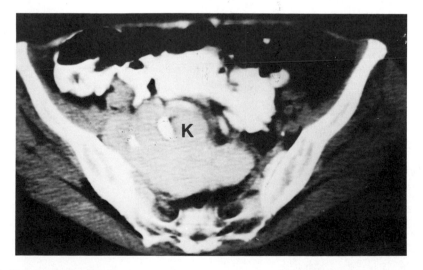

Ref.: Cretler SP, Olsson C, Pfister RC. The anatomic, radiologic and clinical characteristics of the pelvic kidney. An analysis of 86 cases. J Urol 1971; 105:623–627.

*Figure 6–6. **THORACIC KIDNEY.*** A thoracic kidney is situated so that it protrudes through the foramen of Bochdalek, which is essentially a posterior diaphragmatic defect due to failure of the pleuroperitoneal canal to close. Thoracic kidneys are more common on the left than on the right and can be readily identified on computed tomography, frequently without the use of intravenous contrast medium as in this case. Identification of a kidney behind the right hemidiaphragm and extending above it is characteristic.

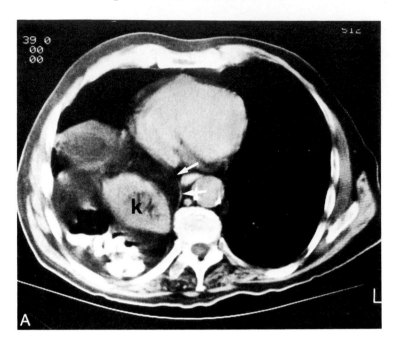

Figure 6–6A. Computed tomography of a chest mass was performed without intravenous contrast medium. This scan through the lower chest demonstrates a kidney (k) above the right hemidiaphragm *(arrows)* Note also the bowel above the right hemidiaphragm.

Figure 6–6B. A scan 2 cm lower demonstrates a staghorn calculus within the right kidney (k). Note the posterior right hemidiaphragm *(straight arrows)* anterior to the kidney, the liver (L) anterior to this structure, and the anterior portion of the right hemidiaphragm *(curved arrows).* The heart (h) is also identified. Note that, as in *A,* bowel can be seen above the right hemidiaphragm.

Illustration continued on opposite page

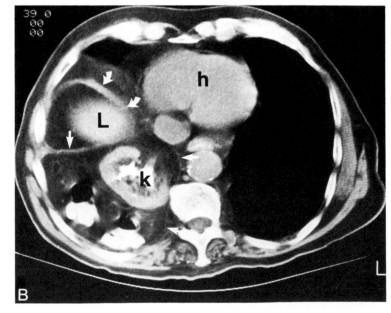

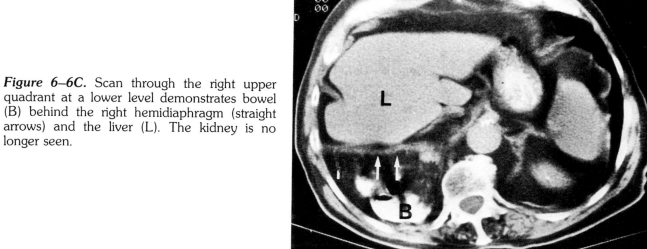

Figure 6–6C. Scan through the right upper quadrant at a lower level demonstrates bowel (B) behind the right hemidiaphragm (straight arrows) and the liver (L). The kidney is no longer seen.

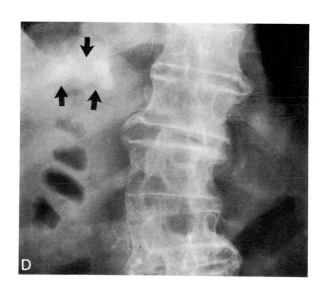

Figure 6–6D. Plain film of the abdomen demonstrates a calcification *(arrows)* high in the right upper quadrant representing the staghorn calculus.

Figure 6–6E. Urography, which was subsequently performed, demonstrates the thoracic kidney.

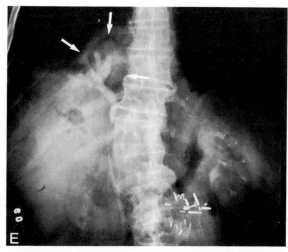

Figure 6–7. HORSESHOE KIDNEY. Horseshoe kidney is a congenital anomaly that is usually an incidental finding. Symptoms may result when the pelves, which cross the kidney anterior, become partially obstructed, thus leading to stasis, stone formation, and infection. Fractures of the isthmus following trauma can also occur. Computed tomography is a rapid way to make the diagnosis of horseshoe kidney. The diagnosis may be missed sonographically because bowel anteriorly and the spine posteriorly can attenuate the beam and obscure the isthmus. If urographic contrast medium is not used, a horseshoe kidney can occasionally be mistaken for extensive adenopathy. It may also be missed on urography and radioisotope scanning if the isthmus does not contain functioning tissue.

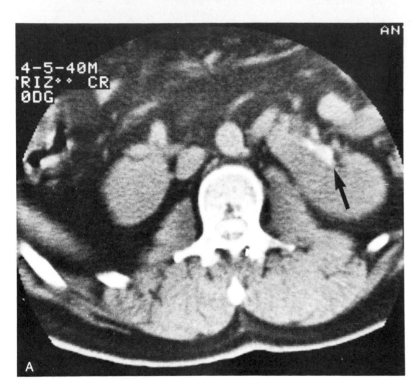

Figure 6–7A. This CT scan of the spine was performed following myelography with water-soluble contrast medium. Incidentally noted were reniform structures in both renal fossae. Note that the pelvis of the left kidney is seen and faces anteriorly (*arrow*) rather than medially.

Illustration continued on opposite page

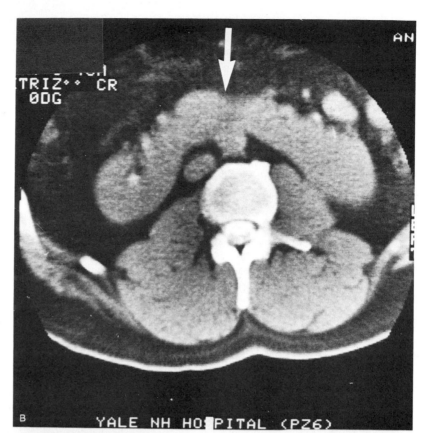

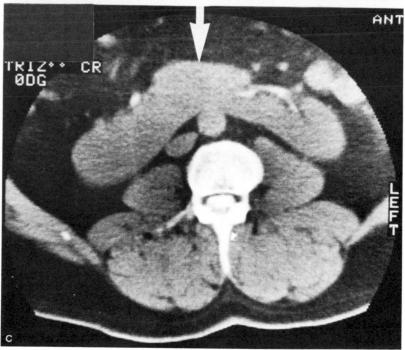

Figure 6–7B and C. Sections taken at the midportion *(B)* and lower portion *(C)* of the kidneys. Anterior pelves bilaterally are appreciated as is an isthmus *(arrows)* between them. These findings are characteristic of horseshoe kidney.

Ref.: Glenn JF. Analysis of 51 patients with horseshoe kidney. N Engl J Med 1959; 261:686–687.

Figure 6–8. CROSSED FUSED RENAL ECTOPIA. Renal ectopia occurs in 1 of 4000 autopsy cases. The fused form is more common than unfused. The lower kidney is usually the one that is ectopic and crossed.

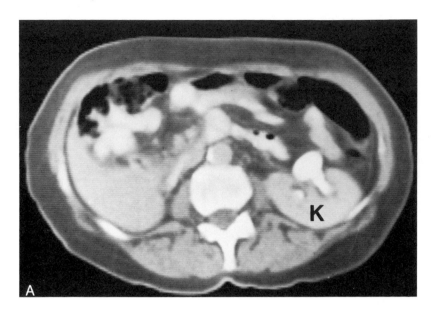

Figure 6–8A. In this CT scan following administration of oral and intravenous contrast material there is no evidence of a right kidney. The left kidney (K) is malrotated.

Figure 6–8B. At a slightly lower level a second kidney (K) was identified with its own collecting system. There was no perceptible separation between the parenchyma of each kidney.

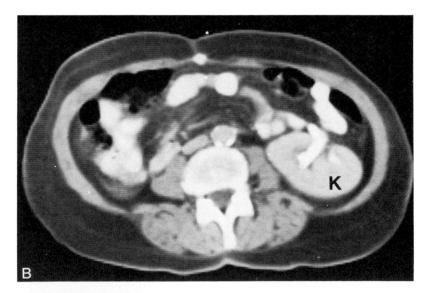

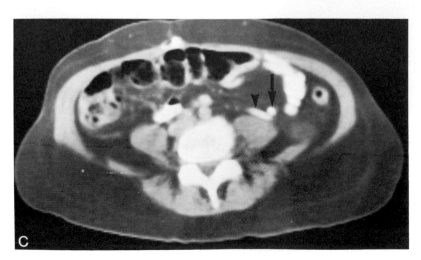

Figure 6–8C. Further caudad, the left ureter *(arrow)* is seen progressing inferiorly, and the ureter from the ectopic right kidney *(arrowhead)* is beginning to cross to the right side of the abdomen.

Illustration continued on opposite page

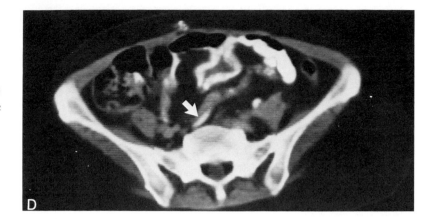

Figure 6–8D. The right ureter *(arrow)* continues to pass to the right side of the abdomen.

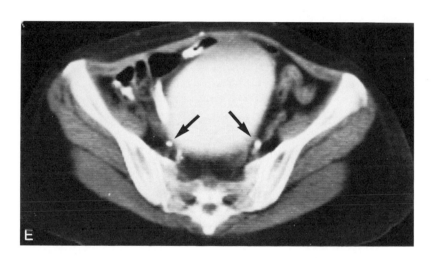

Figure 6–8E. At the level of the bladder, both ureters *(arrows)* are seen in their normal position about to enter each hemitrigone normally.

Figure 6–8F. Excretory urogram illustrates the typical appearance of crossed fused renal ectopia.

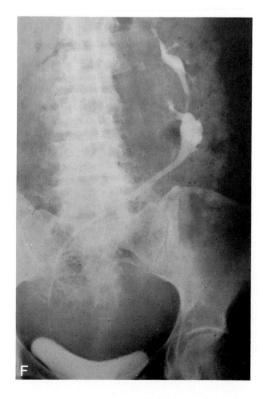

Figure 6–9. **CROSSED UNFUSED RENAL ECTOPIA.** Crossed renal ectopia is a congenital abnormality in which one kidney is crossed to the other side. The kidney may be fused or unfused. If one is not alert to this possibility, it may cause confusion, particularly if the CT scan has been performed without intravenous contrast medium. Both kidneys are on the same side of the abdomen but the ureters always enter normally, with one ureter in each hemitrigone.

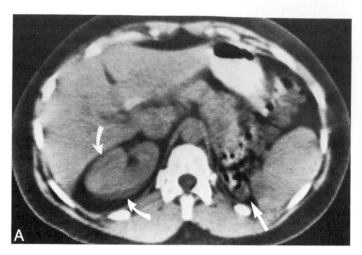

Figure 6–9A. Non–contrast-enhanced scan through the renal fossae demonstrates a normal right kidney in the right renal fossa *(curved arrows)*. The anatomic splenic flexure occupies the left renal fossa *(straight arrow)*.

Figure 6–9B. CT scan through the lower pelvis demonstrates the second kidney in the right lower quadrant *(curved arrows).*

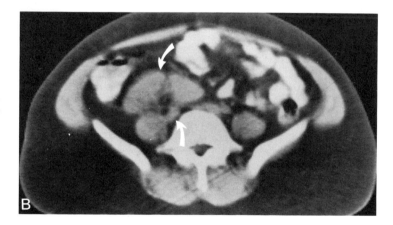

Refs.: (1) Marshall F, Freedman M. Crossed renal ectopia. J Urol 1978; 119:188–191. (2) Myers MA, Whalen JP, Evans JA. Malposition and displacement of bowel in renal agenesis and ectopia: New observations. AJR 1973; 117:323.

Figure 6–10. **DUPLICATED COLLECTING SYSTEM.** A duplicated collecting system is a common anatomic variant. The upper pole moiety is frequently obstructed. When nonfunctioning, the upper pole system may be mistaken for a cystic mass. The identification of the two ureters should prove diagnostic. In addition, the upper pole system frequently exits anteriorly while the lower pole system exits medially, as noted in *D*.

In utero, the kidney is formed from two renunculi. It is common for the upper renunculus to have its renal sinus facing anteriorly and the lower renunculus to have the sinus exiting posteromedially. In the kidney without a duplicated collecting system, a renal vein typically enters the anterior, upper renal sinus while the pelvis exits through the lower, posteromedial renal sinus. When a duplicated system is present, the upper renal collecting system frequently exits anteriorly, as in *B*.

Illustration on opposite page

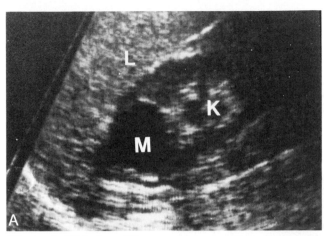

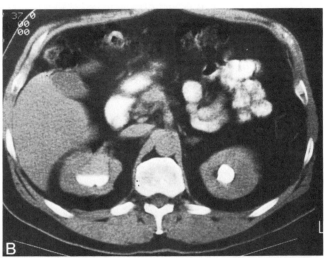

Figure 6–10A. In a 22-year-old man with a duplicated collecting system, sonography demonstrates a fluid-filled mass (M) in the upper pole of the right kidney. The liver (L) and kidney (K) are also identified.

Figure 6–10B. CT scan through the upper portion of the kidneys demonstrates a mildly dilated collecting system on the right. Note contrast-filled urine in the dependent portion of the upper pole system and the upper pole pelvis exiting anteriorly.

Figure 6–10C. In this CT scan through the un-opacified mid-portion of the right renal hilum, a dilated ureter *(arrow)* extending from the upper pole collecting system is seen anterior to a contrast-filled, mildly distended lower pole collecting system.

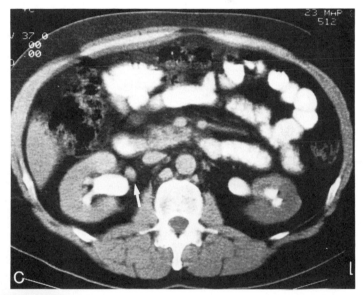

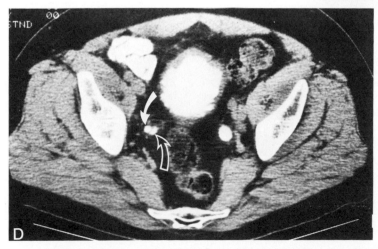

Figure 6–10D. CT scan through the bony pelvis demonstrates a mildly full ureter on the left and two ureters on the right. Some contrast medium now has made its way into the right upper pole ureter *(solid arrow)*. Note also the trabeculated hypertrophied bladder in this patient with a neurogenic bladder. The lower pole ureter is also identified *(open arrow)*.

Refs.: (1) Hartman GW, Hodson CJ. The duplex kidney and related abnormalities. Clin Radiol 1969; 20:387–400. (2) Lindner A, Hertz M, et al. Duplication of the kidney: A potential diagnostic pitfall. Urol Radiol 1981; 3:91–96.

Figure 6–11. "CLASSICAL" SIMPLE RENAL CYST AND NORMAL GEROTA'S FASCIA.

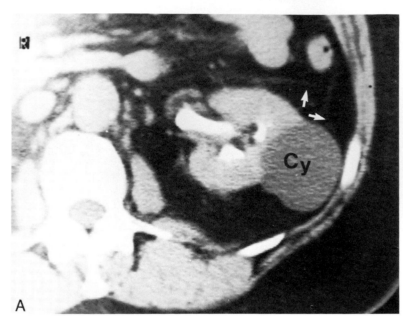

Figure 6–11A. CT scan following administration of oral and intravenous contrast medium demonstrates a large, "classical" renal cyst (Cy) of the lateral left kidney. Note its smooth walls, homogeneous water-density consistency, and sharp "claws." Lesions such as this are a common incidental finding on CT and merit no additional evaluation. This case also nicely illustrates draping of Gerota's fascia *(arrows)* over the cyst.

Figure 6–11B. At a slightly lower level, Gerota's fascia is again clearly seen *(arrow)*. On high-quality CT scans normal Gerota's fascia is often seen. It is usually no more than 1 to 2 mm in thickness. Scattered densities may be seen within the perirenal fat and may represent small lymph nodes or vessels. When multiple perirenal densities are present in association with thickening of Gerota's fascia, pathologic processes such as renal inflammation (acute focal bacterial nephritis or abscess), lymphoma, and pancreatitis must be considered. Collateral vessels secondary to renal vein thrombosis may also be seen in the perirenal fat.

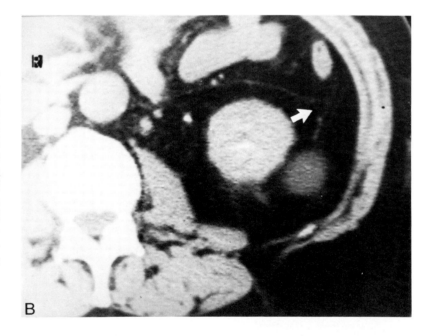

Refs.: (1) Feuerstein, I, Zeman RK, Jaffe MH, et al. Perirenal cobwebs: The expanding CT differential diagnosis. J Comput Assist Tomogr 1984; 8:1128–1130. (2) Zeman RK, Cronan JJ, Viscomi GN, Rosenfield AT. Coordinated imaging in the detection and characterization of renal masses. CRC Crit Rev Diagn Imaging 1981; 15:273–318. (3) McClennan BL, Stanley RJ, Nelson GL. CT for the renal cyst: Is cyst aspiration necessary? AJR 1979; 133:671–675. (4) Parienty RA, Pradel J, Picard J, et al. Visibility and thickening of the renal fascia on computed tomograms. Radiology 1981; 139:119–124.

Figure 6–12. "CLASSICAL" RENAL CELL CARCINOMA.

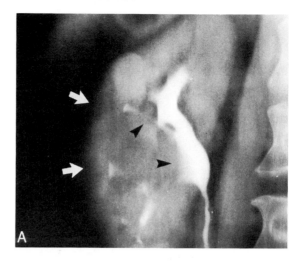

Figure 6–12A. A radiograph of the right kidney obtained during excretory urography demonstrates a large mass *(arrows)* splaying calyces and impinging on the lateral renal pelvis *(arrowheads).*

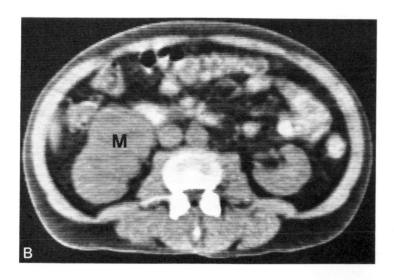

Figure 6–12B. Oral contrast–enhanced CT scan demonstrates the presence of a large soft-tissue mass (M) arising from the anterior margin of the kidney. Even without urographic contrast material it is apparent that this mass is solid and most likely represents a renal cell carcinoma.

Figure 6–12C. Following administration of intravenous contrast medium, the mass is clearly seen impinging on the renal pelvis *(arrowheads).* The mass is surprisingly well defined, with a sharp "claw," but should not be mistaken for a renal cyst because it is neither homogeneous nor of water density. There is no evidence of adenopathy, and at other levels the renal vein was normal. In staging renal cell carcinoma it is important to carefully examine adjacent structures.

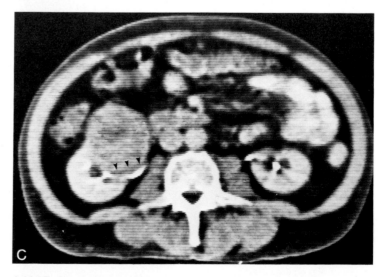

From: (1) Zeman RK, Cronan JJ, Viscomi GN, Rosenfield AT. Coordinated imaging in the detection and characterization of renal masses. CRC Crit Rev Diagn Imaging 1981; 15:273–318. Copyright, CRC Press, Inc., Boca Raton, FL. Reprinted with permission.

Ref.: Cronan JJ, Zeman RK, Rosenfield AT. Comparison of computerized tomography, ultrasound, and angiography in staging renal cell carcinoma. J Urol 1982; 127:712–714.

Figure 6–13. "PSEUDOTUMOR" OF THE KIDNEY.

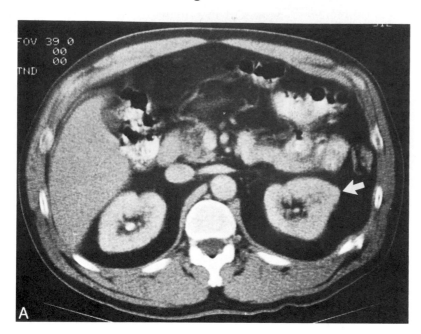

Figure 6–13A. A CT scan obtained immediately following injection of a bolus of contrast medium demonstrates an apparent mass *(arrow)* in the anterolateral aspect of the left kidney (which was read as an abnormal mass on a noncontrast CT study at another institution). This mass has normal nephrogram density.

Figure 6–13B. This scan was made at the same level as in *A* 5 minutes after the injection of contrast medium. Note that there is a calyx *(arrow)* extending into the region of the mass and that the parenchymal thickness is actually normal. A variety of pseudotumors due either to normal variation or to regenerative tissue after an insult to adjacent areas of parenchyma can mimic a mass. By demonstrating normal functioning of tissue, CT can verify that these areas are normal.

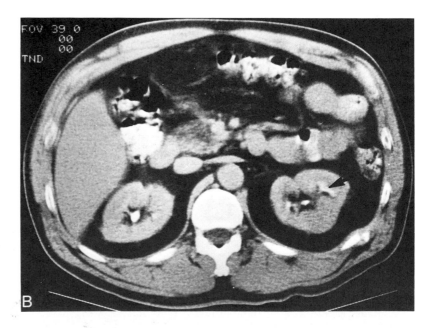

Ref.: Baert AL, Wilms G, Marchal G. Contrast enhancement by bolus technique in the CT examination of the kidney. Radiologe 1980; 20:279–287.

Figure 6–14. RENAL HILAR LIP.

Figure 6–14A. CT scan following administration of oral and intravenous contrast medium in this patient with widely metastatic carcinoma demonstrates a mass (M) medial to the left kidney (K). This mass seems to be of the same density as renal parenchyma. The shape and location is characteristic of a renal hilar-lip pseudotumor. This type of pseudotumor may appear as a focal renal bulge on the medial aspect of the kidney or as an almost completely separate island of renal parenchyma. It is virtually always the upper pole hilar lip that is the cause of difficulty. It results from a fatty cleft extending up into the renal hilum medial to the upper pole infundibulum. Also noted are multiple liver metastases and clip artifacts.

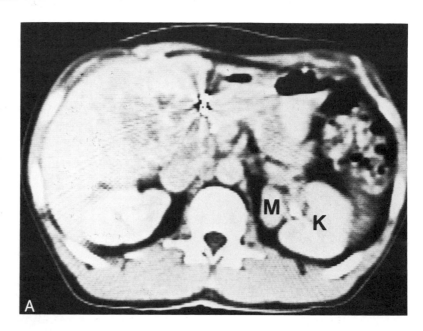

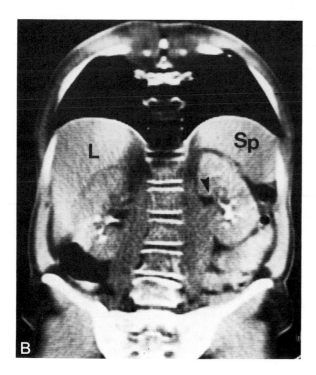

Figure 6–14B. Direct coronal CT or coronal reformatting is helpful in confirming the nature of hilar lip lesions. The fatty cleft *(arrowhead)* is invariably seen and readily explains the axial findings. The spleen (S) and liver (L) are also identified.

Refs.: (1) Zeman RK, Cronan JJ, Viscomi GN, Rosenfield AT. Coordinated imaging in the detection and characterization of renal masses. CRC Crit Rev Diagn Imaging 1981; 15:273–318. (2) Kolbenstuedt A, Lien HH. Isolated renal hilar lip on computed tomography. Radiology 1982; 143:150. (3) Thornbury JR, McCormick TL, Silver TM. Anatomic/radiologic classification of renal cortical nodules. AJR 1980; 134:1–7.

Figure 6–15. BOWEL MIMICKING RENAL MASS.

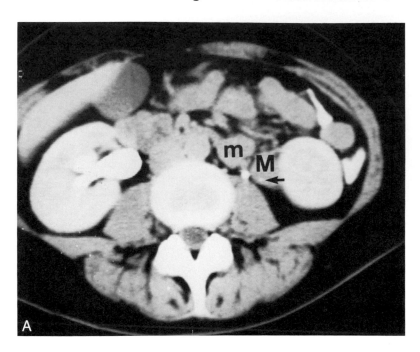

Figure 6–15A. CT scan following administration of oral and intravenous contrast medium demonstrates a soft-tissue mass (M) medial to the kidney with a second "mass" (m) in the para-aortic region. These densities could easily be mistaken for adenopathy or a renal mass with metastatic spread. The presence of a small amount of oral contrast agent *(arrow)* in these so-called masses aids in identifying them as bowel.

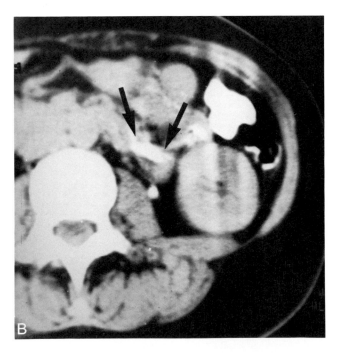

Figure 6–15B. In additional sections obtained several minutes later, the previously seen "masses" *(arrows)* have filled with contrast medium and clearly represent bowel. Giving additional oral contrast agent and bringing the patient back later in the day in addition to reformatting the images can aid in resolving problems such as this.

Ref.: Marincek B, Young SW, Castellino RA. A CT scanning approach to the evaluation of left paraaortic pseudotumor. J Comput Assist Tomogr 1981; 5:723–727.

Figure 6–16. ACCESSORY SPLEEN MIMICKING RENAL MASS.

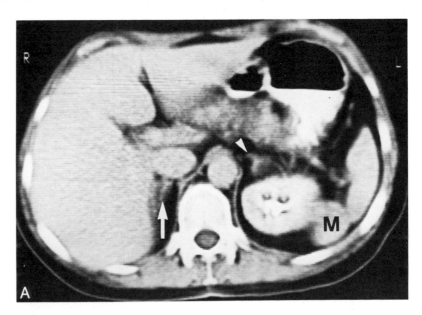

Figure 6–16A. CT scan following administration of oral and intravenous contrast medium demonstrates a soft-tissue mass (M) situated between the upper pole of the left kidney and the spleen. At this level the orgin of the mass is unclear. Note the normal right *(arrow)* and left *(arrowhead)* adrenal glands.

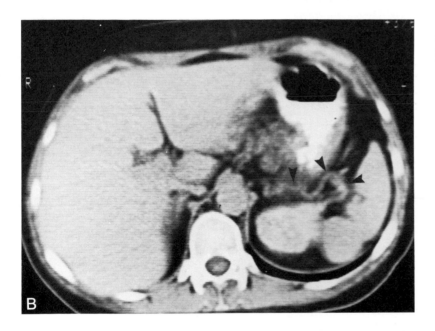

Figure 6–16B. At a slightly higher level, it is apparent that this mass is extrarenal in location. It is the same density as normal splenic tissue and is intimately related to the spleen. Accessory splenic tissue as illustrated in this case can mimic both renal and adrenal pathology. Two of the more popular methods for confirming that left upper quadrant masses are accessory spleens are (1) demonstrating similar enhancement of the questioned mass, compared with normal spleen, and (2) performing a scintigraphic spleen scan with radiolabeled sulfur colloid or heat-damaged red blood cells. Either technique will usually solve most diagnostic dilemmas. Note the normally tortuous splenic artery *(arrowheads)*. (See also Chapter 5, Figure 5–45, for examples of accessory spleens.)

Ref.: Piekarski J, Federle MP, Moss AA, et al. Computed tomography of the spleen. Radiology 1980; 135:683–689.

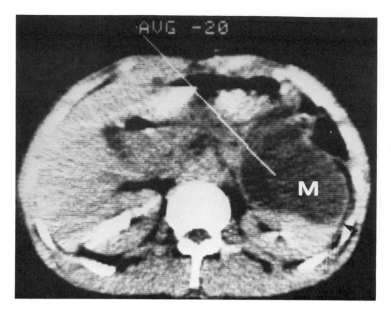

Figure 6–17. PANCREATIC PSEUDOCYST INVOLVING THE PERIRENAL SPACE MIMICKING PRIMARY RENAL DISEASE. CT scan following administration of oral and intravenous contrast medium demonstrates a mass (M) that is near water-density and occupies much of the left upper quadrant. The mass appears to be causing draping of Gerota's fascia *(arrow).* A pancreatic pseudocyst invading the perirenal space was subsequently confirmed.

Only Gerota's fascia and perinephric fat separate the tail of the pancreas from the kidney. It may be difficult to determine the origin of large left upper quadrant cystic masses. Even the more invasive modalities such as endoscopic retrograde cholangiopancreatography may not be that helpful unless actual filling of the pseudocyst is seen. Pseudocysts have also been reported to invade the kidney directly, resulting in subcapsular cystic collections.

Refs.: (1) Zeman RK, Cronan JJ, Viscomi AT, Rosenfield AT. Coordinated imaging in the detection and characterization of renal masses. CRC Crit Rev Diagn Imaging 1981; 15:273–318. (2) Rauch RF, Korobkin M, Silverman PM, Dunnick NR. Subcapsular pancreatic pseudocyst of the kidney. J Comput Assist Tomogr 1983; 7:536–538.

Figure 6–18. PERIPELVIC CYST. CT scan following administration of oral and intravenous contrast medium demonstrates a water-density mass *(arrowheads)* just anterior to the left renal pelvis. This represents the typical appearance of a peripelvic cyst. There is usually little difficulty in differentiating peripheral cysts from sinus lipomatosis or hydronephrosis on images made after the administration of urographic contrast medium. Two smaller cysts *(arrows)* are identified on the right. Peripelvic cysts represent 6 per cent of all renal cysts. They may be single, multiple, or loculated.

Refs.: (1) Jordan WP. Peripelvic cysts of the kidney. J Urol 1962; 87:97–101. (2) Hidalgo H., Dunnick NR, Rosenberg ER, et al. Parapelvic cysts: Appearance on CT and sonography. AJR 1982; 138:667–671.

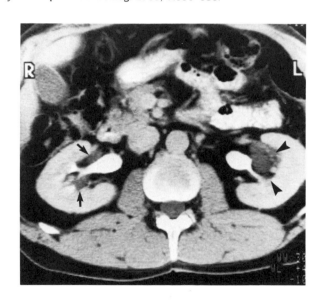

Figure 6–19. PERIPELVIC CYST MIMICKING HYDRONEPHROSIS.

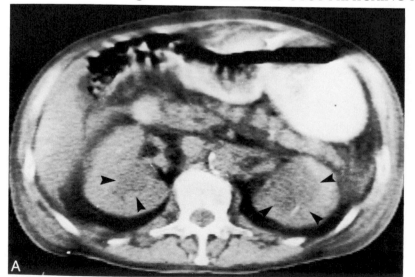

Figure 6–19A. Oral contrast–enhanced CT scan demonstrates water-density masses *(arrowheads)* in the region of the renal hilus. Although these could represent peripelvic cysts, the appearance is indistinguishable from hydronephrosis.

Illustration continued on opposite page

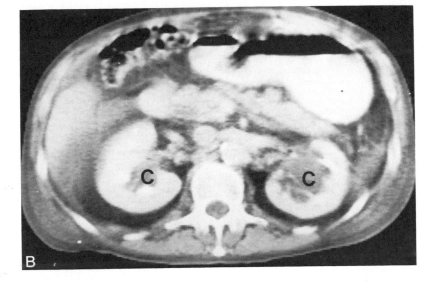

Figure 6–19B. Following the administration of intravenous contrast medium, it is apparent that the collecting system is not dilated but rather is splayed by large peripelvic cysts (C). Note the stretched infundibula bridging the cysts.

Ref.: Amis ES, Cronan JJ, Pfister RC. Pseudohydronephrosis on noncontrast computed tomography. J Comput Assist Tomogr 1982; 6:511–513.

Figure 6–20. PERIPELVIC CYST CAUSING HYDRONEPHROSIS.

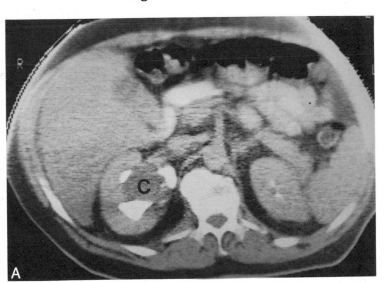

Figure 6–20A. CT scan following administration of oral and intravenous contrast medium demonstrates a large peripelvic cyst (C) splaying the collecting system of the right kidney.

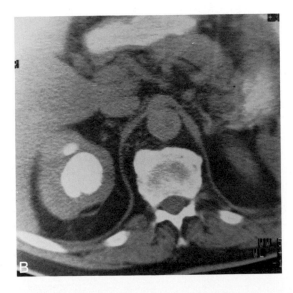

Figure 6–20B. On a slightly more cephalad section, the upper pole calyces are dilated and obstructed due to the compressive effects of the peripelvic cyst. If contrast medium had not been used, it would have been very difficult to make this diagnosis.

Figure 6–21. **SUBCAPSULAR HEMATOMA MIMICKING HYDRONEPHROSIS.**

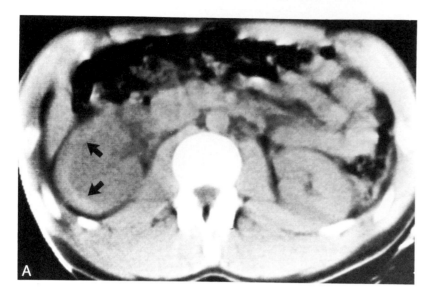

Figure 6–21A. This CT section through the kidneys demonstrates a rim of soft tissue *(arrows)* surrounding a lower-density structure. This appearance could represent a large peripelvic cyst or hydronephrosis.

Figure 6–21B. It is apparent only after intravenous contrast medium has been given that the previously seen lower-density central structure is normal renal parenchyma. On the postcontrast scan, the periphery of the kidney now appears relatively lucent *(arrows)* This inversion of densities is characteristic of the diagnosis of subcapsular hematoma. (Case courtesy of John J. Cronan, M.D., Providence, R.I.)

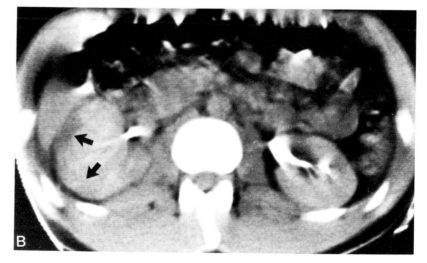

Ref.: Amis ES, Cronan JJ, Pfister RC. Pseudohydronephrosis on noncontrast computed tomography. Comput Assist Tomogr 1982; 6:511–513.

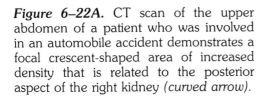

Figure 6–22. SUBCAPSULAR HEMATOMA.

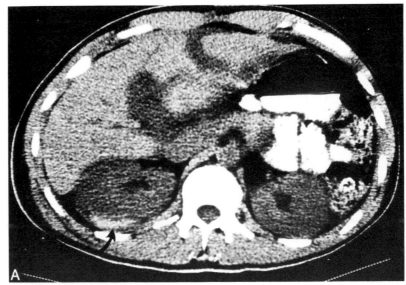

Figure 6–22A. CT scan of the upper abdomen of a patient who was involved in an automobile accident demonstrates a focal crescent-shaped area of increased density that is related to the posterior aspect of the right kidney *(curved arrow).*

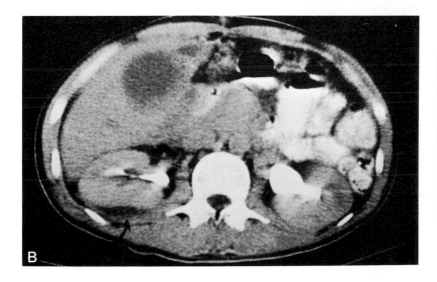

Figure 6–22B. In this scan obtained following the injection of contrast medium, the subcapsular hematoma is now seen to be relatively lucent compared with the denser, functioning renal parenchyma. Note again the length, form and shape. There are also low-density areas in the liver compatible with hepatic hematomas. Recent blood gives an area of increased density initially. This area of increased density may not be apparent if only contrast-enhanced scans are obtained.

Ref.: Swenson SJ, McLeod RA, Stephens DM. CT of extracranial hemorrhage and hematomas. AJR 1984; 143:907–912.

Figure 6–23. **HEMORRHAGIC RENAL CYST.**

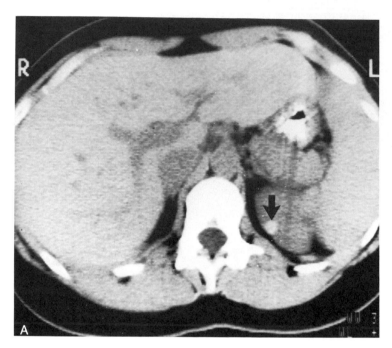

Figure 6–23A. Oral contrast–enhanced CT scan demonstrates a hyperdense, round lesion *(arrow)* in the mid-portion of the left kidney. This appearance is highly suggestive of recent hemorrhage into a renal cyst. A renal hematoma can look quite similar but is often not as smooth and round. The density of the lesion is not high enough to suggest calcification.

Figure 6–23B. Following administration of intravenous contrast medium, the previously dense lesion *(arrow)* appears relatively lucent compared with the surrounding normal nephrogram. The actual CT number was unchanged compared with that of the precontrast study. Several other small cysts are also present in the kidney. If scans are performed with urographic contrast medium only (i.e., direct contrast), hemorrhagic cysts are apt to be missed. Of even greater concern is that, when CT numbers are recorded following administration of contrast medium, these lesions often have greater attenuation than simple cysts. If noncontrast scans were not performed, these lesions might be mistaken as solid masses and approached angiographically instead of more appropriately by percutaneous aspiration to exclude malignancy. Hemorrhage into renal cysts may occur spontaneously, following trauma, or in patients on anticoagulants.

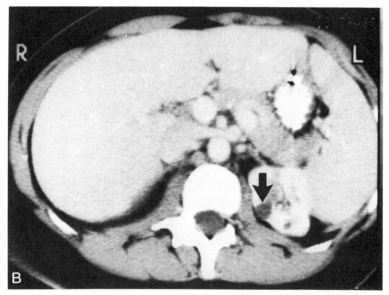

Refs.: (1) Coleman BG, Arger PH, Mintz MC, et al. Hyperdense renal masses: A computed tomographic dilemma. AJR 1984; 143:291–294. (2) Sussman S, Cochran ST, Pagani JJ, et al. Hyperdense renal masses: A CT manifestation of hemorrhagic renal cysts. Radiology 1984; 150:207–211.

Figure 6–24. PSEUDO–THICK-WALLED RENAL CYST.

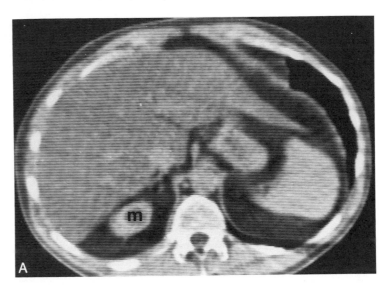

Figure 6–24A. CT scan after administration of intravenous contrast medium demonstrates a thick-walled cystic mass (m) in the upper pole of the right kidney. As the patient had signs of urosepsis, the possibility of an infected cyst or abscess was raised. A large right lower pole renal cyst was also seen.

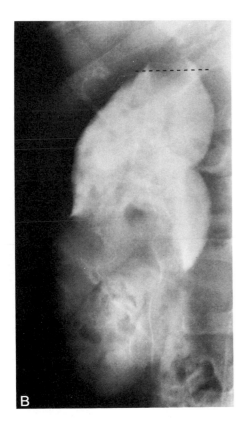

Figure 6–24B. Angiography and subsequently percutaneous aspiration revealed that both lesions were simple cysts. From the capillary phase of this arteriogram it is apparent that a small cyst that is virtually surrounded by renal parenchyma will falsely appear to have thick walls on some sections. Thus, wall thickness cannot be readily assessed in lesions that are predominantly intrarenal.

Ref.: Segal AJ, Spitzer RM. Pseudo thick-walled renal cyst by CT. AJR 1979; 132:827–828.

Figure 6–25. SPLENIC VEIN MIMICKING ADRENAL ABNORMALITY.

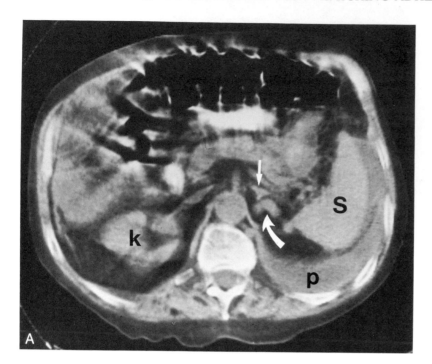

Figure 6–25A. CT scan through the upper abdomen demonstrates a pleural effusion (p). The left adrenal *(straight arrow)* is seen anterior to an apparent mass *(curved arrow).* The scan was performed without intravenous contrast medium.

Figure 6–25B. A section 1 cm lower shows the top of the left kidney behind the apparent pseudomass *(curved arrow).* The true adrenal *(straight arrow)* is seen anterior to this region.

Illustration continued on opposite page

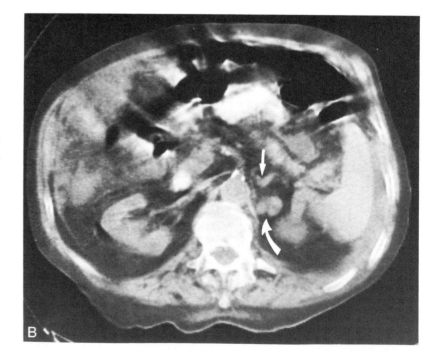

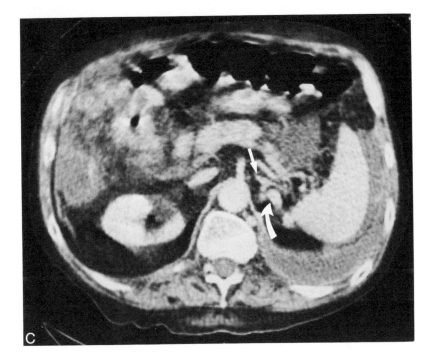

Figure 6–25C. Dynamic scanning through the upper portion of the abdomen after injection of intravenous contrast medium demonstrates the normal left adrenal *(straight arrow)* and the pseudomass *(curved arrow),* which is clearly a vascular structure (probably the splenic vein).

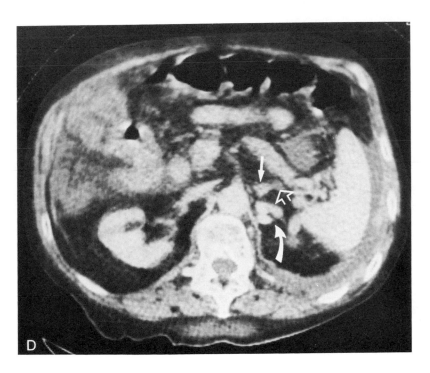

Figure 6–25D. Scan made at a slightly lower level than *C* once again demonstrates the tortuous splenic vessel *(curved arrow)* mimicking a mass. The adrenal gland *(straight arrow)* and a small mass *(open arrowhead),* which is most likely an adenoma, are clearly seen.

Refs.: (1) Berliner L, Bosniak MA, Megibow A. Adrenal pseudotumors on computed tomography. J Comput Assist Tomogr 1982; 6:281–285. (2) Karstaedt N, Sagel SS, Stanley RJ, Melson GL, Levitt RG. Computed tomography of the adrenal gland. Radiology 1978; 129:723–730. (3) Brownlie K, Kreel L. Computer assisted tomography of normal suprarenal glands. J Comput Assist Tomogr 1978; 2:1–10.

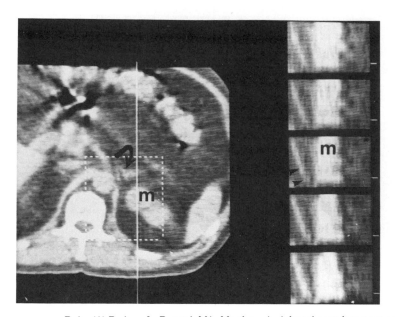

Figure 6–26. UPPER POLE RENAL MASS MIMICKING AN ADRENAL MASS. CT scan following administration of oral and intravenous contrast medium demonstrates a round soft-tissue density mass (m) that appears to project from the upper pole of the left kidney. A normal left adrenal *(curved arrow)* is present. Sagittal reformatting *(right)* again demonstrates the lateral limb of the adrenal *(arrowheads)* anterior to this small renal mass (m). Differentiating renal from adrenal masses is not so much a CT pitfall as a urographic and angiographic pitfall. Since adrenal tumors may be supplied by the renal arteries, they may be difficult to distinguish on arteriography alone. CT can readily differentiate masses of adrenal versus renal origin, especially when a normal adrenal is visualized as in this case.

Refs.: (1) Berliner L, Bosniak MA, Megibow A. Adrenal pseudotumors on computed tomography. J Comput Assist Tomogr 1982: 6:281–285. (2) Shrage GG, McKinnon CM, Clark R. Adrenal tumors simulating intrarenal lesions. AJR 1974, 121:518–522.

Figure 6–27. RIGHT CRUS AND PSOAS MINOR MUSCLES AS PSEUDOMASSES. (See also the section on the diaphragm in Chapter 1.)

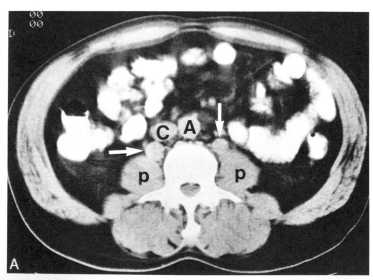

Figure 6–27A. CT scan through the retroperitoneum demonstrates the psoas minor *(arrows)* and major (p) muscles as individual structures. The psoas minor muscles should not be mistaken for adenopathy. (C = inferior vena cava; A = aorta). (See also Chapter 5, Figures 5–10, 5–11, and 5–12, for variations in the psoas muscles.)

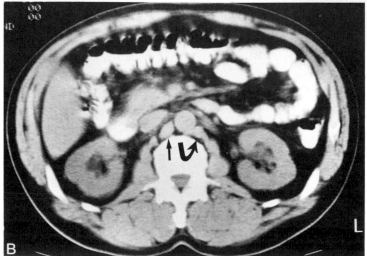

Figure 6–27B. CT scan at the level of the renal hila demonstrates a structure mimicking adenopathy between the aorta and inferior vena cava *(straight arrow)*. This structure is over 1.5 cm in diameter. Note also an additional mass between the aorta and psoas minor muscle *(curved arrow)*.

Illustration continued on opposite page

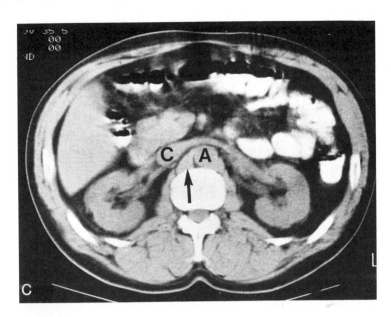

Figure 6–27C. A section 1 cm higher than *B* demonstrates that the structure between the aorta and inferior vena cava is contiguous with the right crus of the diaphragm *(straight arrow)* and is therefore a normal extension of the right crus. Note that the structure between the aorta and psoas minor muscles in *B* is a portion of the left crus (C = inferior vena cava; A = aorta). (See also Chapter 5, Figures 5–18 and 5–19, for examples of diaphragmatic crura.)

Ref.: Donovan PJ, Zerhouni EA, Siegelman SS. CT of the psoas compartment of the retroperitoneum. Semin Roentgenol 1981; 16:241–250.

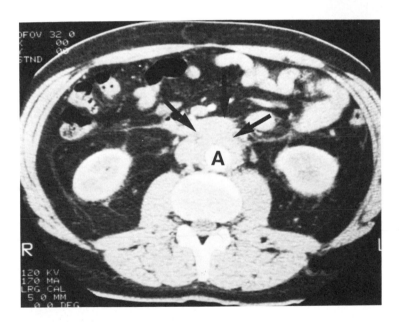

Figure 6–28. RETROPERITONEAL FIBROSIS. CT scan following administration of oral and intravenous contrast medium demonstrates a soft-tissue mass *(arrows)* encasing the aorta (A). There was no evidence of hydronephrosis. The differential diagnosis includes lymphoma, retroperitoneal sarcomas, any cause of adenopathy, and retroperitoneal fibrosis. Retroperitoneal fibrosis typically occurs at and below the level of the renal hilus. Occasionally it is seen in the upper abdomen. The mass may be bulky or sheet-like. In addition to the idiopathic form there are secondary forms resulting from medication (e.g., methysergide), previous radiation therapy, and adjacent retroperitoneal inflammation.

Refs.: (1) Brun B, Laursen K, Sorenson IN, et al. CT in retroperitoneal fibrosis. AJR 1981; 137:535–538. (2) Dalla-Palma L, Rocca-Rosetti S, Pozzi-Mucelli RS, Rizzatto G. Computed tomography in the diagnosis of retroperitoneal fibrosis. Urol Radiol 1981; 3:77–83.

Figure 6–29. NORMAL ADRENAL GLAND. A normal right adrenal gland *(straight arrow)* is demonstrated. Note the slender, curvilinear appearance and its width, which is less than that of the ipsilateral diaphragm. The normal left adrenal gland *(curved arrow)* is also demonstrated. Lack of symmetry of the left and right adrenal glands is not abnormal.

Ref.: Brownlie K, Kreel L. Computer assisted tomography of normal suprarenal glands. Comput Assist Tomogr 1978; 2:1–10.

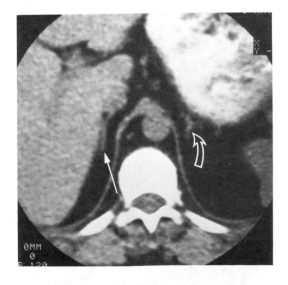

Figure 6–30. NORMAL ADRENAL GLANDS.

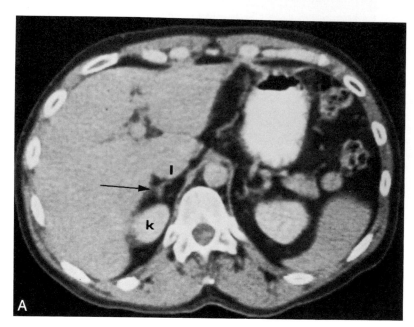

Figure 6–30A. Both a normal right and a normal left adrenal gland are demonstrated. The right adrenal gland *(arrow)* is seen to be posterior to the inferior vena cava (I) and to abut against it, which is normal. It is anterior to the upper pole of the right kidney (k). The left adrenal gland is an inverted V shape in this image.

Figure 6–30B. In this scan, the right adrenal gland has a slightly variant appearance, with an extension of one limb on the lateral aspect *(arrow).*

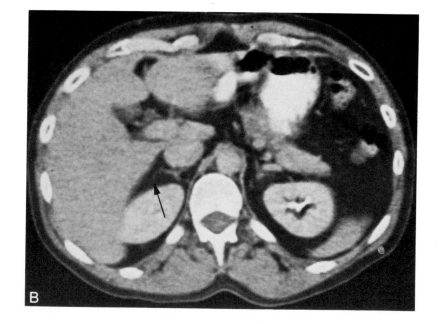

Figure 6–31. NORMAL ADRENAL GLAND.

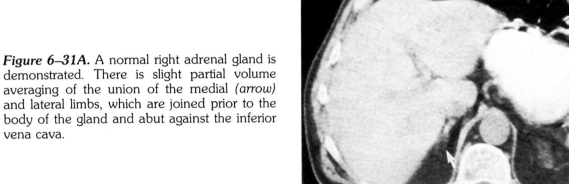

Figure 6–31A. A normal right adrenal gland is demonstrated. There is slight partial volume averaging of the union of the medial *(arrow)* and lateral limbs, which are joined prior to the body of the gland and abut against the inferior vena cava.

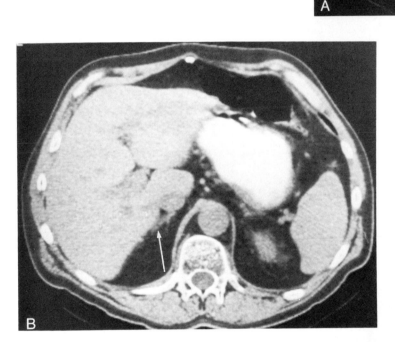

Figure 6–31B. In this scan, the lateral limb *(arrow)* is slightly more apparent than the medial limb.

Figure 6–31C. The normal adrenal gland in this magnified view has common seagull shape *(white arrow)*. The gland is seen posterior to the calcified splenic artery *(black arrow)*. (See also Chapter 5, Figure 5–20, for example of pseudo–adrenal mass.)

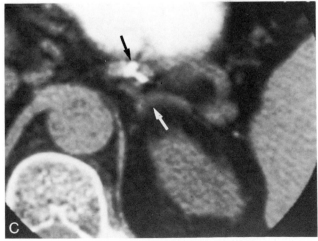

Figure 6–32. RETROCAVAL URETER. Retrocaval ureter is a cause of obstruction of the upper urinary tract on the right. It typically leads to pyelectasis and ureterectasis proximal to the portion of the ureter extending behind the inferior vena cava, and the marked medial course of the ureter on urography or retrograde pyelography, as in *D,* strongly suggests the diagnosis. Until the advent of computed tomography, inferior vena cavography was generally needed to confirm the diagnosis. CT is a rapid, accurate way to diagnose retrocaval ureter. (Case courtesy of David Colley, M.D., Hospital of St. Raphael, New Haven, Conn.)

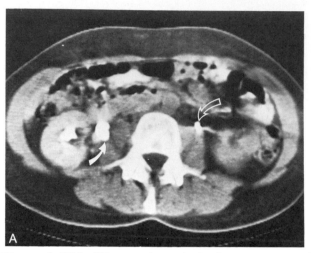

Figure 6–32A. CT scan through the lower portion of the kidneys demonstrates both the right pelvis *(solid curved arrow)* and left ureter *(open arrow).*

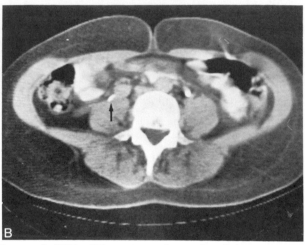

Figure 6–32B. CT scan at a lower level demonstrates both ureters. Note the relatively posterior position of the right ureter *(arrow).*

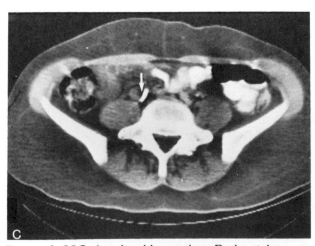

Figure 6–32C. At a level lower than *B,* the right ureter *(arrow)* can be seen going behind the inferior vena cava before beginning its course to the bladder.

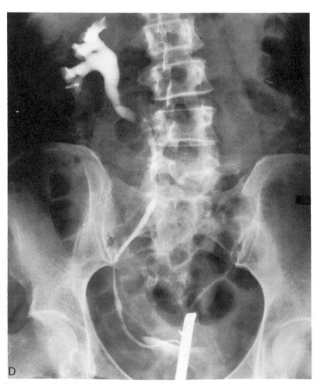

Figure 6–32D. Retrograde pyelogram demonstrates the marked medial course of the upper ureter.

Figure 6–33. LEFT ILIAC VEIN MIMICKING ADENOPATHY. Full reformation of the anatomy from sequential images can frequently indicate whether a structure is vascular or a mass. When indicated, dynamic scanning can be performed to definitely discriminate between vessels and masses. The proximal portion of the left common iliac vein is frequently horizontal and when distended can be confused with adenopathy.

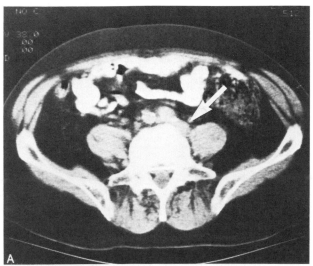

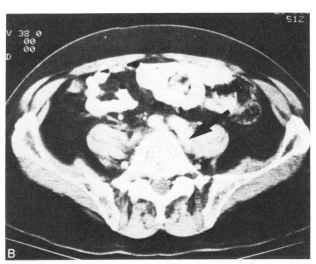

Figure 6–33A. CT section through the true pelvis without the injection of intravenous contrast medium shows an apparent mass *(arrow)* between the aorta and left psoas.

Figure 6–33B. Dynamic scanning demonstrates opacification of the mass, which is the left common iliac vein as it courses horizontally *(arrow).*

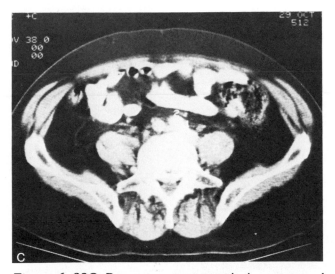

Figure 6–33C. Dynamic scanning with three areas of interest shows that the density of the iliac vein parallels that of the aorta and is significantly greater than that of the psoas (the iliac vein is 77 HU; the aorta, 87 HU; and the psoas, 42 HU).

Ref.: Moncada R, Reynes C, Churchill R, Love L. Normal vascular anatomy of the abdomen on computed tomography. Radiol Clin North Am 1979; 17:25–37.

Figure 6–34. DOUBLE INFERIOR VENA CAVA. In this child with abdominal trauma, the right kidney is congenitally absent. On non-enhanced scans the left inferior vena cava illustrated in this series of figures might be mistaken for retroperitoneal adenopathy. Demonstration of the tubular nature of the structure and its emptying into the left renal vein (or in some cases emptying directly into the right-sided inferior vena cava) excludes that possibility, as would enhancement following injection of contrast medium. The differential diagnosis for left inferior vena cava would include an enlarged gonadal vessel. The double inferior vena cava continues to become the femoral vein, whereas the gonadal vessel extends to the ovary or scrotum. On sequential CT scans, in this case, the left-sided vessel became the left femoral vein. (See also Chapter 5, Figure 5–6.)

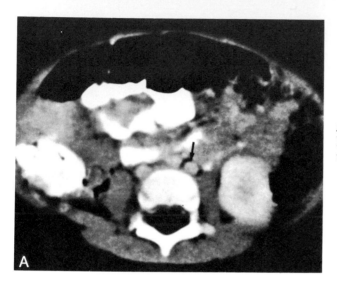

Figure 6–34A. A CT scan through the lower pole of the left kidney demonstrates an enhancing mass *(arrow)* lateral to the aorta and cava.

Figure 6–34B. On a higher section, once again a rounded mass *(arrow)* is seen lateral to the aorta.

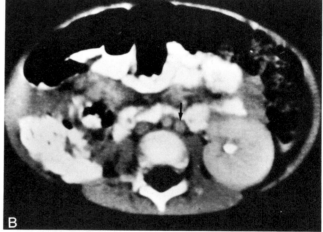

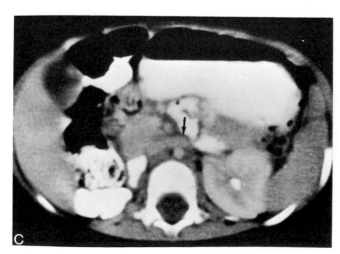

Figure 6–34C. An image at the level of the left renal vein *(arrow)* demonstrates that the mass has emptied into the left renal vein and is no longer apparent.

Illustration continued on opposite page

Figure 6–34D. Anomalies of the inferior vena cava and left renal vein are illustrated in diagrammatic CT sections of the aorta (Ao), inferior vena cava (IVC), and left renal vein (LRV). In transposition and duplication of the inferior vena cava, the venous structure may pass either anterior or posterior *(dashed lines)* to the aorta at the level of the renal veins.

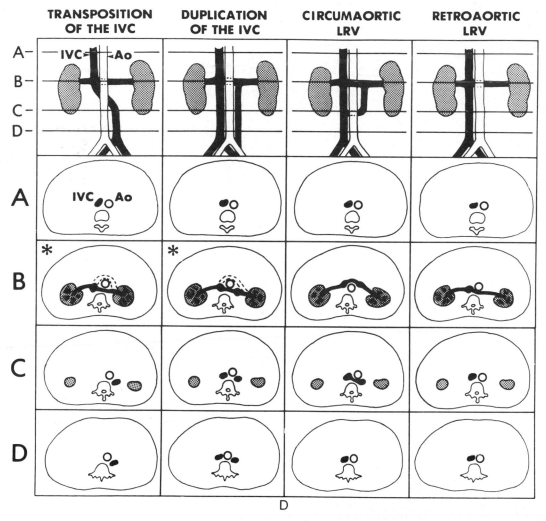

Ref.: Royal SA, Callen PW. Evaluation of the inferior vena cava and left renal vein. AJR 1979; 132:759–763. Reproduced with permission from the American Journal of Roentgenology.

Figure 6–35. INTERRUPTION OF THE INFERIOR VENA CAVA WITH AZYGOS AND HEMIAZYGOS CONTINUATION. The spectrum of vena caval anomalies includes duplication with right- or left-sided predominance as well as interruption with continuation via the azygos or hemiazygos vein or both of these structures.

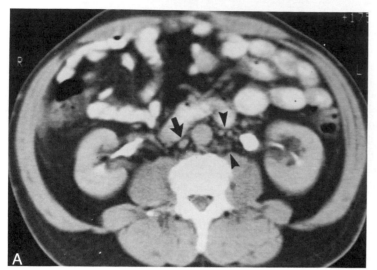

Figure 6–35A. CT scan following administration of oral and intravenous contrast medium demonstrates a small, right-sided inferior vena cava *(arrow)* and multiple, small, enhancing left para-aortic collaterals *(arrowhead).* The infrarenal inferior vena cava appeared normal.

Figure 6–35B. At a higher level, dilation of the azygos (1) and hemiazygos (2) veins is seen. These vessels both carry abdominal and lower extremity venous return to the heart. Their tubular nature and enhancement with contrast medium distinguish them from adenopathy. Hepatic veins are seen converging on a small suprahepatic inferior vena cava.

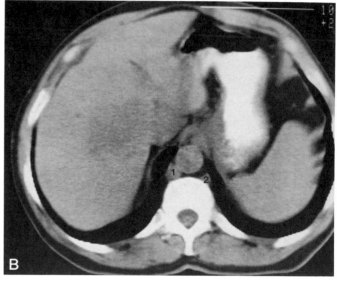

Refs.: (1) Mayo J, Gray R, St. Louis E, et al. Anomalies of the inferior vena cava. AJR 1983; 140:339–345. (2) Breckenridge JW, Kinlaw WB. Azygos continuation of inferior vena cava: CT appearance. AJR 1980; 4:392–397. (3) Chuang VP, Mena CE, Hoskins PA. Congenital anomalies of the inferior vena cava. Review of embryogenesis and presentation of a simplified classification. Br J Radiol 1974; 47:206–213.

Figure 6–36. BOWEL GAS MIMICKING A BLADDER LESION.

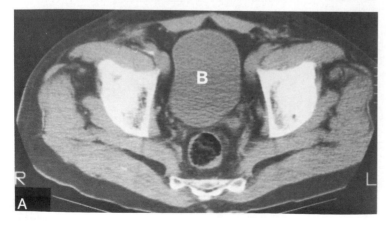

Figure 6–36A. CT section through the true pelvis demonstrates a normal-appearing bladder (B).

Illustration continued on opposite page

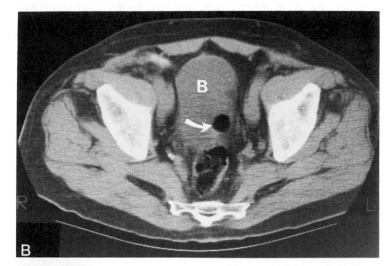

Figure 6–36B. CT section 1 cm cephalad to *A* demonstrates what appears to be a rounded gas collection *(arrow)* within the bladder (B).

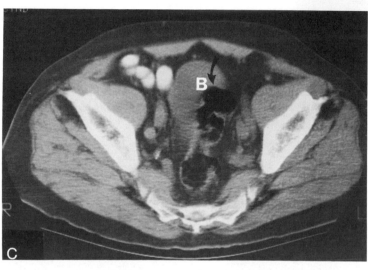

Figure 6–36C. On this section, which is 1 cm cephalad to *B*, gas-filled bowel *(arrow)* is seen contiguous with the bladder (B). Volume averaging of the gas-filled bowel with the urine-filled bladder, in addition to projectional artifact on the axial scan, causes an apparent gas-filled region within the bladder.

Ref.: Goodenough D, Weaver K, Davis D, LaFalce S. Volume averaging limitations of computed tomography. AJR 1982; 138:313–316.

Figure 6–37. URETERAL JET PHENOME-NON. CT scan following administration of intravenous contrast medium demonstrates apparent opaque densities along the anterolateral left bladder wall *(straight arrow)* as well as in the right and mid-portions of the bladder. These were not seen on sections immediately above or below this one. Further observation demonstrates a ureteral jet *(curved arrow)* emanating from the right hemitrigone. The apparent "lesions" in the bladder represent contrast medium seen against unopacified urine present in the bladder. Failure to identify these lesions on contiguous sequential scans verifies that they are transient phenomena. In questionable situations, repeat scanning of the area can be performed to verify that this pseudolesion does not persist after adequate mixing of contrast medium and urine.

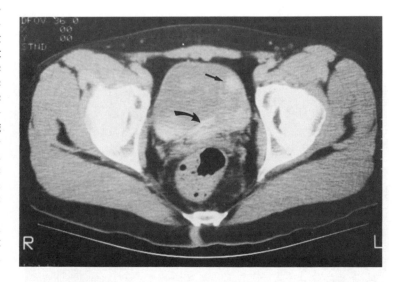

Figure 6–38. PROSTATIC ENLARGEMENT MIMICKING PRIMARY BLADDER MASS.

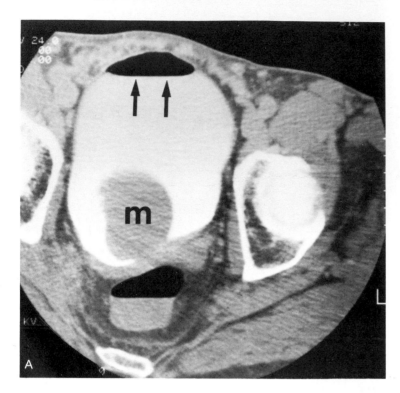

Figure 6–38A. CT scan following injection of intravenous contrast medium demonstrates a large mass (m) projecting into the bladder. Air *(arrows)* from prior catheterization is also identified in the bladder. Although the posterior margins of the mass suggest a primary mucosal lesion of the bladder, this is merely enlargement of the median lobe of the prostate protruding into the bladder. (See also Chapter 5, Figure 5–79.)

Figure 6–38B. Coronal reformation is somewhat helpful in showing the epicenter of the mass (m) arising from the enlarged prostate rather than the bladder wall.

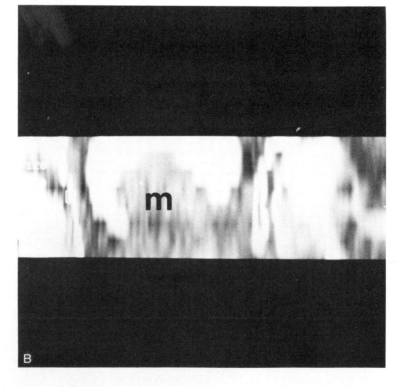

Musculoskeletal System

JAMES B. VOGLER, III, M.D.
CLYDE A. HELMS, M.D.

Figure 7–1. INDISTINCT MEDIAL BORDERS OF THE CLAVICLES. Because of the undulating nature and oblique course of the clavicles, indistinct areas are sometimes identified *(arrows)*. The presence of normal fat planes adjacent to these areas in addition to the bilateral symmetric appearance help to exclude a pathologic process.

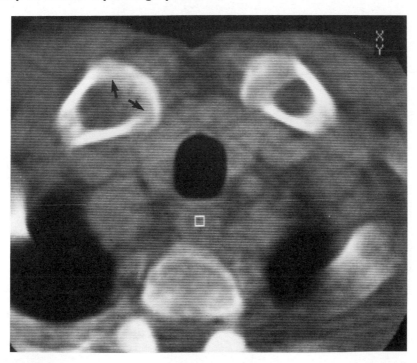

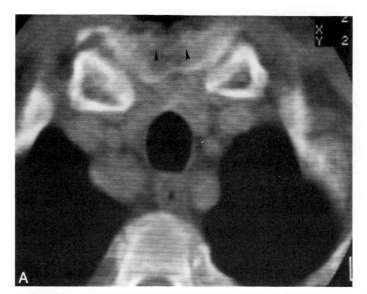

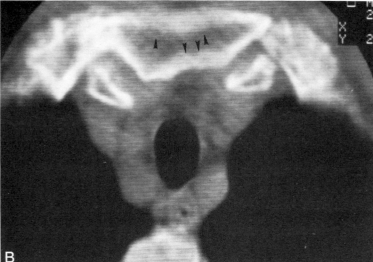

Figure 7–2. ILL-DEFINED CORTICES OF THE MANUBRIUM. Axial scans through the upper *(A)* and mid-portions *(B)* of the manubrium demonstrate indistinct or ill-defined areas *(arrowheads)* of both the anterior and posterior margins of the manubrium. These are normal variations in the CT appearance of the manubrium and are felt to be due, in part, to true variations in the cortical thickness in addition to the slope of the manubrium with respect to the axial scans. These indistinct areas of cortex are most pronounced and seen most commonly in the distal, posterior aspect of the manubrium. The presence of normal fat planes around the manubrium aids in distinguishing these from pathologic processes.

Ref.: Goodman LR, Teplick SK, Kay H. Computed tomography of the normal sternum. AJR 1983; 141:219–223.

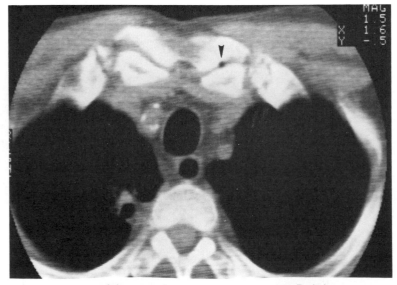

Figure 7–3. VACUUM PHENOMENON. The air density seen in the left sternoclavicular joint *(arrowhead)* is typical of the vacuum phenomenon that can normally occur in these joints.

Ref.: Destouet JM, Gilula LA, Murphy WA. Computed tomography of the sternoclavicular joint and sternum. Radiology 1981; 138:123–128.

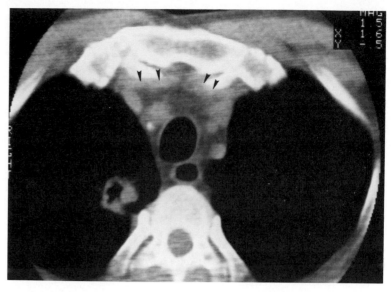

Figure 7–4. POSTERIOR STERNOCLA-VICULAR LIGAMENTS. Soft tissue densities *(arrowheads)* are evident posterior to the clavicles and extending to the manubrium in this patient. These are posterior sternoclavicular ligaments and should not be mistaken for abnormal masses. Note the symmetric appearance and sharply defined adjacent fat planes.

Ref.: Goodman LR, Teplick SK, Kay H. Computed tomography of the normal sternum. AJR 1983; 141:219–223.

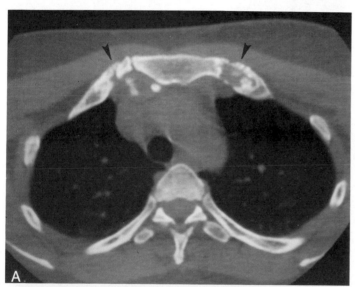

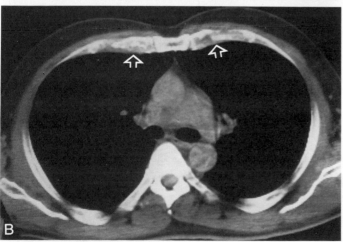

Figure 7–5. IRREGULAR COSTOSTERNAL JUNCTIONS. Costal cartilage *(arrowheads)* in the region of rib insertions on the sternum may appear bulbous, nodular and irregular in normal patients. In the absence of distorted soft-tissue planes or masses these irregular junctions should not be called abnormal.

Ref.: Goodman LR, Teplick SK, Kay H. Computed tomography of the normal sternum. AJR 1983; 141:219–223.

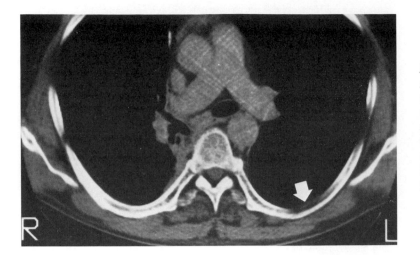

Figure 7–6. INDISTINCT RIB CORTICES.
An area of ill-defined or indistinct cortex is seen in one of the lift ribs *(arrow)*. This is a common finding and is believed to result in part from the non-uniform size of the ribs, the oblique nature in which they are imaged on axial scans, and partial volume averaging. In the absence of adjacent masses this should not be considered abnormal.

Figure 7–7. UNDULATIONS OF THE SCAPULAE. Axial CT scans demonstrate abrupt and gradual undulations of the scapulae *(arrowheads)*. These are common in normal individuals. The scapulae are often symmetric in appearance, which aids in excluding other causes such as occult fractures or scalloped erosions.

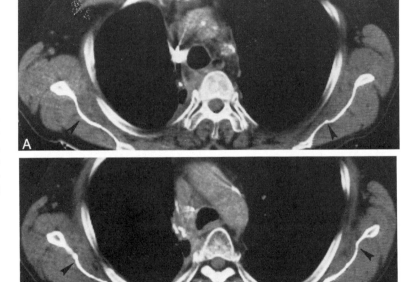

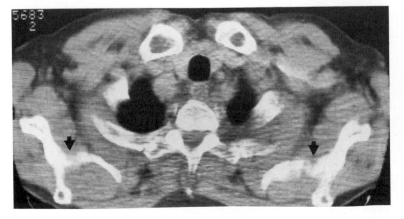

Figure 7–8. APPARENT BONY DEFECTS OF THE SCAPULAE. Indistinct and irregular-appearing areas of both scapular bodies are identified *(arrowheads)*. Similar findings on plain films have been described as developmental defects. The symmetry of these areas helps exclude a pathologic process.

Ref.: Keats, TE. Atlas of Normal Roentgen Variants, 3rd ed. Chicago: Year Book Medical Publishers, 1984; p 313.

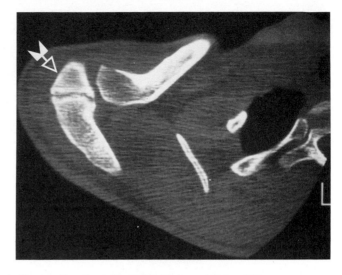

Figure 7–9. OS ACROMIALE. Persistence of a secondary ossification center of the acromion into adult life is termed an os acromiale *(arrow)*. These are often bilateral. The sclerotic margin and characteristic location aid in excluding acute fractures as differential possibilities.

Ref.: Keats, TE. Atlas of Normal Roentgen Variants, 3rd ed. Chicago: Year Book Medical Publishers, 1984; p 308.

Figure 7–10. HUMERAL PSEUDOCYST.

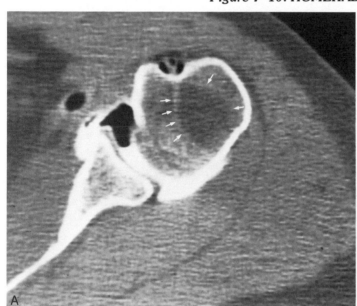

Figure 7–10A. Axial CT scan of the left shoulder taken during a CT arthrogram demonstrates a lucency *(arrows)* in the lateral aspect of the proximal humerus, adjacent to the greater tuberosity. The location and appearance of this lucency are characteristic of a humeral pseudocyst. This well-established plain film normal variant is the result of porous spongiosa in the area of the pseudocyst.

Figure 7–10B. The plain film appearance of the pseudocyst *(arrowheads)* shown in *A* is demonstrated.

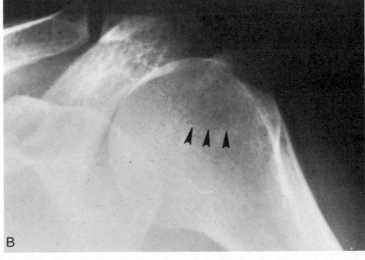

Refs.: (1) Helms, CA. Pseudocysts of the humerus. AJR 1978; 131:287–288. (2) Resnick D, Cone RO III. The nature of humeral pseudocysts. Radiology 1984; 150:27–28.

Figure 7–11. *INSERTIONAL PITS.*

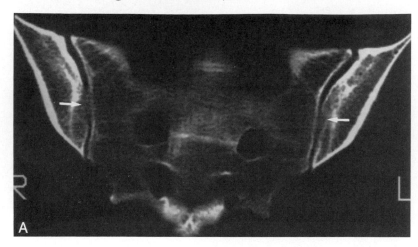

Figure 7–11A. Ill-defined areas *(arrows)* in the subarticular bony plate are frequently encountered in CT studies of the sacroiliac joints. These ill-defined areas may be seen on the iliac side or sacral side or both. They are felt to represent insertional locations for interosseous ligaments and partial volume averaging of different tissue densities included in the CT section. As such, they are most commonly seen at transition zones between the synovial and fibrous portions of the joint. Although these insertional pits may be mistaken for erosions, their characteristic location and the lack of surrounding sclerosis should aid in this differentiation.

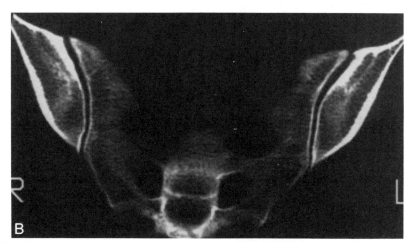

Figure 7–11B. Consecutive sections such as this one typically demonstrate normal-appearing joints and subarticular bony plates.

Ref.: Vogler JB, Brown WH, Helms CA, Genant HK. The normal sacroiliac joint: A CT study of asymptomatic patients. Radiology 1984; 151:433–437.

Figure 7–12. ANTERIOR OSTEOPHYTES. Osteophytes of the sacroiliac joints are typically seen as sclerotic, bony excrescences *(arrows)*. They more commonly occur on the anterior aspect of the joint and are a reflection of degenerative change. Osteophytes do not necessarily indicate sacroiliitis. They can be found in up to 20 per cent of asymptomatic patients.

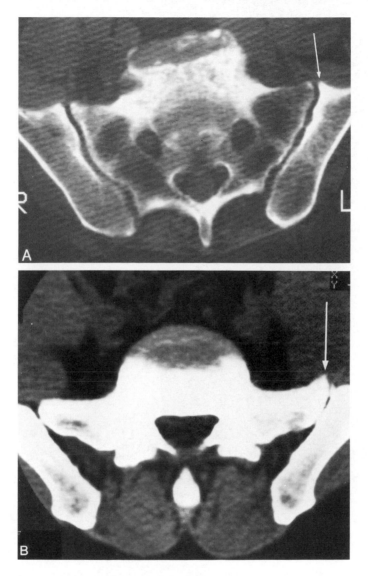

Ref.: Vogler JB, Brown WH, Helms CA, Genant HK. The normal sacroiliac joint. A CT study of asymptomatic patients. Radiology 1984; 151:433–437.

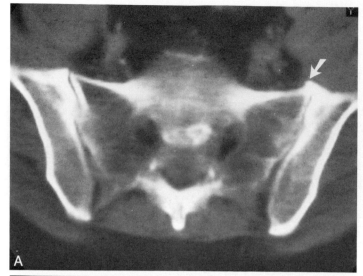

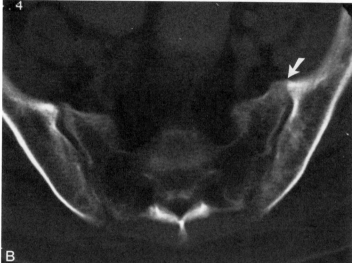

Figure 7–13. BRIDGING ANTERIOR OSTEO-PHYTES. Two examples (A and B) of bridging anterior osteophytes *(arrows)* are demonstrated. This type of para-articular ankylosis can be seen in up to 9 per cent of asymptomatic patients and, by itself, should not be considered evidence of sacroiliitis. Note the absence of intra-articular ankylosis, which is more characteristic of a spondyloarthropathy.

Ref.: Vogler JB, Brown WH, Helms CA, Genant HK. The normal sacroiliac joint: A CT study of asymptomatic patients. Radiology 1984; 151:433–437.

Figure 7–14. ILIAC SUBCHONDRAL SCLE-ROSIS. Focal increased or nonuniform iliac subchondral sclerosis *(arrowheads)*, particularly anteriorly, may be seen in a large portion of asymptomatic patients (83 per cent). This finding alone is not a reliable indicator of sacroiliitis.

Illustration continued on opposite page

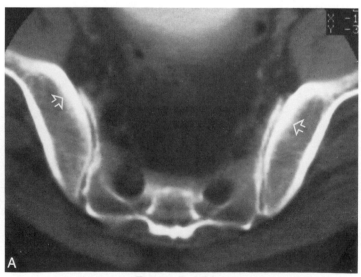

Figure 7–14A

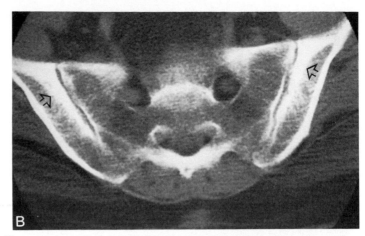

Figure 7–14B

Ref.: Vogler JB, Brown WH, Helms CA, Genant HK. The normal sacroiliac joint: A CT study of asymptomatic patients. Radiology 1984; 151:433–437.

Figure 7–15. APPARENT INTRA-ARTICULAR ANKYLOSIS. These areas of apparent ankylosis are commonly encountered at transition zones between the anteriorly located synovial portion and posteriorly located fibrous portion of the sacroiliac joint. They most probably represent areas of interosseous ligaments and partial volume averaging of different tissue densities on the same CT section. Contiguous CT sections will aid in differentiating these areas from true ankylosis.

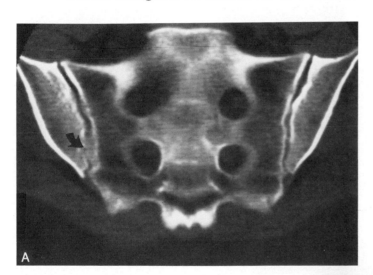

Figure 7–15A. An area of apparent intra-articular ankylosis is visualized in the right sacroiliac joint *(arrow).*

Figure 7–15B. A contiguous CT section demonstrates a normal-appearing sacroiliac joint without evidence of ankylosis.

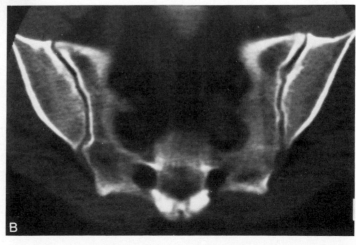

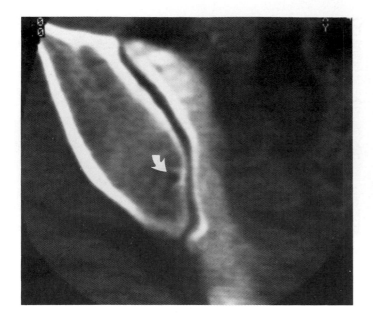

Figure 7–16. SUBCHONDRAL CYST. A subchondral cyst *(arrows)* is identified in the iliac portion of the sacroiliac joint. These cysts generally have a characteristic appearance in that they are rounded lucencies with sclerotic rims. They are often seen in association with other signs of degenerative joint disease such as subchondral sclerosis and joint-space narrowing. Subchondral cysts are relatively infrequent in the sacroiliac joints.

Ref.: Vogler JB, Brown WH, Helms CA, Genant HK. The normal sacroiliac joint: A CT study of asymptomatic patients. Radiology 1984; 151:433–437.

Figure 7–17. FIBROUS (OR LIGAMENTOUS) PORTIONS OF THE SACROILIAC JOINTS. The ligamentous portions of the sacroiliac joints are irregular and wide *(solid arrows)*. The irregular appearance of the fibrous portion is due to the numerous insertion pits for ligaments. These pits should not be misconstrued as erosions, which are discrete disruptions in the subchondral bony plate. The synovial portion of the joint is seen anteriorly *(open arrowheads)* and is normal.

Ref.: Lawson TL, Foley WD, Carrera GF, Berland LL. The sacroiliac joints: Anatomic, plain roentgenographic, and computed tomographic analysis. J Comput Asst Tomogr 1982; 6:307–314.

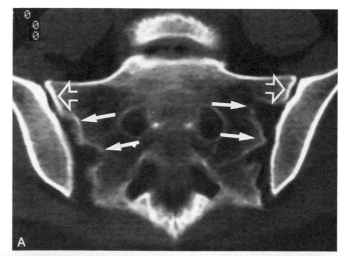

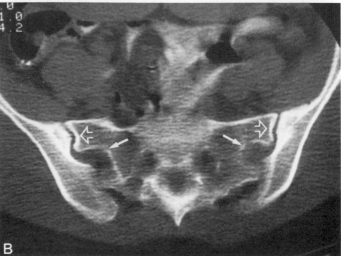

Figure 7–18. **ASYMMETRIC SACROILIAC JOINT SCLEROSIS.** In individuals under the age of 30, the sacroiliac joints usually demonstrate symmetry in the absence of predisposing factors such as scoliosis. Above this age the majority of patients (77 per cent of patients over age 30 and 87 per cent of patients over age 40 in one study) demonstrate subtle or definite asymmetry with respect to sclerosis and joint space. Note that in this 48-year-old asymptomatic patient the joint spaces are non-uniform and there is asymmetric sclerosis of the iliac subarticular bone *(arrow)*. The sacral subchondral bone also shows non-uniform sclerosis from anterior to posterior.

Ref.: Vogler JB, Brown WH, Helms CA, Genant HK. The normal sacroiliac joint: A CT study of asymptomatic patients. Radiology 1984; 151:433–437.

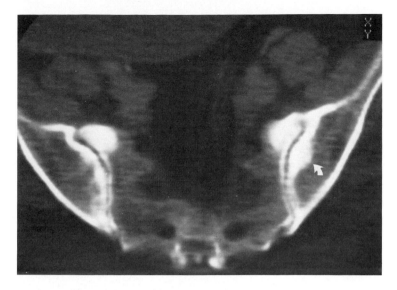

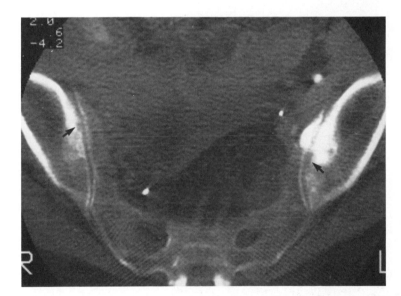

Figure 7–19. **SACROILIAC JOINT EROSIONS.** Bilateral erosions *(arrows)* of the sacroiliac joints are present in this 65-year-old asymptomatic patient. As in this case, erosions characteristically appear as discrete disruptions in the subchondral bone, often associated with sclerosis and joint-space narrowing. In individuals below age 50, erosions are considered a good indicator of sacroiliitis; however, they may be seen in a small percentage of asymptomatic patients older than age 50.

Ref.: Vogler JB, Brown WH, Helms CA, Genant HK. The normal sacroiliac joint: A CT study of asymptomatic patients. Radiology 1984; 151:433–437.

Figure 7–20. **ASYMMETRIC JOINT SPACES.** Although symmetric joint spaces are the rule in patients under age 30, above this age there is an increasing tendency toward asymmetry. This is the case in this 62-year-old patient who demonstrates marked asymmetry of the sacroiliac joint spaces. Thus, asymmetry of the joint spaces should be interpreted with respect to the patient's age, and should be considered a less significant indicator of sacroiliitis with increasing patient age.

Ref.: Vogler JB, Brown WH, Helms CA, Genant HK. The normal sacroiliac joint: A CT study of asymptomatic patients. Radiology 1984; 151:433–437.

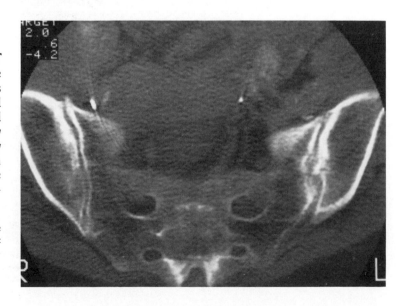

Figure 7–21. NUTRIENT CANALS OF THE ILIUM. Nutrient canals *(arrows)* are often seen traversing the ilium. These usually represent canals for the iliac branch of the iliolumbar artery. Their location, just lateral to the sacroiliac joints, is characteristic as is the circular appearance of the nutrient canal. They are commonly seen bilaterally.

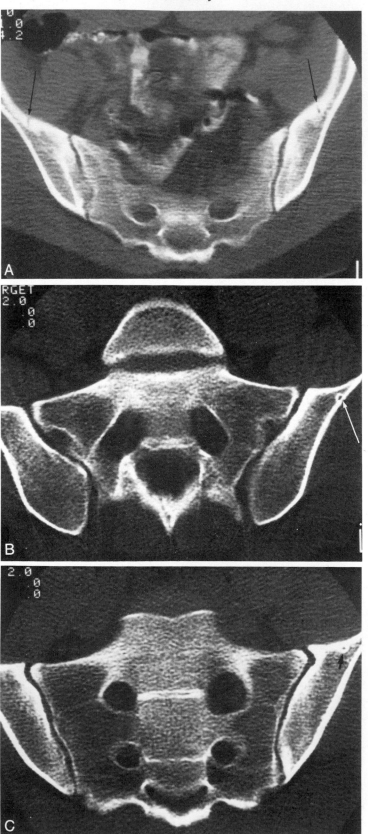

Ref.: Goss CM, ed. Gray's Anatomy, 29th ed. Philadelphia: Lea and Febiger, 1973; p 649.

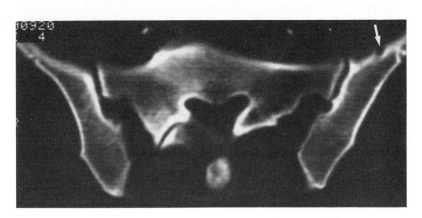

Figure 7–22. ASYMMETRY OF THE SACRAL ALAE. At times there may be asymmetric development of the sacrum, as in this case. Frequently this occurs in patients with scoliosis. By itself, it is not felt to be an indicator of a generalized bony dysplasia. Note also the prominent nutrient canal *(arrow)* in the left ilium.

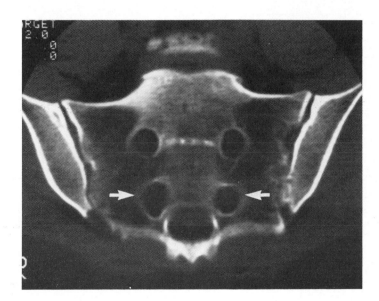

Figure 7–23. ASYMMETRY OF THE SACRAL FORAMINA. The size of the sacral formina is variable and on occasion may appear asymmetric *(arrows)*. This may be a function of patient positioning in some cases; in others, the asymmetry appears to be developmental, as in this example. The presence of normal epidural fat in the neuroforamina excludes a pathologic etiology of the asymmetry.

Figure 7–24. MUSCLE INSERTIONS. At areas of major muscle insertion and curved portions of bones, the bony cortex often appears ill-defined, as can be seen in this example along the posterior-superior iliac spines *(arrows)* where the erector spinal muscles insert. These poorly defined cortical areas are characteristically bilateral. When seen in this context, they should not be confused with pathologic processes that may destroy cortical bone.

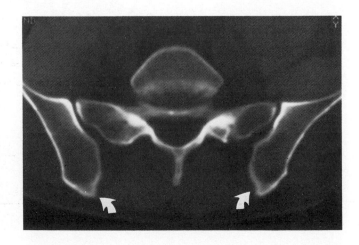

Figure 7–25. PSEUDOTUMORS OF THE SACRUM.

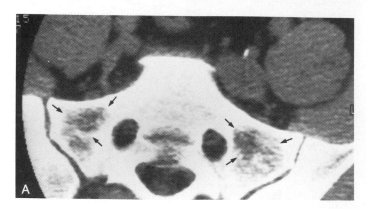

Figure 7–25A. Areas of low density *(arrows)* are identified in both sacral alae. This is a constant finding in regions where trabecular bone predominates or there is abundant marrow. A bilateral symmetric appearance of these "pseudotumors" is important for differentiation from pathologic processes. At times, however, this differentiation may be difficult.

Figure 7–25B. An asymmetric appearance of the pseudotumors may indicate pathology. In this case, the asymmetry in the appearance of the sacral alae was the result of a typical pseudotumor on the left and a blastic prostate metastasis on the right.

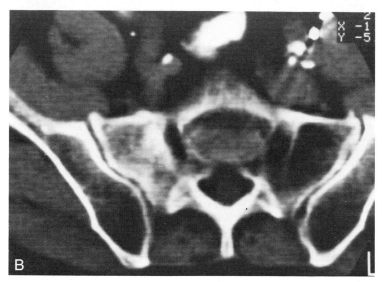

Figure 7–26. FIBROUS DYSPLASIA OF THE SACRUM. Fibrous dysplasia typically appears as a radiolucent lesion with a thick, sclerotic margin. Hazy, radiolucent, or radiopaque areas are often identified in the matrix, reflecting the fibrous and osseous components of the lesion. These characteristic findings are evident in both images shown.

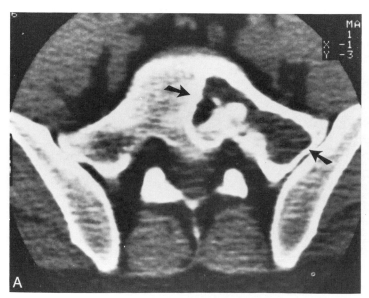

Figure 7–26A. CT scan of a patient with fibrous dysplasia *(arrows)* of the sacrum.

Illustration continued on opposite page

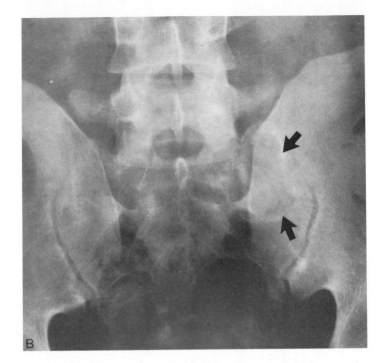

Figure 7–26B. The corresponding plain film of the patient shown in *A*.

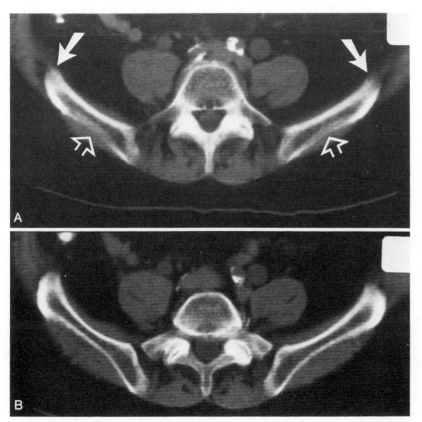

Figure 7–27. INDISTINCT BONY CORTICES. Ill-defined or indistinct bony cortices are commonly seen at muscular insertion sites. Examples of these indistinct cortices are demonstrated in *A*, at the crest of the ilium *(solid arrows)* where the musculus transversus abdominis inserts and along the posterior border of the ilium *(open arrowheads)* where the gluteus medius and maximus muscles originate. Consecutive scans, as in *B*, often demonstrate better definition of these areas. Characteristic locations and symmetry aid in distinguishing these normal areas from aggressive processes.

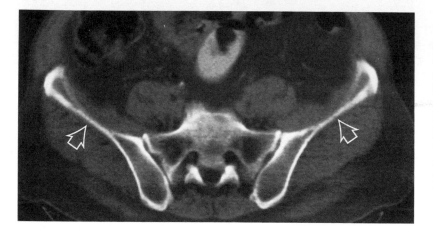

Figure 7–28. THINNING OF THE ILIAC FOSSA. An axial CT scan of the pelvis demonstrates marked thinning of each ilium in the region of the iliac fossae *(arrows)*. This can occur normally, and when bilateral and symmetric, this should not be interpreted as being pathologic. Note also the ill-defined cortex of each ilium in this region, resulting from the origin of the iliac muscles. Pseudotumors are also evident in both sacral alae.

Figure 7–29. PSEUDOTUMORS OF THE ILIUM. Prominent areas of low density *(arrows)* are identified in the iliac wings of this patient. Presumably these represent areas where marrow predominates over osseous tissue.

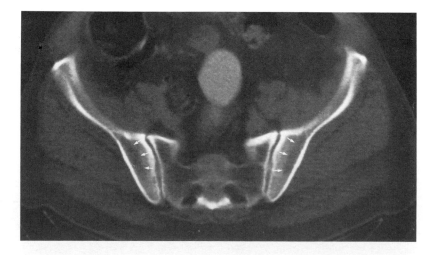

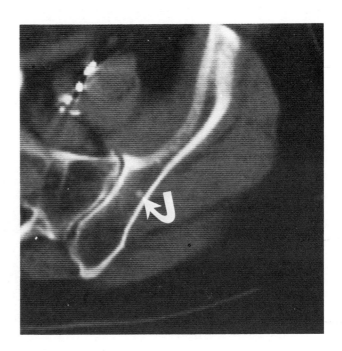

Figure 7–30. SOLITARY BONE ISLAND (ENOSTO-SIS). A small focal density is identified in the left ilium *(arrow)*. The well-defined nature and lack of bony destruction are typical of a bone island. Characteristic radiating bony spicules may be seen emanating from these lesions (not evident in this case). These may range in size from millimeters to centimeters. Bone islands of this size may not be evident on plain films. The ilium is one of the most common locations for these lesions.

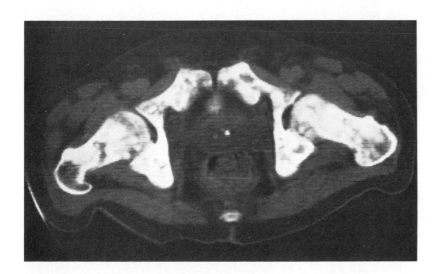

Figure 7–31. OSTEOPOIKILOSIS. Multiple round-to-ovoid sclerotic densities with a periarticular predilection are characteristic of this hereditary benign disorder. The symmetric distribution is also typical. The characteristic distribution and lack of increased activity on radionuclide examination aid in distinguishing this process from more aggressive lesions such as osteoblastic metastases.

Figure 7–32. **ACETABULAR ROOF AND ANTERIOR INFERIOR ILIAC SPINE.**

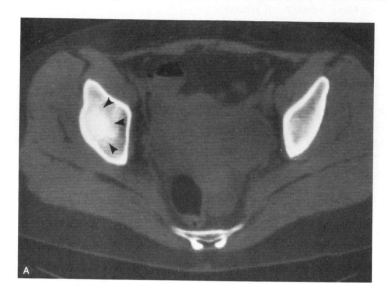

Figure 7–32A. A focal area of high density *(arrowheads)* is present in the body of the right ilium.

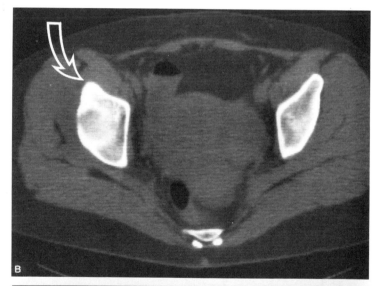

Figure 7–32B and C. Consecutive scans demonstrate this to be normal sclerosis of the acetabular roof, which is only partially imaged on the first scan. The rounded nature of the acetabular roof projects this density into the body of the ilium. When the patient is slightly tilted in the gantry (as in this case), these usually symmetric structures may appear asymmetric. The sclerotic anterior bony projection *(open arrows)* represents the anterior inferior iliac spine and should not be mistaken for osteophyte formation.

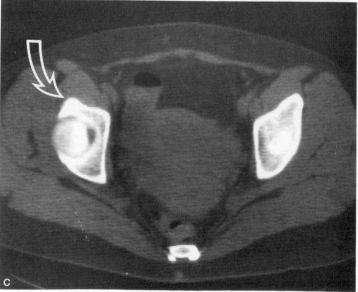

Figure 7–33. ACETABULAR NOTCH. Axial scans through the acetabula at different levels demonstrate the varying appearance of the acetabular notches *(arrows).*

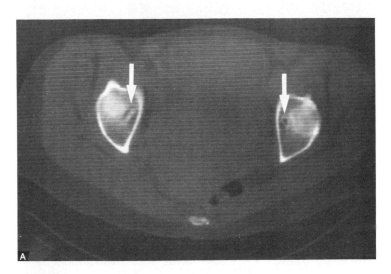

Figure 7–33A. The superior portions of the acetabular notches appear as low density "lesions" with sclerotic margins, on the medial portions of the ilia.

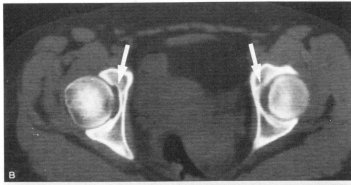

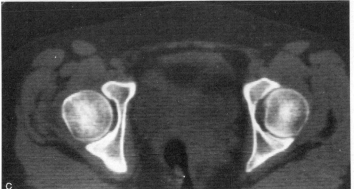

Figure 7–33B and C. Scans thru the mid- and lower portions of the acetabula demonstrate the more characteristic "notch" appearance.

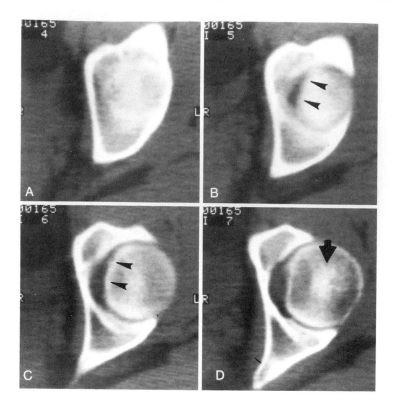

Figure 7–34. "FLATTENING" AND "SCLE-ROTIC" AREAS OF THE FEMORAL HEAD. Consecutive axial scans *(A–D)* through the superior portion of the left femur demonstrate apparent flattening *(arrowheads)* of the medial margin of the femoral head. This appearance can be encountered superior to the fovea. The presence of intact subarticular bone aids in excluding collapse of the articular surface or a compression fracture as a possible etiology of this flattening. Also seen in *D* is an area of high density or sclerosis *(arrow)* in the central portion of the femoral head. This is believed to represent the crossing of compressive and tensile trabeculae of the femoral neck. The characteristic location, absence of bony destruction, and lack of other lesions aid in ruling out a pathologic etiology.

Figure 7–35. FOVEA CAPITIS. The fovea capitis appears as a focal depression on the medial margin of the femoral head *(arrow)*. Due to asymmetric positioning of the patient, the fovea of the left femur is not seen on this CT section. The acetabular ligament attaches at the fovea. The location on the medial border near the acetabular notch is characteristic.

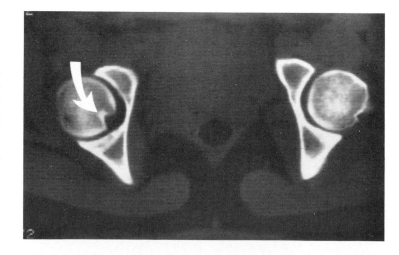

Figure 7–36. HERNIATION PITS.

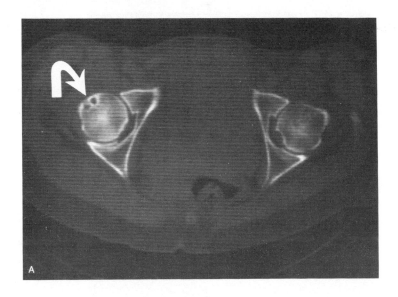

Figure 7–36A. Rounded, subcortical low densities with sclerotic margins *(arrow)* are characteristic of herniation pits. These typically occur in the femoral neck or at the junction of the femoral head and neck. Evidence shows that these subcortical pits result from herniation of synovium through the cortical bone. They occur with increasing frequency in older patients and are of no clinical significance.

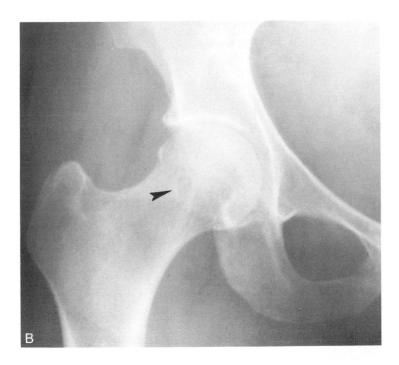

Figure 7–36B. The characteristic plain film appearance is demonstrated *(arrowhead)*.

Ref.: Pitt MJ, Graham AR, Shipman JH, et al. Herniation pit of the femoral neck. AJR 1982; 138:1115.

Figure 7–37. SUBCHONDRAL CYST.

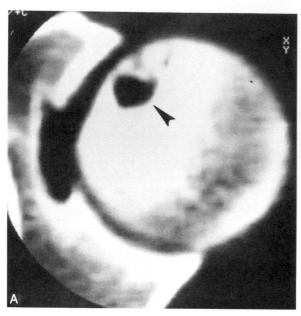

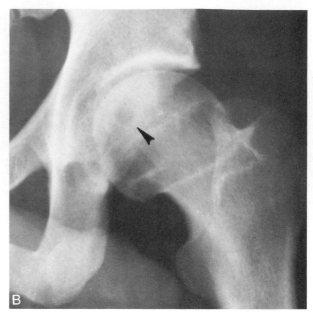

Figure 7–37A. A rounded, subarticular low density *(arrowhead)* with marked reactive sclerosis is seen on the medial portion of the femoral head. This is the typical appearance of a subchondral cyst, which is associated with degenerative joint disease in this patient. The subarticular location and marked reactive sclerosis, often associated with joint space narrowing, aid in distinguishing this benign lesion from a more aggressive process.

Figure 7–37B. Plain film of the same patient shown in A demonstrates the characteristic appearance of the subchondral cyst *(arrowhead).*

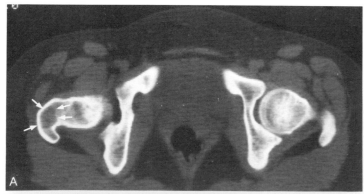

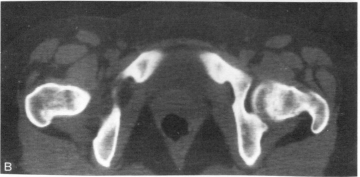

Figure 7–38. PSEUDOCYST OF THE GREATER TROCHANTER. An apparent low-density ''lesion'' is identified in the right greater trochanter *(arrows)* in A. Areas of low density can normally be found in this location, presumably as a result of porous spongiosa in the area of the pseudocyst. This is considered to be analogous to the pseudocyst seen in the greater tuberosity of the humerus. The lucency appears less pronounced away from the greater trochanter *(B).* This, along with the lack of cortical involvement, helps to differentiate these from more aggressive processes.

Figure 7–39. OSTEOCHONDROMAS OF THE FEMUR.

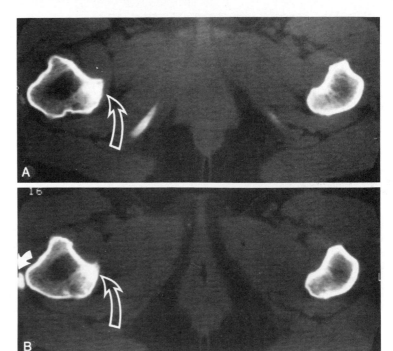

Figure 7–39A and B. Contiguous axial CT scans through the upper femora in a patient with multiple hereditary exostoses demonstrate an osteochondroma *(open arrows)* arising from the medial border of the right femur. Occasionally CT is used to differentiate these lesions from chondrosarcomas. CT characteristics of benign osteochondromas include a thin cartilaginous cap (less than 3 mm), cortex and medullary cavity continuity with parent bone, a peripheral solid cortex with central cancellous bone, and a matrix that is more dense at the periphery than the center. Note the top of another osteochondroma that is partially visualized lateral to the femur *(closed arrow).*

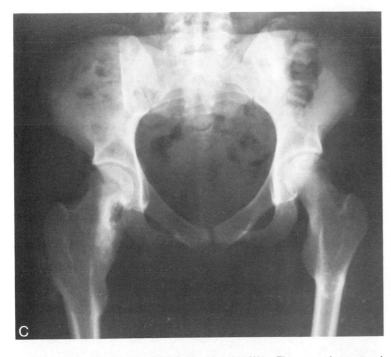

Figure 7–39C. An anteroposterior radiograph of the pelvis in this patient demonstrates the characteristic plain film appearance of these lesions.

Ref.: Kenny PJ, Gilula LA, Murphy WA. The use of computed tomography to distinguish osteochondroma and chondrosarcoma. Radiology 1981; 139:129–137.

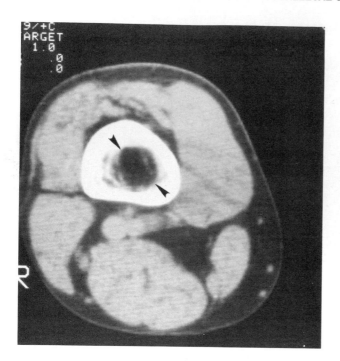

Figure 7–40. PSEUDOTUMOR OF THE DISTAL FE-MUR. A rounded lucency *(arrowheads)* is seen in the central portion of the distal femur. This is a common appearance of the medullary cavity with its fat-containing marrow. Lack of cortical involvement and symmetry with the other side aid in differentiating this from a pathologic process.

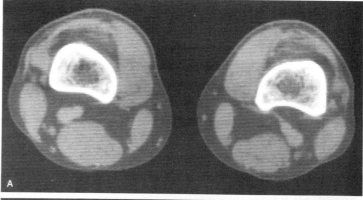

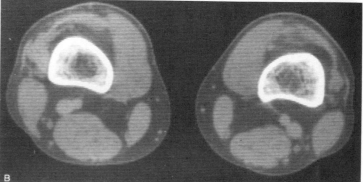

Figure 7–41. NORMAL TRABECULAR PAT-TERN OF THE DISTAL FEMUR. Contiguous axial CT sections *(A–B)* of the distal femora from caudad to cephalad demonstrate sparsity of trabeculae in the medullary portion of the bone. This is a common appearance encountered as one progresses from the metaphysis to the diaphysis. These central lucencies, when symmetric, should not be misconstrued as representing a marrow-infiltrative process.

Figure 7–42. NON-OSSIFYING FIBROMA.

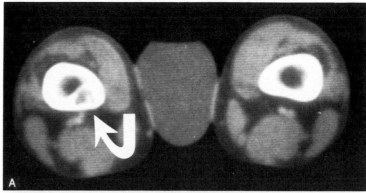

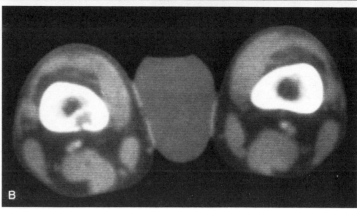

Figure 7–42A and B. Contiguous axial CT scans through the distal femora in a young patient demonstrate a well-circumscribed cortical lucency on the right *(arrow)*. The lack of medullary or soft tissue involvement suggests a benign process, although the CT findings are not diagnostic.

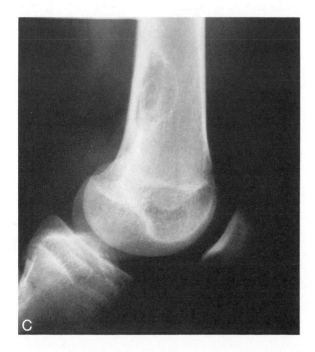

Figure 7–42C. Lateral radiograph of the knee in the same patient as in *A* demonstrates the typical appearance of a non-ossifying fibroma. In the evaluation of bony lesions, it is often necessary to correlate CT findings with plain films to arrive at the correct diagnosis.

Figure 7–43. MUSCLE INSERTION SITES. On contiguous axial CT scans (*A* and *B*) through the distal femora, the cortex often appears ill-defined or irregular at the sites of major muscle insertions *(arrowheads)*. Before these areas are deemed abnormal, other findings such as soft-tissue or medullary changes and lack of symmetry should be present.

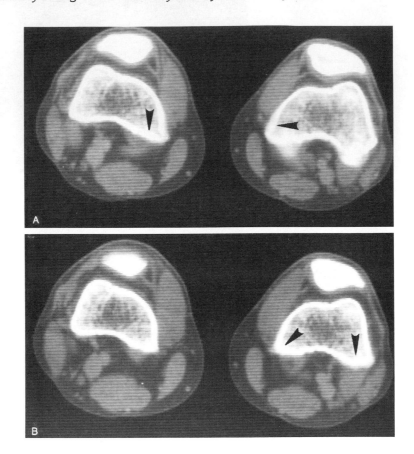

Figure 7–44. ATYPICAL POPLITEAL CYST OF THE KNEE.

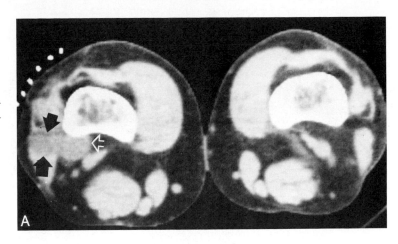

Figure 7–44A. CT scan through the distal femora shows a soft-tissue density *(arrows)* posterolateral to the right femur.

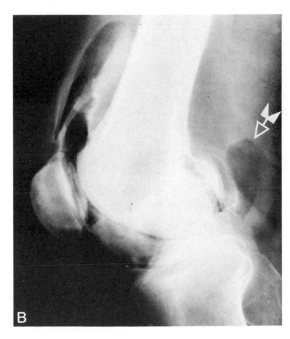

Figure 7–44B. Arthrogram of the right knee shows an atypical popliteal cyst *(arrow)* extending superiorly, which accounted for the soft-tissue mass seen in A. Occasionally, atypical popliteal cysts are seen around the knee and should be considered when soft-tissue masses are seen in this region on CT.

Ref. Shepherd JR, Helms CA. Atypical popliteal cyst due to lateral synovial herniation. Radiology 1981; 140:66. Figure 7–44A reprinted with permission.

Figure 7–45. REMNANT OF THE GROWTH PLATE.

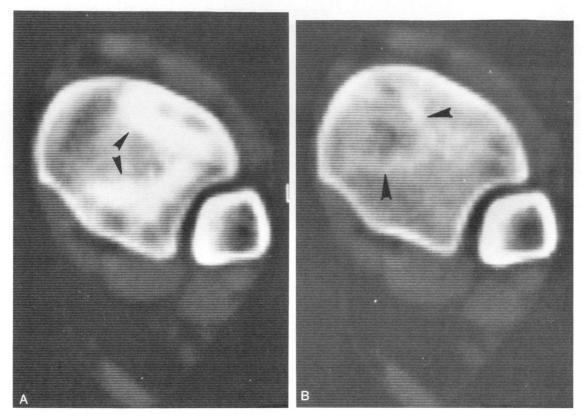

Figure 7–45A and B. Axial scans through the distal left tibia/fibula demonstrate ill-defined sclerotic and lucent areas in the medullary portion of the tibia *(arrowheads)*. When "lesions" such as this are encountered near the ends of a long bone (particularly in younger patients), consideration should be given to their representing remnants of the growth plate, as in this case.

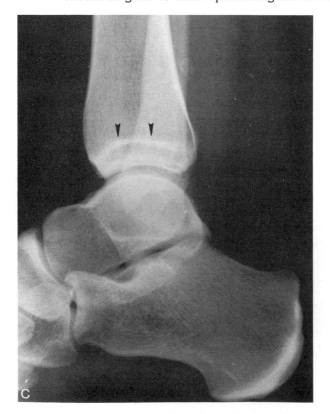

Figure 7–45C. Lateral radiograph of the ankle confirms the presence of growth plate remnants *(arrowheads)* in the distal tibia at the level of CT scanning.

Figure 7–46. PLAFOND OF THE TIBIA.

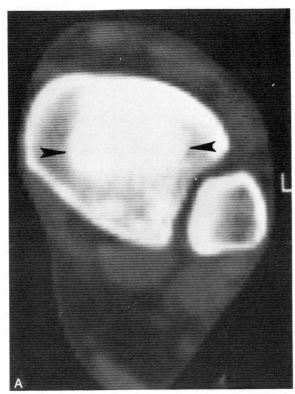

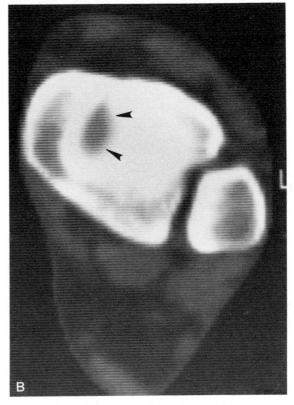

Figure 7–46A. An axial CT section taken at the level of the distal tibial articular surface (plafond) has produced the appearance of a sclerotic lesion in the medullary portion of the tibia *(arrowheads)*. This is a result of partial volume averaging of the undulating articular surface.

Figure 7–46B. On a contiguous caudal section, the joint space *(arrowheads)* becomes evident, confirming that the sclerotic "lesion," in fact, represents the normal subarticular sclerosis of the tibial plafond.

Figure 7–47. ACCESSORY MUSCLE OF THE LOWER CALF. On this CT image of the ankle (at the level of the talus), an asymmetric soft-tissue mass *(arrow)* is identified in the pre–Achilles fat pad on the left. This is a normal variant known as an accessory muscle of the lower calf. These muscles cover the posterior tibial neurovascular bundle and may be unilateral as in this case or bilateral.

Ref.: Nidecker AC, von Hochstetter A, Fredenhagen H. Accessory muscles of the lower calf. Radiology 1984; 151:47–48.

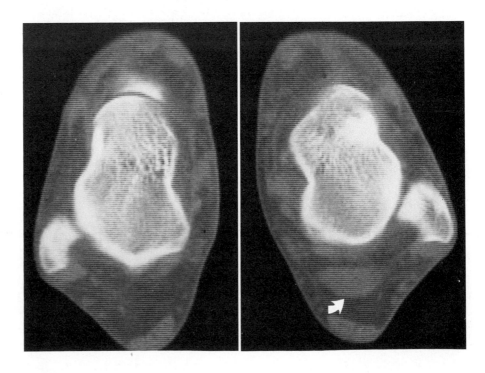

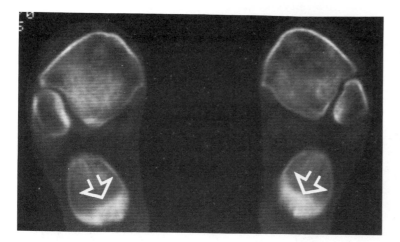

Figure 7–48. ACHILLES TENDON INSERTIONS. On this axial CT scan through the proximal portions of both feet, ill-defined and irregular cortices *(arrows)* are identified in the posterior portions of both calcanei. These represent the insertion sites of the respective Achilles tendons. Cortical involvement by a pathologic process in these locations would be difficult to assess. Lack of symmetry or the presence of soft-tissue changes would be important in identifying pathology.

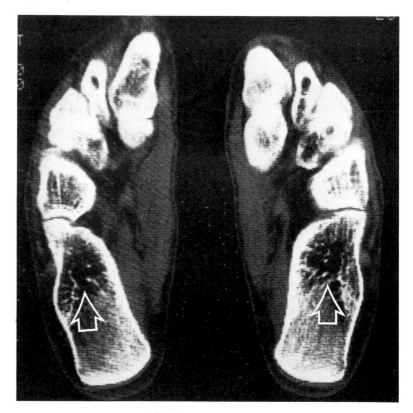

Figure 7–49. PSEUDOCYST OF THE CALCANEUS. An axial CT section through the feet demonstrates prominent lucencies *(arrows)* in both calcanei. These are well-known normal plain film variants and are due to the normal arrangement of the trabecular pattern in this area. The lack of well-defined walls around the lucencies helps to differentiate them from true calcaneal cysts.

Ref.: Keats TE. Atlas of Normal Roentgen Variants, 3rd ed. Chicago: Year Book Medical Publishers, 1984; p 570.

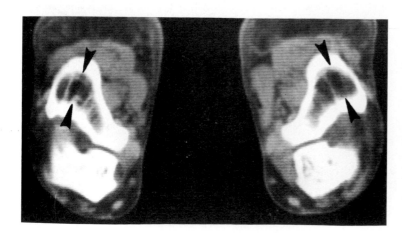

Figure 7–50. PSEUDOTUMOR OF THE TALUS. Axial CT scan taken at the level of the mid-body of the talus in both feet demonstrates prominent lucencies in both talar bones *(arrowheads)*. These lucencies are common findings in the tarsal bones and probably result from the predominance of spongy bone in these structures. Symmetry and the absence of cortical or trabecular bone destruction aid in the exclusion of pathologic etiologies.

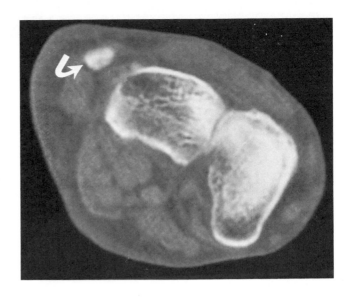

Figure 7–51. ACCESSORY NAVICULAR. Axial CT image through the mid-portion of the left foot demonstrates a rounded, bony density *(arrow)* medial to the tarsal navicular. This represents an accessory navicular. Sesamoid and supernumerary bones are common in the foot. The location, appearance, and lack of donor site are keys in differentiating these from avulsion fractures.

Figure 7–52. ILL-DEFINED CORTICAL MARGINS.

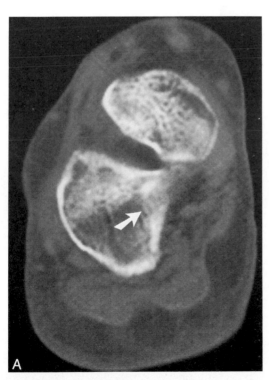

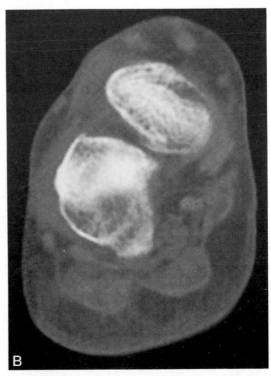

Figure 7–52A. Axial CT section of the foot at the level of the distal calcaneus and talus shows an ill-defined area of cortex along the medial border of the calcaneus *(arrow).* This is a common finding in the tarsus and is believed to result from a number of causes including the undulating nature of the tarsal margins, partial volume averaging, and the numerous sites of ligament and tendon insertions. These areas can be confused with sites of fibrous tarsal coalitions.

Figure 7–52B. A contiguous CT section demonstrates that the cortical margin is intact.

**Figure 7–53. MEDIAL ANTERIOR MENISCUS DISPLACEMENT IN THE TEMPOROMAN-
DIBULAR JOINT.**

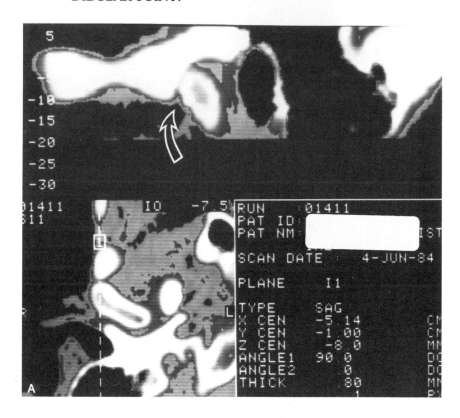

Figure 7–53A. Sagittal reformations through the lateral pole of the right mandibular condyle show no increased soft-tissue density anteriorly *(arrow)*. This would indicate no anteriorly displaced meniscus.

Figure 7–53B. When the reformation is performed through the medial pole of the right mandibular condyle, a definite increased soft-tissue density *(arrow)* is seen anterior to the condyle. This indicates that an anteriorly displaced meniscus is indeed present. As most menisci displace in a medial direction, care should be taken to closely examine the medial pole; otherwise, a displaced meniscus could be missed.

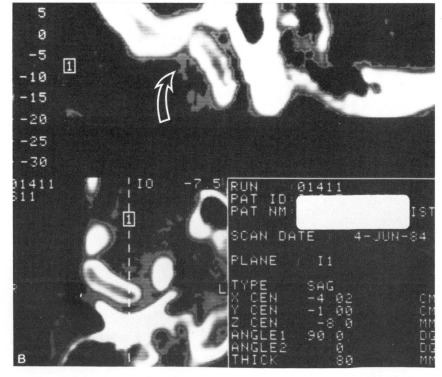

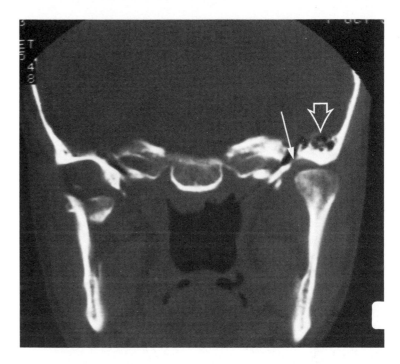

Figure 7–54. SQUAMOTYMPANIC FIS-SURE. Coronal CT scan of the temporomandibular joints in a patient with a fracture of the right mandibular condyle shows apparent thinning of the roof of the left glenoid fossa *(solid arrow)*. This is actually the squamotympanic fissure, a normal anatomic structure. Note also the pneumatization *(open arrow)* extending into the left temporal bone, which can be a normal finding.

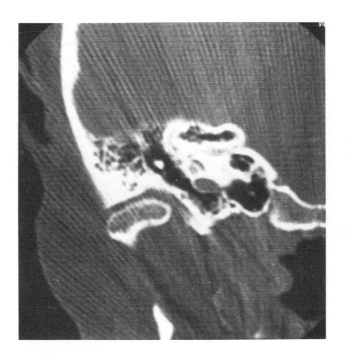

Figure 7–55. STREAK ARTIFACTS SECONDARY TO DENTAL FILLINGS. Coronal CT scan of the right temporomandibular joint shows multiple streak artifacts secondary to dental fillings. This is frequent problem with coronal scans and can be seen also in direct sagittal scans of the temporomandibular joint.

Figure 7–56. EFFECT OF BLINK-MODE WINDOW ON VISUALIZATION OF MENISCUS IN THE TEMPOROMANDIBULAR JOINT.

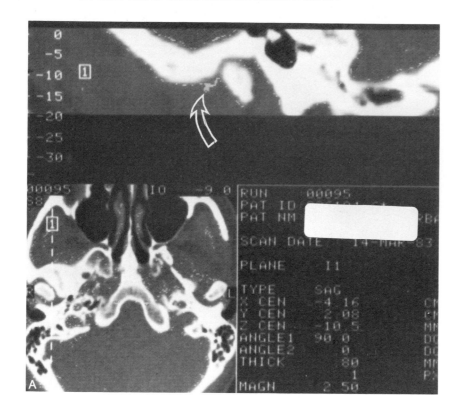

Figure 7–56A. Sagittal reformation of the right temporomandibular joint shows an anteriorly displaced meniscus *(arrow)*, which is indistinct at a narrow blink-mode window setting (9).

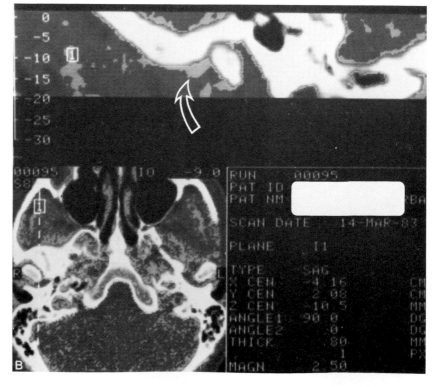

Figure 7–56B. When the blink-mode window is widened to 75, the increased soft-tissue density *(arrow)* is more easily seen than in *A*. If a narrow blink-mode window setting is used, a false-negative reading may result.

Figure 7–57. FALSE-NEGATIVE TEMPOROMANDIBULAR JOINT CT SCAN.

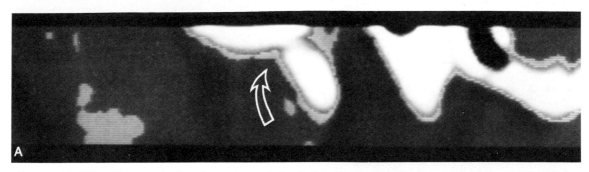

Figure 7–57A. This sagittal reformation of the left temporomandibular joint shows no definite increased soft-tissue density anterior to the condyle at a blink-mode level of approximately 130 HU. The clinical examination did not agree; therefore, an arthrogram was performed, and it showed a definite anteriorly displaced meniscus.

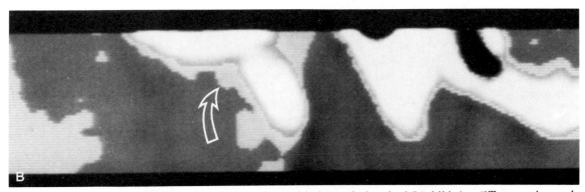

Figure 7–57B. The data was reviewed, and at a blink-mode level of 90 HU the CT scan showed a definite increased soft-tissue density *(arrow)* which conformed to the displaced meniscus evident on the arthrogram. This illustrates that low blink-mode levels (80–120 HU) should be used in searching for displaced menisci, in order to avoid false-negative results.

CHAPTER 8

Pediatrics

CHARLES M. GLASIER, M.D.
JAMES R. McCONNELL, M.D.

Figure 8–1. NORMAL VISUALIZATION OF THE FALX CEREBRI. In this 10-year-old girl with migraine-type headaches, cranial CT shows normal visualization of the falx as a linear high-density structure *(arrow).* This finding should not be confused with subarachnoid hemorrhage when seen on an image generated by a modern CT scanner. (Case courtesy of H. Lynn Magill, M.D., Memphis, Tenn.)

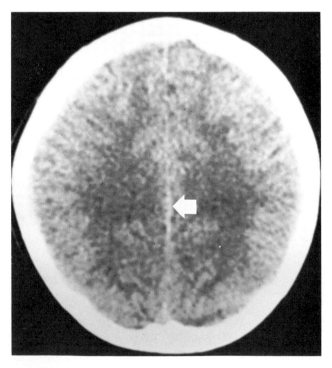

Ref.: Osborn AG, Anderson RE, Wing SD. The false falx sign. Radiology 1980; 134:421–425.

Figure 8–2. METRIZAMIDE OBSCURING METASTATIC BRAIN LESIONS.

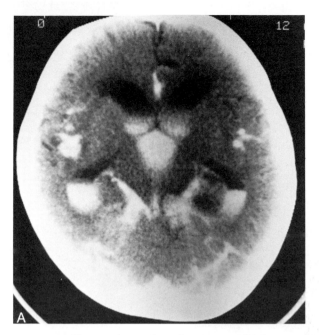

Figure 8–2A. CT post-metrizamide myelography obscures multiple metastatic lesions of neuroblastoma.

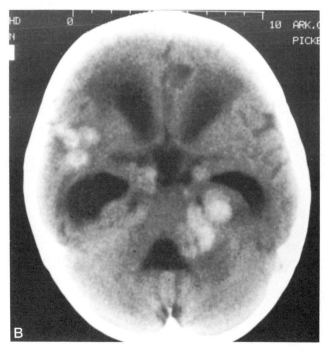

Figure 8–2B. The lesions are clearly seen on this repeat scan made two weeks later, following clearing of metrizamide.

Figure 8–3. NORMALLY HYPERDENSE TENTORIAL VENOUS PLEXUS.

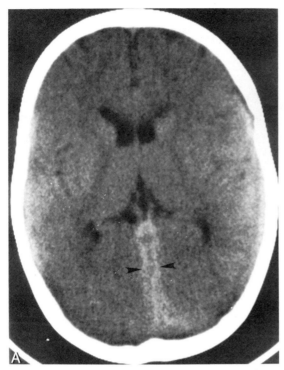

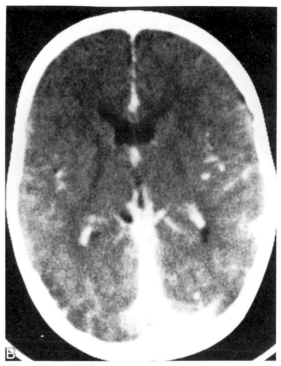

Figure 8–3A. This non-enhanced CT scan shows a dense linear structure *(arrowheads).*

Figure 8–3B. On a post-contrast CT scan this structure is shown to represent a normal vein of Galen and straight sinus. This normal finding should not be confused with subarachnoid or subdural hemorrhage.

Figure 8–4. BENIGN ENLARGEMENT OF THE SUBARACHNOID SPACE.

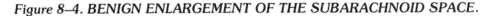

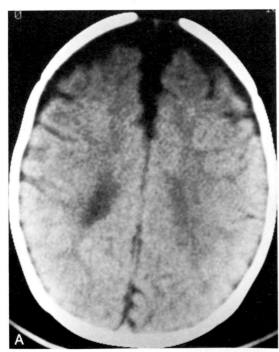

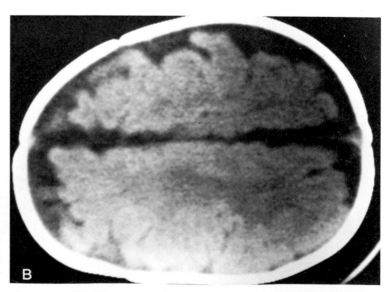

Figure 8–4A. CT scan of a developmentally normal infant with a large head shows prominent extracerebrospinal fluid.

Figure 8–4B. Gravitational view with the infant on the right side shows displacement of the fluid. This is a frequently encountered problem of differentiation of subdural hygroma from subarachnoid fluid. A loculated hygroma would not be expected to disappear with simple changes in patient postion.

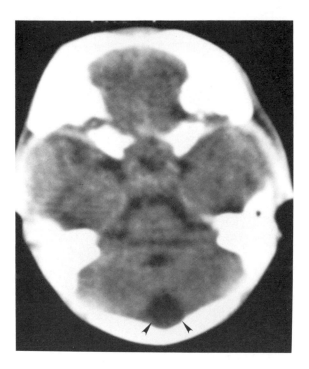

Figure 8–5. PROMINENT CISTERNA MAGNA. This normal cerebrospinal fluid space *(arrowheads)* may be very large and asymmetric and should not be confused with a Dandy-Walker malformation or a posterior fossa subarachnoid cyst, both of which are usually associated with obstructive hydrocephalus. (Case courtesy of H. Lynn Magill, M.D., Memphis, Tenn.)

Ref.: Just NWM, Goldenberg M. Computed tomography of the enlarged cisterna magna. Radiology 1979; 131:385–391.

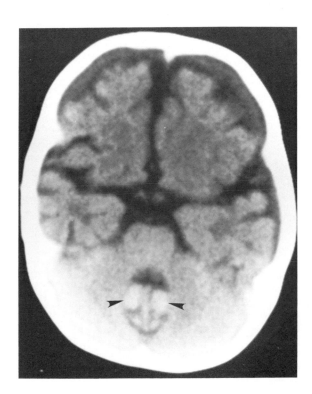

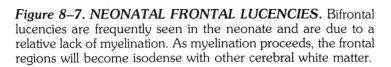

Figure 8–6. PROMINENT NORMAL CEREBELLAR TON- SILS AND NODULUS. The cerebellar tonsils *(arrowheads)* and nodulus appear prominent on this scan and, as in this case, may have higher density than adjacent structures.

Figure 8–7. NEONATAL FRONTAL LUCENCIES. Bifrontal lucencies are frequently seen in the neonate and are due to a relative lack of myelination. As myelination proceeds, the frontal regions will become isodense with other cerebral white matter.

Ref.: Brant-Zawadski M, Enzmann DR. Using computed tomography to correlate low white matter attenuation with early gestational age in neonates. Radiology 1981; 139:105.

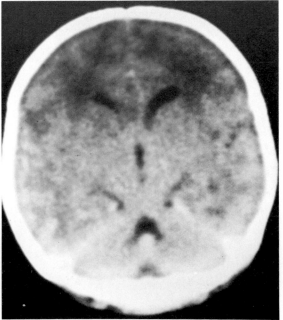

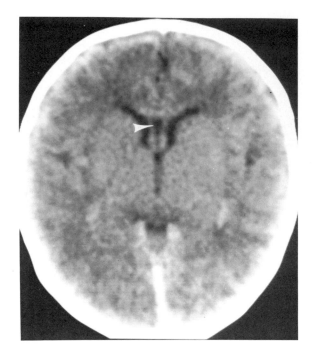

Figure 8–8. CAVUM SEPTI PELLUCIDI. This cerebrospinal fluid–filled space *(arrowhead)* between the leaves of the septum pellucidum is very frequently seen in childhood, especially in pre-term neonates. (Case courtesy of H. Lynn Magill, M.D., Memphis, Tenn.)

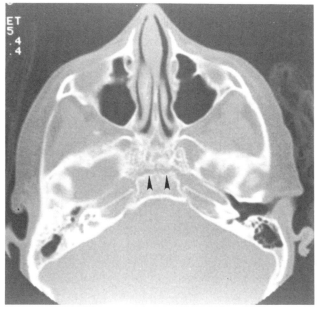

Figure 8–9. SPHENOOCCIPITAL SYNCHONDROSIS. The normal sphenooccipital synchondrosis *(arrowheads)* is seen as a horizontal lucency, frequently with well-corticated margins, joining the body of the sphenoid with the basiocciput. It should not be confused with a basilar skull fracture.

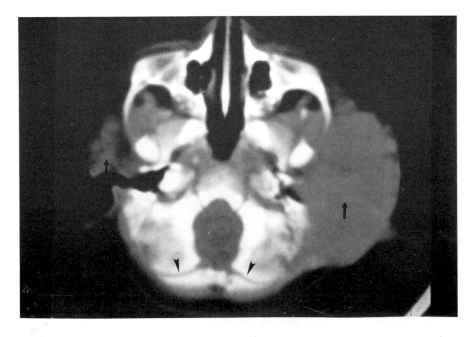

Figure 8–10. OCCIPITAL SYNCHONDROSES. Normal synchondroses *(arrowheads)* between ex-occipital and supra-occipital bones are clearly seen in this infant with multiple facial hemangiomas *(arrows)*.

Ref.: Caffey J. Pediatric X-ray Diagnosis. Chicago: Year Book Medical Publishers, 1978; p 10.

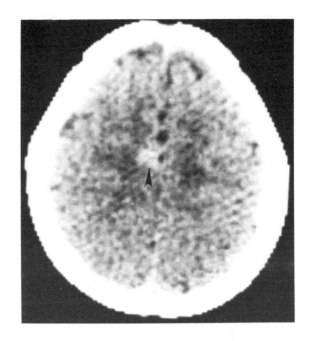

Figure 8–11. DETECTOR ERROR: PSEUDOHEMOR-RHAGE. CT section of the brain of an abused child shows an apparent high-density lesion *(arrowhead)* in the parafalcine cortex. Presence of this artifact on multiple slices and in multiple patients allows recognition of this technical problem.

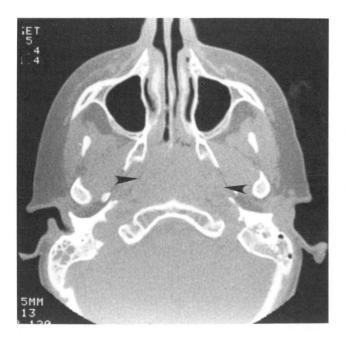

Figure 8–12. PROMINENT ADENOIDS. Normal adenoidal tissue *(arrowheads)* may simulate a nasopharyngeal mass in young children. Correlation with lateral neck films, fluoroscopy, or barium swallow studies may be necessary to exclude a pathologic mass.

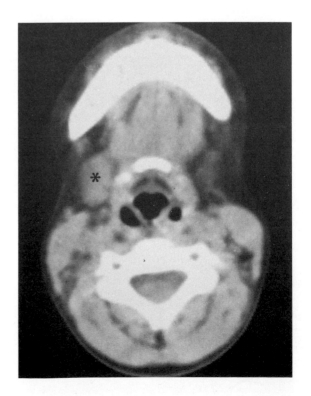

Figure 8–13. HEAD TILT: PSEUDOMASS. A normal right submandibular gland *(asterisk)* can simulate adenopathy or other mass when asymmetry results from a slight head tilt. Sedation may be necessary to assure proper neck positioning even in children who are usually cooperative.

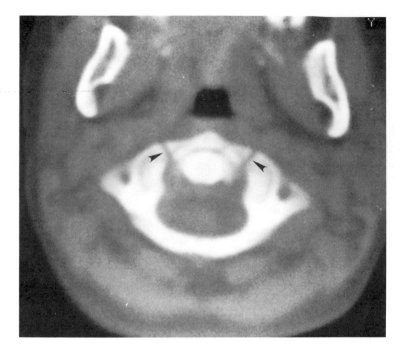

Figure 8–14. NEUROCENTRAL SYNCHONDROSIS (C1). These normal synchondroses *(arrowheads)* were initially mistaken for ring fractures in this child who had severe head trauma. The bilateral symmetry and smooth, straight margins of the synchondroses allow recognition of these normal developmental structures.

Ref.: Caffey J. Pediatric X-ray Diagnosis. Chicago: Year Book Medical Publishers, 1978; p 274.

Figure 8–15. NORMAL BIFID ODONTOID PROCESS. Axial CT scan through the body of C1 and the odontoid shows two bony densities *(arrows)* posterior to the anterior arch of C1 that are the tops of the V-shaped apex of the main mass of the odontoid. A cephalad section would show a single density of the "summit" ossification center when present. Complete ossification to adult configuration occurs by the age 11 to 12 years. (Case courtesy of H. Lynn Magill, M.D., Memphis, Tenn.)

Ref.: Caffey J. Pediatric X-ray Diagnosis. Chicago: Year Book Medical Publishers, 1978; p 274.

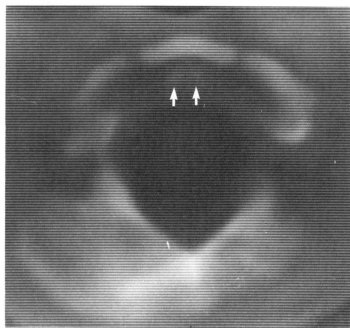

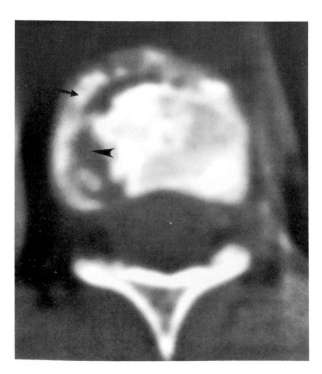

Figure 8–16. SCHMORL'S NODE/RING APOPHYSIS. This CT scan of a lower thoracic vertebral body shows an irregular end plate due to disc protrusion *(arrowhead)* and irregular ossification of normal ring apophysis *(arrow).* Correlation with plain films or tomography is important to exclude pathology. (Case courtesy of H. Lynn Magill, M.D., Memphis, Tenn.)

Figure 8–17. ENLARGED ASCENDING LUMBAR VEINS.

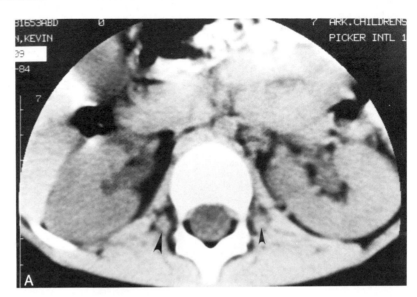

Figure 8–17A. CT section shows apparent paraspinous masses *(arrowheads)* in a child with obstruction of the inferior vena cava at the level of the liver.

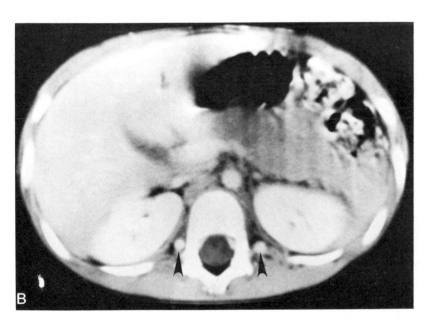

Figure 8–17B. This contrast-enhanced scan demonstrates that the "masses" shown in *A* represent enlarged ascending lumbar veins *(arrowheads)*.

Figure 8–18. DOUBLE AORTIC ARCH: ADOLESCENT.

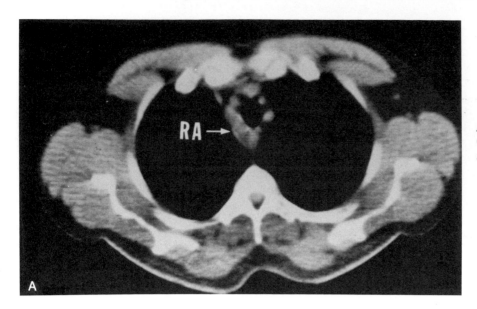

Figure 8–18A. Contrast-enhanced CT study shows a high right aortic arch (RA) on the first section.

Figure 8–18B. A lower left aortic arch (LA) on the second section is seen encircling the trachea and esophagus. In this case, the patient had a very loose vascular ring and was asymptomatic. (Case contributed by Dr. Ina Tonkin, Memphis, Tenn., through H. Lynn Magill, M.D., and Anthony Proto, M.D., Lackland Air Force Base, San Antonio, Tex.)

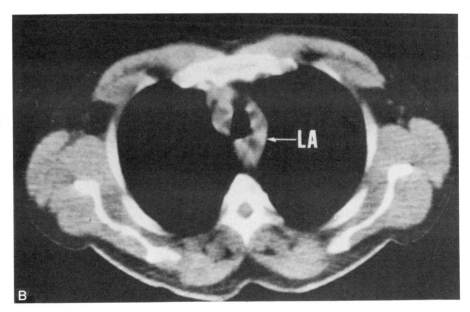

From: Tonkin ILD. Vascular compression of the trachea and esophagus: Newer imaging techniques. In: Margulis AR, Gooding CA, eds. Diagnostic Radiology, 1983; p 38. San Francisco: University of California Press, 1983. Copyright 1983, University of California. Reprinted by permission of the publisher.

Figure 8–19. DOUBLE AORTIC ARCH: INFANT. Computed tomography with contrast enhancement was performed on a 21-month-old male infant with a double aortic arch.

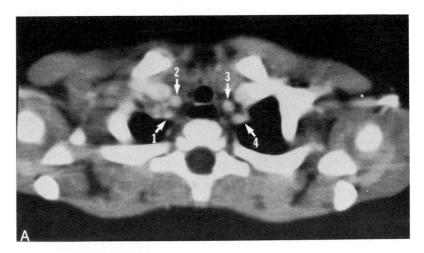

Figure 8–19A. This image shows the four major arteries grouped around the trachea (4 artery sign): (1) right subclavian artery, (2) right carotid artery, (3) left carotid artery, and (4) left subclavian artery.

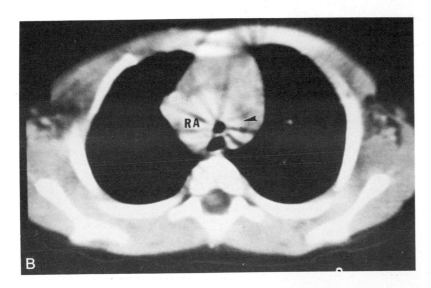

Figure 8–19B. A subsequent caudal cross section shows a large right arch component (RA) with some compression of the trachea and esophagus. Note the presence of the smaller left aortic arch *(arrowhead).*

Figure 8–19C. Another caudal cross section more completely demonstrates the double aortic arch with tracheal and esophageal compression. A large right arch component (RA) and the smaller left arch component (LA) are again noted. (Case courtesy of Ina Tonkin, M.D., LeBonheur Children's Medical Center and the University of Tennessee Center for the Health Sciences, Memphis, Tenn.)

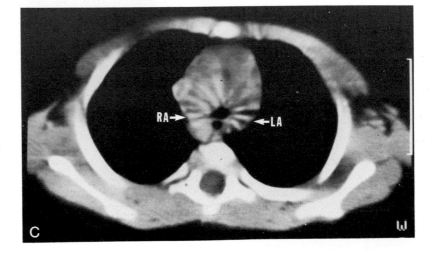

Figure 8–20. LEFT SUPERIOR VENA CAVA.

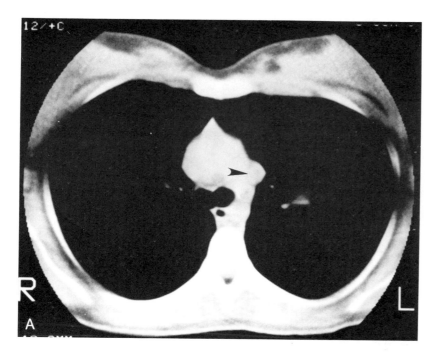

Figure 8–20A. CT scan demonstrates an apparent left-sided mediastinal mass *(arrowhead)* in an adolescent with a left bronchogenic cyst.

Figure 8–20B. On a dynamic CT image, the apparent mass *(arrowhead)* is proved to represent persistence of the left superior vena cava. The tubular nature of the structure and contrast enhancement ensures the diagnosis.

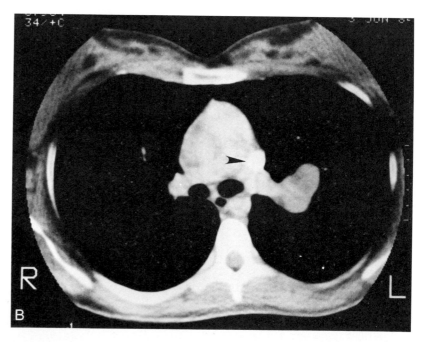

Ref.: Huggins TJ, Lesar ML, Friedman AC, et al. CT appearance of persistent left superior vena cava. J Comput Assist Tomogr 1982; 6:294–297.

Figure 8–21. PULMONARY ARTERY SLING. This contrast-enhanced CT shows the main pulmonary artery (PA) with normal origin of the right pulmonary artery (RPA). An anomalous left pulmonary artery (LPA) arises from the right pulmonary artery and crosses posteriorly to the trachea to the left lung. The ascending aorta (AA) and the descending aorta (DA) are identified. Because of the high incidence of associated congenital heart disease with this lesion, cardiac catheterization and pulmonary arteriography are indicated. (Case courtesy of Ina Tonkin, M.D., LeBonheur Children's Medical Center, Memphis, Tenn., and Bennett Alford, M.D., University of Virginia Medical Center, Charlottesville, Va.)

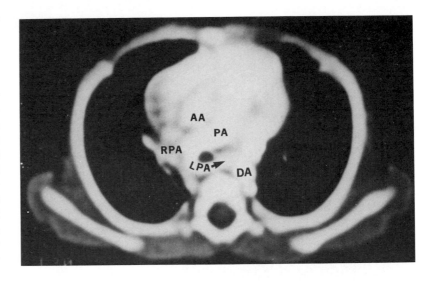

From: Rheuben KS, Ayres N, Still JG, Alford B. Pulmonary artery sling: A new diagnostic tool and clinical review. Pediatrics 1982; 69:472–475. Copyright 1982 by American Academy of Pediatrics. Reprinted by permission of the publisher.

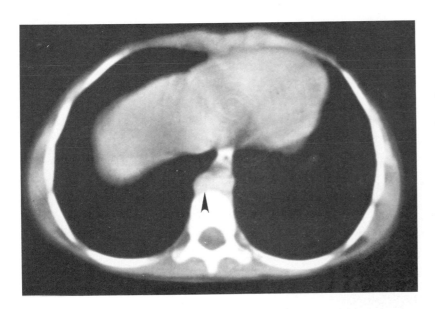

Figure 8–22. AZYGOUS CONTINUATION OF INFERIOR VENA CAVA. The enlarged azygous vein *(arrowhead)* should not be mistaken for retrocarinal adenopathy. Recognition of the density as a tubular structure on contiguous or contrast-enhanced scans establishes the diagnosis. (Case courtesy of Marilyn J. Siegel, M.D., St. Louis, Mo.)

Ref.: Breckenridge JW, Kinlaw WB. Azygous continuation of inferior vena cava: CT appearance. J Comput Assist Tomogr 1980; 4:392–397.

Figure 8–23. ABERRANT RIGHT SUBCLAVIAN ARTERY.

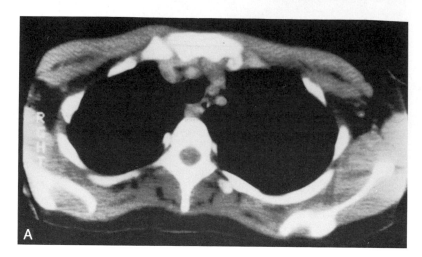

Figure 8–23A. This CT scan of a teenage girl shows normal brachiocephalic vessels with two jugular veins and three great vessels. The esophagus is also visualized.

Figure 8–23B. A contrast-enhanced scan at the same level as A shows large jugular veins *(straight arrows)* with three great vessels. The last branch, which is retro-esophageal, is the aberrant right subclavian artery *(curved arrow).*

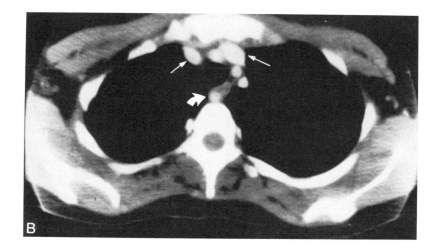

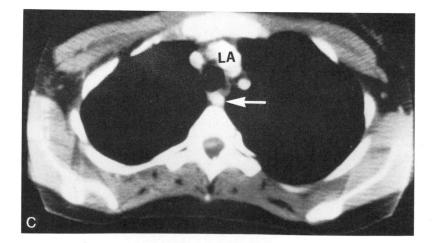

Figure 8–23C. At a lower plane of section, a left aortic arch (LA) is evident with an aberrant retroesophageal vessel *(arrow),* which represents an anomalous right sub-clavian artery. This vessel is passing posterior to the esophagus to reach the right upper extremity.

(Case courtesy of Ina Tonkin, M.D., LeBonheur Children's Medical Center, Memphis, Tenn., and Saskia Hilton, M.D., University of California Medical Center, San Diego, Cal.)

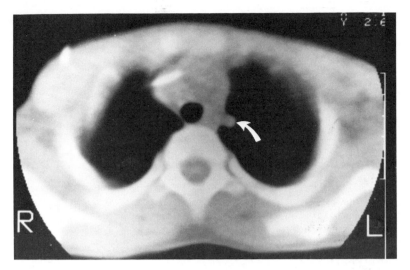

Figure 8–24. LEFT SUBCLAVIAN AR-TERY. The left subclavian artery *(arrow)* as it rises superiorly and laterally over the left pulmonary apex may be surrounded by lung and appear prominent.

Ref.: Zylak CJ, Pallie W, Jackson R. Correlative anatomy and computed tomography: A nodule on the mediastinum. Radiographics 1982; 2:555.

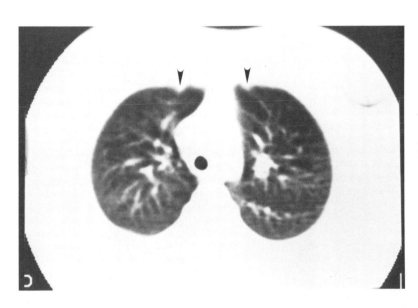

Figure 8–25. INTERNAL MAMMARY VESSELS. Normal internal mammary vessels *(arrowheads)* are seen in a paramedian location bilaterally. Symmetry, small size, and characteristic location prevent confusion with subpleural metastases or adenopathy.

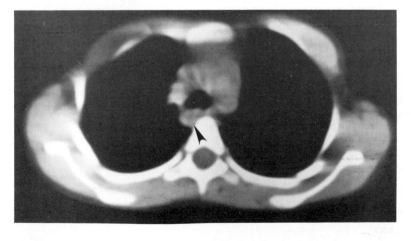

Figure 8–26. ENLARGED AZYGOS VEIN. Prominent azygos vein *(arrowhead)* simulates a posterior mediastinal mass in this child with azygos continuation of the inferior vena cava. (Case courtesy of Marilyn J. Siegel, M.D., St. Louis, Mo.)

Ref.: Webb WR, Gamsu G, Speckman JM. Computed tomographic demonstration of mediastinal venous anomalies. AJR 1982; 139:157–161.

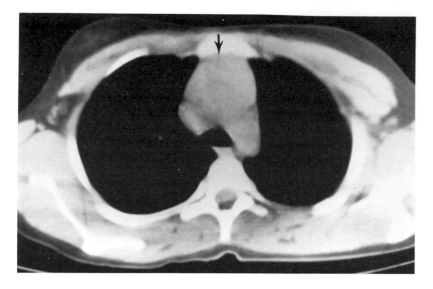

Figure 8–27. PROMINENT NORMAL THYMUS. In a 12-year-old girl with fever and suspected lymphoma, a prominent anterior cleft *(arrow)* is present. An anterior cleft separating left from right lobes is frequently present on CT in the normal thymus. (Case courtesy of Donald R. Kirks, M.D., Durham, N.C.)

Refs.: (1) Moore AV, Korobkin M, Olanow W, et al. Age-related changes in the thymus gland: CT–pathologic correlation. AJR 1983; 141:241–246. (2) Baron RL, Lee JKT, Sagel SS, Peterson RR. Computed tomography of the normal thymus. Radiology 1982; 142:121–125. (3) Heiberg E, Wolverson MK, Sundaram M, et al. Normal thymus, CT characteristics in subjects under age 20. AJR 1982; 138:491–494.

Figure 8–28. POSTERIOR MEDIAS-TINAL THYMUS. Normal thymic tissue extends into the posterior mediastinum in this neonate *(arrowhead).* Similar density to that of the more normally situated thymus anteriorly and lack of a mass effect are useful in distinguishing normal thymic tissue from neoplasm.

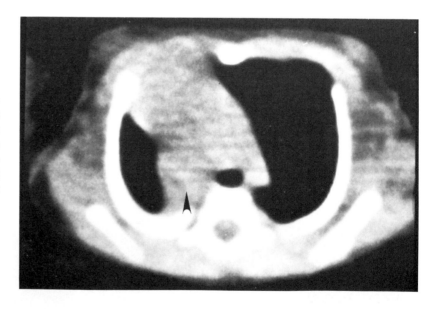

Ref.: Cohen MD, Weber TR, Sequeira FW, et al. Diagnostic dilemma of the posterior mediastinal thymus: CT manifestation. Radiology 1983; 146:691–692.

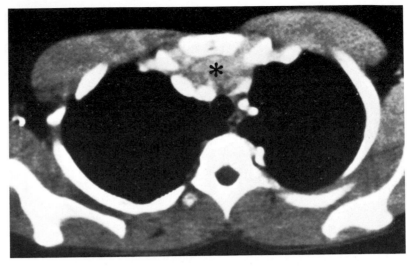

Figure 8–29. MASS-LIKE THYMUS. This surgically proven prominent normal thymus *(asterisk)* is displacing the contrast-enhanced great vessels. When mass effect with vessel or bronchial displacement is present, differentiation of prominent or ectopically placed thymic tissue from neoplasm by CT may be difficult or impossible. (Case courtesy of Donald R. Kirks, M.D., Durham, N.C.)

Ref.: Shackelford GD, McAlister WH. The aberrantly positioned thymus: A cause of mediastinal or neck masses in children. AJR 1974; 120:291–296.

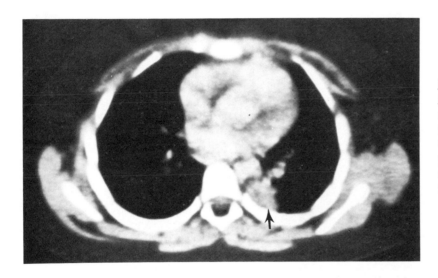

Figure 8–30. PSEUDOTUMOR: PNEUMONIA. Apparent posterior mediastinal mass *(arrow)* was demonstrated on chest radiography (not shown) and CT. Follow-up chest radiograph was normal. "Round pneumonia" should be considered in any small child with a suspected pulmonary or mediastinal mass.

Figure 8–31. ATELECTASIS: APPARENT PULMONARY CAVITY. Peripheral atelectasis *(arrowhead)* in this infant with mediastinal extension of cervical hemangioma *(arrow)* simulates a cavitary pulmonary lesion. Correlation with conventional chest radiography is essential to document the transient nature of atelectasis.

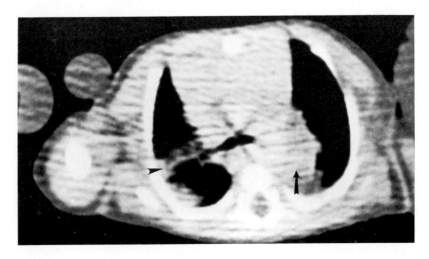

Figure 8–32. CROWDED BASILAR VESSELS SIMULATING NODULES.

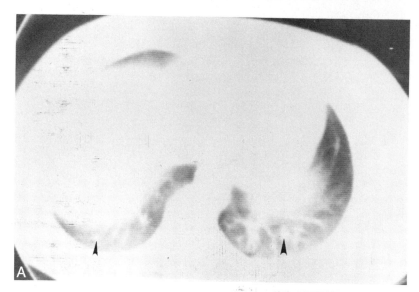

Figure 8–32A. Initial CT scan in expiration shows apparent basilar densities interpreted as nodules *(arrowheads)*.

Figure 8–32B. A scan taken later on the same day in inspiration is normal. (Case courtesy of Marilyn J. Siegel, M.D., St. Louis, Mo.)

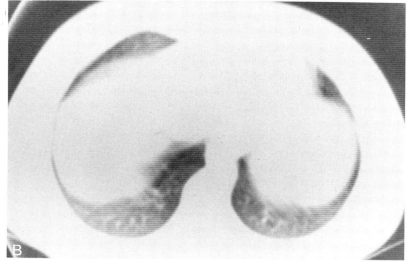

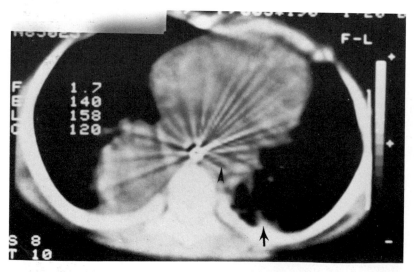

Figure 8–33. BASILAR ATELECTASIS. At surgery, apparent extension across midline *(arrowhead)* of a right posterior mediastinal neuroblastoma was not present. The left "pseudomass" was apparently due to atelectasis. Note peripheral strand of subsegmental atelectasis *(arrow)*, which is a clue to the etiology of this pseudomass.

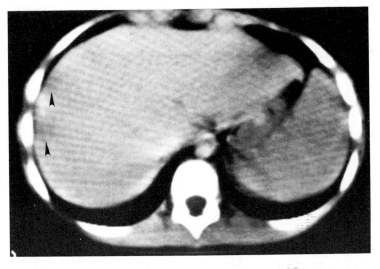

Figure 8–34. BEAM HARDENING ARTI-FACT. Apparent low-density liver lesions *(arrowheads)* are a result of beam hardening and motion from adjacent ribs. (See Chapter 1, Physics and Artifacts.)

Refs: (1) Miraldi F. Imaging principles in computed tomography, pp 1–22. In: Haaga JR, Alfidi RJ, eds. Computed tomography of the whole body. St. Louis: C. V. Mosby, 1983. (2) Young SW, Muller HH, Marshall WH. Computed tomography: Beam hardening and environmental density artifact. Radiology 1983; 148:279–283.

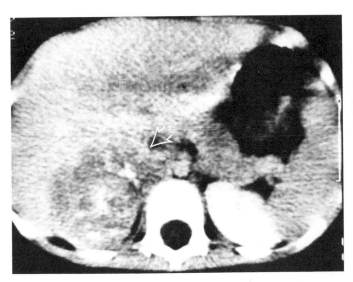

Figure 8–35. APPARENT LIVER INVASION BY NEUROBLASTOMA. A primary calcified right adrenal neuroblastoma *(arrow)* appears to have invaded the liver parenchyma on this contrast-enhanced CT scan. Sonography showed a clear cleavage plane, and at surgery the mass was easily separated from the liver. In children, local tumor extension may be difficult to assess on CT alone due to the sparsity of fat, and other studies are often indicated.

Ref.: Gore RM, Callen PW, Filly RA. Displaced retroperitoneal fat: Sonographic guide to right upper quadrant mass localization. Radiology 1982; 142:701.

Figure 8–36. SPLEEN TIP SIMULATING RENAL MASS. Abdominal CT in this child with known right Wilms' tumor shows an apparent low-density mass *(arrowhead)* involving the anterior-superior border of the left kidney, which proved by ultrasonography and surgery to be a normal spleen tip. (Case courtesy of Marilyn J. Siegel, M.D., St. Louis, Mo.)

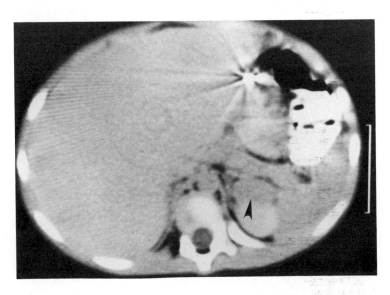

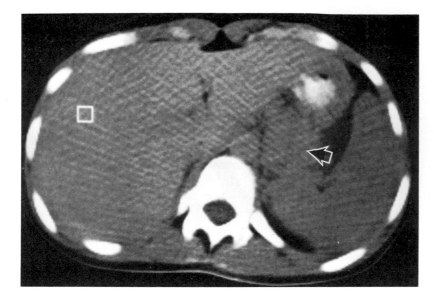

Figure 8–37. PROMINENT GASTRO-ESOPHAGEAL JUNCTION. The normal gastroesophageal junction region *(arrow)* can simulate a left upper quadrant mass. Ingestion of additional oral contrast material and prone or decubitus scanning can be used to prove that the suspicious mass is indeed the gastroesophageal junction.

Ref.: Thompson WM, Halvorsen RA, Williford ME, et al. Computed tomography of the gastroesophageal junction. Radiographics 1982; 2:179–193.

Figure 8–38. MASS-LIKE STOMACH CONTENTS.

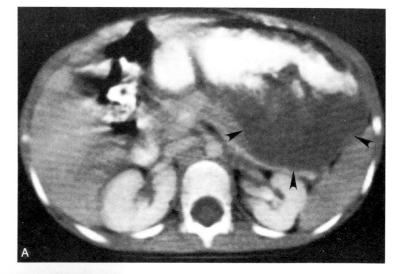

Figure 8–38A. An apparent low-density mass *(arrowheads)* is evident in the left upper quadrant.

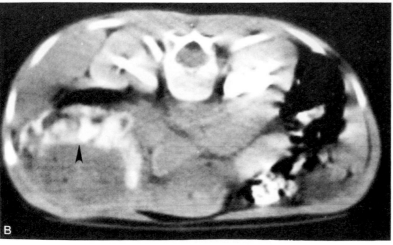

Figure 8–38B. Prone scan taken shortly after *A* shows contrast fluid level in stomach *(arrowhead).* Subsequent investigation revealed that the patient had ingested liquids shortly before entering the scanner.

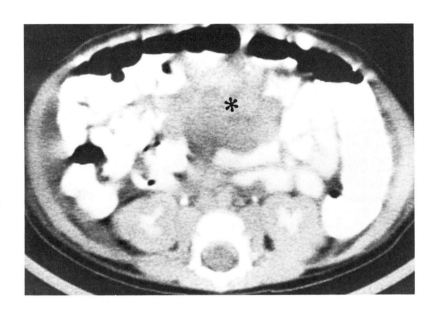

Figure 8–39. BOWEL SIMULATING MASS. In this 13-month-old child with hepatomegaly and ascites, this CT scan shows an apparent mass *(asterisk)* in the midabdomen. At surgery no mass was found. Unopacified loops of bowel were believed to be the cause of the apparent mass seen on the CT scan.

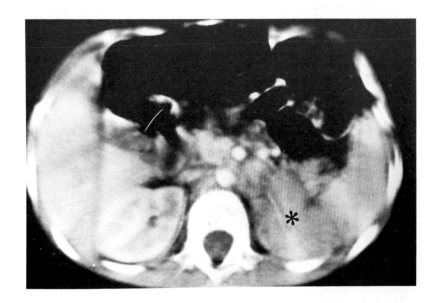

Figure 8–40. BOWEL LOOPS SIMU-LATING TUMOR RECURRENCE. In this child with previous left nephrectomy, normal bowel loops in the left renal fossa *(asterisk)* may simulate recurrent tumor. CT differentiation of pathologic masses from bowel loops often rests on the ability to opacify the bowel with contrast medium.

Figure 8–41. UNOPACIFIED BOWEL LOOP: PSEUDOMASS.

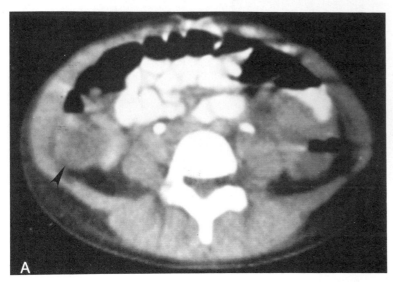

Figure 8–41A. An apparent right paracolic mass *(arrowhead)* is seen on an abdominal CT scan in a 7-year-old child with suspected intra-abdominal abscess.

Figure 8–41B. This was demonstrated to be a normal bowel loop *(arrowhead)* on a delayed scan. (Case courtesy of H. Lynn Magill, M.D., Memphis, Tenn.)

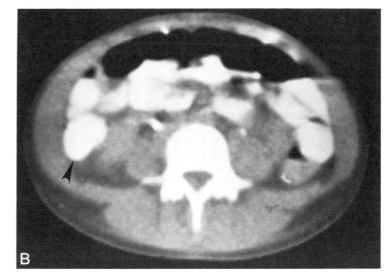

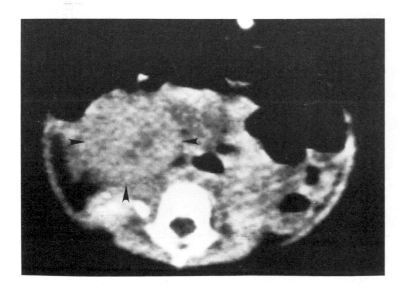

Figure 8–42. ILEOCECAL INTUSSUSCEPTION. Abdominal CT scan demonstrates apparently solid mass *(arrowheads)* in the right lower quadrant. This proved to be an ileocecal intussusception. In the infant or young child with pain and an abdominal mass, a contrast enema should be the first study undertaken, as CT could suggest a solid intra- or retroperitoneal mass as in this case and potentially confuse the diagnosis. (Case courtesy of Edward B. Mewborne, Jr., M.D., Santa Rosa Medical Center, San Antonio, Tex.)

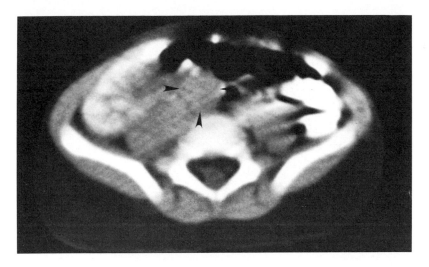

Figure 8–43. METASTATIC NEURO-BLASTOMA. A 3-cm aortic bifurcation lymph node found at surgery *(arrowheads)* was believed to represent poorly opacified bowel loops on the preoperative CT. Paucity of retroperitoneal fat and rapid transit of contrast medium through even an adequately prepared bowel makes evaluation of the retroperitoneum difficult in young children.

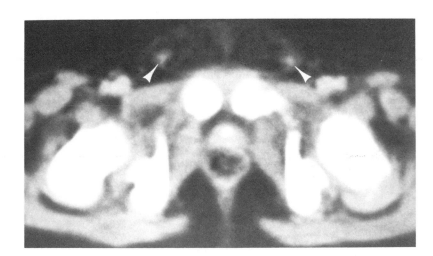

Figure 8–44. SPERMATIC CORDS. The paired spermatic cords *(arrowheads)* should not be mistaken for adenopathy. On contiguous scans they will be seen to course inferiorly into the scrotum.

Figure 8–45. IRREGULAR ACETABU-LAR OSSIFICATION. Mottled appearance of the acetabulum *(arrowheads)* on CT is a normal finding in adolescent patients. This appearance should not be confused with aseptic necrosis or infection.

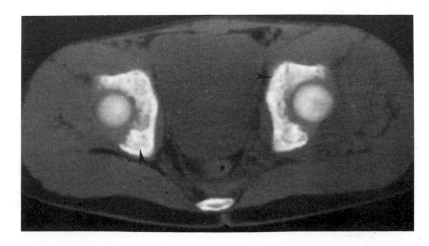

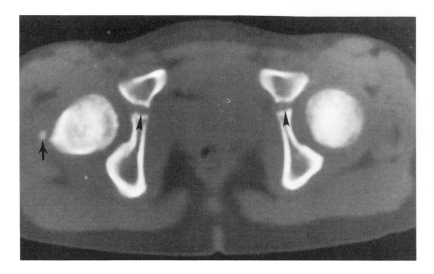

Figure 8–46. NORMAL PELVIC OSSIFICATION. Normal lucent triradiate cartilage *(arrowheads)* is symmetric bilaterally. Note also the most superior portion of the apophysis of the greater trochanter of the femur *(arrow)*, which could simulate a fracture. (Case courtesy of Marilyn J. Siegel, M.D., St. Louis, Mo.)

Figure 8–47. "CORTICAL DESMOID." Cortical irregularity of the medial posterior femoral condyle *(arrow)* at the insertion of the adductor magnus aponeurosis is frequently seen in normal active children.

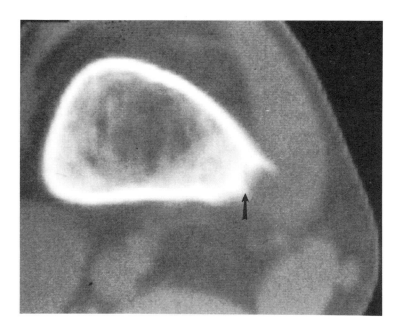

Ref.: Dunham WK, Marcus NW, Enneking WF, Haun C. Developmental defects of the distal femoral metaphysis. J Bone Joint Surg 1980; 62A:801–806.

II

ULTRASOUND

Chest

PETER W. CALLEN, M.D.
BARRY S. MAHONY, M.D.

Figure 9–1. MIRROR-IMAGE ARTIFACT SIMULATING PLEURAL EFFUSION.

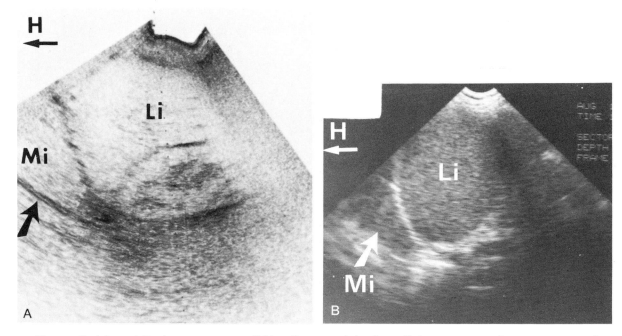

Figure 9–1A and B. A mirror-image (Mi) reflection of the liver (Li) may create the impression of supradiaphragmatic fluid. The upward, anterior angulation of the mirror-image reflection *(arrow)* in *A* helps to distinguish this as an artifact rather than the posterior parietal pleura, which would be more parallel to the table top as in *C* and *D*.

Illustration continued on opposite page

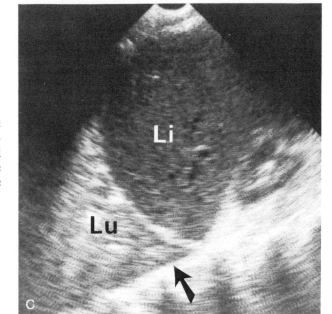

Figure 9–1C. In this patient with lung consolidation, the consolidated lung (Lu) can be differentiated from a mirror-image artifact of the liver (Li) by virtue of the increased echogenicity of the lung as well as by the fact that the posterior aspect of the imaged lung is parallel to the posterior parietal pleura *(arrow).*

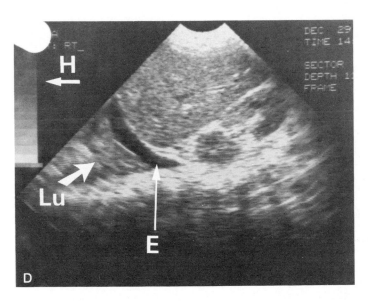

Figure 9–1D. In this patient with consolidated lung (Lu) there is a co-existent pleural effusion (E) extending into the posterior costophrenic sulcus. It can clearly be appreciated as supradiaphragmatic and real for the reasons mentioned above.

Ref.: Gardner FJ, Clark RN, Kozlowski R. A model of a hepatic mirror-image artifact. Med Ultrasound 1980; 4:19–21.

Figure 9–2. RIGHT HEMIDIAPHRAGM SIMULATING PLEURAL OR ASCITIC FLUID.

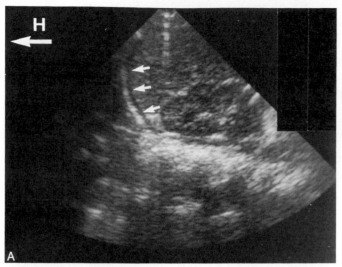

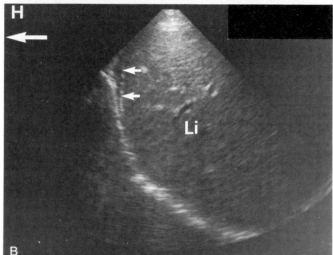

Figure 9–2A, B, and C. In three different patients an anechoic curvilinear region *(arrows)* is seen in the region of the right hemidiaphragm adjacent to the liver (Li). Although this simulates fluid in either the sub- or supradiaphragmatic space, it represents the normal musculature and capsule of the diaphragm and liver.

Illustration continued on opposite page

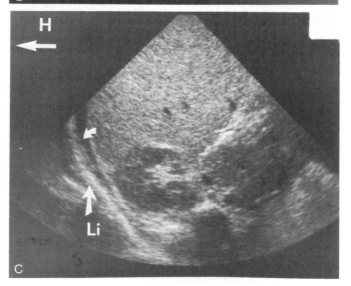

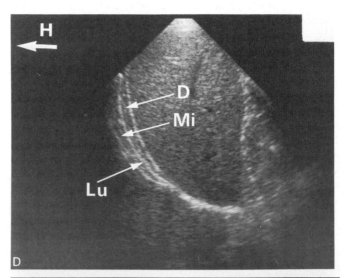

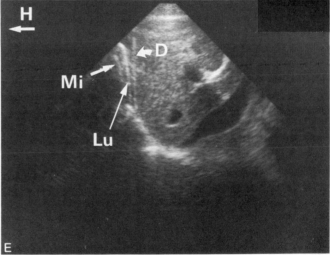

Figure 9–2D and E. In these patients the etiology of the anechoic area can be identified. The initial curvilinear line and its associated poorly echogenic curvilinear area is secondary to the liver capsule and muscle of the right hemidiaphragm (D). The next, more cephalic high-amplitude curvilinear flexion is caused by the interface of the lung itself (Lu). The most superior poorly echogenic curvilinear area is due to a mirror-image (Mi) artifact from the diaphragmatic musculature. Knowledge of this anatomic appearance will avoid misinterpretation of either ascites or pleural effusions.

Ref.: Lewandowski BJ, Winsberg F. Echogenic appearance of the right hemidiaphragm. J Ultrasound Med 1983; 2:243–249.

Figure 9–3. RIGHT CRUS OF THE DIAPHRAGM SIMULATING RETROPERITONEAL ADENOPATHY. On transverse scans (*A* and *B*) of the upper abdomen, the right crus of the diaphragm may appear quite prominent and lobular *(asterisk)*, simulating adenopathy. Knowledge of the normal anatomy and appearance of the crus of the diaphragm as well as evaluation of para-aortic structures elsewhere will help clarify this confusion (Ao = aorta; VC = vena cava).

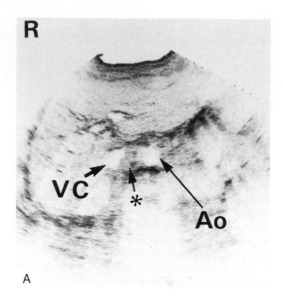

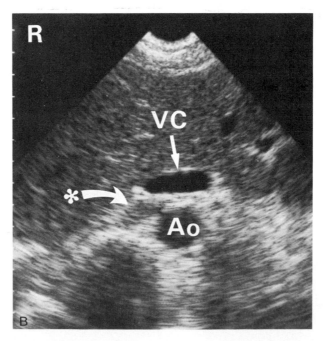

Ref.: Callen PW, Filly RA, Sarti DA, Sample WF. Ultrasonography of the diaphragmatic crura. Radiology 1979; 130:721–724.

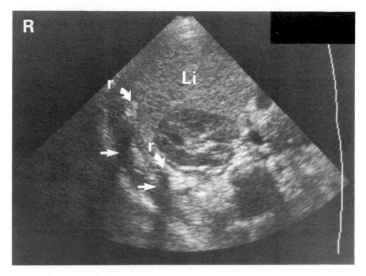

Figure 9–4. RIB ARTIFACT IN ABDOMINAL SCANNING. Scans of the upper and mid abdomen often demonstrate discrete areas of shadowing *(straight arrows)* adjacent to the liver (Li) and the kidney. These areas of shadowing emanate from the ribs and are seen as areas of focally increased echogenicity (r).

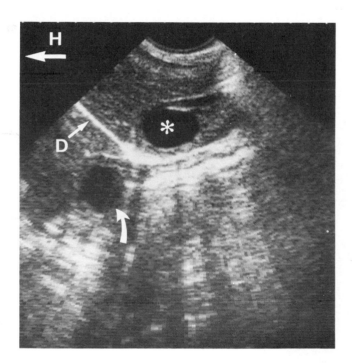

Figure 9–5. MIRROR-IMAGE ARTIFACT SIMULATING A SUPRADIAPHRAGMATIC LESION. In a right parasagittal scan in a child with a large cystic area *(asterisk)* due to an upper pole duplicated collecting system, there appears to be a similarly sized lesion *(curved arrows)* above the right hemidiaphragm *(D)*. This is nothing more than a mirror-image artifact duplicating the renal fluid collection. In this case, in this young child, measurement of the thickness of the body wall will readily clarify this as being positioned outside the patient's body. (Case courtesy of Peter L. Cooperberg, M.D., Vancouver General Hospital.)

Ref.: Gardner FJ, Clark RN, Kozlowski R. A model of a hepatic mirror-image artifact. Ultrasound 1980; 4:19–21.

Figure 9–6. LYMPHOMATOUS MASSES SIMULATING CYSTS. Both normal and abnormal lymph nodes are often quite anechoic and may simulate cysts within the body. At times, many of the features that have been described for cysts (enhanced through-sound transmission, anechogenicity, and a strong posterior wall) may be seen with these masses.

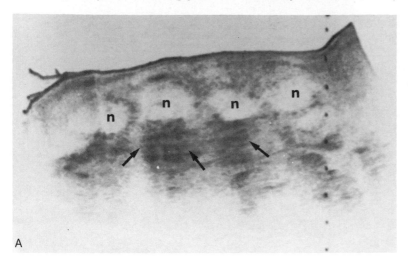

Figure 9–6A. In a 62-year-old woman with a painful right neck mass, longitudinal ultrasonography of the right neck demonstrates multiple poorly echogenic masses (n), which transmit sound well *(arrows).* These features are consistent with fluid-filled lesions; however, this proved to be lymphoma.

Figure 9–6B. Transverse ultrasonography of the right neck with the patient in the left decubitus position shows multiple echo-free masses (n) distorting the anatomy of the right neck (T = trachea).

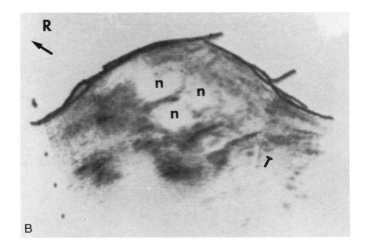

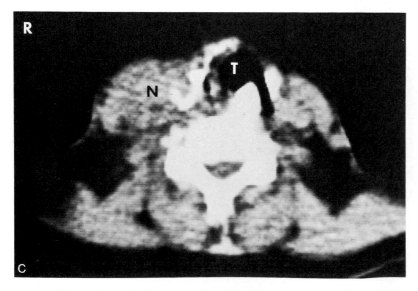

Figure 9–6C. A CT scan of the patient in A and B demonstrates a soft-tissue mass (N) in the right neck. Although the individual nodular masses could not be well differentiated, the high CT number of 41 H was consistent with a solid mass, that is, lymphadenopathy (T = trachea).

From: Callen PW, Marks WM. Lymphomatous masses simulating cysts by ultrasonography. J Can Assoc Radiol 1979; 30:244–246. Reprinted with permission.

Liver and Spleen

PETER W. CALLEN, M.D.
BARRY S. MAHONY, M.D.

Figure 10–1. IMPROPER ULTRASOUND TECHNIQUE RESULTING IN SIMULATED HE-PATIC NEOPLASM.

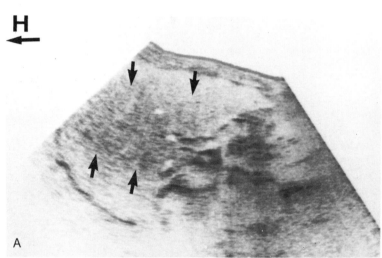

Figure 10–1A. Failure to achieve a "balanced" ultrasonogram of the liver may result in a band of increased echogenicity seen coursing throughout the liver *(arrows)*. This is, in part, also caused by enhanced return of echoes from the "focal zone of the transducer."

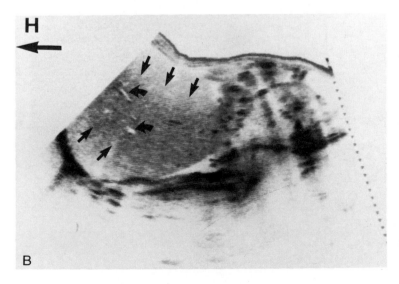

Figure 10–1B. A similar area of increased echogenicity is seen coursing through the central portion of the liver in this patient *(straight arrows)*. The artifactual nature of this finding can be realized by several factors. First, it is very unusual to see neoplasms in the liver that do not distort the normal hepatic and portal veins, which are normally positioned in this case *(curved arrows);* second, this band of increased echogenicity often extends beyond the confines of the liver, making its artifactual nature more apparent; and third, this band of increased echogenicity may be correlated with the focal zone inherent to the transducer.

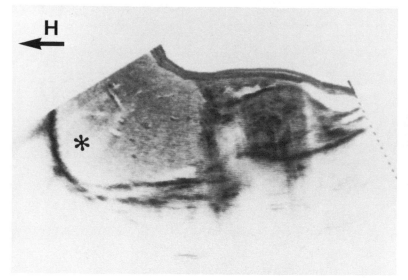

Figure 10–2. POORLY "BALANCED" SONOGRAM OF THE LIVER RESULTING IN SIMULATED CYSTIC OR METASTATIC HEPATIC NEOPLASM. Failure to adjust the time-compensated gain adequately may result in areas of decreased echogenicity in the far field. This is especially common in the posterior aspect of the right lobe of the liver *(asterisk)*. Although this is often readily identified as artifactual, it may be difficult to exclude a poorly echogenic lesion.

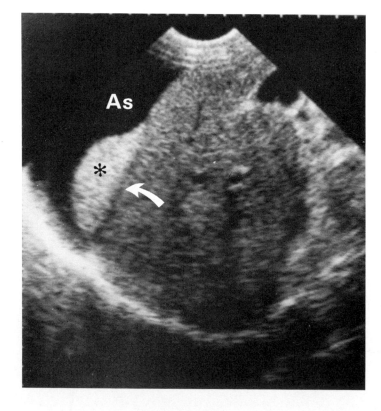

Figure 10–3. PSEUDOLESION OF THE LIVER IN A PATIENT WITH ASCITES. In this patient an echogenic area of the right superior anterior aspect of the liver is identified *(asterisk)*. Although this may simulate an echogenic metastatic lesion, it is likely due to the enhanced through-sound transmission through the large amount of ascites (As) anterior to the liver surface. In addition, the somewhat curved nature of the anterior aspect of the liver may serve as an acoustic lens. One may be further led astray by the sharp delineation from the remainder of the liver, which is secondary to refractive shadowing. Changing the angle of inclination of the ultrasound transducer will often immediately clarify this as normal hepatic tissue. (Case courtesy of Peter L. Cooperberg, M.D., Vancouver General Hospital.)

Ref.: Sommer FG, Filly RA, Minton MJ. Acoustic shadowing due to refractive and reflective effects. Am J Roentgenol 1979; 132:973–977.

Figure 10–4. THE LEFT PORTAL VEIN SIMULATING THE POSTERIOR ASPECT OF THE LIVER.

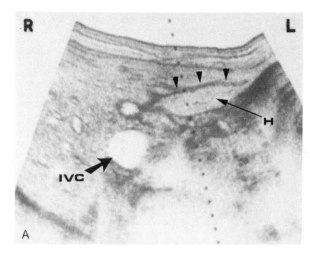

Figure 10–4A. On this transverse ultrasonogram, the left portal vein and connective tissue appear as an echogenic band *(arrowheads)* coursing through the left lobe of the liver. The tissue (H) lying immediately posterior and adjacent to the left portal vein is therefore hepatic in origin (IVC = inferior vena cava).

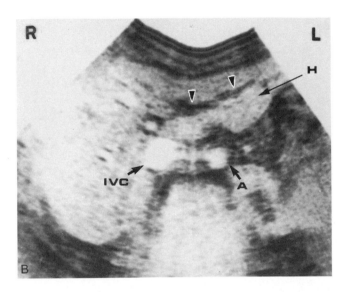

Figure 10–4B. On this limited transverse ultrasonogram, the left portal vein *(arrowheads)* simulates the posterior aspect of the left lobe of the liver. Hepatic tissue (H) could easily be mistaken for extrahepatic tissue (A = aorta; IVC = inferior vena cava).

From: Callen PW, Filly RA, DeMartini WJ. The left portal vein: A possible source of confusion on ultrasonograms. Radiology 1979; 130:205–206. Reproduced with permission.

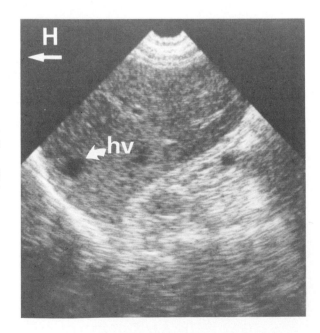

Figure 10–5. VESSEL SIMULATING HEPATIC CYST. When hepatic veins (hv) are seen in their short axis, as in this case, they may simulate the appearance of hepatic cysts. Scanning in a perpendicular plane of section along the long axis of the vessel will alleviate this potential source of confusion.

Figure 10–6. PERINEPHRIC FAT SIMULATING INTRAHEPATIC LESION.

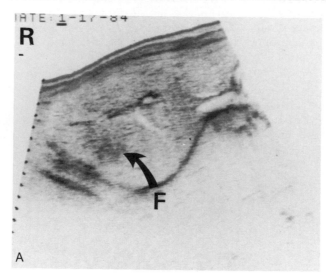

Figure 10–6A. On this transverse scan a focal area of echogenicity (F) is seen, apparently within the right lobe of the liver.

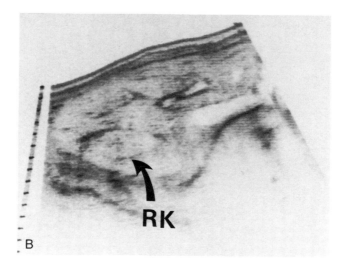

Figure 10–6B. On a plane of section slightly caudal to the one in A, the right kidney (RK) is clearly seen in the same anatomic position. The area of echogenicity in A, represents perinephric fat impressing the right lobe of the liver. Because of partial volume averaging (slice thickness), it artifactually appears as if the perinephric fat is intrahepatic. Longitudinal planes of section will often alleviate this potential source of confusion.

Figure 10–7. LIGAMENTUM TERES SIMULATING HEPATIC NEOPLASM. A focal area of increased echogenicity frequently is seen at the site of the ligamentum teres (*A* and *B, arrows*). Although this appearance may simulate a metastatic neoplasm to the liver (as in *A*), it is most likely due to fibrous or fatty tissue around the ligamentum teres. *B,* Scanning the patient in a longitudinal plane of section demonstrates this area to be present in the left intersegmental fissure dividing the lateral (L) and the medial (M) segments of the left lobe of the liver.

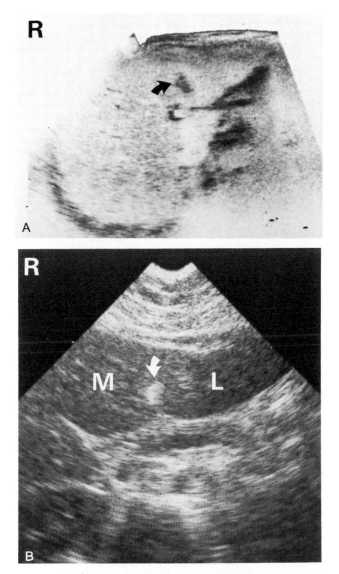

Ref.: Hillman BJ, D'Oris CJ, Smith EH, Bartrum RJ. Ultrasonic appearance of the falciform ligament. AJR 1979; 132:205–206.

Figure 10–8. HEMANGIOMAS SIMULATING HEPATIC NEOPLASMS. Often small focal areas of increased echogenicity (He) may be seen in asymptomatic patients during hepatic ultrasonography *(A–C)*. When unifocal and small in an asymptomatic patient, these almost invariably represent hemangiomas. When they are adjacent to the hemidiaphragm, a mirror image (Mi) of the lesion may be seen on the supradiaphragmatic portion of the scan. These lesions may be followed with ultrasonography or with another imaging modality such as computed tomography.

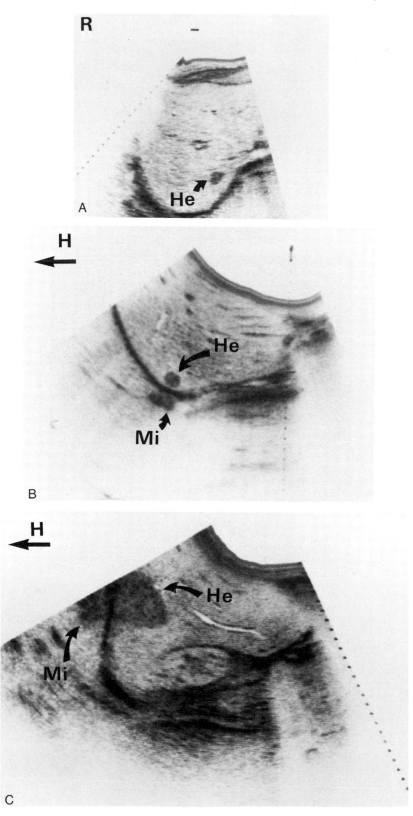

Figure 10–9. LEFT HEPATIC LOBE SIMULATING INTRAHEPATIC OR PANCREATIC MASS. As in these examples (A and B), the posterior aspect of the lateral segment of the left lobe of the liver *(asterisk)* often appears poorly echogenic and may at times be lobular in appearance. This may simulate either an intrahepatic lesion or extrahepatic (i.e., pancreatic) mass. Knowledge that this structure abuts the normal portal vein (PV) will alleviate confusion. The difference in echogenicity between this portion of the liver and the more anterior liver results from reverberation artifact anteriorly (Li = liver).

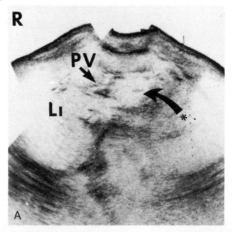

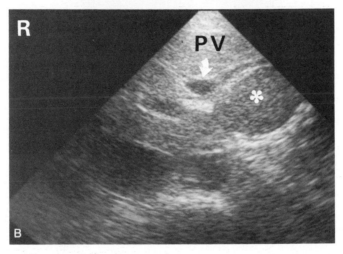

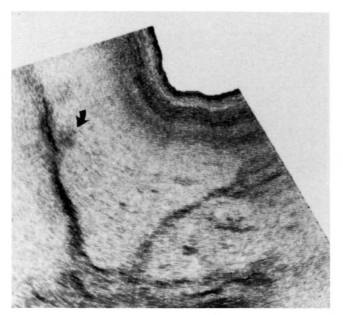

Figure 10–10. HYPERTROPHIC DIAPHRAGMATIC MUSCULAR BUNDLE SIMULATING HEMANGIOMA. Hypertrophic muscular bundles in the tendinous aponeurosis of the diaphragm rarely may be seen. The insinuation of the muscular bundles *(arrow)* is most likely responsible for the so-called hepar lobatum appearance described pathologically. Differentiation of these muscular bundles is difficult, particularly when solitary, but may be distinguished at times on a transverse scan, which may show this insinuation more clearly.

Ref.: Oyen RH, Marchal GJ, Verschakelen JA, Baeret AL. J Clin Ultrasound 1984; 12:121–123.

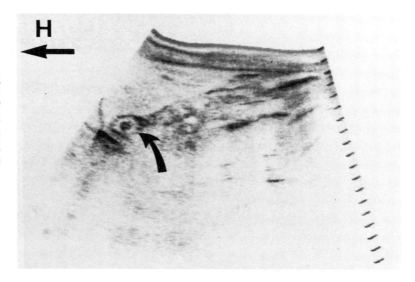

Figure 10–11. GASTROESOPHAGEAL REGION SIMULATING PERIHEPATIC LESION. As the esophagus makes its turn to join the stomach beneath the diaphragm, a target appearance characteristic of bowel can be seen *(arrow)*. This should not be confused with "target-shaped" lesions, which may be seen in hepatic metastatic disease.

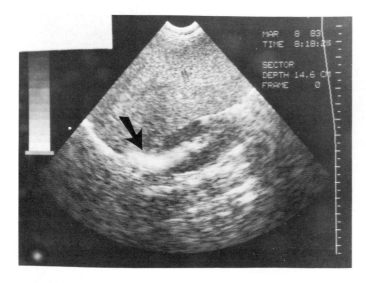

Figure 10–12. PHOTOGRAPHIC ARTIFACT SIMULATING RIGHT UPPER QUADRANT ABNORMALITY. Dust or foreign objects on the photographic lens or mirrors used in obtaining hard-copy images may result in highly echogenic areas *(arrow)* seen on the ultrasonogram. At times, depending on the position of the foreign object, this may simulate abnormalities. Identification of this abnormality at the same location on each image obtained will be a clue to its etiology.

Figure 10–13. FAT IN THE SPLENIC HILUS SIMULATING AN INTRASPLENIC LESION.

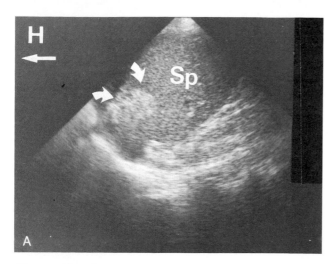

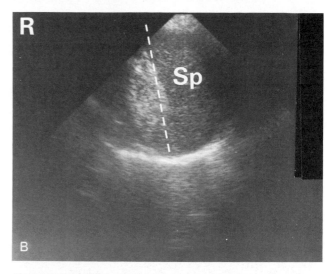

Figure 10–13A. A longitudinal scan along the medial aspect of the spleen may often reveal an echogenic focus *(arrows)* that appears to be within the splenic parenchyma (Sp = spleen).

Figure 10–13B. A transverse scan reveals the true location of this area of increased echogenicity, which lies outside the spleen within the splenic hilus. The dotted lines represent the plane of section that was obtained in *A* (Sp = spleen).

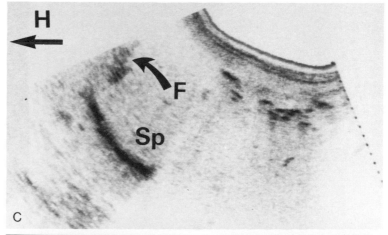

Figure 10–13C and D. In two different patients, longitudinal scans of the left abdomen also reveal echogenic areas representing fat (F) or possibly bowel in the region of the splenic hila, which mimic either a lesion or a calcification within the spleen (Sp).

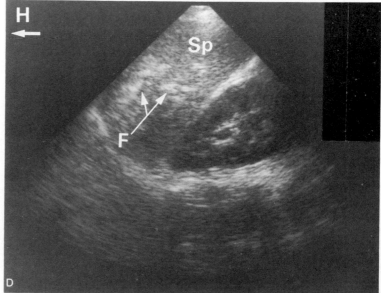

Figure 10–14. LIVER SIMULATING SUBCAPSULAR SPLENIC HEMATOMA.

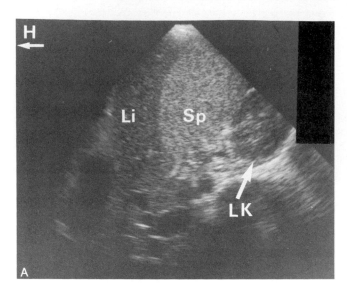

Figure 10–14A. In this patient a longitudinal ultrasonogram of the left upper abdomen reveals the normal spleen (Sp) with a poorly echogenic crescentic area (Li) superior to the spleen beneath the left hemidiaphragm. This crescentic area simulates either a subcapsular splenic hematoma or a subdiaphragmatic fluid collection (LK = left kidney).

Figure 10–14B. In a transverse scan of the same patient as in *A,* the poorly echogenic area can be seen to result from the lateral margin of the left lobe of the liver (Li) insinuating itself anterior to the spleen (Sp) (LK = left kidney).

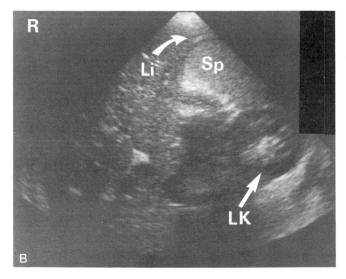

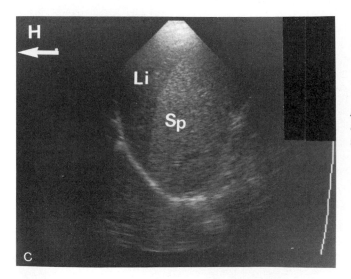

Figure 10–14C. In another patient, a similar finding of a poorly echogenic area (Li) is seen adjacent to the spleen and the left hemidiaphragm (Sp = spleen).

Illustration continued on opposite page

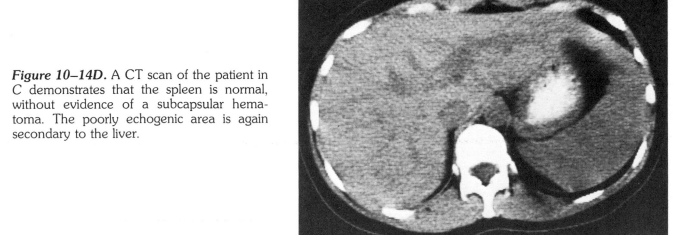

Figure 10–14D. A CT scan of the patient in *C* demonstrates that the spleen is normal, without evidence of a subcapsular hematoma. The poorly echogenic area is again secondary to the liver.

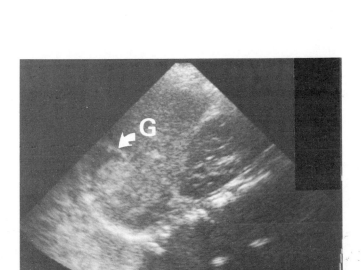

Figure 10–15. GAS AND FLUID IN THE STOMACH SIMULATING INTRASPLENIC OR LEFT SUBPHRENIC LESION. Occasionally, gastric contents may mimic a left subphrenic or splenic lesion (G). Visualization of this region during the administration of water into the stomach will demonstrate microbubbles within the stomach and permit distinction between gastric contents and a splenic or left subphrenic mass.

Gallbladder and Bile Ducts

PETER W. CALLEN, M.D.
BARRY S. MAHONY, M.D.

Figure 11–1. SLUDGE SIMULATING CHOLELITHIASIS. Sludge, seen as low-level echoes lying within the dependent portion of the gallbladder, may be identified in hospitalized patients or patients who are fasting. At times the sludge may be somewhat lobular in configuration and simulate a gallbladder mass or calculus (S). Absence of posterior acoustic shadowing may often alleviate the confusion with calculi.

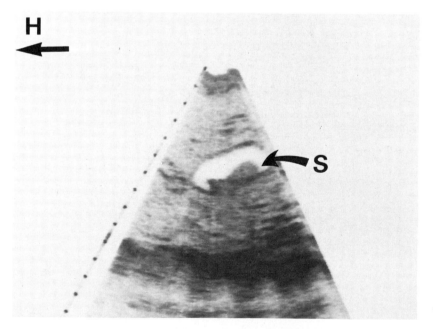

Ref.: Simeone JF, Mueller PR, Ferruci JT Jr, et al. Significance of non-shadowing focal opacities at cholecystosonography. Radiology 1980; 137:181.

Figure 11–2. SLICE THICKNESS ARTIFACT SIMULATING SLUDGE WITHIN THE GALL-BLADDER.

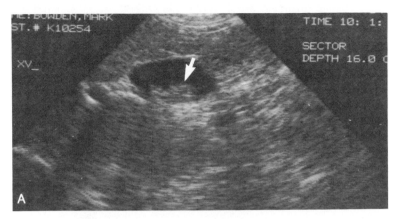

Figure 11–2A. Occasionally an echogenic focus *(arrow)* without posterior shadowing may be seen within the gallbladder and may mimic a collection of sludge.

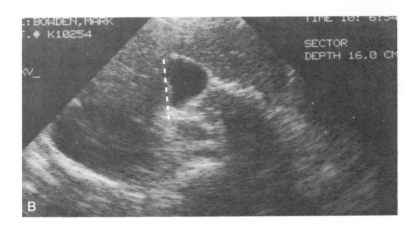

Figure 11–2B. A scan obtained at 90 degrees to A demonstrates hepatic parenchyma indenting the gallbladder slightly but no evidence of sludge. The dashed line demonstrates the plane of section of A that created the "sludge" by slice thickness artifact, which placed the hepatic parenchyma within the gallbladder.

Figure 11–3. GALLBLADDER POLYP SIMULATING CALCULUS. In some patients a moderate-to-high amplitude echo may be seen within the gallbladder *(arrow)*, which may simulate a gallstone. These polyps rarely shadow and this feature may be used to distinguish them from cholelithiasis.

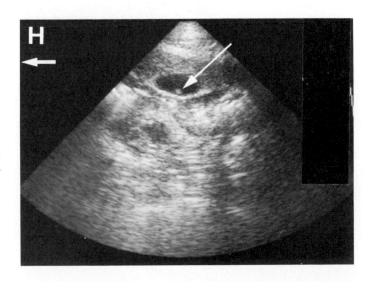

Figure 11–4. GALLBLADDER FOLD SIMULATING A GALLSTONE. Frequently a fold (F) may be seen along the posterior aspect of the gallbladder near the gallbladder neck. This may simulate a gallstone (as in *A*), particularly when it is associated with posterior refractive shadowing. Placing the patient in a left decubitus position and scanning with full inspiration (as in *B*), maneuvers which tend to elongate the gallbladder, will often alleviate this confusion.

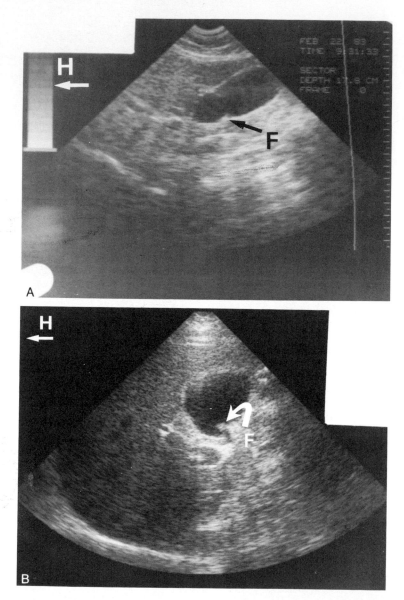

Figure 11–5. THE DUODENUM SIMULATING CHOLELITHIASIS. The gallbladder may often rest anterior to the duodenum (D) or transverse colon.

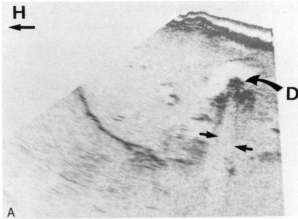

Figure 11–5A and B. When the duodenum contains gas and impresses upon the gallbladder posteriorly, as shown in the longitudinal scans of two different patients, it may simulate intraluminal calculi (*curved arrows, A and B*) with posterior shadowing *(straight arrows, A).*

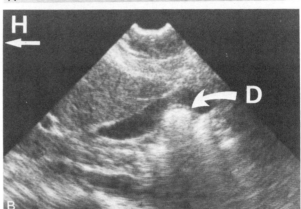

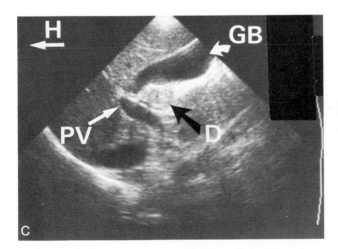

Figure 11–5C. Observation during realtime ultrasound or when air leaves the duodenum may reveal the true etiology of these echoes (GB = gallbladder; PV = portal vein).

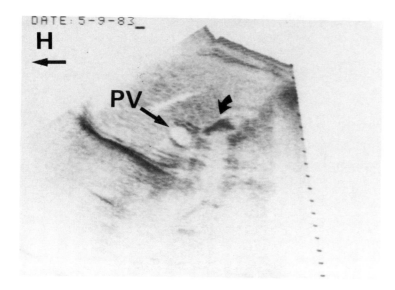

Figure 11–6. BOWEL SIMULATING CHOLELITHIASIS. Frequently, bowel with its echogenic center (arrow) and poorly echogenic wall may simulate a gallbladder containing stones. Observation under realtime ultrasound may often demonstrate peristalsis. Further evaluation of the normal anatomic relationships of the gallbladder will help prevent this confusion. This patient had had a cholecystectomy (PV = portal vein).

Figure 11–7. BOWEL GAS SIMULATING CHOLELITHIASIS IN A CONTRACTED GALLBLADDER. At times an area of echogenicity with shadowing may be seen adjacent to the liver. If the gallbladder is not seen, the area of echogenicity and shadowing may be secondary to a gallbladder that is contracted and filled with gallstones. In other cases, bowel gas adjacent to the liver may simulate this condition (arrow). While several authors have suggested means of differentiating shadowing from calculi versus gas, these are not infallible. In this case the shadowing from the bowel gas in the inferior portion of the left intersegmental fissure might be interpreted as being secondary to calculi. Identification of the gallbladder (GB) adjacent and to the right resolves this potential confusion.

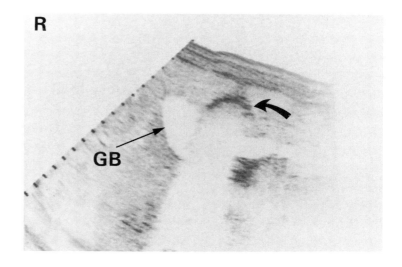

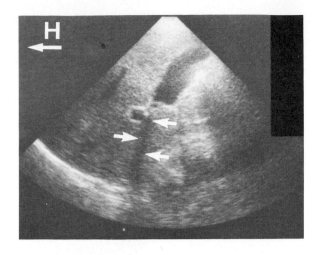

Figure 11–8. REFRACTIVE SHADOWING SIMULATING GALLBLADDER NECK STONE. Often an area of shadowing *(arrows)* may be seen adjacent to the neck of the gallbladder. This represents a refractive shadow which should not be confused with a shadow from a calculus in the gallbladder neck. A refractive shadow occurs when the critical angle of reflection is met or exceeded between two adjacent acoustic media (i.e., gallbladder wall and bile in the gallbladder) with differing velocities of sound.

Ref.: Sommer FG, Filly RA, Minton MJ. Acoustic shadowing due to refractive and reflective effects. AJR 1979; 132:973–979.

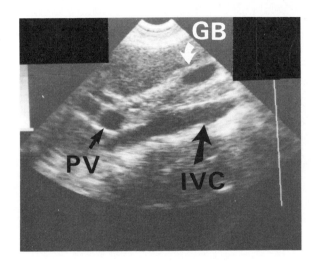

Figure 11–9. GALLBLADDER WALL THICKENING SECONDARY TO A CONTRACTED GALLBLADDER. A number of etiologies of thickened gallbladders have been described in the literature; a common etiology is inadequate distention of the gallbladder (GB). True thickening of the gallbladder wall is only observed in a fasting patient in whom the gallbladder is maximally distended (PV = portal vein; IVC = inferior vena cava).

Figure 11–10. THE GALLBLADDER NECK SIMULATING THE COMMON BILE DUCT.

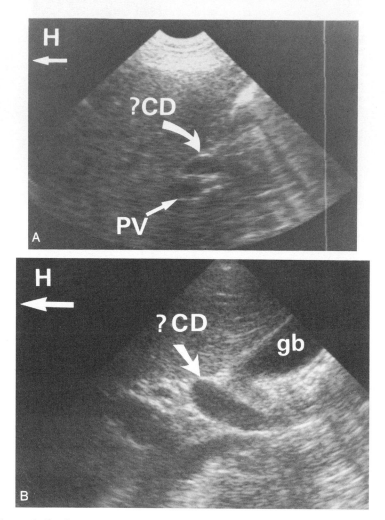

Figure 11–10A and B. In two separate patients a longitudinal scan of the right abdomen demonstrates a dilated tubular fluid-filled structure (?CD) anterior to the portal vein (PV). The gallbladder (gb) is identified in *B*.

Illustration continued on opposite page

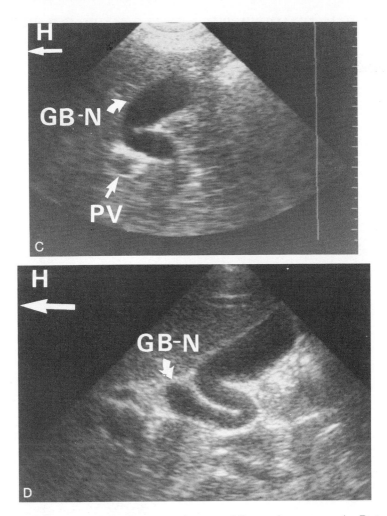

Figure 11–10C and D. Adjacent parasagittal scans (*C* is adjacent to *A; D* is adjacent to *B*) demonstrate that what appeared to be a dilated common bile duct was the neck of the gallbladder (GB-N) anterior to the portal vein (PV).

Ref.: Laing FC, Jeffrey RB. The pseudodilated common bile duct: Ultrasonographic appearance created by the gallbladder neck. Radiology 1980; 135:405.

Figure 11–11. HEPATIC ARTERY SIMULATING DILATED BILE DUCT.

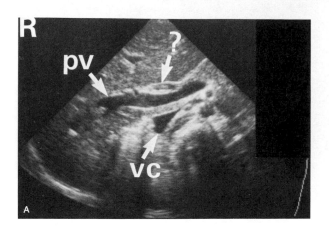

Figure 11–11A. In this transverse scan a dilated tubular structure (?) is seen anterior to the portal vein (pv). Anatomically this structure could either represent the hepatic artery or a dilated bile duct (vc = vena cava).

Figure 11–11B. In another transverse scan from the same patient as in *A*, the tubular structure can be seen to arise from the celiac axis and therefore represents the hepatic artery (ha).

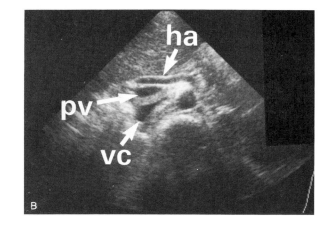

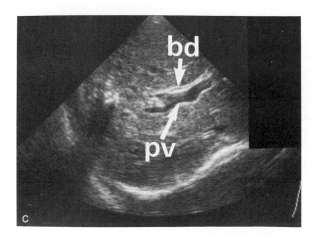

Figure 11–11C. At a slightly more cephalic plane of section, the bile duct (bd), which is normal in size, can be seen intimately associated with the anterior aspect of the portal vein (pv).

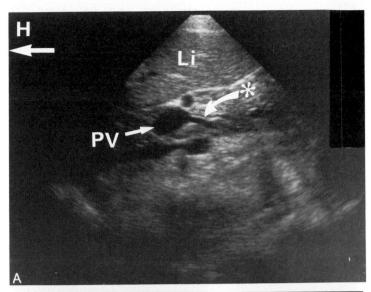

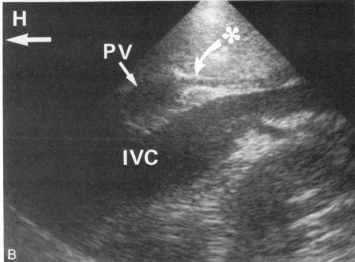

Figure 11–12. COMMON BILE DUCT SIMU-LATING A PORTAL VENOUS BRANCH. The common bile duct normally is located proximally in intimate contact with the portal vein. In its caudal descent the common bile duct turns posteriorly as it goes caudally from the portal vein subsequently to enter the duodenum. Sagittal scans such as *A* and *B* often reveal the common bile duct *(asterisk)* in close apposition with the portal vein (PV). Because of transducer angulation, the interface between these two structures may not be evident and the common duct may appear to represent a venous structure such as the superior mesenteric vein. The characteristic posterior and caudal angulation of the common bile duct makes this structure readily identifiable and separable from the superior mesenteric vein, the course of which more closely parallels that of the inferior vena cava and aorta (Li = liver; IVC = inferior vena cava).

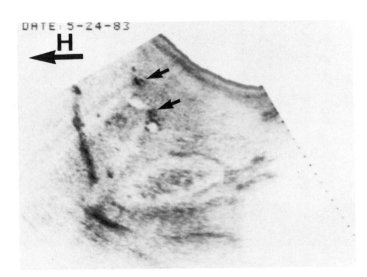

Figure 11–13. AIR IN THE BILIARY TREE SIM-ULATING CALCIFICATION. After surgical procedures that provide patency between the biliary and intestinal tract, air may freely reflux into the biliary tree. This is often seen as areas of high amplitude echoes *(arrows)* within the liver anterior to the portal vein. Often it may be difficult to differentiate gas from calcium in the biliary tree; knowledge of the patient's clinical history may be necessary to differentiate these two possible etiologies.

Retroperitoneum

PETER W. CALLEN, M.D.
BARRY S. MAHONY, M.D.

Figure 12–1. RENAL PSEUDOTUMOR.

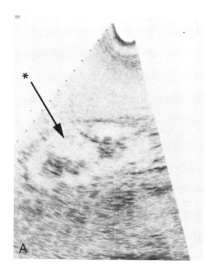

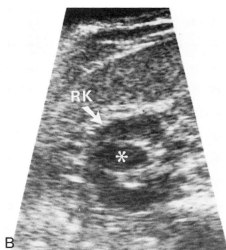

Figure 12–1A and B. In these two patients a renal pseudotumor secondary to a septa of Bertin *(asterisk)* is seen invaginating into the renal sinus. This area of normal renal cortex, because of its mass-like appearance, may be misinterpreted as a renal neoplasm. The characteristic location (splaying the central sinus fat between the upper and middle third of the kidney) as well as echogenicity equal to the normal renal parenchyma and absence of contour irregularity will help distinguish this from a renal cell carcinoma (RK = right kidney).

Figure 12–1C. A CT body scan of the patient in *B* outlines the normally enhancing cortical tissue of a septum of Bertin *(asterisk)*.

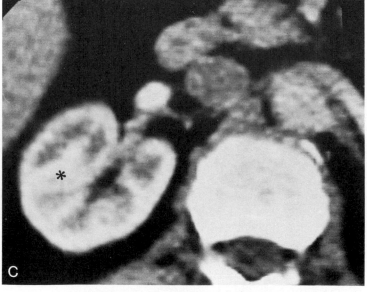

From: Mahony BS, Jeffrey RB, Laing FC. Septa of Bertin: A sonographic pseudotumor. J Clin Ultrasound 1983; 11:317–319. Reproduced with permission.

Figure 12–2. RENAL SINUS FIBROLIPOMATOSIS. In some patients the renal sinus may be extremely echogenic and prominent because of an abundance of fat within this region *(curved arrows).* This should not be mistaken for a mass, as its echogenicity is invariably similar to that of the perinephric fat *(open arrow).*

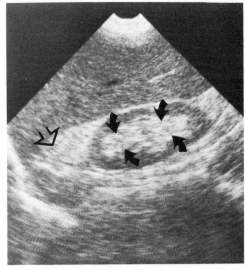

Ref.: Davidson AJ, Hricak H. The myth of anechoic renal sinus fat. Radiology 1983; 147:598.

Figure 12–3. INTERFACE AT THE EDGE OF THE RENAL HILUS SIMULATING AN AREA OF RENAL SCARRING.

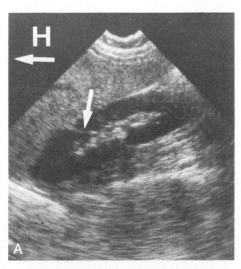

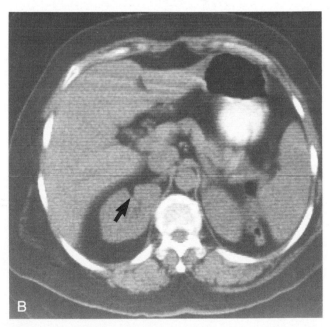

Figure 12–3A. Frequently a linear reflection *(arrow)* may be seen along the anterior aspect of the kidney that may simulate an area of scarring. Careful observation on transverse scans will reveal this to be the edge of the medial aspect of the kidney near the renal hilus.

Figure 12–3B. In this patient a CT scan confirms the explanation for the linear echo *(arrow)* in this slightly more anteriorly positioned renal hilus.

Figure 12–4. MEDULLARY NEPHROCALCINOSIS SIMULATING RENAL SINUS FAT.

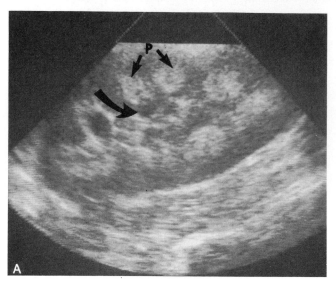

Figure 12–4A. In this renal transplant patient with hyperparathyroidism, numerous echogenic rounded densities (P, *straight arrows*) are positioned radially within the kidney. This indicates medullary nephrocalcinosis, which affects the renal pyramids. In medullary nephrocalcinosis the renal pyramids become echogenic and may resemble renal sinus fat. This differentiation may be made by virtue of the peripheral position of the echogenic pyramids rather than the more central position of the renal sinus fat. The central sinus fat *(curved arrow)* is diminished in this patient, suggesting transplant rejection.

Figure 12–4B. In this patient with renal tubular acidosis and medullary nephrocalcinosis, focal echogenic densities *(straight arrows)* occupy part of the normally poorly echogenic renal pyramids. Posterior acoustic shadowing *(arrowheads)* emanate form the pyramids (RK = right kidney).

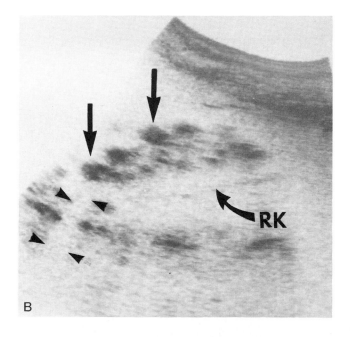

From: Glazer GM, Callen PW, Filly RA. Medullary nephrocalcinosis: Sonographic evaluation. AJR 1982; 138:55–57. Reproduced with permission.

Figure 12–5. NEONATAL RENAL PYRAMIDS SIMULATING CYSTS.

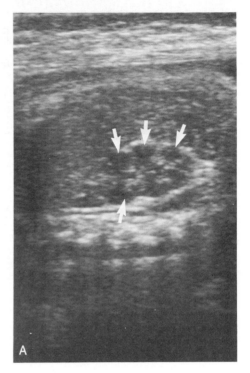

Figure 12–5A. The renal pyramids in neonates are poorly echogenic and often quite prominent *(arrows)*, in contrast to the adult kidney (see *B*).

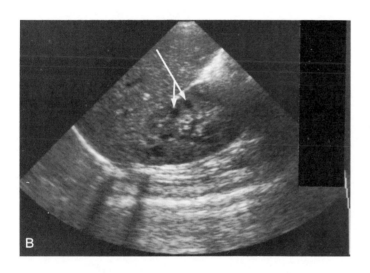

Figure 12–5B. In the adult kidney the renal pyramids *(arrows)* are also poorly echogenic but are significantly smaller in relative size.

Figure 12–5C. In the normal neonatal kidney the echogenic cortex outlines relatively large hypoechoic medullae, which may appear cystlike. Observation of the normal anatomic arrangement of the medullae in anterior and posterior rows *(arrows)* permits distinction from cysts. The increased echogenicity of the normal neonatal renal cortex probably results from the relatively large number of anatomic structures (and thus, more tissue interfaces) in the neonatal renal cortex compared with that of an adult.

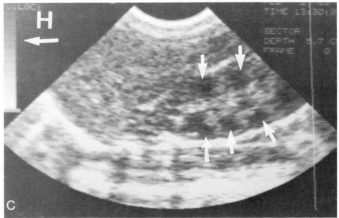

Ref.: Hricak H, Slovis TL, Callen PW, Romanski RN. Neonatal kidneys: Sonographic anatomic correlation. Radiology 1983; 147:699–702.

Figure 12–6. **TOMOGRAPHIC SECTION THROUGH THE RENAL CORTEX SIMULATING A RETROPERITONEAL MASS.**

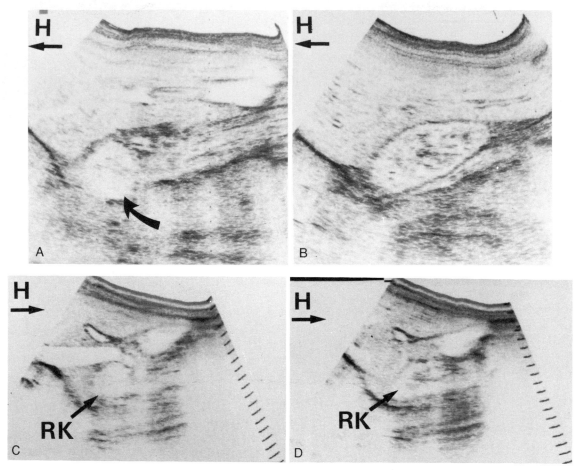

Figure 12–6A–D. *A,* A parasagittal tomographic plane of section through the medial aspect of the right renal cortex demonstrates a solid but poorly echogenic "mass" *(arrow)*. *B,* In the same patient a scan slightly more leftward and medial, demonstrates this pseudomass to be in the same anatomic position as the remainder of the kidney and of the same echogenicity. *C,* In another patient a similar finding of a poorly echogenic mass (RK, *arrow*) posterior to the inferior vena cava is seen. *D,* A slightly more medial, leftward scan again demonstrates this to be of the same echogenicity as the right kidney (RK, *arrow*).

Illustration continued on opposite page

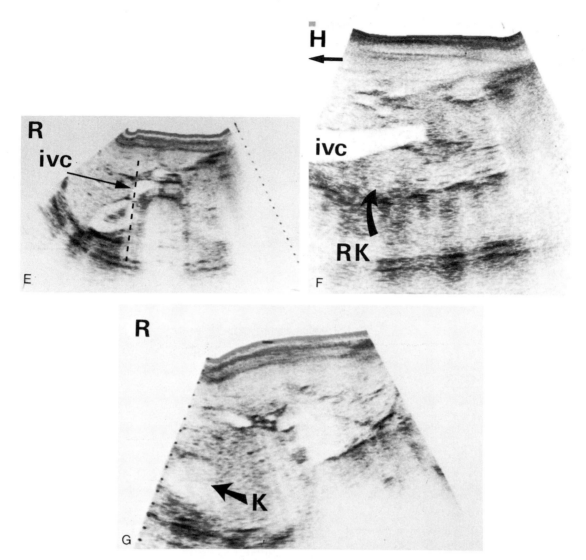

Figure 12–6E–G. *E,* A transverse plane of section through the mid-abdomen reveals the etiology of this pseudomass. A tomographic plane of section obtained in the same plane as is represented by the dashed line would reveal the poorly echogenic renal cortex posterior to the inferior vena cava (ivc) as seen in *A* and *C. F,* A parasagittal scan of another patient demonstrates a solid area (RK, *arrow*) posterior to the inferior vena cava (ivc). This also results from a plane of section through the renal cortex at the medial aspect of the right kidney. Pathologic structures that might have a similar location include abnormal lymph nodes or an enlarged right adrenal gland. *G,* A transverse plane of section through the superior aspect of the right kidney (K) will produce the same effect as in *F.* In this patient the scan appears to show a mass in the right upper abdomen (K); however, scans somewhat more caudal showed continuity with the right kidney, which had a similar echogenicity.

Figure 12–7. MULTIPLE PARAPELVIC CYSTS MIMICKING HYDRONEPHROSIS.

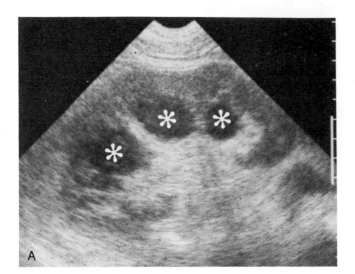

Figure 12–7A. Scans of the kidney occasionally reveal multiple, hypoechoic structures *(asterisks)* apparently emanating from the renal pelvis. These structures may resemble dilated infundibula and calyces. Although the absence of associated dilation of the renal pelvis may suggest the diagnosis of multiple parapelvic cysts, especially if the walls between these cysts are not apparent, the sonographic distinction between multiple parapelvic cysts and hydronephrosis may be very difficult.

Figure 12–7B and C. CT scans through the level of the kidneys following intravenous administration of contrast medium demonstrate the multiple parapelvic cysts (cy) in *B* and non-dilated collecting systems (p) in *C*. Incidentally noted is a small left renal cortical cyst. (Case courtesy of Mark E. Baker, M.D., Duke University Medical Center, Durham, N.C.).

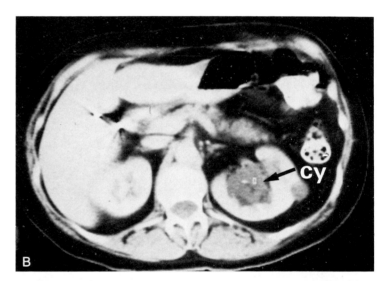

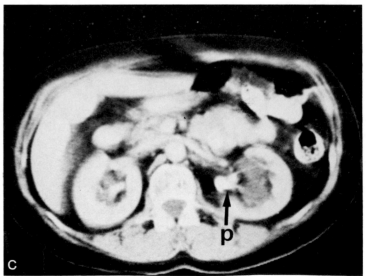

Figure 12–8. BOWEL SIMULATING THE NORMAL KIDNEY. The normal and abnormal intestine has a characteristic target configuration. This is seen with an echogenic center representing either mucus or microbubbles surrounded by the more sonolucent bowel wall. Frequently the morphology of bowel, especially when abnormal, may simulate the appearance of the kidney.

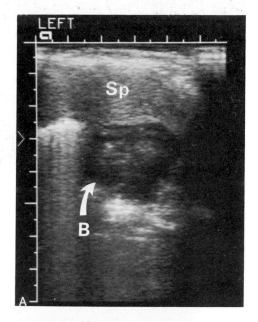

Figure 12–8A. In this patient status–post left nephrectomy, bowel (B) has filled the left renal fossa simulating the appearance of the left kidney (Sp = spleen).

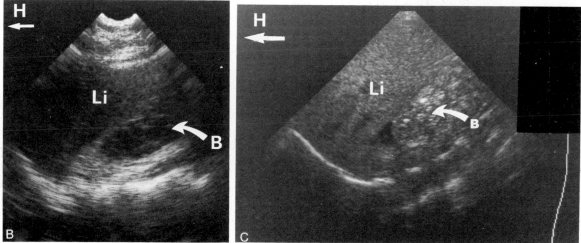

Figure 12–8B and C. Similarly, in two other patients status–post right nephrectomy, bowel (B) has filled the space normally occupied by the kidney, simulating a right kidney. Visualization of hypoechoic pyramids arranged in anterior and posterior rows provides convincing evidence of renal tissue. In the absence of this finding, other structures residing in the renal fossa may be mistaken for a kidney (Li = liver).

Ref.: Fakhry JR, Berke RN. The 'target' pattern: Characteristic sonographic feature of stomach and bowel abnormalities. AJR 1981; 137:969–972.

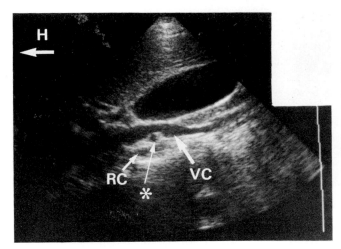

Figure 12–9. RIGHT RENAL ARTERY SIMULATING LYMPH NODE. Longitudinal scans of the right abdomen often reveal a small rounded structure *(asterisk)* posterior to the inferior vena cava (VC) and anterior to the right crus of the diaphragm (RC). Although this may simulate a lymph node, it represents the right renal artery seen in its short axis. Transverse scans through this plane of section will clearly reveal this to be a normal arterial structure.

Figure 12–10. LYMPHOMATOUS MASSES SIMULATING CYSTS.

Figure 12–10A. A 61-year-old man with known lymphoma presented with an abdominal mass. A longitudinal ultrasonogram through the mid-abdomen demonstrates a poorly echogenic mass (M) that transmits sound well *(arrows)*.

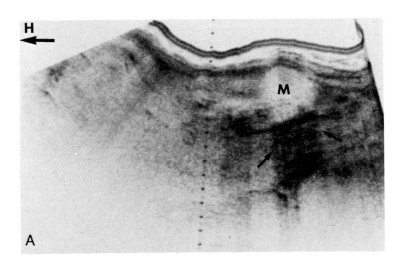

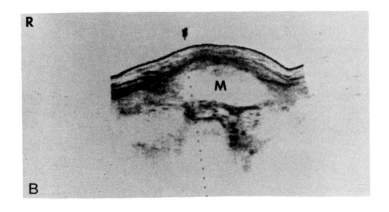

Figure 12–10B. A transverse ultrasonogram again demonstrates an anechoic mass (M) within the mesentery anterior to the great vessels. This proved to be a lymphomatous mass.

Illustration continued on opposite page

Figure 12–10C. An 8-year-old boy with an immune disorder presented with abdominal pain and a right lower quadrant mass. A longitudinal ultrasonogram through the right abdomen demonstrates an anechoic mass (m) caudal to the liver (Li) with a strong posterior wall reflection *(curved arrow)* and enhanced through-sound transmission *(small arrows)*. On the basis of the ultrasonogram, this was thought to represent a fluid-filled mass, but it was caused by lymphadenopathy.

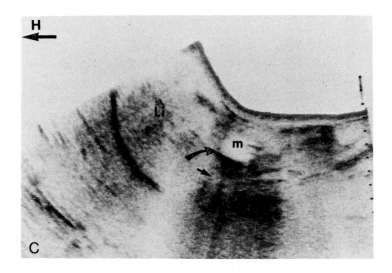

From: Callen PW, Marks WM. Lymphomatous masses simulating cysts by ultrasonography. J Can Assoc Radiol 1979; 30:244–246. Reproduced with permission.

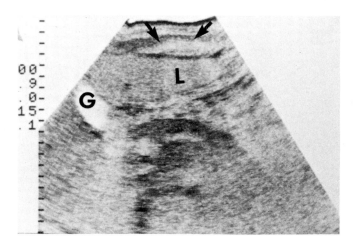

Figure 12–11. SUBXIPHOID ABDOMINAL WALL FAT SIMULATING ABNORMAL FLUID COLLECTION OR MASS. In many patients a poorly echogenic crescentic area *(arrows)* may be seen adjacent to the anterior abdominal wall. This is normal fat and should not be mistaken for an abnormal mass or fluid collection (G = gallbladder: L = liver).

***Figure 12–12. THE QUADRATUS LUMBORUM MUSCLE SIMULATING A PATHOLOGIC
FLUID COLLECTION.*** The quadratus lumborum muscle has been noted to appear as a
hypoechoic structure on sonograms of the abdomen. On occasion its appearance may simulate a
pathologic fluid collection such as an abscess or a retroperitoneal hematoma.

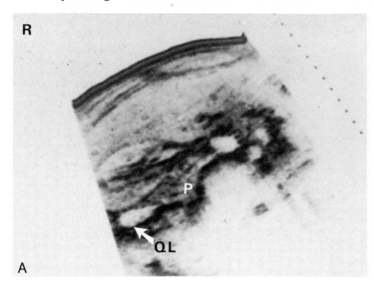

Figure 12–12A. A 27-year-old man was evaluated
by sonography because of a suspected abscess or
hematoma. On a limited transverse sonogram of
the right mid-abdomen, the quadratus lumborum
muscle (QL) appears as a poorly echogenic ovoid
structure that could easily be confused with an
abdominal fluid collection posterior to the right
kidney (P = psoas muscle).

Figure 12–12B. On a right parasagittal sonogram
obtained with the patient in the prone position, the
quadratus lumborum muscle (QL) appears as a
cephalically tapering elliptical structure posterior to
the right kidney.

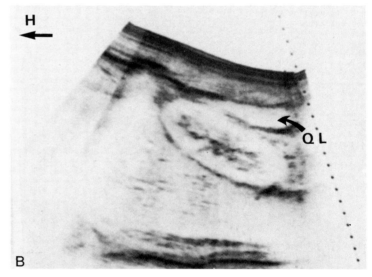

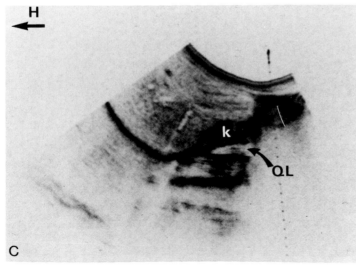

Figure 12–12C. A 34-year-old woman with
chronic renal failure was evaluated by sonography
because of intermittent fevers and suspected abscess. In this right parasagittal sonogram the quadratus muscle (QL) appears as a hypoechoic elliptical structure posterior to the right kidney (k). The
markedly hypoechoic appearance of this muscle
results in part from the abnormal increased echogenicity of the adjacent right kidney secondary to
renal disease.

From: Callen PW, Filly RA, Marks WM. The quadratus lumborum muscle: A possible source of confusion in sonographic
evaluation of the retroperitoneum. J Clin Ultrasound 1979; 7:349–352. Reproduced with permission.

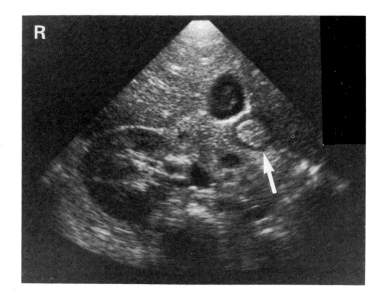

Figure 12–13. NORMAL INTESTINE SIMU-LATING A METASTATIC LESION. Character-istically, intestine has a target-shaped appearance *(arrow)*. While this appearance is typical of meta-static disease when seen within the hepatic paren-chyma, it is very characteristic of normal bowel seen within the abdomen.

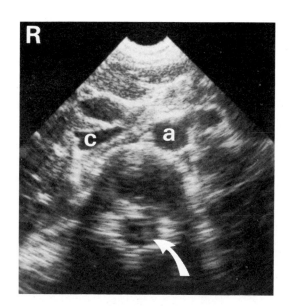

Figure 12–14. SPINAL CANAL SIMULATING POSTERIOR RETROPERITONEAL MASS. A transverse plane of section at a level through the intervertebral disc space will often reveal the spinal canal *(arrow)* posteriorly. Identification of the normal ana-tomic landmarks more anteriorly, specifically the aorta (a) and the inferior vena cava (c), assists in the correct identification of the spinal canal.

Figure 12–15. INTERFACE ECHO SIMULATING AOR-TIC THROMBUS CALCIFICATION. A high-amplitude specular reflection frequently may be seen at the interface between thrombus in the aorta and free-flowing blood. This high-amplitude specular reflection *(arrows)* is secondary to the interface between two differing acoustic media—free flowing blood and thrombus (th). This should not be mistaken for calcification at the intimal surface, associated with an aortic dissection.

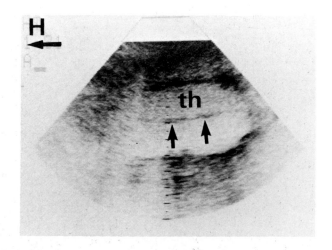

From: Harter LP, Gross BH, Callen PW, Barth RA. Ultrasonic evaluation of abdominal aortic thrombus. J Ultrasound Med 1982; 1:315–318. Reproduced with permission.

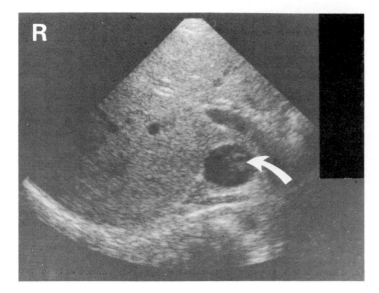

Figure 12–16. SIDE-LOBE ARTIFACT AND SLICE THICKNESS ARTIFACTS SIMULATING INTRAVASCULAR THROMBUS. During a Valsalva maneuver in this young normal patient, echoes are seen *(arrow)* projecting into the inferior vena cava on this transverse scan. The movement of these echoes was seen to correlate with adjacent duodenal peristalsis rather than with blood flow.

Ref.: Laing FC, Kurtz A. The importance of ultrasonic side-lobe artifacts. Radiology 1982; 145:763.

Figure 12–17. PSEUDOPANCREATIC DUCT SECONDARY TO GASTRIC WALL.

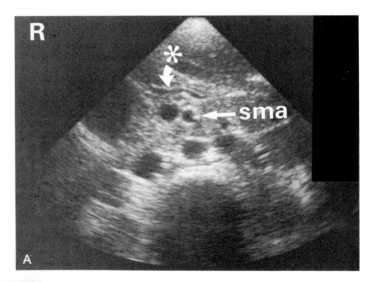

Figure 12–17A. Transverse scans of the upper abdomen occasionally demonstrate an anechoic tubular structure *(asterisk)* in the region of the pancreas anterior to the superior mesenteric vessels (sma = superior mesenteric artery). Although this may simulate the pancreatic duct, it actually represents the posterior muscular wall of the gastric antrum.

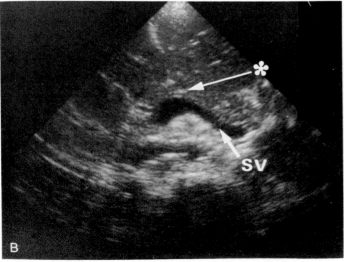

Figure 12–17B. On an adjacent transverse scan to A, the true pancreatic duct *(asterisk)* may be seen in the substance of the pancreas anterior to the splenic vein (sv).

Figure 12–18. SPLENIC ARTERY MIMICKING DILATED PANCREATIC DUCT.

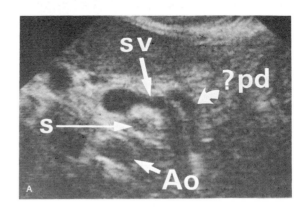

Figure 12–18A. Occasionally on a transverse sonogram in the region of the pancreas a tubular structure is seen anterior to the splenic vein (sv) and may mimic a dilated pancreated duct (?pd) in the tail of the pancreas (Ao = aorta; s = superior mesenteric artery).

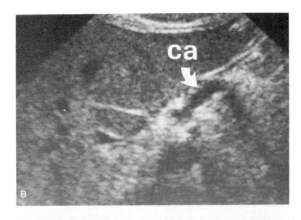

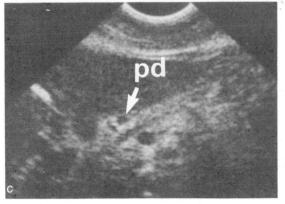

Figure 12–18B and C. Documentation that the tubular structure arises from the celiac axis (ca) as well as visualization of the true pancreatic duct (pd) in the substance of the pancreas confirm that the structure in question represents the splenic artery rather than the pancreatic duct.

Figure 12–19. FLUID IN THE LESSER SAC SIMULATING A DILATED PANCREATIC DUCT. Occasionally fluid in the lesser sac (F) may be confused with a dilated pancreatic duct. Recognition that the fluid lies anterior to the pancreas rather than in the substance of the pancreas permits an accurate diagnosis (S = collapsed stomach; SV = splenic vein; A = small amount of fluid in the left anterior subhepatic space).

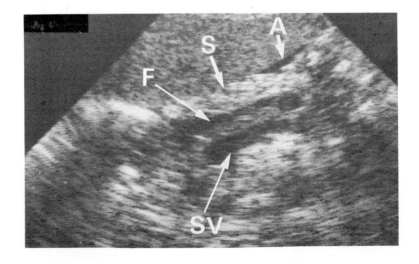

Figure 12–20. **DILATED FLUID-FILLED STOMACH SIMULATING LEFT UPPER QUAD-RANT MASS.** Patients with gastric outlet obstruction, or patients who have ingested a large amount of fluid in preparation for bladder ultrasonography, may have a large fluid-filled stomach resembling a cystic mass in the left upper quadrant, as in these examples (*A* and *B*). By carefully observing peristalsis within this structure, one can identify that it represents the stomach (St). At times it may be necessary to have the patient swallow a cup of water to notice the microbubbles swirling in the stomach. This may be the only way of differentiating this structure from a pancreatic pseudocyst (Sp = spleen).

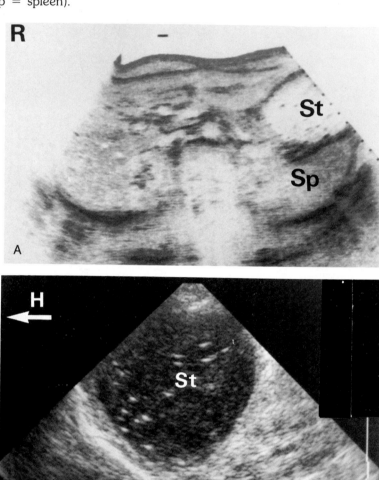

Figure 12–21. *FLUID-FILLED DUODENUM MIMICKING A RIGHT ANTERIOR SUB-HEPATIC FLUID COLLECTION.*

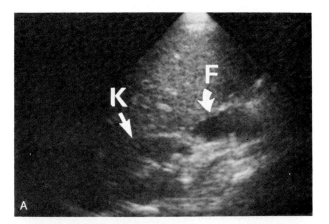

Figure 12–21A and B. Longitudinal (A) and transverse (B) sonograms of the right upper quadrant show a fluid collection (F in A; *arrow* in B) in the region of the anterior subhepatic space (K = kidney).

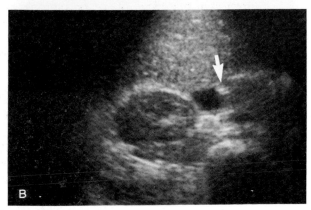

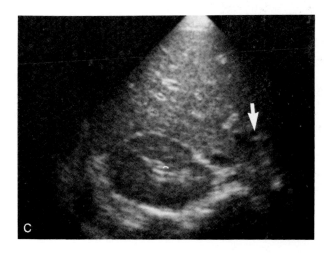

Figure 12–21C. Following the oral administration of water, microbubbles within the ingested water are seen moving by peristalsis through the duodenum *(arrow)*. The administration of water permitted distinction between normal duodenum and an anterior subhepatic fluid collection.

Pelvis

PETER W. CALLEN, M.D.
BARRY S. MAHONY, M.D.

Figure 13–1. DOUBLE-IMAGE ARTIFACT MIMICKING TWIN GESTATIONS. Occasionally, when scanning a singleton pregnancy one may see two apparent intrauterine gestational sacs *(arrows)* in one plane of section but only one gestational sac when scanning at a slightly different angle. The artifact usually occurs when scanning with a mechanical sector transducer over the midline and probably results from refraction of the sound by the rectus abdominis muscle. Scans obtained away from the maternal midline will confirm the presence of a singleton pregnancy.

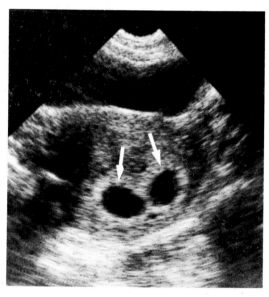

Ref.: Muller N, Cooperberg PL, Rowley VA, et al. Ultrasonic refraction by the rectus abdominis muscles: The double image artifact. J Ultrasound Med 1984; 3:515–519.

Figure 13–2. BICORNUATE UTERUS SIMULATING A UTERINE MYOMA. In patients with a bicornuate uterus the non-gravid horn may simulate a myoma adjacent to the pregnant horn containing the gestational sac. In this patient a soft tissue mass is identified to the right of the gestational sac (gs). The characteristic features that define this as a bicornuate uterus rather than a myoma are (1) the similar appearance of the echogenicity of the soft tissue to the myometrium surrounding the gestational sac and (2) a decidual reaction *(asterisk)* seen within the uterine cavity of the non-gravid horn.

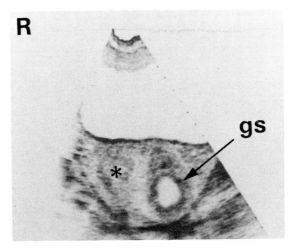

Ref.: Gross BH, Callen PW. Ultrasound of the uterus. In: Callen PW, ed. Ultrasonography in Obstetrics and Gynecology. Philadelphia: W. B. Saunders, 1983.

Figure 13–3. BOWEL GAS ARTIFACT SIMULATING THE UTERUS. In this patient status–post hysterectomy, a pseudomass *(asterisk)* is seen at the end of the vagina (V). This pseudomass is related to bowel gas artifact and only appears somewhat solid because of artifactual low-level echoes within the area of shadowing. In addition, a specular reflection representing side-lobe artifact is seen posteriorly (A).

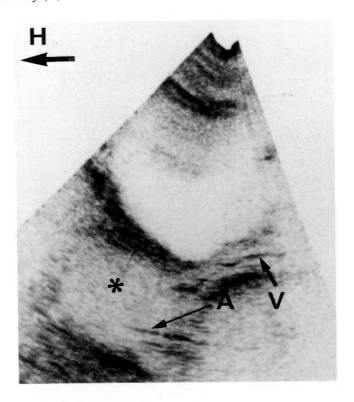

Figure 13–4. RETROPOSITIONED UTERUS SIMULATING UTERINE MYOMA OR CUL-DE-SAC MASS.

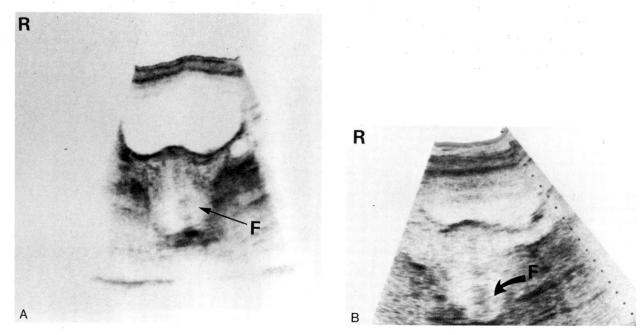

Figure 13–4A and B. In patients who have a retropositioned uterus, the fundic portion of the uterus may appear lobular with decreased echogenicity (F). This region of decreased echogenicity, which may resemble a uterine fibroid, most likely results from attenuation anteriorly.

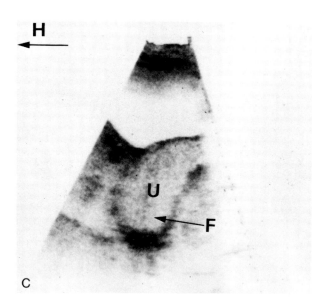

Figure 13–4C. Correlation with a longitudinal scan, as in this case, often clearly demonstrates that the hypoechoic lobular area (F) is part of the retropositioned uterus (U).

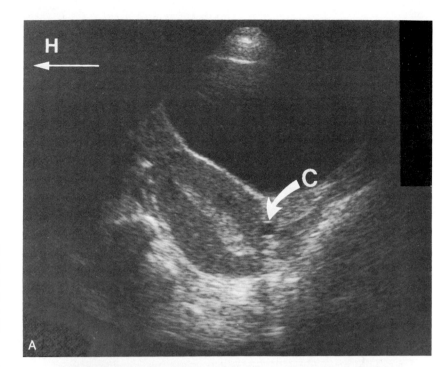

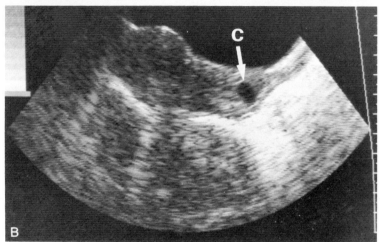

Figure 13–5. NABOTHIAN CYSTS SIMULATING CERVICAL FLUID. In these scans of two different patients a small cystic area (C) is seen in the cervix. This is characteristic of a nabothian cyst and should not be confused with other pathological lesions.

Ref.: Fogel SR, Slasky BS. Sonography of nabothian cyst. AJR 1982; 138:927–930.

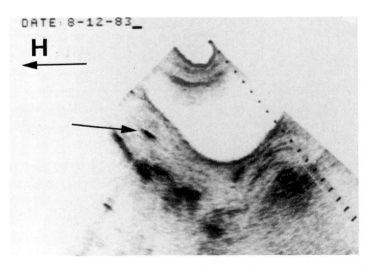

Figure 13–6. INTRAUTERINE AIR AFTER DILATION AND CURETTAGE, SIMULATING INTRAUTERINE CONTRACEPTIVE DEVICE (IUD). During uterine manipulation (i.e., dilation and curettage), air may be introduced into the uterine cavity. This may be seen as an intensely echogenic area *(arrow)*, occasionally associated with posterior acoustic shadowing. The lack of resemblance to the normal morphology of an IUD will help to differentiate retained air from an IUD.

Ref.: Gross BH, Callen PW. Ultrasonography in the detection of intrauterine contraceptive devices. In: Callen PW, ed. Ultrasonography in Obstetrics and Gynecology. Philadelphia: W. B. Saunders Co., 1983.

Figure 13–7. OVARIAN MASS SIMULATING AN ENLARGED UTERUS.

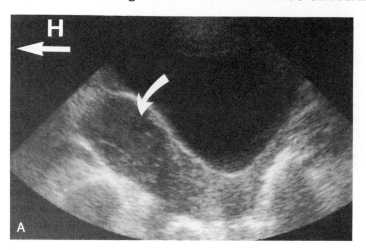

Figure 13–7A. On this longitudinal ultrasonogram through the pelvis, the uterus appears to have a bulbous contour in its fundic portion *(arrow)*. This scan was obtained in the midline and might lead one to believe that all structures seen on this scan are part of the uterus.

Figure 13–7B. On an adjacent longitudinal scan somewhat to the left of midline, the normal uterus (U) can be identified with its normal size and contour. The endometrial cavity echo (c), which further clarifies the structure as the normal uterus, can be seen. This case reminds us that a structure should not be assumed to be uterine if it appears in the midline and is inseparable from the uterus on a longitudinal scan. Ovarian masses, as in this case, may displace the uterus, particularly in the fundic portion to one side, and may mimic the appearance of a uterine myoma.

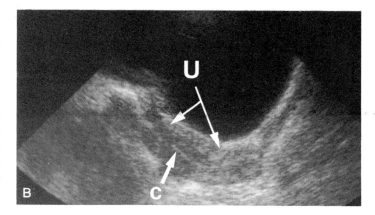

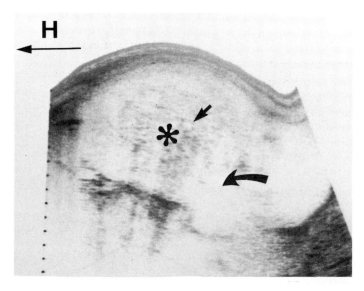

Figure 13–8. DEGENERATING UTERINE MYOMA SIMULATING HYDATIDIFORM MOLE. In this patient with a large degenerating myoma, numerous small, fluid-containing spaces *(small arrow)* can be seen within the large solid mass *(asterisk)*. The differentiation between this myoma and trophoblastic disease may be made by virtue of the marked attenuation of sound by this mass *(large arrow)* characteristic of a myoma. Trophoblastic disease would characteristically be more echogenic than is seen in this case.

Ref.: Callen PW: Ultrasonography in the evaluation of gestational trophoblastic disease. In: Callen PW, ed. Ultrasonography in Obstetrics and Gynecology. Philadelphia: W. B. Saunders Co., 1983.

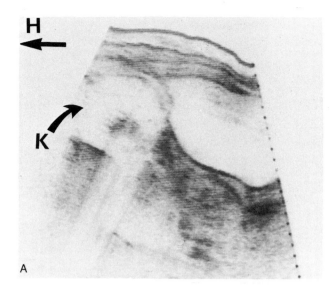

Figure 13–9. PELVIC KIDNEY SIMU-LATING A PELVIC MASS. In these two patients a large mass (K) was seen adjacent to the urinary bladder. The echogenic center of this mass should make one suspicious that this represents either bowel or kidney. Searching for the kidney in the renal fossa bilaterally will alleviate this potential confusion.

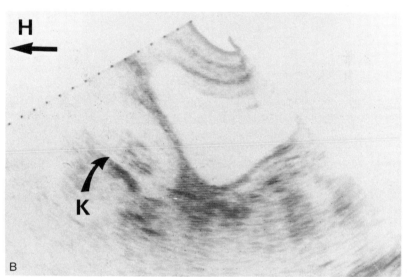

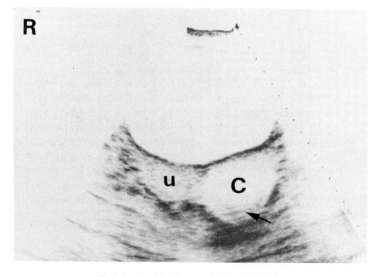

Figure 13–10. PSEUDODEBRIS WITHIN AN OVARIAN CYST. Occasionally low-level echoes *(arrow)* may be seen intraluminally within a cyst (C). Although this may simulate the appearance of intraluminal debris or perhaps blood, it often represents an artifact, either from slice thickness or from side-lobe artifact. Scanning in varying planes of section will often clear up this confusion (u = uterus).

Ref.: Laing FC, Kurtz AB. The importance of ultrasonic side-lobe artifacts. Radiology 1982; 145:763–768.

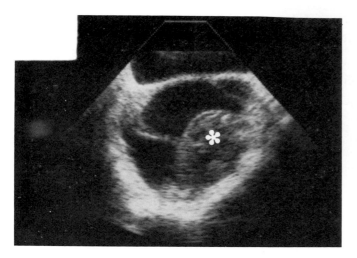

Figure 13–11. BENIGN INFLAMMATORY MASS SIMULATING AN OVARIAN NEOPLASM. Inflammatory masses within the pelvis, such as endometriomas, may simulate an ovarian neoplasm. In this case a large, complex, predominantly cystic mass is seen within the pelvis. The mass contains a large solid component *(asterisk)*. If the clinical history is not characteristic, at times only laparoscopy will help differentiate a benign mass from neoplasia.

Ref.: Callen PW, Gross BH. Ultrasound evaluation of benign and malignant ovarian disease. Clin Diagn Ultrasound 1984; 12:31–147.

Figure 13–12. BOWEL GAS SIMULATING ADNEXAL MASS (DERMOID). In this transverse scan, gas-containing sigmoid colon *(curved arrow)* creates the appearance of an echogenic adnexal mass. Failure to demonstrate a posterior wall of this "mass" helps to distinguish it from a true adnexal mass. The left ovary (O) can be seen positioned slightly posterior to the uterus (u).

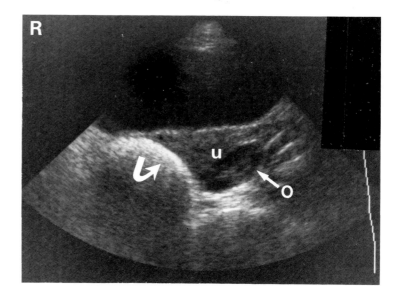

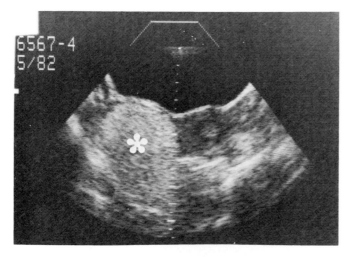

Figure 13–13. DERMOID SIMULATING BOWEL WITHIN THE PELVIS. Some dermoid tumors present as characteristic areas of increased echogenicity that tend to shadow posteriorly. While echogenic regions within the adnexal areas are often secondary to bowel gas, in this case the echogenic area can be seen *(asterisk)* as a more discrete mass than would be seen with bowel. Cases that are not as clear as this one may need plain film radiography to confirm the diagnosis.

Ref.: Laing FC, Van Dolsom V, Marks W, et al. Dermoid cysts of the ovary: Their ultrasonographic appearance. Obstet Gynecol 1981; 57:99–104.

Figure 13–14. BOWEL SIMULATING A PELVIC MASS. In three different patients bowel within the pelvis has created the appearance of a large pelvic mass *(asterisk)*. This is often confusing because there appears to be a posterior wall to the mass. This wall represents a mirror-image duplication artifact from reflection of the strong interface of the bowel gas anteriorly (B). Scanning in various planes of section or, if necessary, after a water enema may help elucidate the etiology of this pseudomass.

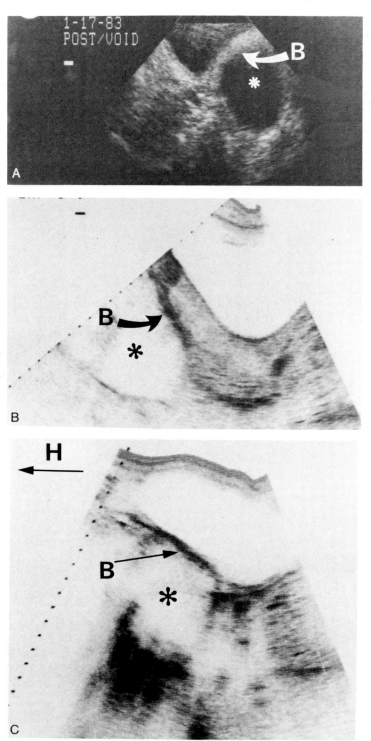

Figure 13–15. FLUID COLLECTION SIMULATING THE URINARY BLADDER.

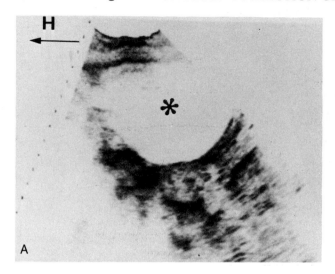

Figure 13–15A. On a longitudinal sonogram of a 32-year-old woman with a large palpable pelvic mass, a large, fluid-filled cystic structure *(asterisk)* within the pelvis was presumed to be the urinary bladder.

Figure 13–15B. One week later, distention of the urinary bladder (Bl) permits identification of a large cystic mass (C) separate from the bladder. An ovarian cystadenoma was found at surgery.

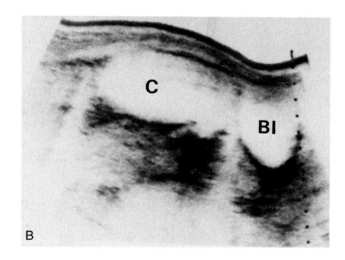

From: Fiske CE, Callen PW. Ultrasonography in the evaluation of cystic lesions and fluid collections within the pelvis simulating urinary bladder. J Can Assoc Radiol 1981; 31:254–255. Reproduced with permission.

Figure 13–16. LYMPHOCELE SIMULATING THE URINARY BLADDER.

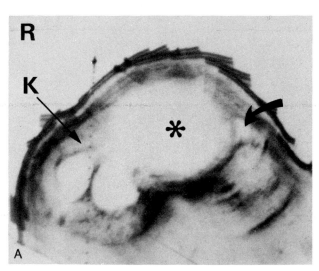

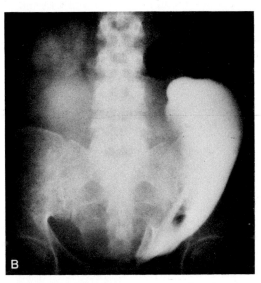

Figure 13–16A. A palpable pelvic mass was seen in this patient approximately two months after renal transplantation. A transverse ultrasonogram reveals a large midline cystic mass *(asterisk)* that appeared to be continuous with the hydrocalyces of the renal transplant (K) in the right iliac fossa. What might be considered to be extravesical fluid proved to be the patient's urinary bladder *(curved arrow)* displaced to the left.

Figure 13–16B. Intravenous urography demonstrated a large pelvic mass, which proved to be a lymphocele displacing the urinary bladder to the left.

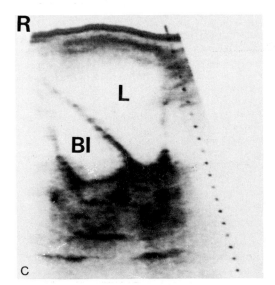

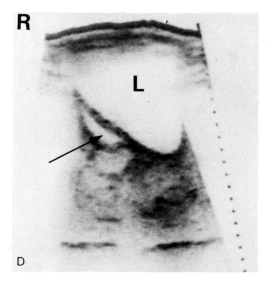

Figure 13–16C. A renal transplant patient presented with an enlarging pelvic mass. A transverse ultrasonogram demonstrated two similar fluid-filled structures within the pelvis, making the accurate distinction of the urinary bladder (Bl) and lymphocele (L) difficult.

Figure 13–16D. A postvoid ultrasonogram clearly demonstrates the lymphocele (L) to be the more anterior structure, with the collapsed urinary bladder seen to its right *(arrow)*.

From: Fiske CE, Callen PW. Ultrasonography in the evaluation of cystic lesions and fluid collections within the pelvis simulating urinary bladder. J Can Assoc Radiol 1981; 31:254–255. Reproduced with permission.

Figure 13–17. ASCITES SIMULATING THE URINARY BLADDER. A 46-year-old man presented with diffuse abdominal pain.

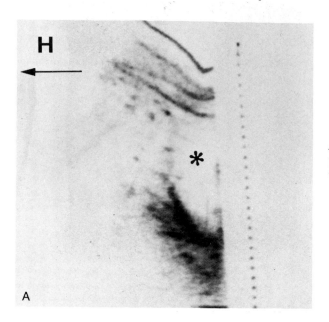

Figure 13–17A. A longitudinal midline ultrasonogram of the pelvis demonstrated a large, fluid-filled structure *(asterisk),* which has the appearance of the urinary bladder.

Figure 13–17B. When a scan through the same plane of section is continued caudally, the distinction can be seen between the pelvic ascites *(asterisk)* and the urinary bladder (Bl). Another clue to the true nature of the ascites is the angulation of the fluid as it interdigitates between bowel loops *(arrows).*

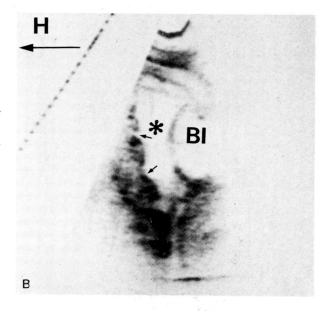

From: Fiske CE, Callen PW. Ultrasonography in the evaluation of cystic lesions and fluid collections within the pelvis simulating urinary bladder. J Can Assoc Radiol 1981; 31:254–255. Reproduced with permission.

Figure 13–18. URETERAL JET SIMULATING BLADDER MASS.

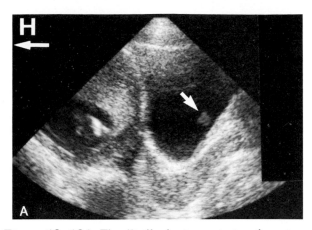

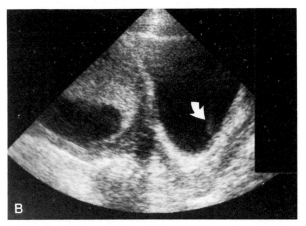

Figure 13–18A. The "jet" of urine entering the urinary bladder may simulate an intravesical mass *(arrow).*

Figure 13–18B. Constant observation of this area using realtime ultrasonography will clear up the confusion as the characteristic stream-like configuration can be seen *(arrow)* as the urine enters the bladder.

Ref.: Elejalde BR, Elejalde MM. Ureteral ejaculation of urine visualized by ultrasound. J Clin Ultrasound 1983; 11:475–476.

Figure 13–19. SLICE THICKNESS ARTIFACT FROM THE UTERUS SIMULATING BLADDER MASS.

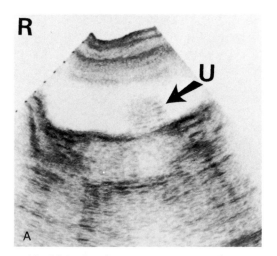

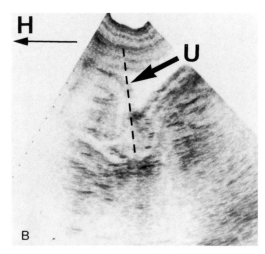

Figure 13–19A. On this transverse scan there appears to be a soft tissue mass (U) projecting into the urinary bladder.

Figure 13–19B. On this longitudinal scan the etiology of this "mass" is clearly seen. It is secondary to the uterus (U) which is projecting anteriorly into the urinary bladder. This is a normal finding and occurs when the tomographic plane of section occurs at the edge of two adjacent structures.

Figure 13–20. LARGE CYSTADENOMA SIMULATING THE URINARY BLADDER.

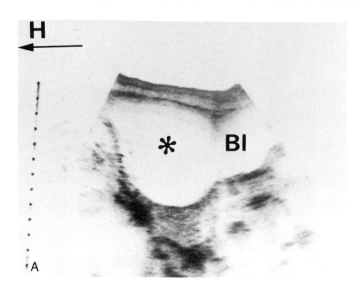

Figure 13–20A. All fluid collections within the pelvis should be specifically identified as representing either the urinary bladder or a separate cystic mass. In this case the interface between the urinary bladder (Bl) and the cystic mass *(asterisk)* is not well seen because this interface is parallel rather than perpendicular to the ultrasound beam. This may create the impression that the bladder is markedly distended. Scanning in various planes of section as well as emptying of the urinary bladder will help alleviate this confusion.

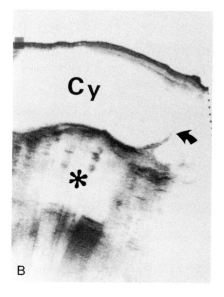

Figure 13–20B. In another patient, a large cystic mass arises out of the true and false pelvis (Cy). Identification of the superior aspect of the urinary bladder wall *(arrow)* delineates the mass from the bladder. Additionally noted is an area of shadowing from bowel gas, with a pseudomass *(asterisk)* created by a duplication mirror-image artifact (see Fig. 13–14).

Figure 13–21. IMPRESSION FROM PELVIC SIDEWALL SIMULATING BLADDER MASS.

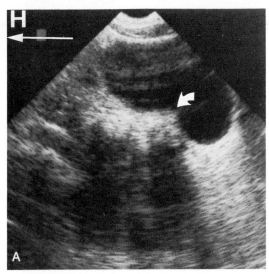

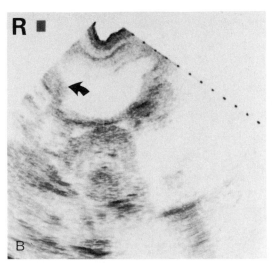

Figure 13–21A. On a longitudinal scan of the pelvis, an angulated mass *(arrow)* is seen projecting into the urinary bladder.

Figure 13–21B. On a transverse scan of the same patient, the etiology of this "mass" can be identified as a slight indentation of the pelvic sidewall into the distended urinary bladder. This is a normal finding.

Figure 13–22. SPINAL CANAL SIMULATING A POSTERIOR CYSTIC MASS. A transverse scan obtained at the level of the intervertebral disc space (V) permits visualization of the normal spinal canal (S). This should not be mistaken for a cystic mass or other pathology.

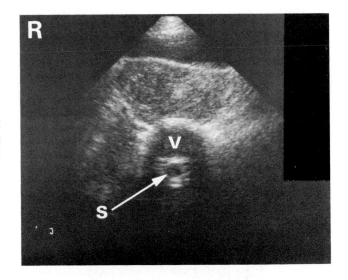

CHAPTER 14

Testis

PETER W. CALLEN, M.D.
BARRY S. MAHONY, M.D.

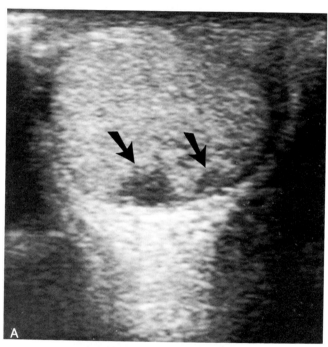

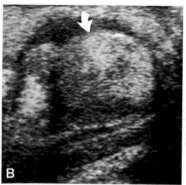

Figure 14–1. ORCHITIS SIMULATING TESTICU-LAR NEOPLASM. Patients with a severe epididymitis, as shown in these two examples, often have a co-existent orchitis. The areas of inflammation of the testicle may appear as hypoechoic regions *(arrow)*, which may simulate a testicular neoplasm. Knowledge of the patient's clinical history as well as correlative findings of an enlarged tender epididymis that suggest epididymitis help to distinguish orchitis from testicular neoplasm. In addition, follow-up scans may be helpful to differentiate these two entities.

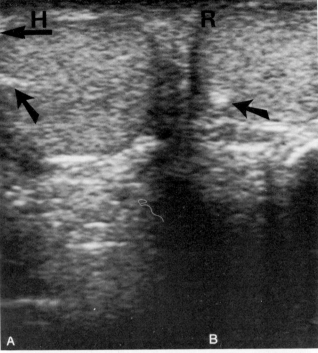

Figure 14–2. MEDIASTINUM TESTIS SIMULATING TESTICULAR PATHOLOGY. Ultrasonograms taken in either the transverse or longitudinal plane of section may often reveal a high amplitude echo within the testes *(arrows)*. This represents the mediastinum testis, a fascial covering seen in the posterolateral aspect of the testicle. Scans obtained in the transverse plane of the testis *(B)* demonstrate the mediastinum testis as a round echogenic focus. Rotation of the transducer into the longitudinal axis of the testis *(A, C, and D)* confirms the linear nature of the mediastinum testis.

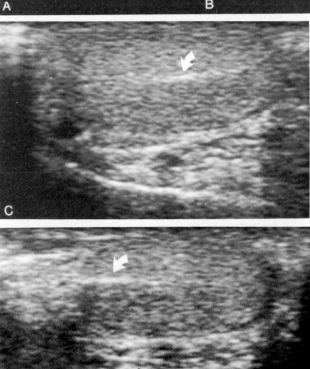

Figure 14–3. TESTICULAR CLEFT SIMULATING LACERATION. In some patients, as in these examples, a poorly echogenic linear region *(arrow)* may be seen coursing through the testicle. While the etiology of this "cleft" is uncertain, it is not a pathological lesion and in most instances may be differentiated from a true laceration on the basis of history.

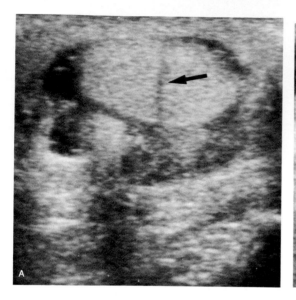
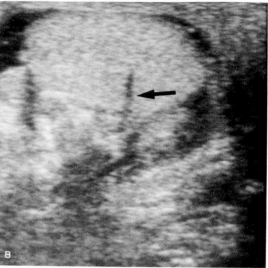

Neonatal Brain

PETER W. CALLEN, M.D.
BARRY S. MAHONY, M.D.

Figure 15–1. CEREBELLAR VERMIS SIMULATING INTRACEREBRAL HEMORRHAGE.
The cerebellar vermis often appears quite echogenic on parasagittal scans of the neonatal head. This represents the normal cerebellum (C) and should not be mistaken for intracerebral hemorrhage.

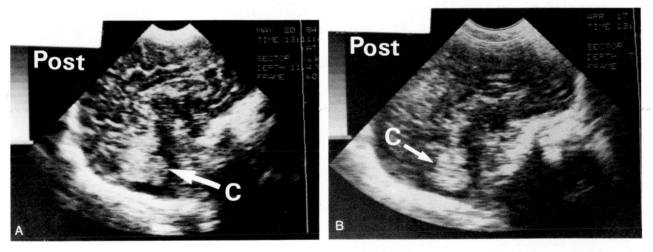

Ref.: Grant EG, Schellinger D, Richardson JD. Realtime ultrasonography of the posterior fossa. J Ultrasound Med 1983; 2:73.

Figure 15–2. LOBULARITY OF THE CHOROID PLEXUS SIMULATING CHOROIDAL HEMORRHAGE.
The choroid plexus in the region of the atrium of the lateral ventricle may often appear quite lobular in configuration (C). While this may simulate bleeding within the ventricle it is invariably a variation of the choroid plexus morphology and may be followed for serial change, if clinically indicated.

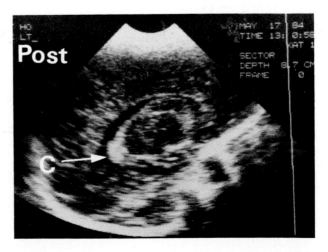

Figure 15–3. CAVUM SEPTI PELLUCIDI SIMULATING HYDROCEPHALUS. The cavum septi pellucidi and cavum Vergae are seen in approximately 60 per cent of preterm infants. On coronal scans such as *A* and *C* the cavum may appear as a large, fluid-filled structure in the midline between the lateral ventricles.

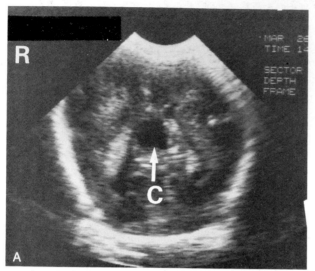

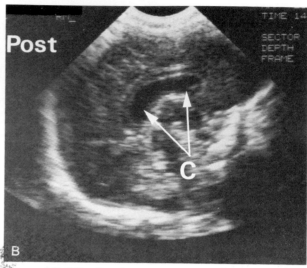

Figure 15–3A. Coronal scan of the neonatal head demonstrating the cavum septi pellucidi (C).

Figure 15–3B. On this sagittal scan of the neonatal head taken in the midline, the anterior and posterior locations of the cavum septi pellucidi (C) can be identified.

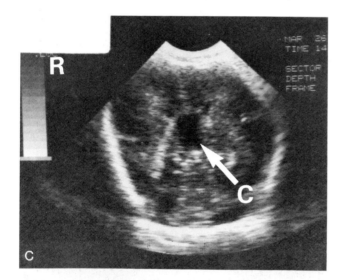

Figure 15–3C. Coronal scan, similar to *A*, of the neonatal head showing the cavum septi pellucidi (C).

Ref.: Farruggia S, Babcock DS. The cavum septi pellucidi: Its appearance and incidence with cranial ultrasonography in infancy. Radiology 1979; 139:147.

Figure 15–4. ABSENCE OF THE SEPTUM PELLUCIDUM SIMULATING CONGENITAL ANOMALY. As a variant, the septum pellucidum may not be seen in some patients with dilated ventricles. This may occur with hydrocephalus following disruption of the septum pellucidum. Its absence *(arrow)* should not imply either a congenital anomaly or more serious intracranial damage.

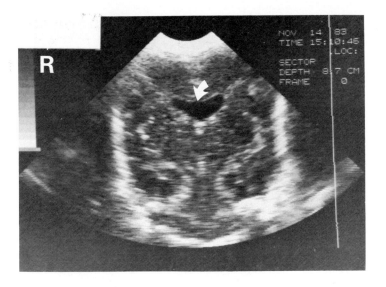

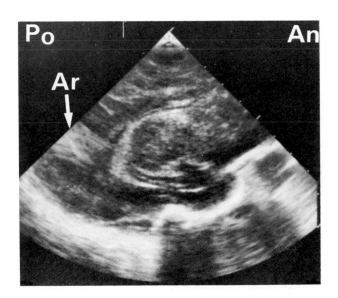

Figure 15–5. SIDE-LOBE ARTIFACT SIMULATING INTRACRANIAL HEMORRHAGE. Occasionally artifact (Ar) from areas peripheral to the area of interest may be placed within the image scan. These represent side-lobe artifacts and their etiology may be identified more clearly with repositioning of the ultrasound transducer.

Ref.: Laing FC, Kurtz AB. The importance of ultrasonic side-lobe artifacts. Radiology 1982; 145:763.

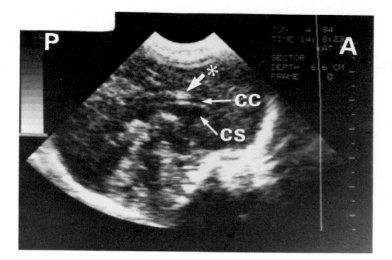

Figure 15–6. SPECULAR REFLECTION FROM THE CORPUS CALLOSUM OR ROOF OF THE LATERAL VENTRICLE SIMULATING INTRACRANIAL HEMORRHAGE. At times an area of bright reflection may mimic an intracranial hemorrhage *(asterisk).* This artifact results from a prominent specular reflection created when the ultrasound beam is perpendicular to either the corpus callosum (CC) or the roof of the lateral ventricle. These are rarely seen on perpendicular, coronal scans and usually are more cephalic in location than are true germinal matrix hemorrhages (CS = cavum septi pellucidi).

Ref.: Siedler DE, Mahony BS, Hoddick WK, Callen PW. A specular reflection arising from the ventricular wall: A potential pitfall in the diagnosis of germinal matrix hemorrhage. J Ultrasound Med 1985; 4:109–112.

Figure 15–7. ECHOGENIC THALAMUS AND CORPUS STRIATUM COMPLEX SIMULATING INTRACRANIAL HEMORRHAGE. Frequently in more mature neonates areas of increased echogenicity may be seen in the region of the thalamus and corpus striatum *(arrows).* Although this may appear identical to the appearance of cerebral hemorrhage, the lack of deformation of normal structures as well as the symmetry will help distinguish these normal structures from cerebral hemorrhage.

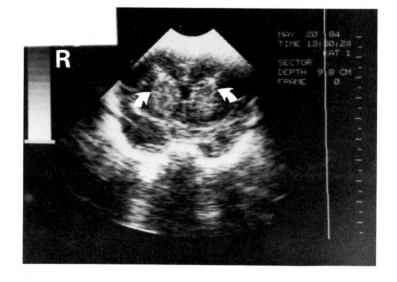

CHAPTER 16

Obstetrics

PETER W. CALLEN, M.D.
BARRY S. MAHONY, M.D.

Figure 16–1. AMNIOTIC MEMBRANE SIMULATING AMNIOTIC BAND. In the first trimester of pregnancy, the amniotic membrane (A) frequently may be identified. This is a normal structure and does not imply pathologic disruption of the amnion. This membrane may be apparent until 16 weeks, at which time there is usually apposition of the amnion and chorion.

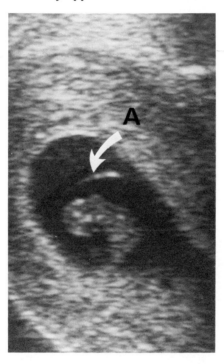

Ref.: Burrows PE, Lyons EA, Philips HJ, Oates I. Intrauterine membranes: Sonographic findings and clinical significance. J Clin Ultrasound 1982; 10:1–8.

Figure 16–2. NORMAL LOBULATION OF THE MYOMETRIUM EARLY IN THE FIRST TRIMESTER OF PREGNANCY. In early first trimester pregnancies, there is often a lobularity of the myometrium *(asterisk),* usually beneath the site of implantation. This is a normal finding and should not be mistaken for a myoma.

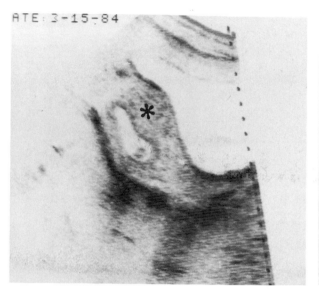
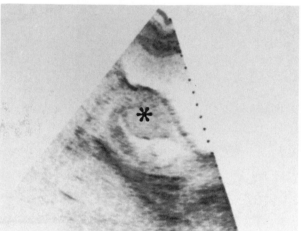

Figure 16–3. YOLK SAC SIMULATING FETAL BODY PART. With the improved resolution of ultrasound equipment, the yolk sac (YS) can usually be identified in most first trimester pregnancies. This structure should not be included in measurements of the fetus (F) obtained for the crown rump length and should not be mistaken for an abnormal twin pregnancy.

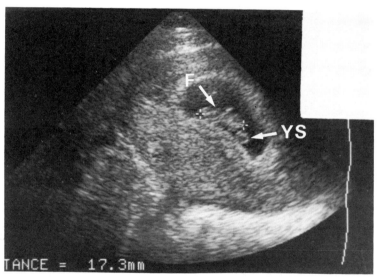

Ref.: Mantoni M, Pedersen JF. Ultrasound visualization of the human yolk sac. J Clin Ultrasound 1979; 7:459–460.

Figure 16–4. **DISTENDED URINARY BLADDER SIMULATING FLUID IN THE CERVICAL CANAL.** Marked distention of the maternal urinary bladder (B) has caused near apposition of the anterior and posterior walls (arrows) of the lower uterine segment, simulating the cervical canal. Normal amniotic fluid *(asterisk)* is trapped between the lower uterine segment walls and appears to lie within the cervix. A post-void scan will help alleviate this confusion.

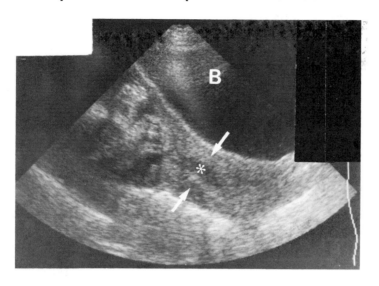

Figure 16–5. **PSEUDO-UTERINE MYOMA SECONDARY TO MATERNAL UMBILICUS.** Scanning over the umbilicus often produces an artifact in the uterine wall resembling a myoma *(arrows).* Marking the umbilicus at the time of scanning will often avoid this dilemma.

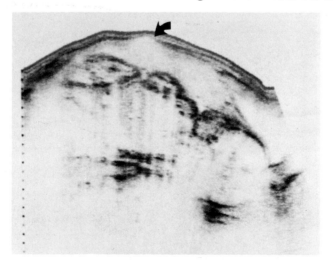

Figure 16–6. OVERDISTENDED MATERNAL URINARY BLADDER SIMULATING A PLA-CENTA PREVIA.

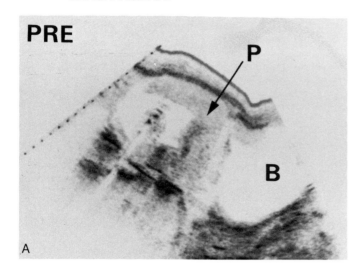

Figure 16–6A. In this pre-void scan, the distended urinary bladder (B) has pushed the placenta (P) across the endocervical canal simulating a placenta previa.

Figure 16–6B. In this post-void scan the placenta (P) can be seen to end cephalad to the cervical canal.

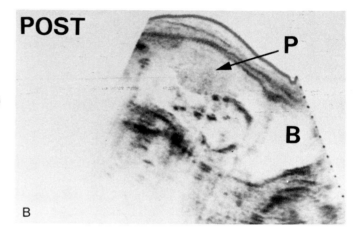

Ref.: Zemlyn S. The effect of the urinary bladder in obstetrical sonography. Radiology 1978; 128:169–175.

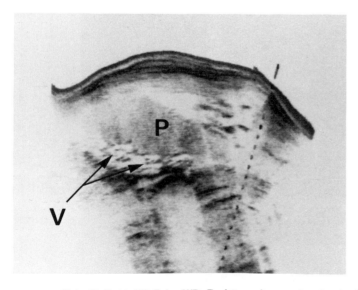

Figure 16–7. PROMINENT RETROPLACENTAL VEINS SIMULATING ARTERIOVENOUS MAL-FORMATION OR ABRUPTION. Normal dilated decidual and myometrial veins (V) may be seen beneath the placenta (P) from the second trimester onward. These veins are usually seen posteriorly and, when the interfaces between the individual veins are not seen, may appear as a large anechoic area simulating an abruption. Focused transducers with higher frequencies may, at times, alleviate this confusion.

Ref.: (1) Smith DF, Foley WD. Real-time ultrasound and pulse Doppler evaluation of the retroplacental clear area. J Clin Ultrasound 1982; 10:215–219. (2) McGahan AP, Phillips HE, Reid MH. The anacholic retroplacental area. Radiology 1980; 134:475–478.

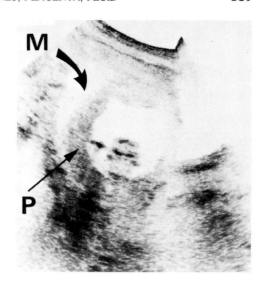

Figure 16–8. NORMAL MYOMETRIUM SIMULATING ABRUP-TIO PLACENTAE. The subplacental myometrium (M) may often appear anechoic, simulating abruptio placentae. This appearance may result from a combination of the normal subplacental uterine veins and refractive shadowing, particularly when the placenta is located adjacent to a curved surface, such as the fundus or the lateral uterine walls (P = placenta).

Ref.: Callen PW, Filly RA. The placental-subplacental complex: A specific indicator of placental position on ultrasound. J Clin Ultrasound 1980; 8:21–26.

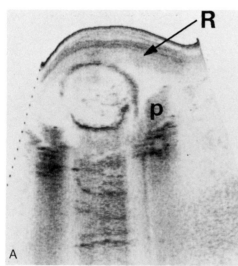

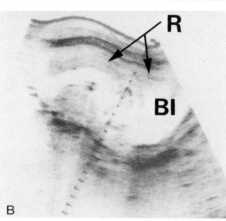

Figure 16–9. REVERBERATION ARTIFACT SIMULATING THE PLACENTA. Reverberation artifact (R) in the near field may simulate the placenta. Two features may allow one to make the distinction between this artifact and the normally appearing placenta. First, reverberation artifact can be specifically identified when it extends outside the confines of the uterus into the maternal urinary bladder (Bl). Second, the two may be distinguished when the placenta (P) can be recognized on the opposing uterine wall by virtue of its differing echogenicity and placental-subplacental complex.

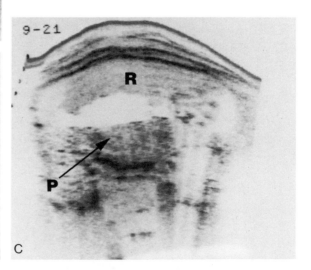

Ref.: Callen PW, Filly, RA. The placental-subplacental complex: A specific indicator of placental position on ultrasound. J Clin Ultrasound 1980; 8:21–26.

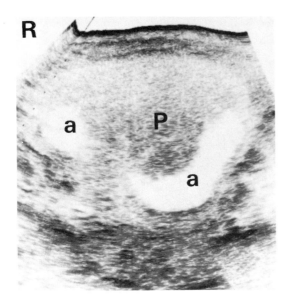

Figure 16–10. **PSEUDO–BICORNUATE UTERUS.** In cases in which an extreme degree of cephalocaudad angulation of the transducer is used, particularly in the fundic portion of the uterus, the placenta (P) may create the appearance of a bicornuate uterus. When a placenta with a short insertion site contacts the opposing wall it may also appear to divide the amniotic cavities into two compartments. Alternate planes of section at 90 degrees to the one obtained in the scan will often alleviate this potential confusion (a = amniotic fluid).

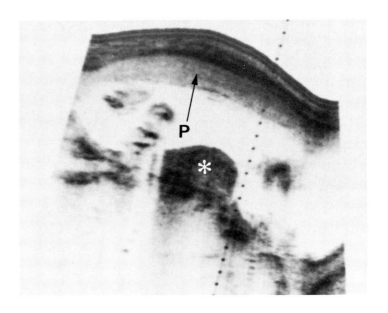

Figure 16–11. **TRANSIENT MYOMETRIAL CONTRACTION SIMULATING THE PLACENTA.** Transient myometrial contractions of the uterus *(asterisk)* may simulate the echogenicity of the placenta (P). These may be differentiated by virtue of the contraction's focal nature and its absence of a normal placental-subplacental complex of echoes.

Ref.: Callen PW, Filly RA. The placental-subplacental complex: A specific indicator of placental position on ultrasound. J Clin Ultrasound 1980; 8:21–26.

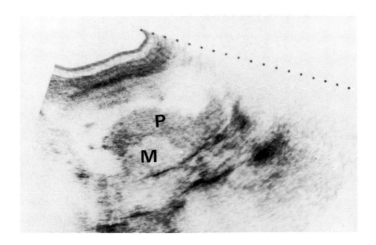

Figure 16–12. **TRANSIENT MYOMETRIAL CONTRACTION SIMULATING UTERINE MYOMA.** Focal contractions of the myometrium (M) may cause deformation of the inner aspect of the uterus and placenta (P). The transient nature of the contraction, as well as the failure to deform the outer contour of the uterus helps differentiate this contraction from a myoma.

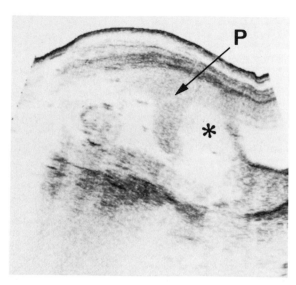

Figure 16–13. TRANSIENT MYOMETRIAL CONTRACTION SIMULATING ABRUPTIO PLACENTAE. Prominent myometrial contractions *(asterisk),* especially when seen in a subplacental location, may simulate abruptio placentae. The transient nature of the contraction, as well as the patient symptomatology, may help alleviate this confusion (P = placenta).

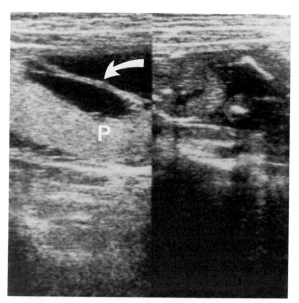

Figure 16–14. PROBABLE UTERINE SYNECHIA SIMULATING AMNIOTIC BAND. At times, a sheet of tissue *(arrow)* may be seen crossing the amniotic fluid, extending from one area of the uterine wall to another. This tissue probably represents a partial uterine septation or synechia and, as such, has intact amnion covering its surface. The ability of the fetal parts to move on either side of this tissue, as well as the absence of disruption of the amnion, are features that characterize this as a benign process which is unlikely to cause fetal deformity (P = placenta).

Ref.: Mahony BS, Filly RA, Callen PW, Golbus MS. The amniotic band syndrome: Antenatal sonographic diagnosis and potential pitfalls. Am J Obstet Gynecol 1985; 152:63–68.

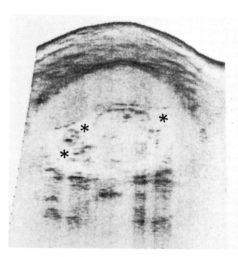

Figure 16–15. ARTIFACTUAL ECHOES WITHIN THE AMNIOTIC FLUID SIMULATING OLIGOHYDRAMNIOS. In obese patients, because of increasing gain levels that are used in scanning, artifactual echoes may be seen within the amniotic fluid *(asterisks).* These may simulate the appearance of oligohydramnios. Scanning with a lower frequency transducer at lower levels of receiver sensitivity will reveal the amniotic fluid to be appropriate in amount.

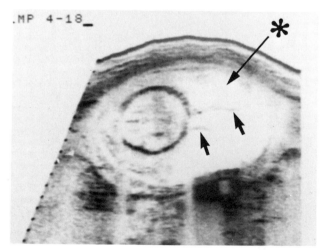

Figure 16–16. CYSTIC MASS SIMULATING AMNIOTIC FLUID. Cystic masses about the fetal head or fetal spine, especially when adjacent to the myometrium, may simulate pockets of amniotic fluid. In this patient, a large cystic hygroma extending from the fetal head may at first appear to represent amniotic fluid. With careful scanning, one can determine that the fluid *(asterisk)* is contained within multiple areas of loculation and septations *(arrows)* and therefore represents a cystic mass associated with the fetus rather than amniotic fluid.

Figure 16–17. NORMAL CHOROID PLEXUS SIMULATING CRANIAL MASS. Scans (*A* and *C* = axial; *B* = parasagittal) of the fetal head in three different patients in the early second trimester of pregnancy demonstrate echogenic soft-tissue structures (CP) seen within the fetal calvarium. These represent the choroid plexus of the lateral ventricle. The choroid plexus is a rich vascular network that fills the body of the lateral ventricle from its medial to its lateral wall. It is useful in identifying the lateral ventricle and excluding the diagnosis of hydrocephalus. The choroid plexus does not extend into the occipital horn or the anterior horns of the lateral ventricle.

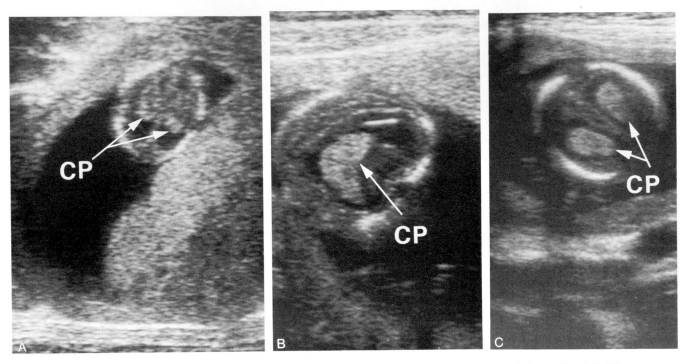

Ref.: Chinn DH, Callen PW, Filly RA. The lateral cerebral ventricle in early second trimester. Radiology 1983; 148:529–531.

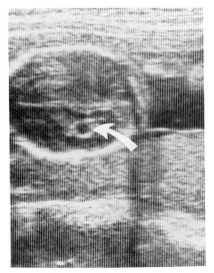

Figure 16–18. CHOROID PLEXUS CYST SIMULATING INTERCRANIAL CYSTIC MASS. Rarely, cysts of the choroid plexus may be identified *(arrow)* during routine obstetrical scanning. These usually disappear during the pregnancy and are of no clinical significance.

Ref.: Chudleigh P, Pearce JM, Campbell S. The prenatal diagnosis of transient cysts of the fetal choroid plexus. Prenat Diagn 1984; 4:135–137.

Figure 16–19. NORMAL FETAL BRAIN SIMULATING DILATED LATERAL VENTRICLES.

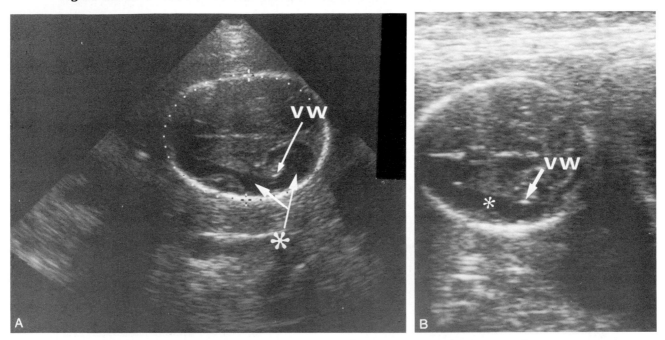

Figure 16–19A and B. In two separate patients during the second trimester of pregnancy, an anechoic space *(asterisk)* is seen adjacent to the calvarium. Although this simulates the appearance of fluid (that is, hydrocephalus), the true nature of this area, which represents extraventricular normal brain, can be seen by virtue of the identification of the lateral wall of the lateral ventricle (VW).

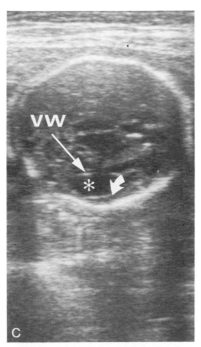

Figure 16–19C. In another patient with a similar finding of anechoic normal brain *(asterisk)* adjacent to the lateral ventricular wall (VW), tissue is seen adjacent to the calvarium *(arrow)*. This does not represent compressed brain from dilated ventricles, but, rather, the normal pia-arachnoid.

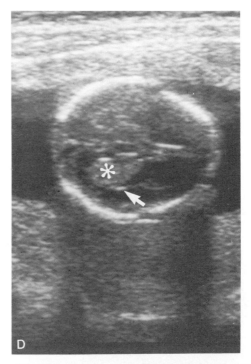

Figure 16–19D. Further resolution of the question of the normal position and size of the ventricle will occur if one identifies the normal choroid plexus *(asterisk)*, filling the body of the lateral ventricle from its medial wall to its lateral wall *(arrow)*.

Ref.: Chinn DH, Callen PW, Filly RA. The lateral cerebral ventricle in early second trimester. Radiology 1983; 148:529–531.

Figure 16–20. OCCIPITAL HORN SIMULATING AN INTRACEREBRAL CYSTIC MASS.

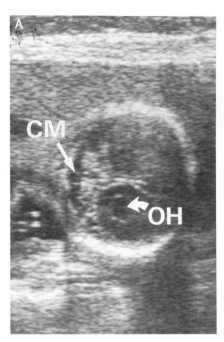

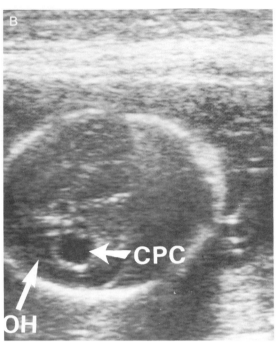

Figure 16–20A. When the fetal head is sectioned in an oblique coronal plane, the occipital horn may appear as a spherical structure (OH). When one obtains scans in a more transverse axial plane, similar to that obtained for the measurement of the biparietal diameter, the more characteristic appearance of the occipital horn will be seen (CM = cisterna magna).

Figure 16–20B. In a true axial plane of section, a choroid plexus cyst (CPC) can be seen residing within the choroid plexus in the lateral ventricle. This can be differentiated from occipital horn shown in A by virtue of the ability to see the occipital horn (OH) projecting beyond the margins of this structure. (See Figure 16–8.)

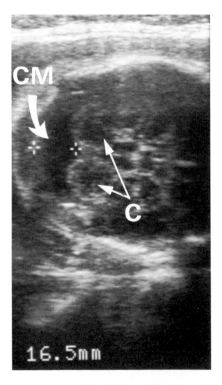

Figure 16–21. NORMAL CISTERNA MAGNA SIMULATING DANDY-WALKER MALFORMATION. The fluid-filled cisterna magna (CM) can be identified in most obstetrical sonograms in the third trimester. The cisterna magna may be quite prominent, however, and should not be misinterpreted as a Dandy-Walker malformation or cellebellar atrophy (C = cerebellar hemispheres).

Ref.: Mahony BS, Callen PW, Filly RA, Hoddick WK. The fetal cisterna magna. Radiology 1984; 153:773–776.

Figure 16–22. DOLICHOCEPHALY RE-SULTING IN INACCURATE PREDIC-TION OF MENSTRUAL AGE. The fetal head has a variable shape, and at times it may be dolichocephalic in configuration. This may result from compression in cases in which there is decreased amniotic fluid. In other cases it may be a result of normal biological variation. If the shape of the head is not taken into consideration, the menstrual age based upon the biparietal diameter will result in underestimation of the gestational age.

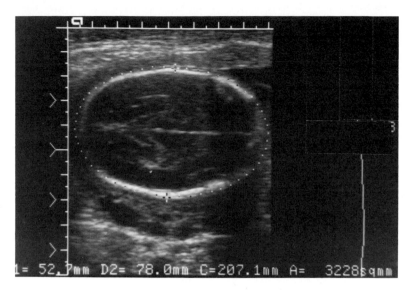

Figure 16–23. FETAL MOVEMENT SIMULATING ABNORMAL CRANIAL MORPHOLOGY.

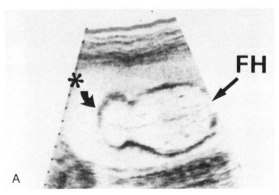

Figure 16–23A. When static articulated arm scans of the fetal head are obtained, movement may be represented either by a double calvarium suggesting edema or by an area of lobularity *(asterisk),* as in this case. Scanning with a realtime scanner often will resolve this confusion.

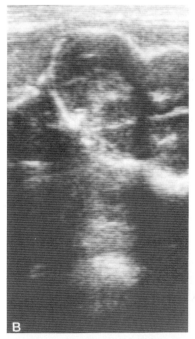

Figure 16–23B. The scan shown in A should be compared with this case of "cloverleaf skull," in which there is a marked deformity of the fetal calvarium, secondary to premature closure of the sutures.

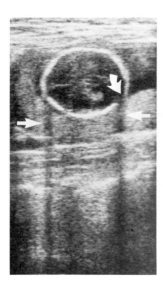

Figure 16–24. DISRUPTION OF THE FETAL CALVARIUM BY REFLECTIVE ACOUSTIC SHADOWING. Acoustic shadowing that interrupts the normal continuity of the fetal calvarium *(curved arrow)* is commonly seen during obstetrical ultrasonography. This shadowing *(straight arrows)* occurs where a solid structure of high acoustic velocity (fetal calvarium) is immersed in a medium of lower acoustic velocity (amniotic fluid). As the ultrasound beam path crosses the margin of soft tissue–fluid, shadows are generated at points where the critical angle is met or exceeded. This is often referred to as the critical angle of reflection.

Ref.: Sommer FG, Filly RA, Minton MJ. Acoustic shadowing due to refractive and reflective effects. AJR 1979; 132:973–977.

Figure 16–25. REFRACTION OF SOUND FROM THE FETAL HEAD SIMULATING CALVARIAL OVERLAP. Refraction of sound at the edge of the fetal head will result in artifactual displacement of the fetal calvarium *(arrows)* along the vector in the direction in which the transducer was pointing at the time of scanning. This same phenomenon is seen when the diaphragm is artifactually displaced due to refraction from the sound passing through the liver.

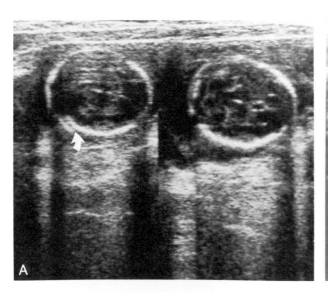
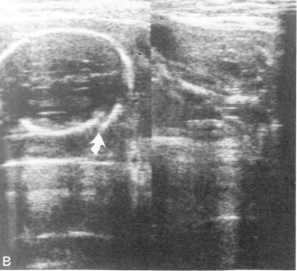

Ref.: Mayo J, Cooperberg PL. Displacement of the diaphragmatic echo by hepatic cysts. J Ultrasound Med 1984; 3:337–340.

Figure 16–26. NORMAL FETAL EAR SIMULATING A MASS. A knowledge of the plane of section during scanning and the normal anatomy of the ear will prevent confusion regarding this structure.

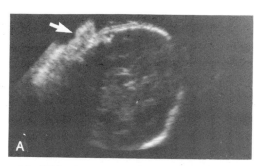

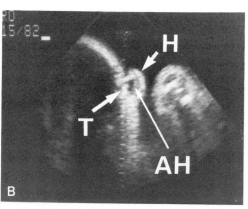

Figure 16–26A. A coronal image of the head demonstrates soft tissue *(arrow)* along the lateral aspect of the head, suggesting a parietal encephalocele.

Figure 16–26B. Parasagittal image of the lateral aspect of the fetal head shows the characteristic helix (H), antihelix (AH), and Tragus (T) of the ear.

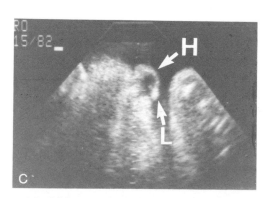

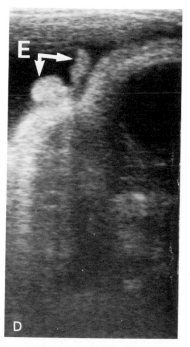

Figure 16–26C. A minor change in transducer angulation from that used in *B* demonstrates the helix (H) and the lobule (L) of the pinna.

Figure 16–26D. When the ear (E) is more tangential to the calvarium, its characteristic morphology may be recognized, thereby avoiding confusion with other pathologic entities.

A–C from: Fink IJ, Chinn DH, Callen PW. A potential pitfall in the ultrasonographic diagnosis of fetal encephalocele. J Ultrasound Med 1983; 2:313–314. Reproduced with permission.

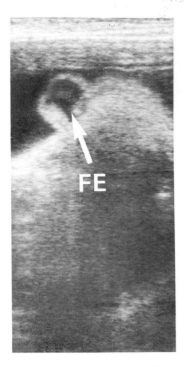

FE

Figure 16–27. FETAL EAR SIMULATING AN ENCEPHALOCELE. At times the fetal ear may project perpendicular to the calvarium into the amniotic fluid and simulate a cystic mass projecting from the fetal head (i.e., an encephalocele). The rare occurrence of encephaloceles in the parietal area and the characteristic morphology of the fetal ear will help to avoid this confusion.

Ref.: Fink IJ, Chinn EH, Callen PW. A potential pitfall in the ultrasonic graphic diagnosis of fetal encephalocele. J Ultrasound Med 1983; 2:303:314.

Figure 16–28. INADEQUATE "GAIN" SETTINGS SIMU-LATING HYDROCEPHALUS. If the time-compensated gain is inappropriately set, an inadequate number of echoes will be seen from the normal brain. This may create the appearance of large fluid-filled collections in the calvarium *(asterisk)* (i.e., hydrocephalus). Attention to adequate technique will prevent this confusion in all cases.

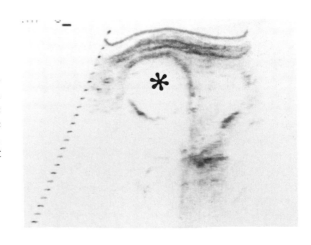

Figure 16–29. SIDE-LOBE AND DUPLICATION ARTIFACT SIMULATING FETAL MASSES, MOTION, AND SKIN EDEMA. When the ultrasound transducer is placed on the midline of the abdominal wall, refraction of sound at the muscle–fat interface may result in a double image effect. In addition, transducer side-lobe artifacts, although more commonly seen with single-element transducers and sector scanners, also can be seen with linear array transducers. Side-lobe artifacts result from multiple low-intensity sound beams located outside of the main ultrasound beam.

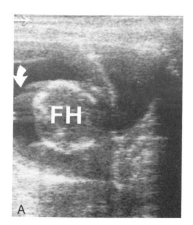

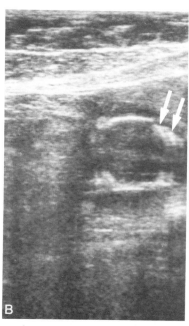

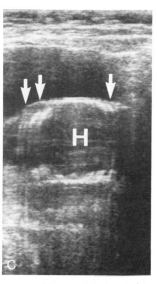

Figure 16–29A. Side-lobe artifacts create the impression of extra tissue *(arrow)* emanating from the fetal head (FH).

Figure 16–29B. Although there was no fetal motion at the time of this scan, two distinct specular reflections *(arrows)* representing the fetal calvarium are seen secondary to this same phenomenon.

Figure 16–29C. Double-image artifacts *(arrows)* create impression of soft-tissue edema surrounding the fetal head (H).

Refs.: (1) Laing FC, Kurtz AB. The importance of ultrasonic side-lobe artifacts. Radiology 1982; 145:763–768. (2) Sauerbrei EE. The split-image artifact in pelvic ultrasonography: The anatomy and physics. J Ultrasound Med 1985; 4:29–34.

Figure 16–30. PSEUDOEDEMA AND MASS AT THE FETAL CALVARIUM. Transverse planes of section in a fetus in a longitudinal lie in a cephalic presentation may often demonstrate a portion of the calvarium (C) that may look abnormal. Scans slightly more caudal in the fetus will show that this is contiguous with the remainder of the fetal head. What appears to be thickening about the fetal calvarium is often secondary to the maternal bladder wall *(BW)* and adjacent myometrium; this should not be mistaken for scalp edema.

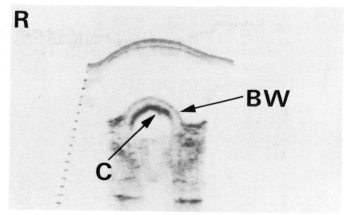

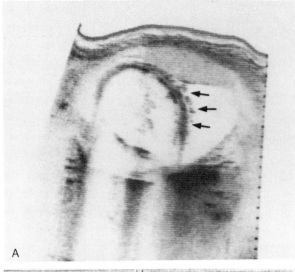

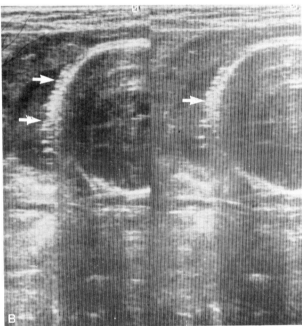

Figure 16–31. NORMAL FETAL HAIR. In the third trimester, especially when there are adequate amounts of amniotic fluid, fetal hair can be identified *(arrows)* in the sonogram. This should not be mistaken for abnormal projections from the fetal calvarium.

Figure 16–32. NORMAL NUCHAL INTEGUMENT SIMULATING SKIN EDEMA. When the fetal head (H) is extended, there is often prominence of the skin and subcutaneous tissue in the region about the neck *(arrow)*. This is a normal finding and will become less prominent with degree of fetal flexion. This should not be mistaken for focal edema or other abnormalities such as cystic hygroma (Sp = spine).

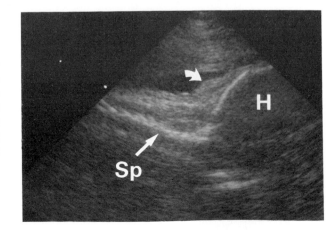

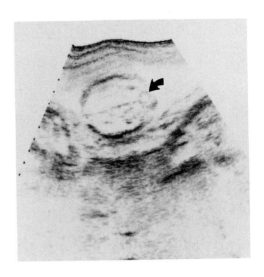

Figure 16–33. **ANGLED SCAN THROUGH THE CRANIAL VERTEBRAL JUNCTION SIMULATING A POSTERIOR FETAL CYSTIC MASS.** An oblique coronal scan through the posterior aspect of the fetal head demonstrates a cystic-appearing area *(arrow)* that probably is secondary to a scan through the cranial vertebral junction. Altering the plane of section will reveal this to be a normal structure.

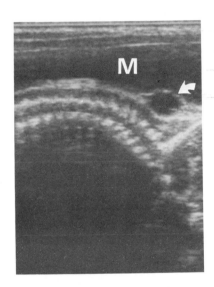

Figure 16–34. **"TRAPPED" AMNIOTIC FLUID SIMULATING A FETAL CYSTIC MASS.** When the fetus lies adjacent to the myometrium or placenta, small amounts of amniotic fluid that are trapped between the fetus and the uterine wall (M) may simulate a cystic mass *(arrow)*. Having the mother turn to a decubitus position will often alter fetal position relative to the myometrium (M) and reveal this area to be normal.

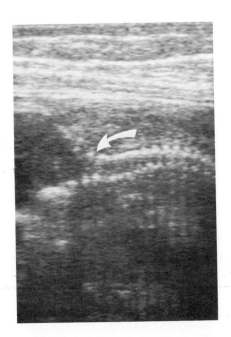

Figure 16–35. **NORMAL FLARING OF THE CRANIAL VERTEBRAL JUNCTION, SIMULATING A SPINA BIFIDA.** Normally the cephalic aspect of the cervical spine flares *(arrow)* at the junction of the spine and calvarium. This is normal and should not be mistaken for flaring due to a meningomyelocele or intraspinal mass.

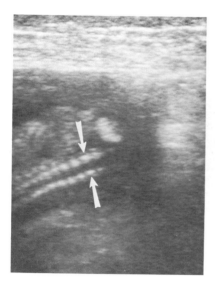

Figure 16–36. NORMAL FLARING OF THE FETAL SPINE, MIMICKING A NEURAL TUBE DEFECT. A normal fetal spine frequently demonstrates slight flaring of the lumbar region *(arrows)* with flexion. Scanning of the fetus transversely with demonstration of the spinal laminae pointing medially will confirm the absence of spinal dysraphism.

Figure 16–37. FETAL FLEXION SIMU-LATING SPINAL ABNORMALITY. If a plane of section is obtained through the fetal spine parallel to the long axis during flexion, there may be apparent widening of the posterior elements, simulating a mass *(arrow).* Observation of the fetus when it is in a more neutral position will avoid this confusion.

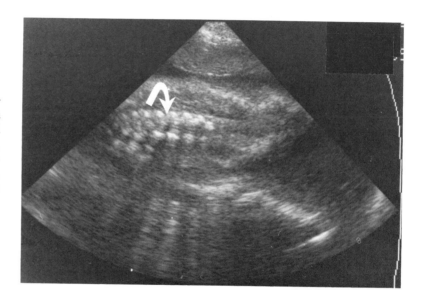

Figure 16–38. FETAL FLEXION SIMULATING A FETAL VERTEBRAL ABNORMALITY RESULTING IN KYPHOSIS. Varying degrees of fetal flexion may reveal acute angulation of the spine. Although this should always be investigated to exclude a serious vertebral abnormality, such a finding often is secondary to normal flexion. Observation over an extended period of time with visualization of gentle curvature of the fetal spine will often clarify this concern.

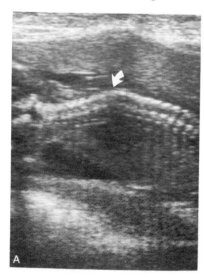

Figure 16–38A. This scan shows apparent acute angulation of the fetal spine *(arrow).*

Illustration continued on opposite page

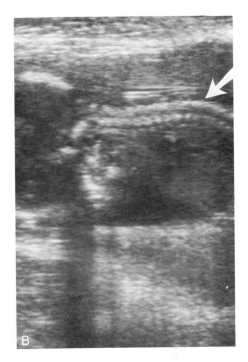

Figure 16–38B. In this sonogram taken several minutes after A, gentle curvature of the spine *(arrow)* is evident.

Figure 16–39. NORMAL UMBILICAL CORD SIMULATING A NEURAL TUBE DEFECT. *A,* If a portion of the umbilical cord (U) localizes posterior to the fetal spine (S), it may mimic a neural tube defect, such as a meningocele or meningomyelocele. *B,* By altering the plane of section slightly, the normal umbilical cord anatomy, including an artery (a) and veins (v), is visualized. *C,* The lack of spinal dysraphism at this level, documented by medial angulation of the spinal lamina (l), confirms that there is no neural tube defect.

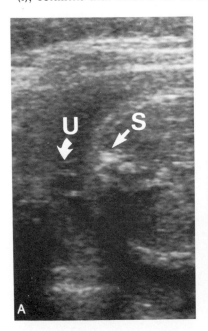
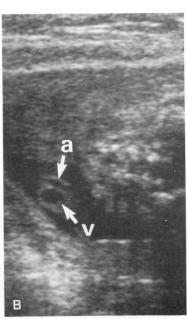
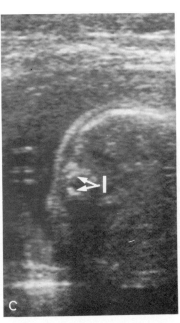

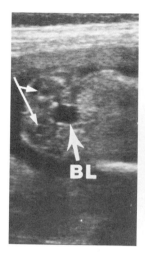
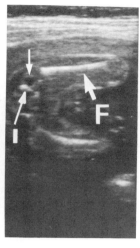

Figure 16–40. NORMAL FEMORAL HEADS MIMICKING CYSTIC MASSES. The fetal cartilage is normally hypoechoic. Occasionally when scanning the fetal pelvis the cartilaginous femoral heads may be seen *(arrows)*. The confirmation that the hypoechoic structures localize between the ossified ischium (I) and the primary ossification center of the femur (F) enables distinction between the normal cartilaginous femoral heads and a cystic mass in this region (BL = bladder).

Ref.: Mahony BS, Filly RA: High-resolution sonographic assessment of the fetal extremities. J Ultrasound Med 1984; 3:489–498.

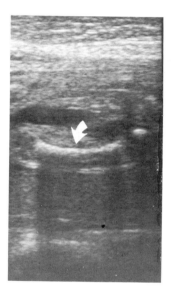

Figure 16–41. NORMAL PLANE OF SECTION THROUGH THE FETAL FEMUR, SIMULATING BOWING. Normal flaring of the distal ends of the femur may not be seen if the plane of section is truly sagittal. Scans that are somewhat more coronal *(arrow)*, as in this case, will often reveal what appears to be bowing of the femur. This is secondary to the opposite side of the femur being shadowed by the near aspect of the femur and by the normal flaring of the metadiaphysis as it joins the relatively prominent fetal femoral epiphyses. Scans in varying planes of section will often reveal this to be a normal finding.

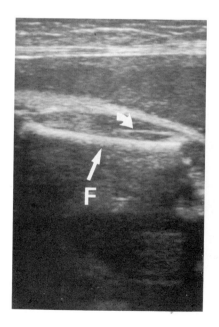

Figure 16–42. NORMAL FASCIAL PLANE SIMULATING SOFT-TISSUE ABNORMALITY IN THE FETUS. A high-amplitude linear echo frequently may be seen *(arrow)* adjacent to the femur (F) or other muscles of the upper or lower extremity. This probably results from the fascial plane interface between muscle groups.

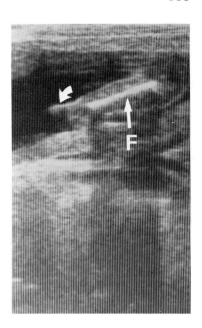

Figure 16–43. SIDE-LOBE ARTIFACT FROM THE FEMUR, SIMULATING SOFT-TISSUE ABNORMALITY. Side-lobe artifacts, as in this sonogram *(arrow)*, may simulate soft-tissue abnormality projecting from the femur (F). This will usually be seen in a single plane of section and cannot be verified when scanning is performed at 90 degrees.

Ref.: Laing FC, Kurtz AB. The Importance of ultrasonic side-lobe artifacts. Radiology 1982; 145:763–768.

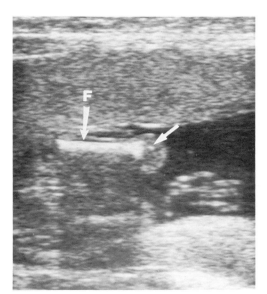

Figure 16–44. ARTIFACT SIMULATING DISTAL FEMORAL EPIPHYSEAL OSSIFICATION CENTER. The ossification center of the distal femoral epiphyses appears at approximately 29 to 35 menstrual weeks. Occasionally during the middle of the second trimester of pregnancy, many weeks before the appearance of the ossification center of the distal femoral epiphysis, one may see an echogenic focus *(arrow)* distal to the primary ossification center of the femur (F). While the etiology of this echogenic focus is uncertain in this 19–menstrual week fetus, it should not be mistaken for the distal femoral epiphyseal ossification center.

Ref.: Mahony BS, Callen PW, Filly RA. Sonographic identification and measurement of the distal femoral epiphyseal ossification center in the assessment of third-trimester menstrual age. Radiology 1985; 155:201–204.

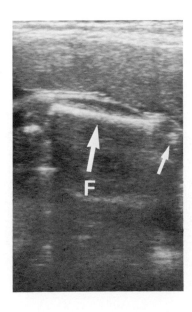

Figure 16–45. NORMAL ECHOGENICITY FROM THE SYNOVIUM, SIMULATING THE DISTAL FEMORAL EPIPHYSIS. The echogenicity of the synovium at the intercondylar notch (arrow) simulates ossification of the distal femoral cartilaginous epiphysial center. However, this is too large for a normally ossified epiphysis at this stage of gestation and is more distal from the end of the femur (F) than is usually seen with the normal epiphysial ossification center.

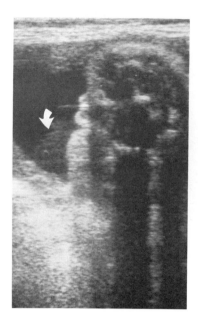

Figure 16–46. DOUBLE-IMAGE ARTIFACT SIMULATING SOFT-TISSUE MASS OF THE FETAL THIGH. When the ultrasound transducer is placed on the midline of the abdominal wall, refraction of sound at the muscle–fat interface may result in a double-image effect *(arrow)* (see also Fig. 16–29).

Ref.: Sauerbrei EE. The split image artifact in pelvic ultrasonography. J Ultrasound Med 1985; 4:29–34.

Figure 16–47. MODERATOR BAND SIMULATING INTRACARDIAC LESION.

Figure 16–47A. Four-chamber view of the fetal heart demonstrates an apparent soft-tissue mass (MB) within the right ventricle (RV). The tissue imaged represents the normal moderator band (MB), which is a useful landmark for identifying the right ventricle and should not be mistaken for mural thrombus. Also seen in this view are the right atrium (RA), aortic root (Ao), and left ventricle (LV).

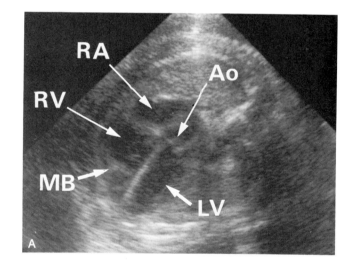

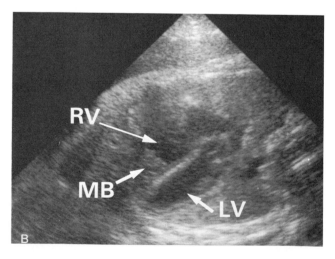

Figure 16–47B. A slightly anterior angulation from the view in A demonstrates the moderator band (MB) clearly seen within the right ventricle (RV). The left ventricle (LV) is also seen.

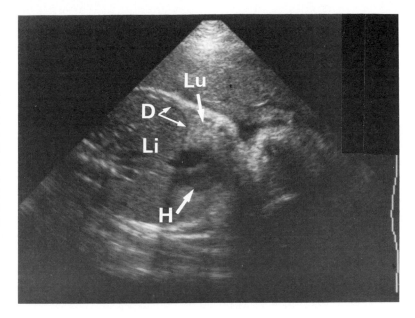

Figure 16–48. NORMAL FETAL DIA-PHRAGM SIMULATING ASCITES OR PLEURAL FLUID. The diaphragm is often poorly echogenic, as is true of various other normal muscles within the fetus and adult patient. In this case, the diaphragm (D) appears as a curvilinear anechoic region. It will be seen to move during normal fetal breathing movements and can be clearly seen to separate the fetal lung (Lu) from the liver (Li). The heart (H) can be seen resting on the hemidiaphragm, obliterating the echo at its point of contact.

Figure 16–49. FETAL-BOWEL OBSTRUCTION MIMICKING BILATERAL RENAL CYSTS. The multiple, distended fluid-filled segments of small bowel in a fetus with small-bowel obstruction *(small arrows)* may superficially resemble large multicystic dysplastic kidneys. Documentation that the "cysts" do not touch the fetal spine *(open arrows)* as well as the presence of polyhydramnios (p) permits this distinction (s = stomach).

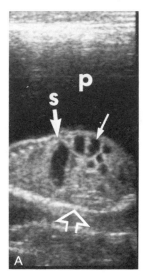

Figure 16–49A. Sagittal sonogram of the thorax and abdomen in a fetus demonstrates small bowel obstruction.

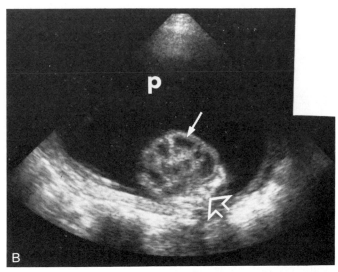

Figure 16–49B. Axial view of the fetal abdomen documents that the fluid-filled segments of small bowel *(small solid arrow)* do not touch the fetal spine *(large open arrow)* (p = polyhydramnios).

Figure 16–50. GASTROSCHISIS SIMULATING THE NORMAL UMBILICAL CORD.

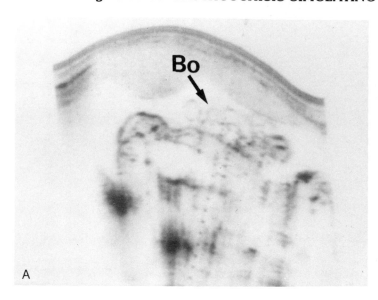

Figure 16–50A. Abdominal wall defects in the developing fetus may allow the fetal intestines to protrude into the amniotic fluid. When adjacent to the anterior abdominal wall, the bowel (Bo) may simulate the appearance of the normal umbilical cord.

Figure 16–50B. The normal umbilical cord (UC) can be identified by the multiple vessels within this structure and its entry into the midportion of the fetal abdomen. Note also the fetal ascites *(asterisk)* seen incidentally.

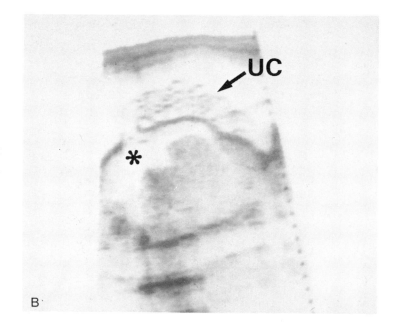

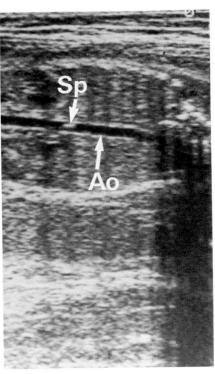

Figure 16–51. VOLUME AVERAGING SIMULATING INTRA-AORTIC ECHO. A near-coronal scan of the fetal chest and abdomen demonstrates the descending and abdominal aorta (Ao). A high amplitude echo that appears intra-aortic (Sp) is secondary to volume averaging from the adjacent ossification center of the vertebral body of the fetal spine.

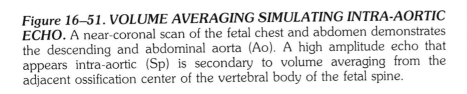

Figure 16–52. REFRACTION AND SHADOWING SIMULATING HYDRONEPHROSIS.

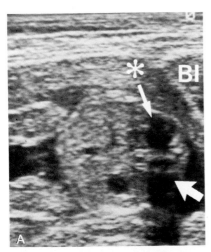

Figure 16–52A. In this longitudinal scan of a fetus in transverse lie, a sonolucent area *(asterisk)* is seen in the "up" side of the fetus while another sonolucent area is seen adjacent to the spine *(arrow)* on the "down" side of the fetus. On this scan, this might be mistaken for bilateral hydronephrosis. The lucent area adjacent to the fetal spine in the near field is probably secondary to refractive shadowing from the bladder-myometrial junction as well as normal fetal musculature. (Bl = bladder). The paraspinal sonolucent area in the far field is probably related to shadowing from the fetal spine.

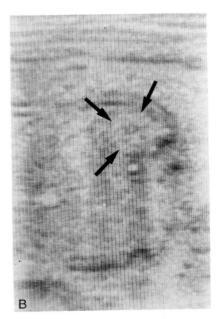

Figure 16–52B. Scanning the same fetus from a slightly different plane of section demonstrates the normal kidney *(arrow)* in the near field, thus verifying the appearance on *A* as being artifactual in nature.

Figure 16–53. FETAL GALLBLADDER SIMULATING THE UMBILICAL VEIN; PSEUDO-ASCITES.

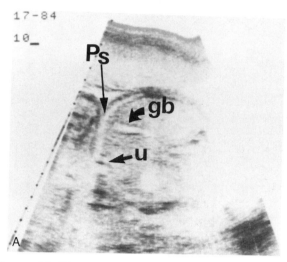

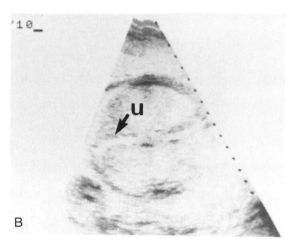

Figure 16–53A. In this axial scan through the fetal abdomen, the fetal gallbladder (gb) appears as a tubular fluid-filled, structure adjacent to the anterior abdominal wall. The differentiation between this structure and the umbilical vein (U) is best made when both are seen in the same plane of section. Also noted in this scan is a sonolucent curvilinear area adjacent to the anterior abdominal wall, which is termed pseudoascites (Ps). This results from refractive shadowing and from the normal poorly echogenic subcutaneous tissues of the anterior wall.

Figure 16–53B. The umbilical portion of the left portal vein (U) can be seen in this patient. Its differentiation from the gallbladder can be made by identifying both structures on the same plane of section as in A.

Refs.: (1) Chinn DH, Filly RA, Callen PW. Ultrasonic evaluation of fetal umbilical and hepatic vascular anatomy. Radiology 1982; 144:153–157. (2) Rosenthal SJ, Filly RA, Callen, PW, Sommer FG. Fetal Pseudo-Ascites. Radiology 1979; 131:195–197.

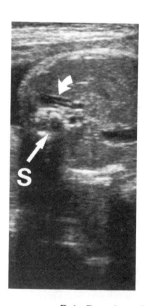

Figure 16–54. NORMAL FETAL ADRENAL GLAND SIMULATING PARASPINAL FLUID. The normal fetal adrenal is now being recognized with increased frequency. The adrenal gland *(arrow)* is often poorly echogenic and may simulate either fluid or even the normal fetal kidney adjacent to the spine. The characteristic elongated morphology, as well as an internal linear echo within the adrenal gland, are findings that will help to correctly identify the structure (S = spine).

Ref.: Rosenberg ER, Bowie JD, Andreotti RF, Fields, SI, Sonographic evaluation of fetal adrenal glands. AJR 1982; 139:1145–1147.

Figure 16–55. PROMINENT FETAL RENAL PELVES SIMULATING HYDRONEPHROSIS.
At times, the fetal renal pelves (*arrows, A; P, B*) may be somewhat prominent and simulate moderate hydronephrosis secondary to obstruction of ureteropelvic junctions or distal urethral obstruction. This degree of dilation (P, in view *B*) is usually benign, especially when the amniotic fluid and fetal bladder are normal in appearance.

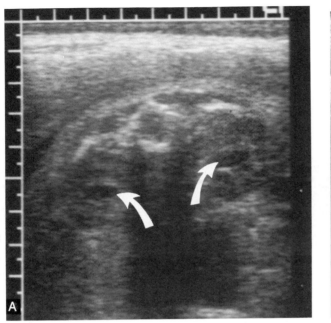
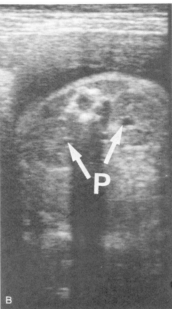

Ref.: Hoddick WK, Filly RA, Mahony BS, and Callen PW. Minimal fetal renal pyelectasis. J Ultrasound Med 1985; 4:85–90.

Figure 16–56. GREATER OMENTUM SIMULATING INTESTINAL DILATION FROM OBSTRUCTION. In the presence of fetal ascites (A), fluid may be seen on either side of the greater omentum (O) and simulate a dilated viscus. The characteristic lobular configuration of this structure and its undulating appearance during fetal movement will distinguish this from intestinal obstruction. The structure is only seen in the presence of fetal intraperitoneal fluid.

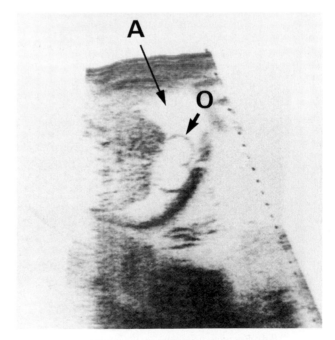

From: Gross BH, Callen PW, Filly, RA. Ultrasonic appearance of the fetal greater omentum. J Ultrasound Med 1982; 1:67–69.

Figure 16–57. **ABDOMINAL WALL MUSCULATURE AND SOFT TISSUE SIMULATING ANASARCA.** With the improved resolution of ultrasound equipment, the musculature of the body wall and the adjacent soft tissues may be seen with increased frequency. These structures are often poorly echogenic (arrows) and may simulate intraperitoneal fluid. Their location, either posterially adjacent to the spine or at prominent areas of normal musculature, will help differentiate these structures from either soft-tissue edema or intraperitoneal fluid.

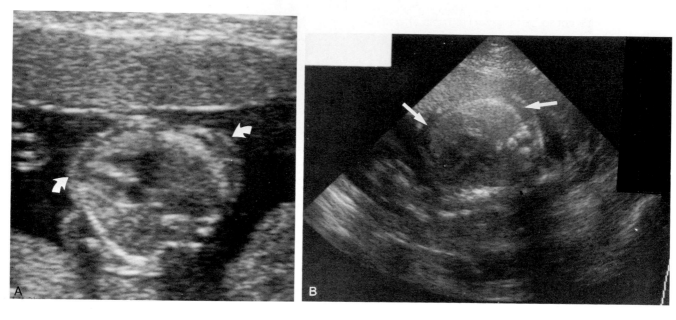

Figure 16–58. **SPECULAR REFLECTION ARTIFACT SIMULATING SKIN THICKENING OR NEURAL TUBE DEFECT.** In A, a curvilinear echo *(arrows)* parallel to the fetal skin surface mimics focal skin thickening. In B, a bright linear echo *(arrows)* is generated over the fetal spine, mimicking a neural tube defect. This artifact results from specular reflection of the sound beam from the fetal skin surface, which is nearly perpendicular to the incident angle of the sound beam. Changes in transducer angulation will shift or eliminate the reflection and reveal its artifactual nature.

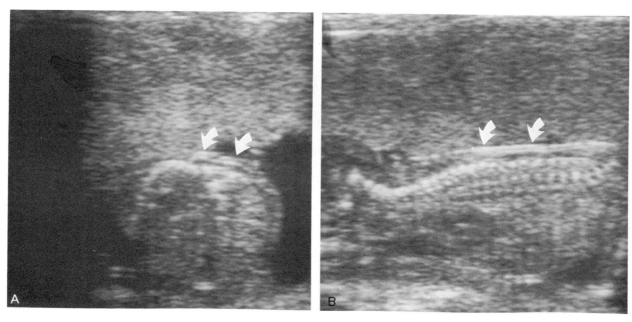

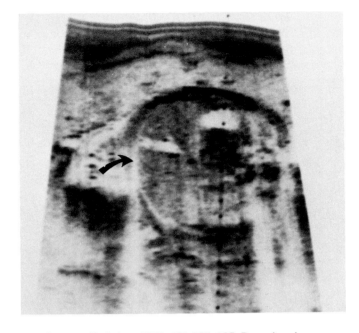

Figure 16–59. FETAL PSUEDOASCITES. A lucency seen adjacent to the anterior abdominal wall of the fetus may be seen in a large percentage of normal patients. This lucent area is partly due to refraction at the edge of the body wall *(arrow)*, and partly due to the normal abdominal wall. It should not be confused with intraperitoneal fluid.

From: Rosenthal SJ, Filly RA, Callen PW, Sommer FG. Fetal pseudoascites. Radiology 1979; 131:195–197. Reproduced with permission.

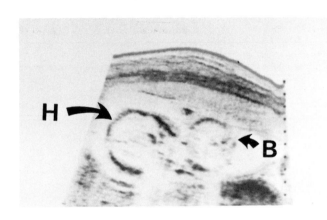

Figure 16–60. OFF-AXIS SECTION THROUGH THE FETUS, SIMULATING HEAD–BODY DISCORDANCE. Discordance between the measurements and appearance of the fetal head (H) and the fetal body (B) will allow one to make the diagnosis of either intrauterine growth retardation or hydrocephalus. In this case, the scan plane contains the central portion of the fetal head but images the edge of the fetal body, mimicking head–body discordance. A comparison of similarly obtained transverse axial scans of the fetal head and body will alleviate this potential confusion.

Figure 16–61. FILM ARTIFACT SIMULATING FETAL PATHOLOGY. Dust on either the camera lens or mirror used in ultrasonography may often simulate an intracranial or intra-abdominal mass *(arrows)*. Similar location of the abnormality in each film obtained of the fetus, regardless of the plane of section, will elucidate the etiology of this artifact.

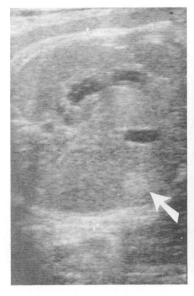
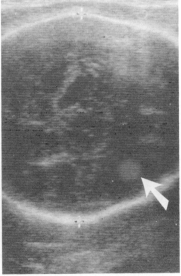

III

NUCLEAR
MEDICINE

17

Quality Control

DONALD E. JACKSON, M.D.
CHARLES E. PETERSON, M.D.

Figure 17–1. CONTAMINATED COLLIMATOR.

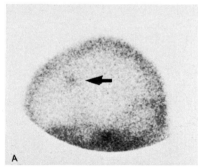

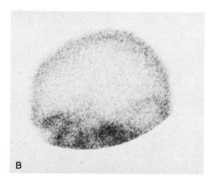

Figure 17–1A. The solitary focus of radioactivity *(arrows)* seen on a lateral brain scan was seen in the same location relative to the crystal face in all views.

Figure 17–1B. A repeat view after the collimator was cleaned demonstrates the artifactual nature of the activity. Contamination of the crystal/collimator should be suspected any time that an area of activity remains in the same location relative to the crystal face on multiple views.

Ref.: Datz FL. Gamuts in Nuclear Medicine. Norwalk, CT: Appleton-Century-Crofts, 1983; p 43.

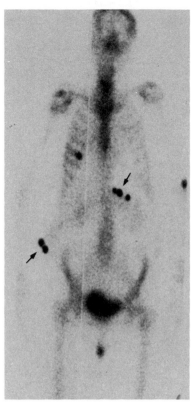

Figure 17–2. SKIN CONTAMINATION—BLOOD. Multiple areas of tracer activity are seen in atypical areas on this bone scan *(arrows).* Upon examination, it was discovered that the patient had contaminated multiple skin areas with blood oozing from the injection site. Any area of atypical deposition of tracer must be considered as possible contamination. Re-imaging in another obliquity, or after skin decontamination, may be necessary to prove the nature of the activity. (The area of increased tracer activity in the right anterior rib represents a true lesion—a rib fracture.)

Ref.: Brill DR. Radionuclide imaging of nonneoplastic soft tissue disorders. Semin Nucl Med 1981; 11:277–288.

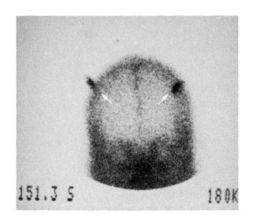

Figure 17–3. SKIN CONTAMINATION—BLOOD. This scan demonstrates an unusual case of skin contamination *(arrows)* by blood from the injection site.

Figure 17–4. SKIN CONTAMINATION—URINE. The urinary system is the major route of excretion of many radiopharmaceuticals; thus, urine contamination is a major source of potential errors. Urine contamination of the blanket *(arrow)* by an infant undergoing a bone scan may mask an underlying bony abnormality.

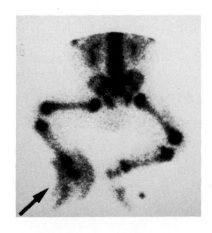

Ref.: Wells, LD, Berner, DR. Radionuclide Imaging Artifacts, Chicago: Year Book Medical Publishers, 1980; p 98.

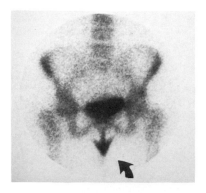

Figure 17–5. SKIN CONTAMINATION—URINE. In women, urinary incontinence may produce significant contamination of the perineal region *(arrow)*, potentially masking pelvic pathology. In men, activity at the tip of the penis may overlie the pelvis or proximal femur.

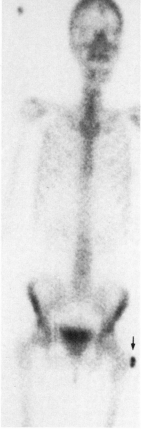

Figure 17–6. BANDAGE CONTAMINATION. The gauze or bandage used after venipuncture will become contaminated with radioactive blood. If not properly disposed, it is a source of potential misinterpretation. In this bone scan, the activity is obviously extraosseous *(arrow)*, and a repeat image after emptying the patient's pockets would reveal the true nature of this artifact.

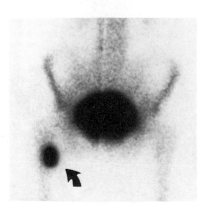

Figure 17–7. BANDAGE CONTAMINATION. The fact that the area of increased activity in this patient's proximal femur is a contaminated gauze *(arrow)* is much less obvious than in Figure 17–6. The area of contamination appears much larger than the one in Figure 17–6 due to the "blooming" effect in a concentrated area of radioactivity.

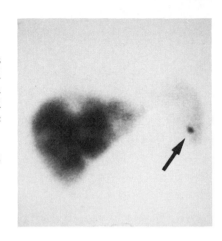

Figure 17–8. BANDAGE CONTAMINATION. Contaminated gauze simulates a "hot spot" in the patient's spleen *(arrow)* on this technetium sulfur colloid scan. This artifact mimics the appearance of an accessory spleen on a radiocolloid spleen scan. Splenosis, a post-traumatic disorder, is usually detected after the normal splenic tissue has been removed. (The defects in the liver are from metastatic lung carcinoma.)

Ref.: Jacobson SJ, De Nardo GL. Splenosis demonstrated by splenic scan. J Nucl Med 1970; 12:570–572.

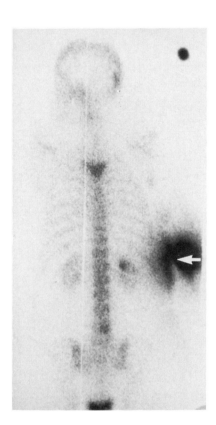

Figure 17–9. EXTRAVASATION. Extravasation of a quantity of the radiopharmaceutical will cause an area of increased radioactivity. If it is sufficiently large, it will cause an artifactual apparent increase in the activity of adjacent soft tissues by narrow-angle Compton scatter *(arrow)*. Re-imaging the patient after moving the site of the extravasation farther away from the body will reveal the artifactual nature of this finding.

Ref.: Sprawls P. The Physics and Instrumentation of Nuclear Medicine. Baltimore, MD: University Park Press, 1981; p 56.

Figure 17–10. EXTRAVASATION. If the area of the extravasation is not included in the image, the source of the apparent increased soft-tissue activity is less obvious *(arrow)*.

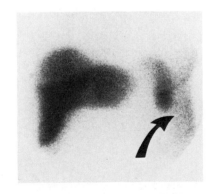

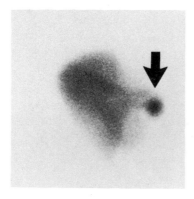

Figure 17–11. EXTRAVASATION. The extravasation in this patient's elbow simulates an area of increased activity in the liver *(arrow)*. The true nature of this artifact would be revealed upon imaging in other obliquities.

Ref.: Stadalnik RC. "Hot spots"—liver imaging. Semin Nucl Med 1979; 9:220–221.

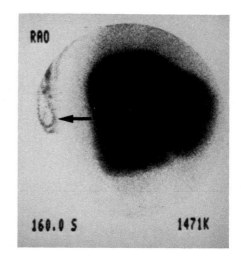

Figure 17–12. INJECTION OF RADIOPHARMACEUTICAL INTO AN INTRAVENOUS LINE. Injection of a radiopharmaceutical into an intravenous line *(arrow)* should be avoided, as less than the intended dose reaches the target organ. If the injected line overlies the area of interest, it could simulate a lesion.

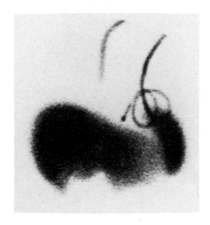

Figure 17–13. INJECTION OF RADIOPHARMACEUTICAL INTO AN INTRAVENOUS LINE. In this patient, the indwelling central line was used for the injection of the radiocolloid.

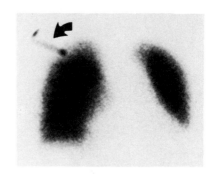

Figure 17–14. **INJECTION OF RADIOPHARMACEUTICAL INTO AN INTRAVENOUS LINE.** The macroaggregated albumin used in this perfusion lung scan was injected through a peripheral intravenous line *(arrow).* Injection through a central line in the pulmonary artery has been reported to be a cause of simulating decreased perfusion to an entire lung.

Ref.: Brachman M, Tanasescw D, Ramanna L, et al. False-positive lung imaging: Inadvertent injection into a pulmonary artery catheter. Clin Nucl Med 1979; 4:415–416.

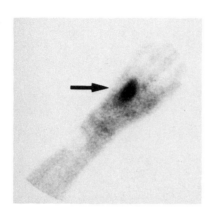

Figure 17–15. **INJECTION OF RADIOPHARMACEUTICAL INTO AN INTRAVENOUS LINE.** Injection into the heparin-filled reservoir of an intravenous catheter *(arrow)* resulted in a simulated bone lesion in this bone scan. Only a high index of suspicion and further examination of the patient allowed detection of this artifact.

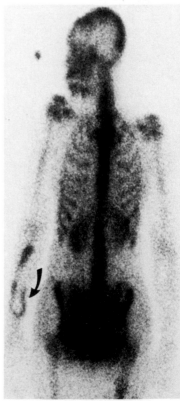

Figure 17–16. **INJECTION OF RADIOPHARMACEUTICAL INTO AN INTRAVENOUS LINE.** Injection into this patient's intravenous tubing *(arrow)* does overlie the bone but is less likely to be mistaken for a bony lesion.

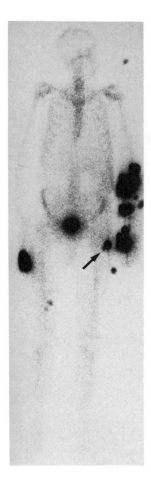

Figure 17–17. MULTIPLE EXTRAVASATION SITES. When multiple extravasations occur following unsuccessful attempts at intravenous injection, a technician may long for an intravenous line into which to inject! The arrow indicates a "hot" gauze in the patient's pocket. The remainder of the extremely hot areas represent extravasations. Note the poor quality of the bone scan, as little of the radiopharmaceutical was injected.

Figure 17–18. ATTENUATION BY OVERLYING BREAST. Any extraneous material (for example, soft tissue) placed between the target organ and the crystal face will attenuate the photons emitted from the organ.

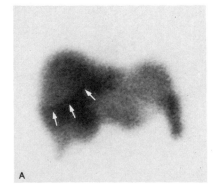

Figure 17–18A. This scan demonstrates an ill-defined defect superiorly in the liver *(arrows)* that is caused by the attenuation of a pendulous breast. The half-value layer for the attenuation of the 140 keV photons of technetium in soft tissue is approximately 5 cm. This makes elevation of the breast necessary prior to radiocolloid examination of the liver in women.

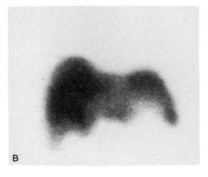

Figure 17–18B. A repeat image after elevation of the breast demonstrates that there is no underlying abnormality.

Ref.: Sprawls P. The Physics and Instrumentation of Nuclear Medicine. Baltimore, MD: University Park Press, 1981; p 65.

Figure 17–19. BREAST PROSTHESIS.

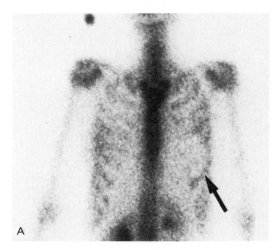

Figure 17–19A. This patient had had a mastectomy but was not asked to remove her breast prosthesis before bone imaging. The attenuation of the prosthesis caused an ill-defined photopenic area in the left chest *(arrow).*

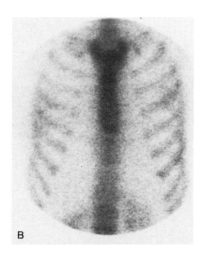

Figure 17–19B. A repeat image after the removal of the prosthesis demonstrates that the underlying bones are normal.

Ref.: Buchignani JS, Rochett JF. Effects of breast prosthesis on 99m Tc-stannous-polyphosphate bone scans. J Nucl Med 1973; 14:878.

Figure 17–20. SKIN FOLDS.

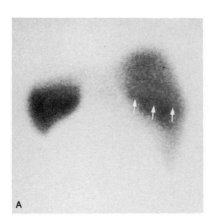

Figure 17–20A. In a patient with excess adipose tissue, skin folds may be a significant source of photon attenuation. The posterior image in this radiocolloid liver exam was obtained without removal of the patient's bra. The resultant skin fold caused an ill-defined photopenic line *(arrows)*.

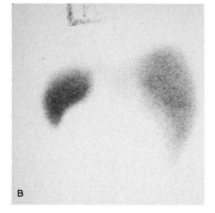

Figure 17–20B. A repeat image after removal of the bra reveals the artifactual nature of this finding.

Ref.: McCauley D, Braumstein P. Unusual artifact in lateral liver scans. J. Nucl Med 1974; 15:1201–1202.

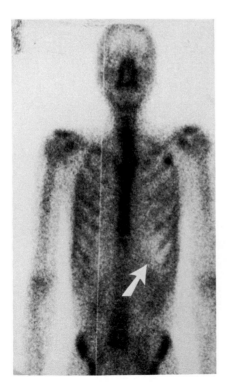

Figure 17–21. "LUNCH" DEFECT. The presence of food in the stomach will displace the normal blood pool and will also attenuate the photons that arise posterior to the fundus of the stomach, causing a left upper-quadrant photopenic defect *(arrow)*. Oral ingestion of a radionuclide such as technetium-labeled sulfur colloid will allow identification of the source of the defect. However, in most cases, awareness of the cause of the defect is sufficient to allow recognition.

Ref.: Manlio FL, Mehan KP. Photopenic area in Tc-99m MDP bone scan. Clin Nucl Med 1982; 7:479.

Figure 17–22. **BUCKLES.** These three examples demonstrate the necessity for removing all metallic objects, such as jewelry and clasps, prior to radionuclide imaging. Defects caused by various buckles and clasps *(arrows)* are identified.

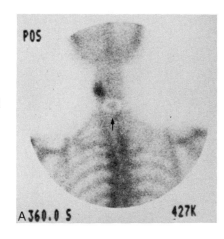

Figure 17–22A. Photopenic defect *(arrow)* on this bone spot image is caused by a metallic artifact.

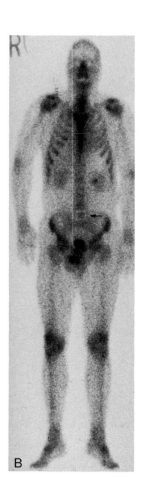

Figure 17–22B. Metallic artifact *(arrow)* is demonstrated on this whole body bone scan.

Figure 17–22C. Photopenic defect *(arrow)* caused by a metal object is seen on this liver/spleen scan.

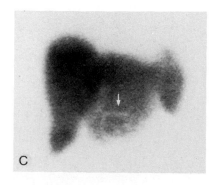

Ref.: Wells LD, Bernier DR. Radionuclide Imaging Artifacts. Chicago: Year Book Medical Publishers, 1980; p 88.

Figure 17–23. **COINS IN POCKET.** These five examples of photopenic defects demonstrate the importance of removing all metallic objects from the patient's pockets prior to imaging.

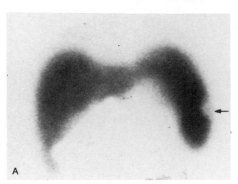

Figure 17–23A. Liver/spleen scan demonstrates a cold defect *(arrow)* in the spleen.

Figure 17–23B. A cold defect *(arrow)* over the left chest is apparent on this bone scan.

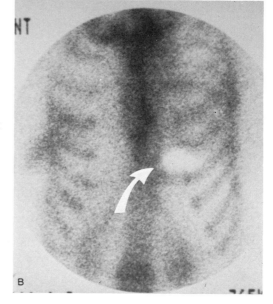

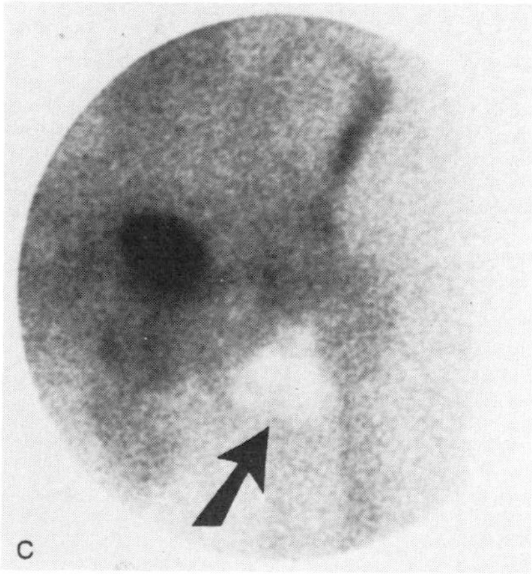

Figure 17–23C. Bone scan demonstrates a cold defect *(arrow)* over the left femur.

Figure 17–23D. In this bone scan a cold defect *(arrow)* is seen over the right scrotum.

Illustration continued on opposite page

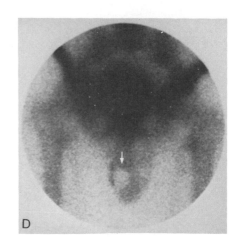

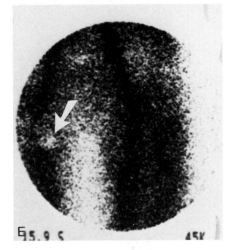

Figure 17–23E. In this flow study a cold area *(arrow)* can be seen over the right thigh.

Ref.: Wells DL, Bernier DR. Radionuclide Imaging Activity. Chicago: Year Book Medical Publishers, 1980; p 86.

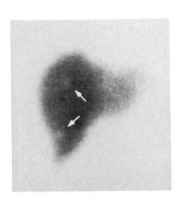

Figure 17–24. GOWN SNAP. When hospital inpatients are imaged, special care must be taken to ensure that the metallic gown snaps are not overlying target organs. This liver image demonstrates two artifacts *(arrows)* from snaps.

Ref.: Wells DL, Bernier DR. Radionuclide Imaging Artifacts. Chicago: Year Book Medical Publishers, 1980; p 116.

Figure 17–25. BULLET. Not all metallic artifacts are on the skin surface. This patient has a bullet *(arrow)* lodged in the liver parenchyma. Only adequate clinical history will allow identification of this pitfall.

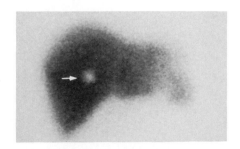

Figure 17–26. BARIUM IN THE GUT.

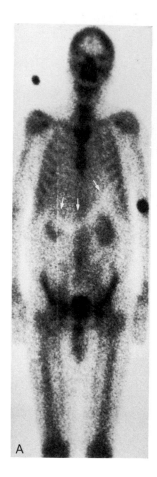

Figure 17–26A. This whole body scan illustrates the photon absorption caused by the presence of barium in the gut at the time of imaging *(arrows)*. Whenever possible, all radionuclide imaging procedures should be completed before barium studies are carried out.

Figure 17–26B. Recognition of the artifact *(arrows)* is not difficult when the barium takes on the typical shape of the gut, as in the bone spot image, but may be more difficult in cases of isolated retention of barium in a small area of bowel.

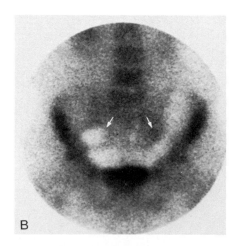

Ref.: Wells DL, Bernier DR. Radionuclide Imaging Artifacts. Chicago: Year Book Medical Publishers, 1980; p 99.

Figure 17–27. PATIENT MOTION. Because of the sometimes long imaging times necessary to produce studies, it is absolutely essential that the patient remain motionless in order not to obscure potential areas of abnormality. These whole body bone scans illustrate the problem of gross patient motion. Lesser degrees of motion will degrade image contrast and lesion detectability but may be more difficult to detect.

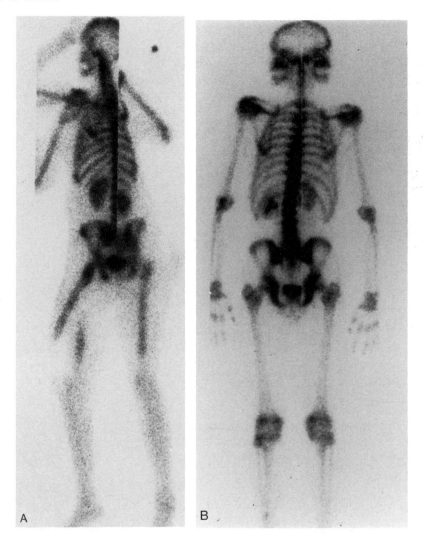

Ref.: Wells DL, Bernier DR. Radionuclide Imaging Artifacts. Chicago: Year Book Medical Publishers, 1980; p 114.

Figure 17–28. "CORNER SHOT"—RIB LESION.

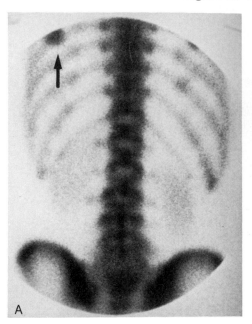

Figure 17–28A. When imaged at the periphery of the crystal face, normal areas of increased tracer deposition, such as the tip of the scapula *(arrow)*, may simulate abnormalities (in the rib in this instance).

Figure 17–28B. When re-imaging is done with the camera more centered over the suspicious area, the normal anatomic relationships are seen and allow identification of the true nature of the increased activity, that is, the scapular tip *(arrow)*.

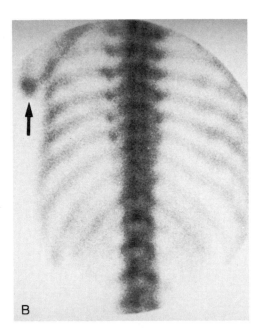

Instrumentation

DONALD E. JACKSON, M.D.
CHARLES E. PETERSON, M.D.

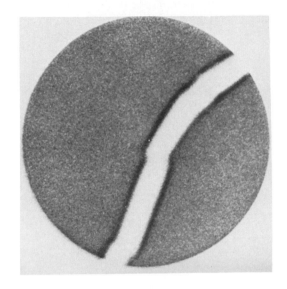

Figure 18–1. CRACKED CRYSTAL. Although encased in a protective cover, the NaI(Tl) crystal is very sensitive to direct physical force, as well as to sudden changes in temperature and humidity. This crystal was cracked by accidentally bringing the tube head down onto a fixed object, using the motor drive.

Ref.: Wells LD, Bernier DR. Radionuclide Imaging Artifacts. Chicago: Year Book Medical Publishers, 1980; p 2.

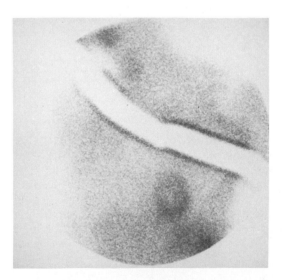

Figure 18–2. CRACKED CRYSTAL. This patient had a thallium stress test, and the image was made using the cracked crystal shown in Figure 18–1. Note the edge packing seen at the edges of the crack, caused by the more efficient collection of scintillations near the edge of the crystal. Reflection of the events occurring near the edge will cause this apparent increase in activity.

Ref.: Turner DA, Silverstein EA. Instrumentation quality control Case 2. In: Alderman PO, Coleman RE, Grove RB, et al., eds. Nuclear Radiology (Third Series) Syllabus, American College of Radiology, 1983.

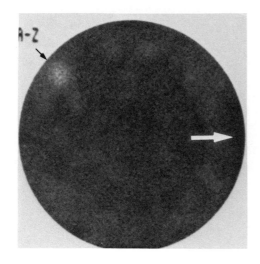

Figure 18–3. **UNBALANCED PHOTOMULTIPLIER TUBE.** This flood field image, obtained without any uniformity correction, demonstrates an unbalanced photomultiplier tube *(black arrow).* Note the edge packing *(white arrow)* due to asymmetric placement of the electronic "iris."

Ref.: Rollo FD. Nuclear Medicine Physics. Instrumentation and Agents. St. Louis: C. V. Mosby, 1977; p 343.

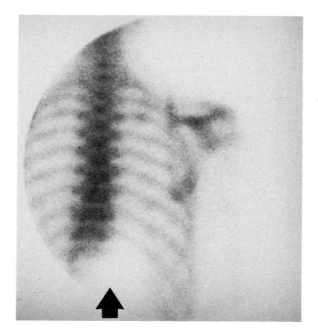

Figure 18–4. **NONFUNCTIONAL PHOTOMULTIPLIER TUBE.** Bone scan demonstrates a cold defect *(arrow)* that is due to a nonfunctioning photomultiplier tube. This defect should not be a source of error, as it will be detected on the routine quality control flood field images.

Ref.: Wells LD, Bernier DR. Radionuclide imaging artifacts. Chicago: Year Book Medical Publishers, 1980; p 17.

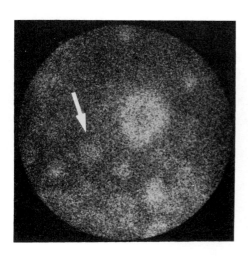

Figure 18–5. **MULTIPLE UNBALANCED PHOTOMULTIPLIER TUBES.** Thallium scan demonstrates multiple artifactual areas of apparent increased activity that are caused by multiple tubes being unbalanced. (A typical example is indicated by the arrow.) If one of these areas were to overlie an area of ischemia or infarct in the myocardium, it could potentially mask the defect and cause an error in interpretation. This problem can be avoided by careful attention to the quality control flood field images.

Figure 18–6. OFF-PEAK IMAGE.

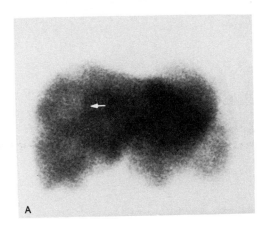

Figure 18–6A. Liver scan demonstrates multiple cold areas within the right lobe. (The arrow indicates one of these defects.) These cold areas remained in the same position relative to the crystal face in all projections. Investigation revealed that the pulse height analyzer had been centered on the 80 keV photopeak from a xenon-133 ventilation study done immediately prior to the liver scan.

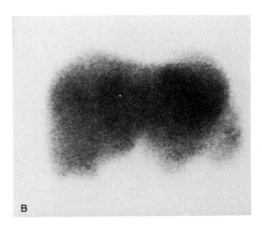

Figure 18–6B. Re-imaging the patient after centering the pulse height analyzer on the 140 keV photopeak of technetium-99m demonstrated the artifactual nature of these defects.

Ref.: Mettler FA, Guiberteau MJ. Essentials of Nuclear Medicine Imaging. New York: Grune & Stratton, 1983; p 37.

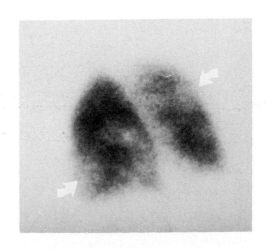

Figure 18–7. OFF-PEAK IMAGE. This patient underwent a perfusion lung scan with the pulse height analyzer set on the 80 keV photopeak of xenon-133 from the ventilation performed immediately prior to the perfusion scan. The scan demonstrates the same photopenic areas as in Figure 18–6A. To prevent an error in diagnosis, strict attention must be paid to setting the pulse height analyzer on the proper photopeak.

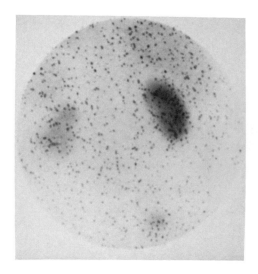

Figure 18–8. ELECTRICAL NOISE. In this renal scan, a myriad of tiny dots seen over the entire image are the result of electrical noise in the line between the camera and the imager. This artifact can be suspected by its intermittent nature and the relationship between its appearance and the operation of the interfering device. Electrical line filters or relocation of the offending equipment should solve the problem.

Ref.: Wells LD, Bernier DR. Radionuclide Imaging Artifacts. Chicago: Year Book Medical Publishers, 1980; p 42.

Figure 18–9. STATIC ELECTRICAL DISCHARGE. This spot image from a bone scan is barely recognizable due to the artifact caused by the discharge of static electricity, and the resultant exposure of the film. The artifact is not a difficult one to detect and can be prevented by careful grounding of all equipment; also, discharge of any built-up charge in the body can be prevented by touching a grounded object before handling the film.

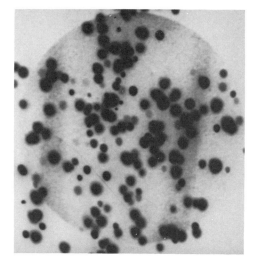

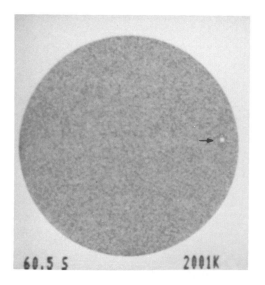

Figure 18–10. NONFUNCTIONAL PIXEL. On a uniformity corrected flood field image, a cold area *(arrow)* is seen, which is due to the failure of a single memory element in the image matrix of the camera's uniformity correction device, resulting in a square pixel defect.

Ref.: Erickson JJ, Rollo FD. Digital Nuclear Medicine. Philadelphia; J. B. Lippincott, 1982; p 194.

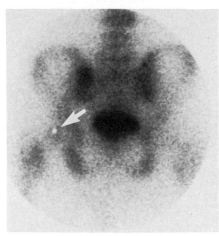

Figure 18–11. NONFUNCTIONAL PIXEL. This spot image from a bone scan demonstrates the effect of the nonfunctional pixel *(arrow)* seen on the flood image in Figure 18–10.

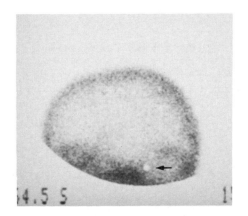

Figure 18–12. NONFUNCTIONAL PIXEL. Image from a brain scan demonstrates the same nonfunctional pixel *(arrow)* seen on the flood image in Figure 18–10.

Figure 18–13. NONFUNCTIONAL PIXELS. This bone scan spot image shows the effect of losing multiple memory elements within the matrix. Multiple square cold areas represent the nonfunctional picture elements.

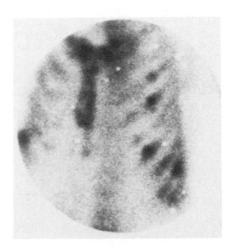

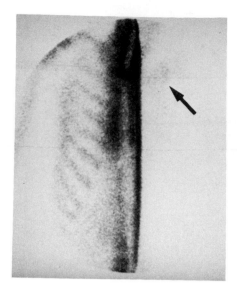

**Figure 18–14. LOSS OF SIGNAL FROM CAMERA DURING IMAG-
ING.** This spot image from a bone scan demonstrates the effect of the loss
of x^+ output from the camera during the acquisition of an image. Note the
faint image of the left side of the patient's chest *(arrow),* acquired before
the loss of signal.

Ref.: Chandra R. Introductory Physics of Nuclear Medicine, 2nd ed. Philadelphia: Lea &
      Febiger, 1982; p 154.

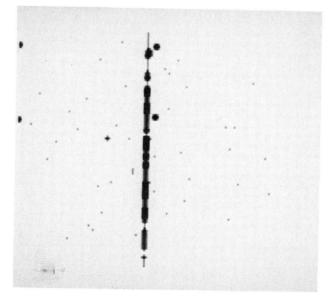

**Figure 18–15. LOSS OF SIGNAL FROM CAMERA
DURING IMAGING.** During the acquisition of a renogram,
the line carrying the x output from the camera to the
computer became disconnected. As a result, all the data
acquired had a valid y coordinate but had 0 for the x
coordinate, producing the dark stripe in the center of the
image. The smaller dots scattered around the image are
valid data that were recorded before the loss of signal.

Ref.: Chandra R. Introductory Physics of Nuclear Medicine, 2nd ed.
      Philadelphia: Lea & Febiger, 1982; p 154.

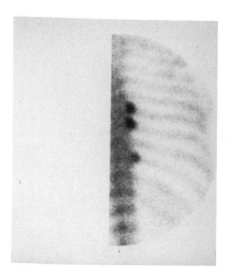

Figure 18–16. FAILURE TO REMOVE OPAQUE SLIDE. This artifact
simulates the loss of x^- output, but in this case the cause was failure to
completely remove the opaque slide from the film cassette prior to imaging.

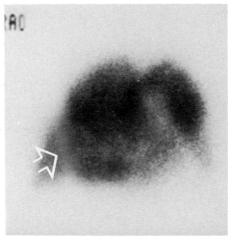

Figure 18–17. SCRATCH IN THE CATHODE RAY TUBE COVER.
In this perfusion lung scan image, an ill-defined oblique line can be seen
running through the right lung *(arrow)*. It is caused by a scratch in the
cover of the output phosphor of the cathode ray tube.

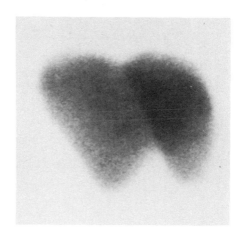

Figure 18–18. DOUBLE EXPOSURE. The apparent hepatomegaly seen
in this radiocolloid liver scan is caused by a double exposure as a result of
a failure of the image formatter to index.

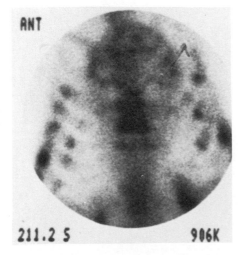

Figure 18–19. DOUBLE EXPOSURE. The double exposure seen here
is not hard to detect, but both images should be repeated to exclude the
possibility that a lesion is being masked.

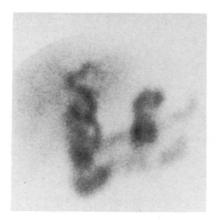

Figure 18–20. APPARENT DOUBLE EXPOSURE. Apparent double exposure on a hepatobiliary scan was the result of repeated deep sighing by the patient during imaging.

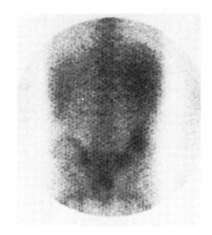

Figure 18–21. VISUALIZATION OF COLLIMATOR SEPTA. The long imaging time used in the formation of this gallium scan image resulted in the imaging of the hexagonal collimator septa of the medium energy collimator. (The septa cause the image to have a "grainy" appearance.) Termination of the image collection at an earlier time would not have allowed imaging of the collimator septa.

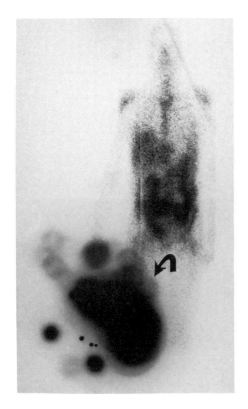

Figure 18–22. POWER FAILURE. During the imaging of this whole body bone scan, there was a power failure. The unexpected power loss resulted in the return of the output cathode ray tube in the image formatter to a neutral position. This was also associated with flaring of the cathode ray tube due to the power surge during the failure, which resulted in the exposure of the film in an undesirable fashion *(arrow).*

Ref.: Wells LD, Bernier DR. Radionuclide Imaging Artifacts. Chicago: Year Book Medical Publishers, 1980; p 4.

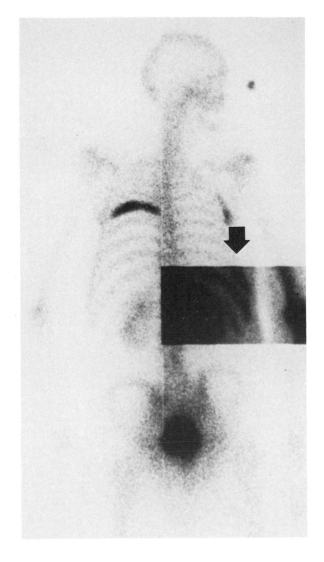

Figure 18–23. OBSTRUCTION OF WHOLE BODY IMAGING TABLE. During the performance of this patient's whole body bone scan, the moving table top became temporarily obstructed in its passage. The slowing of the table resulted in the collection of a larger than usual number of counts in the area being scanned. This resulted in a "hot square" *(arrow)*. The obstruction was noticed by the technical staff and was corrected, allowing normal completion of the scan.

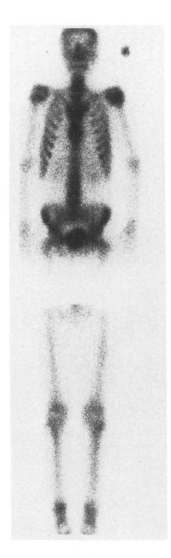

Figure 18–24. MALADJUSTMENT OF IMAGE FORMATTER. In this whole body bone scan, the image formatter was incorrectly adjusted, resulting in an artifactual separation of the upper half of the image from the lower.

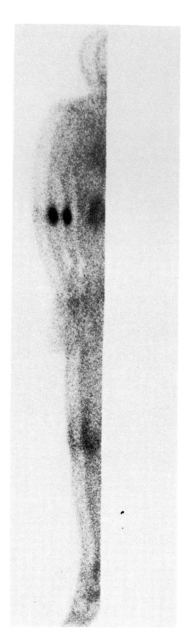

Figure 18–25. WHOLE BODY IMAGING TABLE MALFUNCTION. The two-pass whole body imaging table malfunctioned, with the result that on the second pass the same side of the patient's body was imaged.

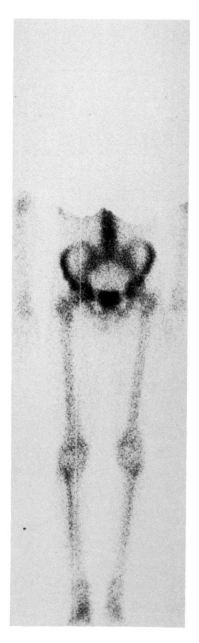

Figure 18–26. FOREIGN OBJECT IN IMAGE FORMATTER. A foreign object was inadvertently dropped inside the image formatter, thus obscuring part of this whole body bone scan.

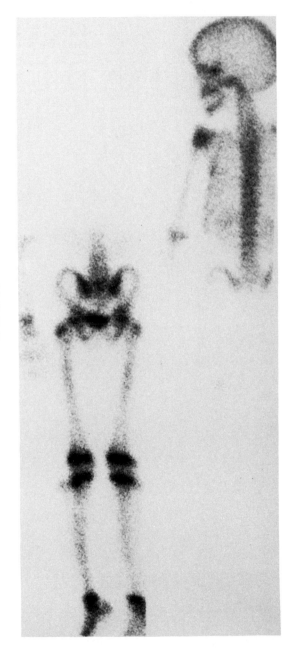

Figure 18–27. MISALIGNMENT OF OUTPUT CATHODE RAY TUBE IN IMAGE FORMATTER. Misalignment of the output cathode ray tube in the whole body image formatter resulted in disconnected upper and lower images in the total body view.

Figure 18–28. **OFF-PEAK WHOLE BODY IMAGE.**

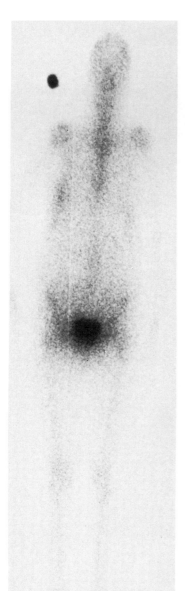

Figure 18–28A. This whole body bone image was acquired with the pulse height analyzer peaked 20 per cent below the 140 keV photopeak of technetium-99m.

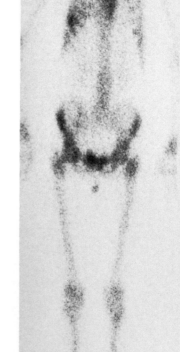

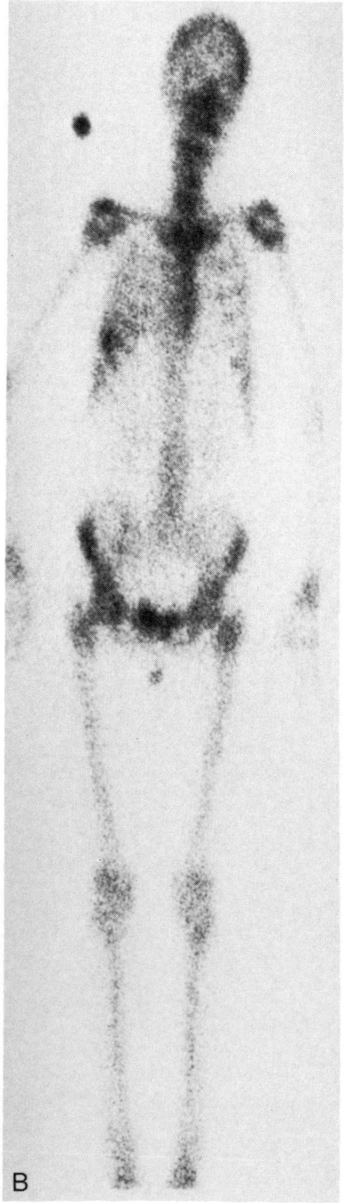

Figure 18–28B. A repeat bone scan obtained using the proper window setting demonstrates a dramatic improvement in image quality. A right rib lesion is detected that could only be suspected on the first study.

Ref.: Turner DA, Silverstein, EA. Instrumentation quality control, Case 2. In: Alderman PO, Coleman RE, Grove RB, et al., eds. Nuclear Radiology (Third Series) Syllabus, American College of Radiology, 1983.

Figure 18–29. WIDE WINDOW. This whole body bone image was produced with the window of the pulse height analyzer centered on the 140 keV photopeak of technetium-99m, but the window width was 40 per cent. Thus, energies from 112 to 168 keV would be accepted. The acceptance of the large amount of scattered radiation seriously degrades the image, rendering it diagnostically useless.

Ref.: Turner DA, Silverstein EA. Instrumentation quality control, Case 2. In: Alderman PO, Coleman RE, Grove RB, et al., eds. Nuclear Radiology (Third Series) Syllabus, American College of Radiology, 1983; p 24.

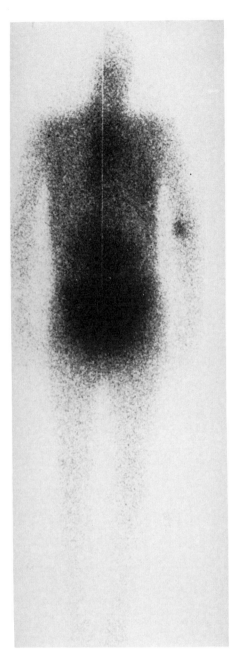

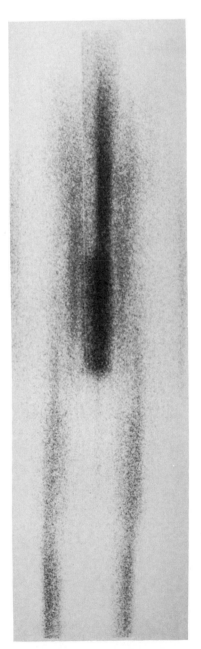

Figure 18–30. OVER/UNDER SWITCH CONFUSION. The camera orientation switch on the whole body imaging system was left in the "over table" position, but the camera head was positioned beneath the table. This resulted in a malplacement of all the collected data, and a totally uninterpretable image.

CHAPTER 19

Radiopharmaceuticals

DONALD E. JACKSON, M.D.
CHARLES E. PETERSON, M.D.

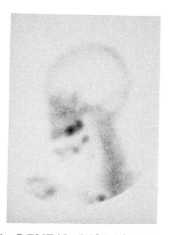

Figure 19–1. DENTAL DISEASE. Dental disease, while not a normal variant per se, is imaged on bone scans quite frequently, as in the lateral bone spot image, and should be recognized as such.

Ref.: Lyons KP, Jensen JL. Dental lesions causing abnormalities on skeletal scintigraphy. Clin Nucl Med 1979; 4:509–512.

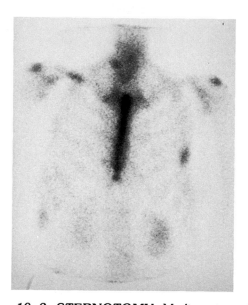

Figure 19–2. STERNOTOMY. Median sternotomies are very common operative procedures. During the healing phase of the sternum, increased bone tracer deposition may be seen. The characteristic linear nature of the uptake, and its location, will allow ready identification of the source and should not be confused with malignant pathology.

Ref.: Thrall JH, Ghaed N, Geslien G, et al. Pitfalls in Tc99m polyphosphate skeletal imaging. AJR 1974; 121:739–747.

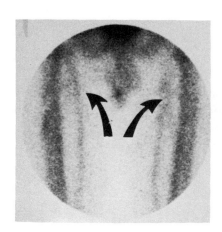

Figure 19–3. VASCULAR CALCIFICATION. Vascular calcification is extremely common in persons over the age of 40. Deposition of bone tracer can occur in vascular calcifications that are not radiographically visible. It should be recognized because of its characteristic location, most commonly in the femoral vessels *(arrows)*, and by its symmetry. Radiolabeled blood pool could be mistaken for vascular calcification, but imaging over the heart should allow visualization of any blood pool activity.

Ref.: Thrall JH, Ghaed N, Geslien G, et al. Pitfalls in Tc99m polyphosphate skeletal imaging. AJR 1974; 121:739–747.

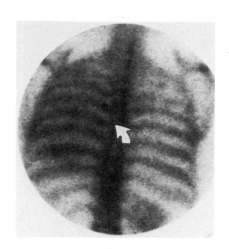

Figure 19–4. PLEURAL EFFUSION. Bone tracer (methylene diphosphonate) has been reported to deposit in the pleural effusions secondary to malignant and non-malignant causes. The tracer is present in the non-cellular component of the fluid. Upright imaging may reveal the dependent nature of tracer-laden fluid. Effusion *(arrow)* is seen in this supine image of a patient with metastatic breast carcinoma.

Ref.: Lamki L, Cohen P, Driedger A. Malignant pleural effusion and Tc99m-MDP accumulation. Clin Nucl Med 1982; 7:331–333.

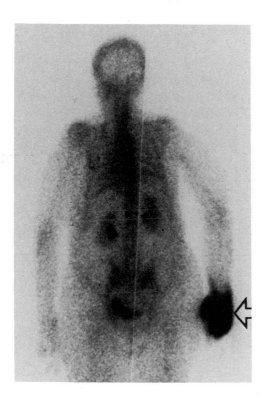

Figure 19–5. ARTERIAL INJECTION. Bone tracer, when injected intra-arterially, deposits in a typical distribution. This has been termed the "gauntlet sign." This scan illustrates an injection made inadvertently into the radial artery *(arrow)*.

Ref.: Andrews GA, Theocheung JL, Andrews E, Tyler KR. Unintentional intra-arterial injection of a bone-imaging agent. Clin Nucl Med 1980; 5:499–501.

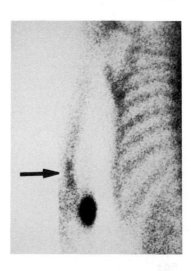

Figure 19–6. INTERSTITIAL INJECTION. After extravasation, bone tracer may find its way into the lymphatic channels *(arrow)*. This is a potential source of misinterpretation as abnormal bony deposition unless the entity is recognized. Lateral views will demonstrate the true soft-tissue location of the tracer in most instances.

Ref.: Penney HF, Styles CB. Fortuitous lymph node visualization after interstitial injection of Tc-99m-MDP. Clin Nucl Med 1982; 7:84–85.

Figure 19–7. WOUND LOCALIZATION OF BONE TRACER. Bone tracer may localize in both acute hematomas as well as in healing scars. When these areas of tracer deposition overlap bone, a potential source of error exists. Orthogonal views and clinical history will aid in the discovery of the true nature of the lesion. The following three scans illustrate tracer deposition.

Ref.: Thrall JH, Ghaed N, Geslien G, et al. Pitfalls in Tc99m polyphosphate skeletal imaging. AJR 1974; 121:739–747.

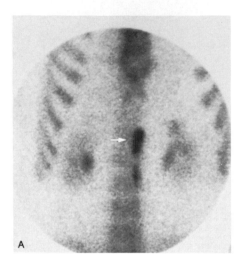

Figure 19–7A. Bone tracer deposition in a wound hematoma *(arrow)*.

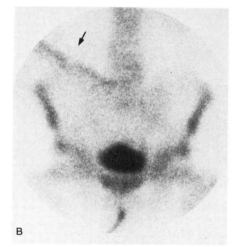

Figure 19–7B. Bone tracer deposition in a healing scar *(arrow)*.

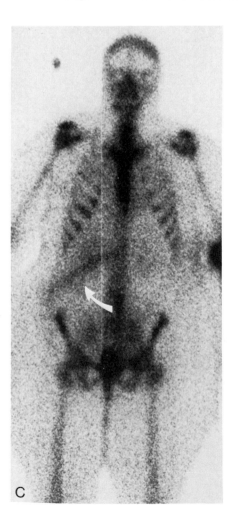

Figure 19–7C. Bone tracer deposition in an old cholecystectomy scar *(arrow)*.

Figure 19–8. LIVER ACTIVITY ON BONE SCAN. When the liver is visualized on a bone scan, a number of possible causes exist, including a prior liver scan without adequate decay interval. Pathologic processes that calcify in the liver, such as metastases from mucinous adenocarcinoma of the colon should also be considered. This scan demonstrates a third cause—colloid formation in the radiopharmaceutical, with localization in the liver *(curved solid arrow)*. In addition, free pertechnetate is present, as evidenced by the activity present in the colon (open arrow). Whenever the apparent biodistribution of a radiopharmaceutical is altered from normal, considerations should include abnormalities from iatrogenic causes and poor radiopharmaceutical preparation as well as pathologic processes within the patient.

Ref.: Coleman RE, Petry NA, Wang TST. Nuclear Radiology (Third Series) Syllabus, American College of Radiology, 1983; p 2.

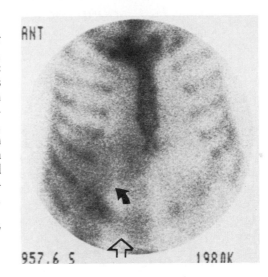

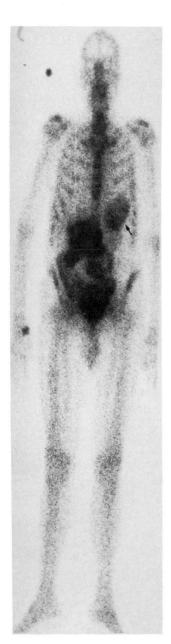

Figure 19–9. GUT ACTIVITY ON BONE SCAN. In this patient, there is tracer activity present in the stomach *(arrow)* as well as in the small bowel. This represents an alteration of the usual biodistribution of the radiopharmaceutical due, in this case, to a large percentage of free pertechnetate in the bone agent. (Paper chromatography can be used to determine the percentage of radiochemical purity.) Note also the rather poor quality of the bone scan due to the less than usual amount of deposition of the tracer in the bones.

Ref.: Wilson MA, Pollack MJ. Gastric visualization and image quality in the radionuclide bone scanning: Concise communication. J Nucl Med 1981; 22:518–521.

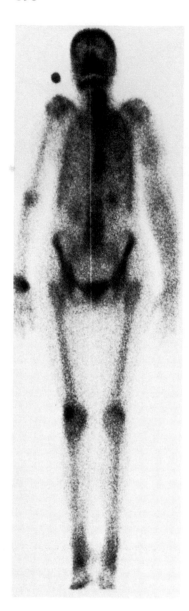

Figure 19–10. SOFT-TISSUE ACTIVITY ON BONE SCAN. This patient has had chronic edema in the left arm after a left radical mastectomy. The bone agent accumulated in the edema fluid and potentially could mask underlying bone pathology.

Ref.: Thrall JH, Ghaed N, Gelien G. Pitfalls in Tc99m polyphosphate skeletal imaging. AJR 1974; 121:739–747.

Figure 19–11. NORMAL BREAST ACTIVITY.

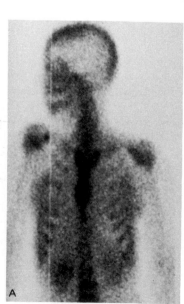

Figure 19–11A. On the anterior image, this patient demonstrates normal, symmetric activity in the breast tissue. Pathologic uptake within inflammatory or neoplastic lesions will be asymmetric and should not be considered a normal finding, unless the patient has had a mastectomy.

Illustration continued on opposite page

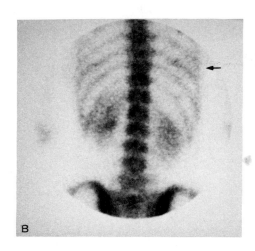

Figure 19–11B. Note that the breast activity is intense enough to "shine" through to the posterior image of the thorax. This should not be confused with thoracic pathology.

Ref.: Brill DR. Radionuclide imaging of nonneoplastic soft tissue disorders. Semin Nucl Med 1981; 11:277–288.

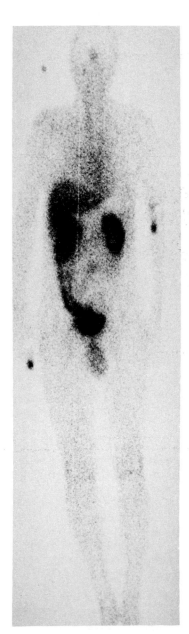

Figure 19–12. MISADMINISTRATION OF PHARMACEUTICAL. This patient was scheduled for a bone scan. However, glucoheptonate was inadvertently administered. This fact could be suspected from the images, due to the observed biodistribution of the radiopharmaceutical. Note the predominant renal excretion of the tracer, with less excretion via the hepatobiliary system. (The hepatobiliary system/gastrointestinal tract appears more prominent because of the overexposure of the study.)

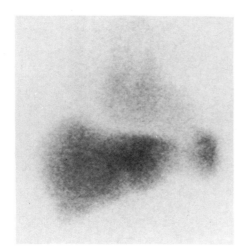

Figure 19–13. BLOOD POOL ON RADIOCOLLOID IMAGE. Radiocolloid image of the liver demonstrates excessive blood pool activity in the heart. The disappearance half-time from the blood of technetium sulfur colloid is 2 to 3 minutes in normal patients but may be prolonged in patients with hepatocellular dysfunction. This patient was imaged immediately after injection, rather than after the usual delay of 15 to 20 minutes. Hepatocellular disease can be excluded by the normal appearance of the liver and spleen as well as by the normal distribution of the radiopharmaceutical.

Ref.: Phan T, Wasnich, R. Practical Nuclear Pharmacy. Honolulu: Banyan Enterprises Ltd., 1981; p 59.

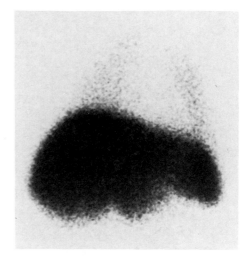

Figure 19–14. LUNG ACTIVITY ON RADIOCOLLOID IMAGE. Radiocolloid scan in an infant demonstrates faint lung activity, a normal finding at this age.

Ref.: Stadalnik RC. Diffuse lung uptake of Tc-99m sulfur colloid. Semin Nucl Med 1980; 10:106–107.

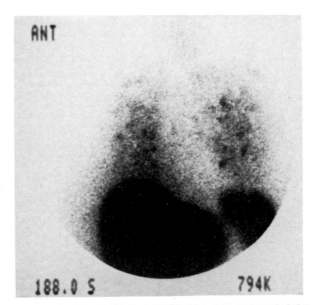

Figure 19–16. LUNG ACTIVITY ON RADIOCOLLOID IMAGE. The lung activity in this scan of another patient is less homogeneous than that seen in Figure 19–15, with distinct "clumps." The production of aggregates large enough to be trapped in the capillary bed of the lung may occur during improper kit preparation or may be due to increased serum aluminum or to aluminum contamination of the generator eluate. It is possible to test for the presence of aluminum in the eluate using a readily available test kit. If poor kit preparation was the cause of the problem, then presumably all the liver scans made on the same day and using the same kit would demonstrate the finding.

Ref.: Klingensmith WC III, Yang SL, Wagner HN Jr. Lung uptake of Tc-99m sulfur colloid in liver and spleen imaging. J Nucl Med 1978; 19:31–35.

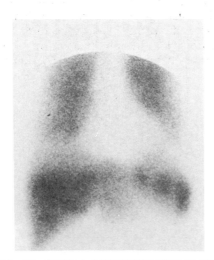

Figure 19–15. LUNG ACTIVITY ON RADIOCOLLOID IMAGE. Anterior radiocolloid scan demonstrates lung activity in a patient with breast cancer and diffuse lung metastasis.

Ref.: Imarisio JJ. Liver scan showing intense lung uptake in neoplasia and infection. J Nucl Med 1975; 16:188–190.

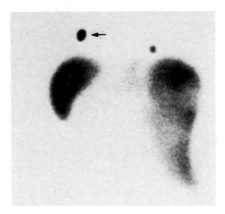

Figure 19–17. LUNG ACTIVITY ON RADIOCOL-LOID IMAGE. The lung activity present in this patient is localized to distinct "clumps" only. The cause of this activity is poor injection technique, with the formation of radiolabeled microemboli *(arrow).* Incidentally seen are multiple photopenic defects within the liver from metastatic breast carcinoma.

Ref.: Keye JW Jr, Wilson GA, Quinonest JD. An evaluation of lung uptake of colloid during liver imaging. J Nucl Med 1973; 14:687–691.

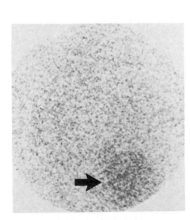

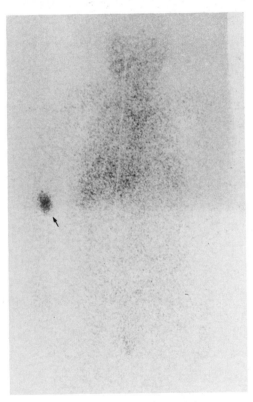

Figure 19–18. XENON ACCUMULATION IN THE LIVER. In this patient, after undergoing a Xenon-133 ventilation study, accumulation of the xenon was seen in the liver *(arrow).* Fatty infiltration is the postulated cause for this finding in most cases. Xenon is lipophilic and thus will accumulate in areas of fatty deposition.

Ref.: Cary J. Localization of xenon in the liver during ventilation studies. J Nucl Med 1974; 15:1178.

Figure 19–19. GALLIUM ACCUMULATION IN A WOUND HEMATOMA. This patient was noted clinically to have an infected injection site *(arrow)* upon return for routine 48-hour imaging.

Ref.: Carter JE, Joo KG. Gallium accumulation in intramuscular injection sites. Clin Nucl Med 1979; 4:304.

CHAPTER 20

Thyroid Imaging

DONALD E. JACKSON, M.D.
CHARLES E. PETERSON, M.D.

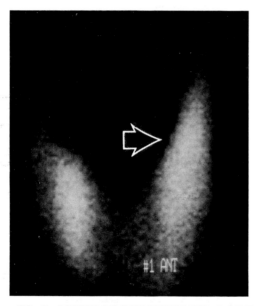

Figure 20–1. ASYMMETRIC THYROID LOBE SIMULATES NODULE. This patient had a "fullness" to the left lobe that clinically suggested a nodule. The I-123 scan reveals asymmetry of the lobes *(arrow),* a common finding. No nodule was seen on this image or on the oblique scans. Asymmetry is a common finding, with the right lobe generally being the larger.

Ref.: Mettler FA, Guiberteau MJ. Essentials of Nuclear Medicine Imaging. New York: Grune & Stratton, 1983; p 89.

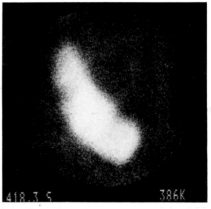

Figure 20–2. THYROID HEMIAGENESIS SIMULATES A NODULE. During clinical examination, a "nodule" was palpated on the right side of this patient's neck. The I-123 scan reveals the true nature of the "nodule"—hemiagenesis of the left lobe. The resultant absence of tissue on the left side made the remaining normal tissue in the right neck seem abnormally prominent. Thyroid hemiagenesis is relatively rare. Careful correlation with palpation findings and possibly a thyroid-stimulation hormone test may be necessary in some cases to differentiate this entity from a hot nodule with suppression of the remainder of the gland.

Ref.: Melnick JC, Stemkowski PE. Thyroid hemiagenesis (hockey stick sign): A review of the world literature and a report of four cases. J Clin Endocrinol Metab 1981; 52:247–251.

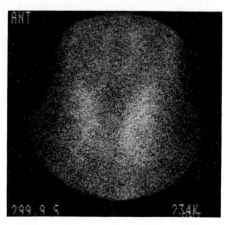

Figure 20–3. THYROID SCAN AFTER IODINE LOAD. This patient was inadvertently scheduled for a technetium thyroid scan on the same day and immediately following computed tomography of the neck in which the patient received 27 grams of iodine intravenously. It can be seen from the scan that trapping of the technetium by the gland has been greatly reduced, hampering the formation of an interpretable image. Of course, the results of a radioiodine uptake test would also be invalidated by the iodine load. Great care must be taken in scheduling patients for thyroid scan and uptake tests prior to the administration of iodinated contrast materials.

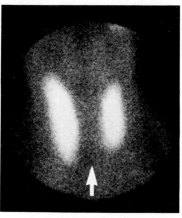

Figure 20–4. ABSENCE OF TISSUE IN THE THYROID ISTHMUS, SIMULATING A COLD NODULE. This I-124 scan demonstrates an area of decreased photon activity in the region of the thyroid isthmus (arrow). No clinically palpable nodule was present. The thyroid isthmus may demonstrate relatively decreased activity compared with the remainder of the gland. This case illustrates the importance of correlation of the scan with the findings on palpation.

Ref.: Mettler FA, Guiberteau MJ. Essentials of Nuclear Medicine Imaging. New York: Grune & Stratton, 1983; p 89.

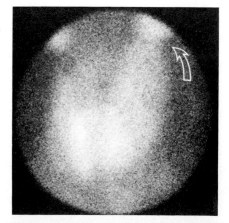

Figure 20–5. SUBMANDIBULAR GLAND SIMULATING A HOT NODULE. This scan illustrates the potential for confusion between the normal activity seen in the salivary glands (arrow) on both technetium and I-123 scans and a hot nodule located superiorly in the thyroid. Oblique views and awareness of the normal distribution of the radioisotope will prevent an error in diagnosis.

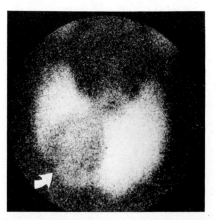

Figure 20–6. COLD NODULE SIMULATED BY A METALLIC MEDALLION. In this scan a cold nodule (arrow) is seen that is caused by attenuation from an overlying metallic medallion. Errors in diagnosis can be avoided by removal of all overlying material from the neck before imaging.

Ref.: Cold nodule—thyroid scan. Semin Nucl Med 1981; 11:320–321.

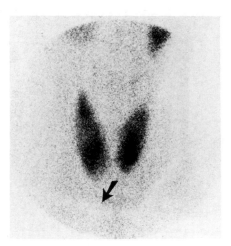

Figure 20–7. ARTIFACT CAUSED BY JEWELRY.
The photopenic artifact *(arrow)* in this scan is caused
by a metallic necklace worn during imaging. Although
it did not interfere with thyroid imaging in this case, all
overlying material should be removed before thyroid
imaging is performed.

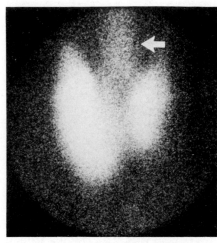

Figure 20–8. PYRAMIDAL LOBE. On this scan, a
pyramidal lobe *(arrow)* is visualized. This should not
be confused with esophageal activity that is seen on
I-123 and, more often, technetium scans. Re-imaging
after clearing the esophagus with water, and also
oblique views, should allow differentiation of these two
entities.

Ref.: Levy HA, Sziklas JJ, Rosenberg RJ, Spencer RP. Incidence of
a pyramidal lobe on thyroid scans. Clin Nucl Med 1982; 7:560–
561.

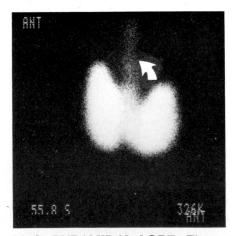

Figure 20–9. PYRAMIDAL LOBE. This scan of a
patient with Graves' disease demonstrates a pyramidal
lobe *(arrow)* that bears a striking resemblance to esophageal activity. However, oblique views and persistence
of the activity after water ingestion to clear the esophagus demonstrated the true nature of the finding.

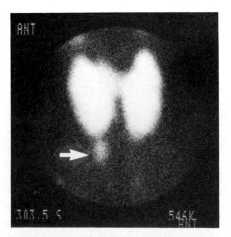

Figure 20–10. ACCESSORY THYROID TISSUE. In
this scan, a small amount of accessory thyroid tissue
(arrow) is demonstrated just inferior to the right lobe.
This was initially mistaken for esophageal activity until
oblique views and clearing of the esophagus with water
ingestion revealed its true nature.

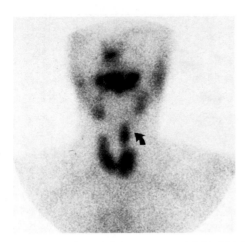

Figure 20–11. ACCESSORY THYROID TISSUE. A bit of accessory thyroid tissue (or a pyramidal lobe) *(arrow)* is seen just superior to the left lobe on this scan. This should not be confused with esophageal activity.

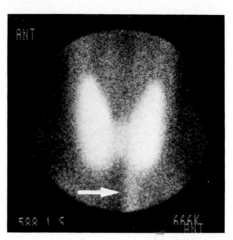

Figure 20–12. ESOPHAGEAL ACTIVITY. Activity within the esophagus is demonstrated on this technetium scan *(arrow)*. Re-imaging after water ingestion demonstrated the true nature of the finding. Gastroesophageal reflux may also be a potential source of confusion, especially if the patient is supine when imaged, as is usually the case. Awareness of the problem, and re-imaging with oblique views should prevent misinterpretation.

Ref.: Grossman M. Gastroesophageal reflux: A potential source of confusion in technetium thyroid scanning. J Nucl Med 1977; 18:548.

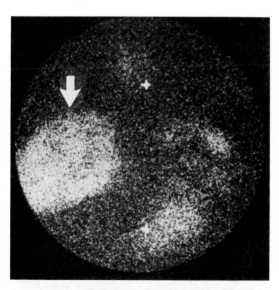

Figure 20–13. BREAST ACTIVITY AFTER I-131 METASCAN. This I-131 metascan was performed in a nursing mother, who nursed her infant predominantly with the right breast *(arrow)*. Significant amounts of I-131, I-123, and technetium will be secreted into breast milk. Nursing mothers should avoid breast-feeding for 72 hours after technetium scanning, for 6 weeks following I-131 scans, and for 1 week following I-123 scans.

Ref.: Wybur JR. Human breast milk excretion of radionuclides following administration of radiopharmaceuticals. J Nucl Med 1972; 14:115.

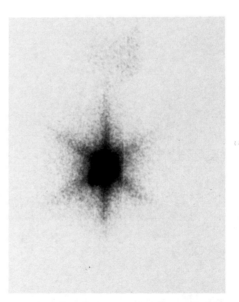

Figure 20–14. RESIDUAL THYROID ACTIVITY ON METASCAN. This patient with thyroid carcinoma demonstrates residual thyroid tissue imaged by administration of 5 mCi of I-131. The star-shaped pattern is created by the septal penetrations of the 364 keV photons of I-131 through the medium-energy collimator.

Ref.: Turner DA, Silverstein EA. Instrumentation quality control, Case 2. In: Alderman PO, Coleman RE, Grove RB, et al., eds. Nuclear Radiology (Third Series) Syllabus, American College of Radiology, 1983.

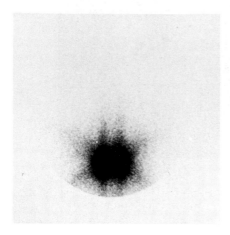

Figure 20–15. RESIDUAL THYROID TISSUE ON METASCAN. In this patient with thyroid carcinoma, residual thyroid tissue is demonstrated after administration of 5 mCi of I-131 for a metascan. The star-shaped pattern is caused by septal penetration of the medium-energy collimator. The residual thyroid tissue is bilobed, causing two stellate patterns side-by-side.

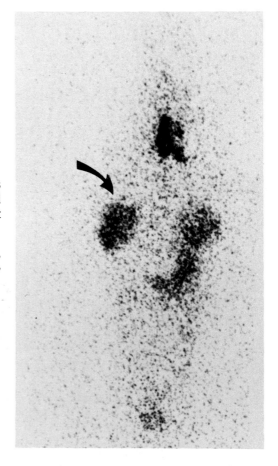

Figure 20–16. BREAST ACTIVITY ON METASCAN. In this patient with thyroid cancer, bilateral breast uptake of I-131 (a normal finding) is demonstrated. Note the activity within the right breast *(arrow)*.

Ref.: Coleman RE, Workman JR. Thyroid carcinoma, Case 36. In: Alderman PO, Coleman RE, Grove RB, et al., eds. Nuclear Radiology (Third Series) Syllabus, American College of Radiology, 1983.

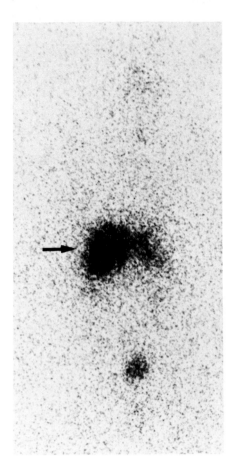

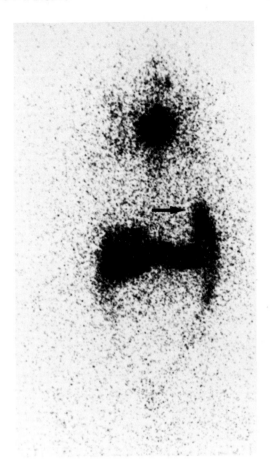

Figure 20–17. LIVER ACTIVITY ON METASCAN. Activity within the right upper quadrant *(arrow)*, which is demonstrated on this scan of a patient with thyroid carcinoma, represents I-131 within the liver, a normal finding if the patient has functioning residual thyroid tissue. Spot views of the patient's neck revealed a small thyroid remnant. The I-131 is incorporated into thyroid hormone and the liver is the major degradation site for thyroxine. The focal area of tracer accumulation seen inferiorly represents fecal activity in the rectum.

Ref.: Coleman RE, Workman JB. Thyroid carcinoma, Case 36. In: Alderman PO, Coleman RE, Grove RB, et al., eds. Nuclear Radiology (Third Series) Syllabus, American College of Radiology, 1983.

Figure 20–18. COLONIC ACTIVITY ON META-SCAN. In this scan of a patient with thyroid carcinoma, normal accumulation of I-131 is seen within the colon. The splenic flexure *(arrow)* is also demonstrated. Other sites of physiologic accumulation include the salivary glands, the nasopharynx, the stomach, and bladder as well as the breast and liver, in which accumulation was previously demonstrated. (This patient also has a large amount of residual thyroid in the neck.)

Figure 20–19. STOMACH ACTIVITY ON METASCAN. This patient with thyroid carcinoma has no residual thyroid bed activity; however, on the edge of the crystal there is an area of activity in the right upper quadrant *(arrow)*. This represents normal accumulation within the stomach.

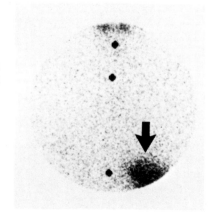

21

Renal Imaging

DONALD E. JACKSON, M.D.
CHARLES E. PETERSON, M.D.

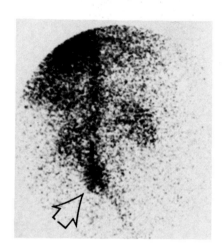

Figure 21–1. DETECTION OF AORTIC ANEURYSM ON RENAL FLOW STUDY. This patient was undergoing renal scanning in the evaluation of hypertension. On the flow study, an area of increased activity is seen in the region of the distal aorta *(arrow)*. Angiography proved this to be due to an atherosclerotic aneurysm.

Figure 21–2. HYPERVASCULAR BONE METASTASES DETECTED ON RENAL FLOW STUDY. This patient was undergoing routine evaluation after nephrectomy renal cell carcinoma.

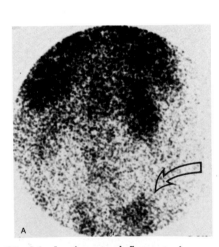

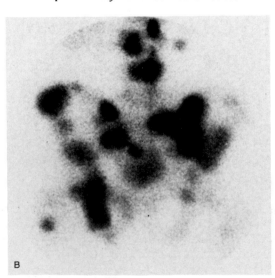

Figure 21–2A. In the renal flow study, several hypervascular regions are identified in the region of the sacrum *(arrow)*.

Figure 21–2B. Correlation with this bone scan revealed the metastatic deposits that were the cause of the hypervascularity seen in A.

Ref.: Simon H. Metastatic recurrent hypernephroma demonstrated by isotope angiography. Clin Nucl Med 1977; 2:214.

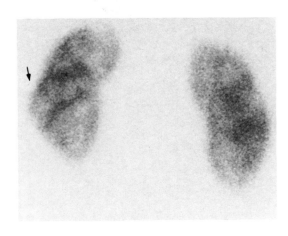

Figure 21–3. DROMEDARY HUMP. An excretory urogram performed in this patient was considered suspicious for the presence of a renal mass lesion in the left kidney. Technetium glucoheptonate renal imaging (posterior view) reveals an area of normal renal tissue laterally *(arrow)*, known as a *"dromedary hump,"* and excludes the presence of a space-occupying lesion.

Ref.: Older RA, Korobkin M, Workman J, et al. Accuracy of radionuclide imaging in distinguishing renal masses from normal variants. Radiology 1980; 136:443–448.

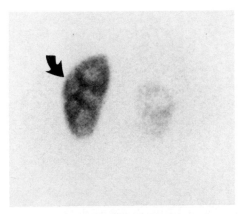

Figure 21–4. PHOTOPENIC RENAL PYRAMIDS. This patient underwent renal scanning with technetium-labeled dimercaptosuccinic acid (DMSA). This image demonstrates the fact that the renal pyramids are normally photopenic *(arrow)* compared with the renal cortex, and they should not be mistaken for space-occupying pathology or hydronephrosis.

Ref.: Leonard JC, Allen EW, Goin J, Smith CW. Renal cortical imaging and the detection of renal mass lesions. J Nucl Med 1979; 20:1018–1022.

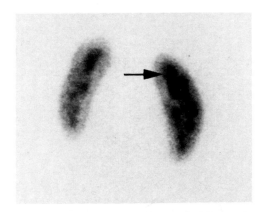

Figure 21–5. PROMINENT COLLECTING SYSTEM. Very prominent collecting structures *(arrow)* can be seen in this image. Careful construction of the renal regions of interest will be necessary for accurate evaluation of renal cortical function. The administration of a diuretic may help to distinguish obstructive uropathy from prominent collecting structures.

Ref.: Thrall JH, Koff SA, Keyes JW Jr. Diuretic radionuclide renography and scintigraphy in the differential diagnosis of hydro-ureteronephrosis. Semin Nucl Med 1981; 11:89–104.

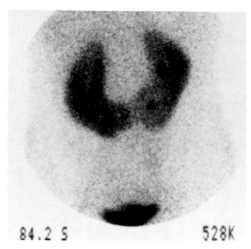

Figure 21–6. HORSESHOE KIDNEY. The horse-shoe kidney illustrated on this scan is the most common form of fusion anomaly.

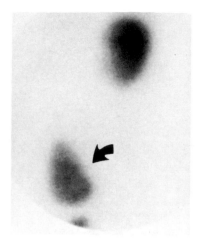

Figure 21–7. PELVIC KIDNEY. The anomalous pelvic kidney *(arrow)* is a potential source of error, as it may not be included in the routine posterior view and therefore may be interpreted as absent. If the patient is being evaluated for trauma, the finding of a pelvic kidney may be misinterpreted as a renal pedicle avulsion. Routine imaging of the pelvis should be performed in the anterior position in any patient without a history of nephrectomy who demonstrates an absence of one kidney.

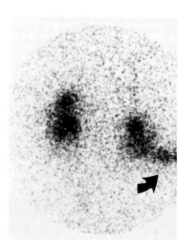

Figure 21–8. PERCUTANEOUS NEPHROSTOMY. This I-131–labeled hippuran renogram demonstrates an area of tracer activity *(arrow)* lateral to the right kidney. This activity is due to the presence of a renal drainage catheter placed through a percutaneous nephrostomy. Knowledge of any iatrogenic alterations of the renal system is vital for accurate interpretation of the renogram.

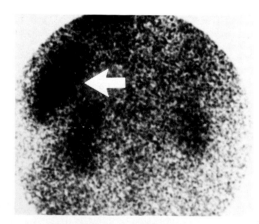

Figure 21–9. NORMAL SPLENIC BLUSH ON RENAL FLOW STUDY. Renal flow study demonstrates a normal splenic blush *(arrow)* arising superior to the left kidney. This must be differentiated from a hypervascular renal or suprarenal mass.

Ref.: Ball JD, Cowan RJ, Maynard CD. Splenic simulation of a renal mass [letter]. J Nucl Med 1976; 17:1104–1105.

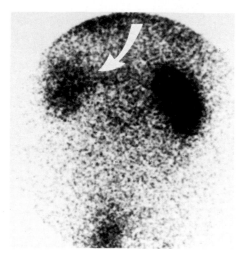

Figure 21–10. SPLENIC PSEUDOKIDNEY. This patient has undergone a left nephrectomy. The activity in the left renal fossa *(arrow)* on the flow study (posterior view) is caused by the spleen. In a post nephrectomy patient, the bowel may also simulate renal perfusion on a flow study. Both of these entities may be distinguished from normal renal flow by the fact that the activity fades on post-dynamic images.

Ref.: Freeman LM, Lutzker LG. The kidneys. In: Freeman LM, ed. Freeman and Johnson's Clinical Radionuclide Imaging. New York: Grune & Stratton, 1984; p 749.

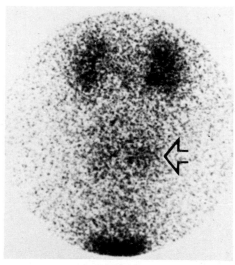

Figure 21–11. PSEUDOKIDNEY DUE TO COINCIDENCE SUMMING. In this I-131–labeled hippuran scan, two areas of increased activity (arrow) are visualized inferior to both kidneys. These are ghost images produced by coincidence summing of technetium photons from the prior injection of glucoheptonate. These artifacts may be minimized by the use of a gamma camera with good pulse pile-up rejection schemes, the use of a narrow window centered on the 364 photopeak of I-131, and waiting until the technetium clears from the kidney before injection of the hippuran.

Ref.: Harris CC, Wilkinson RH Jr, Schuler FR. Artifacts in iodine-131 renal images due to coincidence summing of technetium-99m photons. Radiology 1983; 146:505–507.

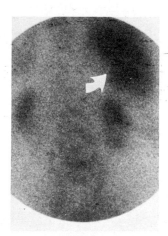

Figure 21–12. PROMINENT LIVER ACTIVITY ON GLUCOHEPTONATE SCAN. Scan of a patient with renal insufficiency demonstrates the vicarious excretion of glucoheptonate through the liver *(arrow)*, with prominent visualization of the liver on the posterior view.

Ref.: Freeman LM, Lutzker LG. The kidneys. In: Freeman LM, ed. Freeman and Johnson's Clinical Radionuclide Imaging. New York: Grune & Stratton, 1984; p 751.

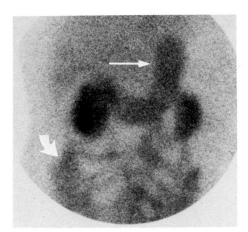

Figure 21–13. GUT VISUALIZATION ON GLUCO-HEPTONATE SCAN. For this scan, the patient was imaged using glucoheptonate that had been prepared 8 hours prior to injection, resulting in an excessive amount of free pertechnetate in the kit. Careful attention to the preparation and administration of radiopharmaceuticals is necessary to prevent such errors. The stomach *(straight arrow)* and the colon *(curved arrow)* are demonstrated.

Figure 21–14. I-131–LABELED HIPPURAN STUDY OFF PEAK. This patient had been injected with technetium glucoheptonate for a flow study, and then with I-131–labeled hippuran for a renogram. However, the camera was left on the 140 keV photopeak of technetium for the first 5 minutes of the hippuran study.

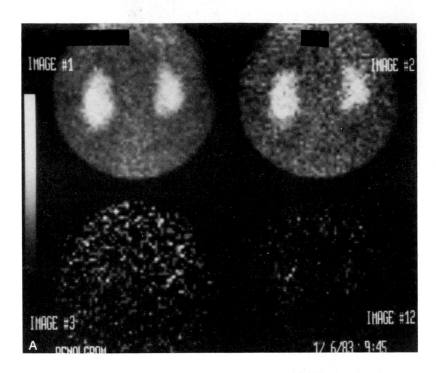

Figure 21–14A. The images demonstrate the dramatic change in counts when the technician noticed the error and switched to the 364 keV photopeak.

Figure 21–14B. The time-activity curve reflects the dramatic drop in count rate *(arrow)*. If the curve is re-plotted on a smaller scale, the remainder of the reno-gram can be viewed (it is compressed into a straight line on the scale in the figure).

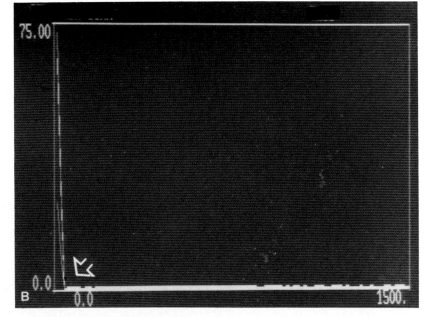

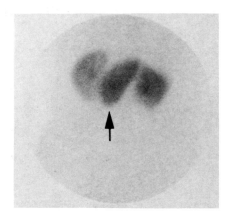

Figure 21–15. DOUBLE EXPOSURE. In a glucoheptonate renal scan, this patient, who has only two kidneys, appears to have three. This appearance is the result of an inadvertent double exposure *(arrow).* The cause could be suspected by the lack of a constant spatial relationship between the three kidneys on various views.

Figure 21–16. RENAL ACTIVITY SIMULATED BY BONE DISEASE.

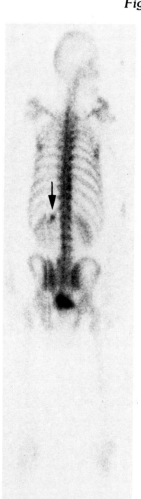

Figure 21–16A. Whole body image of a bone scan demonstrates an apparent area of abnormal tracer activity within a renal collecting structure *(arrow).*

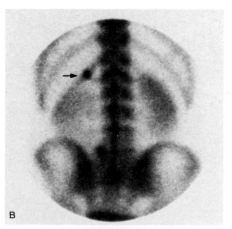

Figure 21–16B. An upright posterior spot view reveals the true nature of the finding—a rib lesion *(arrow).* Renal activity may simulate bone disease and vice versa. Imaging in a variety of positions and obliquities will prevent confusion of one pathology with the other.

Ref.: Williamson BR, Teates CD, Bray, ST, et al. Renal excretion simulating bone disease on bone scans—a technique for solving this problem. Clin Nucl Med 1979; 4:200–201.

A

Figure 21–17. BLADDER ACTIVITY SIMULATING BONE DISEASE.

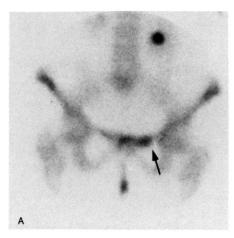

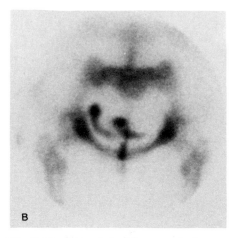

Figure 21–17A. Anterior bone spot image demonstrates an apparent increase in tracer activity within the superior ramus of the left pubis *(arrow)*.

Figure 21–17B. A caudal view reveals the true nature of the activity—retention within the bladder.

Ref.: Ham HR, Verelst J, Vandivere J. Caudal view on bone scan to visualize coccygeal and pubic lesions. Clin Nucl Med 1982; 7:41.

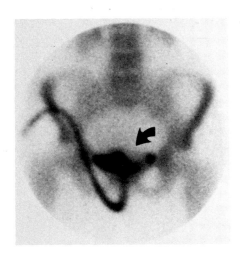

Figure 21–18. URINARY CATHETER SIMULATING A BLADDER MASS. A bladder mass can be visualized on bone scans if the mass is large enough and there is sufficient activity in the patient's bladder. However, the "mass" *(arrow)* seen in the bladder of this patient is actually the inflated balloon of a urinary drainage catheter.

Ref.: Duong RB, Gelfand MJ, Volarich DT, et al. Urinary tract imaging—filling defect in the urinary bladder. Semin Nucl Med 1983; 13:383.

CHAPTER 22

Gated Cardiac Imaging

DONALD E. JACKSON, M.D.
CHARLES E. PETERSON, M.D.

Figure 22–1. PACEMAKER DEFECT ON GATED EQUILIBRIUM BLOOD POOL CARDIAC STUDY.

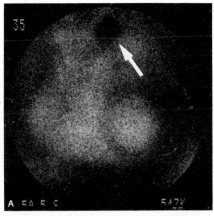

Figure 22–1A. This blood pool image demonstrates a photopenic defect in the upper chest due to a pacemaker *(arrow)*.

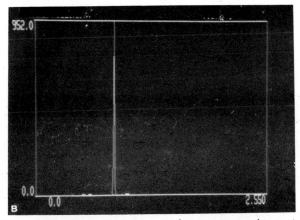

Figure 22–1B. R-R histogram demonstrates the typical narrow "spike" due to little variation in the R-R interval of the paced beats.

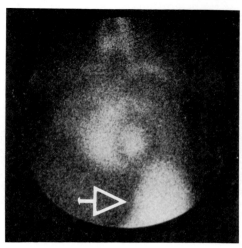

Figure 22–2. SPLENOMEGALY ON GATED CARDIAC STUDY. Labeled red blood cell equilibrium cardiac study demonstrates a very large spleen *(arrow)*. To prevent a falsely high estimation of the ejection fraction, care must be taken to avoid including part of the spleen in the background region of interest.

Ref.: Shih W, Domstad PA, DeLand FH, et al. Demonstration of splenomegaly by gated cardiac blood pool imaging. Clin Nucl Med 1982; 7:568–569.

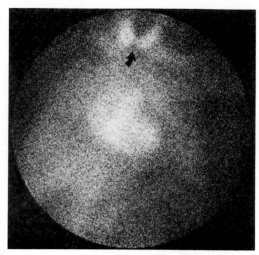

Figure 22–3. THYROID ACTIVITY ON LABELED BLOOD POOL CARDIAC STUDY. This patient underwent a gated blood pool cardiac study. However, the background activity was excessively high and the thyroid was visualized *(arrow)*. Examination of the patient's blood revealed a tagging efficiency of only 70 per cent. Careful attention must be paid to the tagging methodology, and efficiencies of greater than 90 to 95 per cent should be obtained.

Ref.: Van Nostrand D, Smallridge R. Thyroid trapping technetium during in vivo labeling of RBCs [letter]. J Nucl Med 1982; 23:1146–1147.

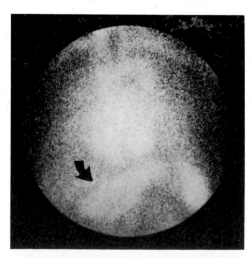

Figure 22–4. STOMACH VISUALIZATION ON GATED BLOOD POOL CARDIAC STUDY. This image shows gastric activity *(arrow)* due to the presence of free pertechnetate secondary to poor tagging efficiency.

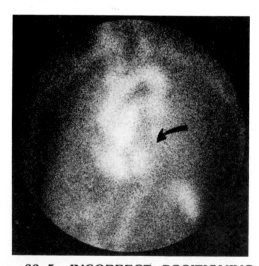

Figure 22–5. INCORRECT POSITIONING ON GATED BLOOD POOL CARDIAC STUDY. The left anterior oblique position results in the projection of the aorta behind the left ventricle *(arrow)*. This should be avoided, as the counts contributed to the left ventricle region of interest will falsely lower the calculated ejection fraction.

Ref.: Mettler FA, Guiberteau MJ, Essentials of Nuclear Medicine Imaging. New York: Grune & Stratton, 1983; p 127.

Figure 22–6. INCORRECT BACKGROUND PLACEMENT RESULTING IN FALSELY HIGH EJECTION FRACTION ON GATED CARDIAC STUDY. Gated blood pool cardiac study images demonstrate the effect of incorrect placement of the background region of interest over the aorta on the calculated ejection fraction. Note that the ejection fraction drops from a normal value with the incorrect background to an abnormally low value with correct placement. This emphasizes the need for accurate placement of the backround region of interest to avoid the great vessels and other chambers and the spleen.

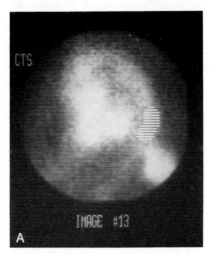

Figure 22–6A. Left anterior oblique view with incorrect background.

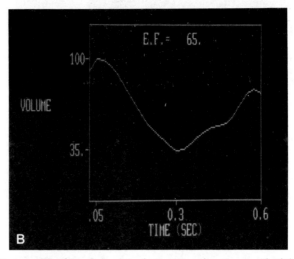

Figure 22–6B. Calculated ejection fraction with false background.

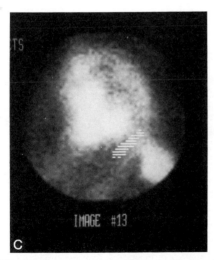

Figure 22–6C. Left anterior oblique view with correct background.

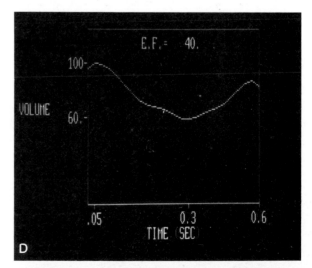

Figure 22–D. Calculated ejection fraction with good background.

Ref.: Berger HJ, Zaret BL. Radionuclide assessment of cardiovascular performance. In: Freeman LM, ed. New York: Freeman and Johnson's Clinical Radionuclide Imaging. Grune & Stratton, 1984; p 405.

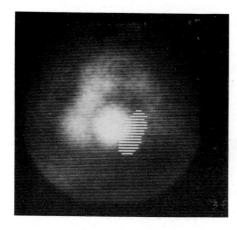

Figure 22–7. EXAMPLE OF BAD BACKGROUND REGION OF IN-TEREST INVOLVING THE LEFT VENTRICLE. This image demonstrates the inclusion of the left ventricular edge in the region of interest for the background. This results in a falsely high background count and a falsely high ejection fraction.

Figure 22–8. R-R HISTOGRAM DEMONSTRATING SIGNIFICANT ECTOPY. The patient had significant ectopy during this gated blood pool cardiac study, which was acquired using the frame mode without beat length exclusion. The calculated ejection fraction will be artifactually low and the resultant volume curve will be severely disorted.

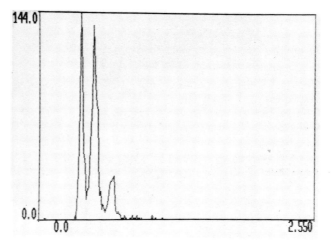

Ref.: Berger HJ, Zaret BL. Radionuclide assessment of cardiovascular performance. In: Freeman LM, ed. Freeman and Johnson's Clinical Radionuclide Imaging. New York, Grune & Stratton, 1984, p 374.

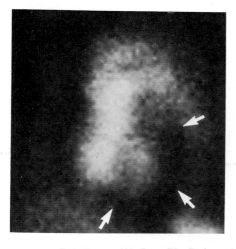

Figure 22–9. PHOTOPENIC HALO AROUND VENTRICLE. A photopenic halo can be seen around the heart secondary to a malignant pericardial effusion *(arrows)*. This must be differentiated from the "halo" caused by concentric myocardial thickening. The latter can usually be identified by the involvement of the ventricular septum in the hypertrophy.

Ref.: Berger HJ, Zaret BL. Radionuclide assessment of cardiovascular performance. In: Freeman LM, ed. Freeman and Johnson's Clinical Radionuclide Imaging. New York: Grune & Stratton, 1984, p 383.

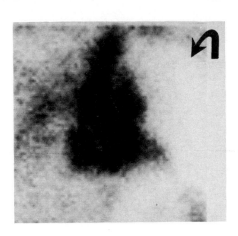

Figure 22–10. PHOTOPENIC REGION DUE TO PNEUMONEC-TOMY. In this image a photopenic region adjacent to the left ventricle extends into the left chest *(arrow)*. This is due to a pneumonectomy, with the subsequent loss of the blood pool activity contributed by the left lung. This can be differentiated from a pericardial effusion by its extent and by the lack of involvement of the right side of the heart.

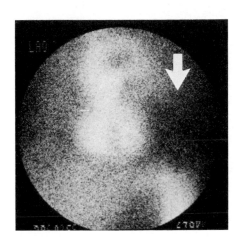

Figure 22–11. PHOTOPENIC REGION DUE TO PLEURAL EFFU-SION. Lateral anterior oblique view demonstrates a photopenic region adjacent to the left ventricle secondary to a left pleural effusion *(arrow)*. This can be differentiated from other causes of cardiac "halo" by its location and the lack of involvement of the right heart. An image acquired in a different position (decubitus, upright) may reveal the true nature of the finding.

CHAPTER — 23

Thallium Cardiac Imaging

DONALD E. JACKSON, M.D.
CHARLES E. PETERSON, M.D.

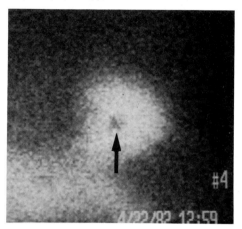

Figure 23–1. CHEST LEAD CAUSING PHOTO-PENIC DEFECT. The low-energy 80 keV photons of thallium-201 are easily attenuated by any overlying absorber. In this case, the EKG monitor leads were not removed prior to imaging, resulting in a photopenic defect *(arrow)* in the region of the left ventricular myocardium. Potential misdiagnosis as infarct or ischemia can be avoided by prior removal of any overlying material between the patient and the gamma camera crystal.

Ref.: Berman DS, Garcia EV, Maddahi J. Role of thallium-201 imaging in the diagnosis of myocardial ischemia and infarction. In: Freeman L, Weissmann H, eds. Nuclear Medicine Annual, 1980. New York: Raven Press, 1980; p 1.

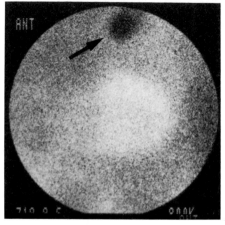

Figure 23–2. PACEMAKER CAUSING PHOTO-PENIC DEFECT. The photopenic defect *(arrow)* caused by the pacemaker in this patient should not present a diagnostic problem. However, in patients with pacers implanted slightly lower, part of the myocardium could be obscured.

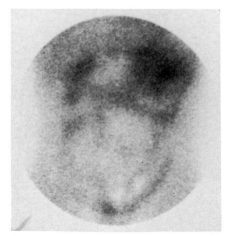

Figure 23–3. NORMAL THALLIUM ACTIVITY IN THE GUT. This is an image over the abdomen in a patient who was injected with thallium when at rest. It illustrates the large amount of thallium activity present within abdominal structures such as the gut and the liver.

Ref.: Atkins HL, Budinger TF, Lebowitz E, et al. Thallium-201 for medical use. Part 3: Human distribution and physical imaging properties. J Nucl Med 1977; 18:133–140.

Figure 23–4. THALLIUM UPTAKE IN AN ARM VEIN.

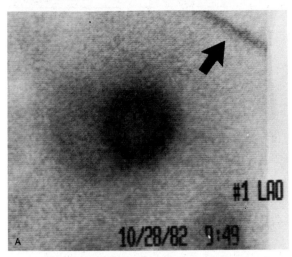

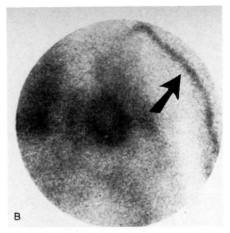

Figure 23–4A. Magnified spot thallium study demonstrates an oblique line of activity *(arrow)* in the left upper quadrant of the image.

Figure 23–4B. A view that includes more of the patient's body reveals that this activity is in an arm vein *(arrow)*. This may be caused by injection into the arm with a blood pressure cuff partially occluding the blood flow, allowing more thallium uptake in the wall of the vein.

Ref.: Atkins HL, Budinger TF, Lebowitz E, et al. Thallium-201 for medical use. Part 3: Human distribution and physical imaging properties. J Nucl Med 1977; 18:133–140.

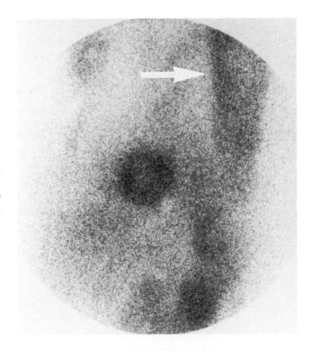

Figure 23–5. THALLIUM IN MUSCULATURE OF THE SHOULDER GIRDLE. Left anterior oblique thallium image demonstrates thallium activity *(arrow)* in the muscles of the shoulder girdle. Although blood is usually shunted to the muscles of the lower extremities during treadmill exercise testing, flow may also increase to the upper extremities and potentially obscure the view of the myocardium in a patient with well-developed musculature.

Ref.: Atkins HL, Budinger TF, Lebowitz E, et al. Thallium-201 for medical use. Part 3. Human distribution and physical imaging properties. J Nucl Med 1977; 18:133–140.

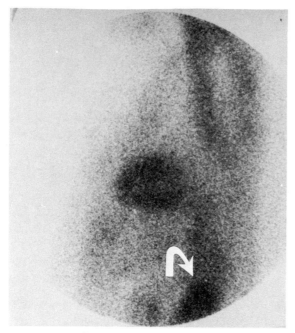

Figure 23–6. THALLIUM IN THE KIDNEY. Thallium is excreted by the kidneys normally; about 5 per cent of the injected dose is present in the kidney *(arrow)* 10 minutes post-injection. Awareness of the normal distribution of thallium-201 is necessary to prevent errors of interpretation.

Ref.: Atkins HL, Budinger TF, Lebowitz E, et al. Thallium-201 for medical use. Part 3: Human distribution and physical imaging properties. J Nucl Med 1977; 18:133–140.

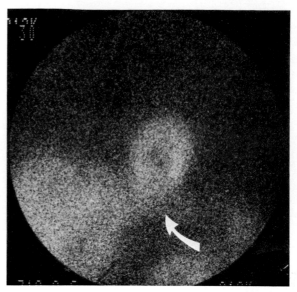

Figure 23–7. ATTENUATION OF THALLIUM BY THE EDGE OF THE LIVER. This image demonstrates an area of decreased photon activity inferiorly. Notice, however, that the edge of the liver overlies this part of the myocardium *(arrow)* and attenuates the activity. This could be a source of misinterpretation, either by producing a photopenic defect or by masking one.

Ref.: Gordon DG, Pfisterer M, Williams R, et al. The effect of diaphragmatic attenuation on 201Ti images. Clin Nucl Med 1979; 4:150–151.

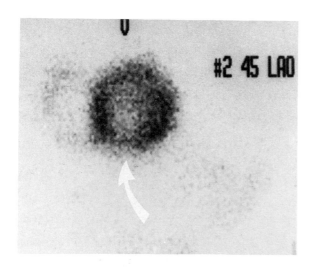

Figure 23–8. APICAL THINNING SIMULATING DEFECT. The apex of the heart is an area that normally has decreased photon activity. This area *(arrow)* should not be interpreted as abnormal when it is small in extent and demonstrates no change from stress to redistribution images.

Ref.: Cook DJ, Bailey I, Strauss HW, et al. Thallium-201 for myocardial imaging: Appearance of the normal heart. J Nucl Med 1976; 17:583–589.

Figure 23–9. RIGHT VENTRICULAR VISUALIZATION.

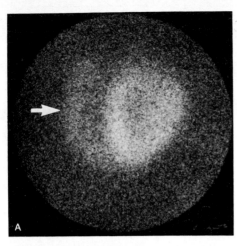

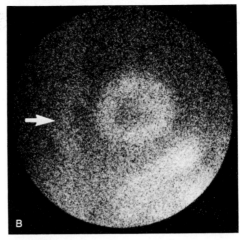

Figure 23–9A. The appearance of right ventricular activity on thallium imaging is a normal finding after stress *(arrow).*

Figure 23–9B. If the right ventricle is seen after an injection made while the patient was at rest *(arrow),* it indicates increased blood flow or increased muscle mass or both.

Ref.: Ohsuzu F, Handa S, Kondo M, et al. Thallium-201 myocardial imaging to evaluate right ventricular overloading. Circulation 1980; 61:620–625.

Figure 23–10. INCREASED LUNG ACTIVITY ON STRESS THALLIUM IMAGING. This patient demonstrates an increased amount of thallium activity in the lungs *(arrow)* on imaging after exercise. This indicates the presence of volume or pressure overload to the heart.

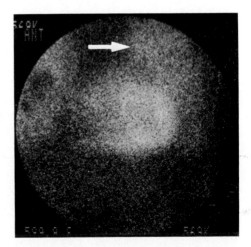

Ref.: Boucher CA, Zir LM, Beller GA, et al. Increased lung uptake of thallium-201 during exercise myocardial imaging: Clinical, hemodynamic and angiographic implications in patients with coronary artery disease. Am J Cardiol 1980; 46:189–196.

Pyrophosphate Cardiac Imaging

DONALD E. JACKSON, M.D.
CHARLES E. PETERSON, M.D.

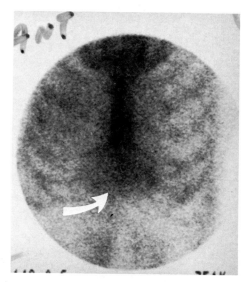

Figure 24–1. EXCESSIVE BLOOD POOL ACTIVITY. This patient underwent a pyrophosphate infarct scan. This image, taken at 2.5 hours after injection, demonstrates diffuse activity in the region of the heart *(arrow)*. While this can be related to myocardial pathology, in this case re-imaging at 4 hours revealed a significant decrease in the blood pool activity. Other causes for increased blood pool activity besides early imaging would include a prior gated equilibrium study, delayed clearance due to decreased renal function, and excessive free pertechnetate in the injected kit, with resultant labeling of red blood cells.

Ref.: Klein MS, Coleman RE, Roberts R, et al. False positive pyrophosphate myocardial infarct images related to delayed blood pool clearance. Clin Nucl Med 1976; 1:45–46.

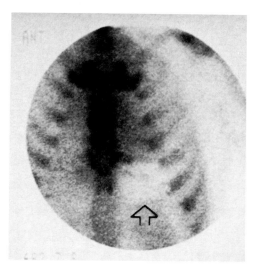

Figure 24–2. CASE 13: PHOTOPENIC AREA. This patient ate lunch just prior to the scan, which resulted in the photopenic area *(arrow)* in the left upper quadrant on this pyrophosphate image.

Ref.: Font D. Stomach artifact in bone scintigraphy. J Nucl Med 1978; 19:974–975.

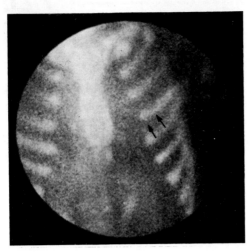

Figure 24–3. RIB ACTIVITY. The prominent pyrophosphate uptake by the ribs *(arrows)* seen in this image could potentially obscure uptake by an infarct. Oblique views should reveal the true nature of the defect.

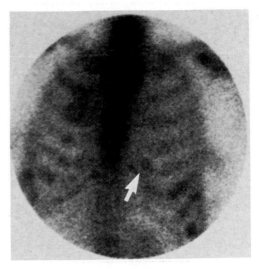

Figure 24–4. COSTAL CARTILAGE UPTAKE. The prominent pyrophosphate uptake by costal cartilages *(arrow)* seen in this image could potentially simulate or obscure myocardial uptake of the pyrophosphate. Oblique views may reveal the true nature of the finding.

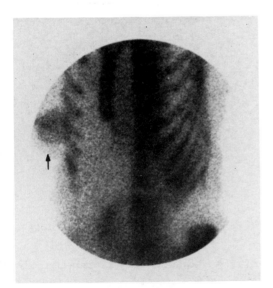

Figure 24–5. BREAST ACTIVITY. This image demonstrates prominent pyrophosphate tracer activity within the breast *(arrow)*, a normal variant.

Ref.: Landgarten S. Uptake of Tc-99m pyrophosphate by the lactating breast [letter]. J Nucl Med 1977; 18:943.

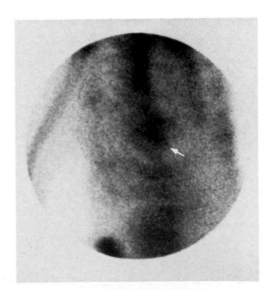

Figure 24–6. BREAST ACTIVITY. The phyrophosphate activity in the breast that is seen in this image overlies the area of the heart *(arrow)* and potentially could be misinterpreted as myocardial activity. Oblique views should reveal the true nature of the finding.

Ref.: Meyer-Pavel C, Clark JK, Parel DG. Incidence and consequence of breast artifacts in radionuclide cardiac studies. Clin Nucl Med 1982; 7:53–57.

Pulmonary Imaging

DONALD E. JACKSON, M.D.
CHARLES E. PETERSON, M.D.

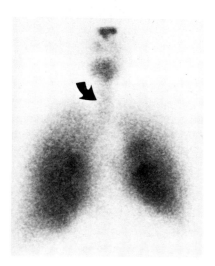

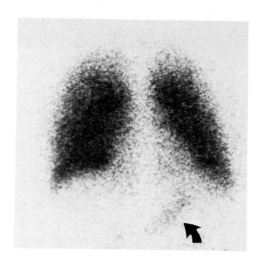

Figure 25–1. AEROSOL VENTILATION WITH TRACHEAL DEPOSITION. This patient underwent an inhalational aerosol ventilation study using technetium DTPA aerosol. The aerosol normally will impact to a small extent in the larger airways, and this does not represent a pathologic process. Note deposition in the trachea *(arrow)*.

Ref.: Usselman RA. An improved technique for inhalation imaging. Clin Nucl Med 1982; 7:180.

Figure 25–2. FREE PERTECHNETATE ON PULMONARY PERFUSION SCAN. This patient underwent a technetium-labeled macroaggregated albumin perfusion lung scan. The activity seen below the heart on the left side *(arrow)* represents free pertechnetate secretion in the stomach resulting from poor tag efficiency.

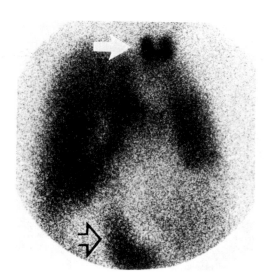

Figure 25–3. FREE PERTECHNETATE IN THE THYROID AND STOMACH ON PERFUSION SCAN. Perfusion scan image demonstrates free pertechnetate in both the stomach *(open arrowhead)* and the thyroid *(white arrow)*. Careful preparation of the radiopharmaceutical kit according to the manufacturer's instructions is necessary to prevent a poor tag. Delayed scanning beyond 1 hour post-injection will often demonstrate thyroid, stomach, and renal tracer activity due to breakdown and dissociation of the pertechnetate from the macroaggregated albumin particles.

Ref.: McAfee JG, Subramanian G. In: Freeman LM, ed. Freeman and Johnson's Clinical Radionuclide Imaging. New York: Grune & Stratton, 1984; p 123.

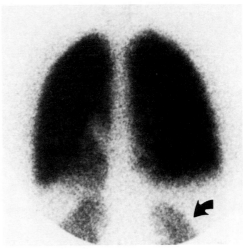

Figure 25–4. FREE PERTECHNETATE IN THE KIDNEYS ON PERFUSION SCAN. This image demonstrates free pertechnetate excreted in the kidneys *(arrow)* after a perfusion lung scan due to poor tag efficiency.

Figure 25–5. PROMINENT HILA ON PERFUSION SCAN. These two patients had perfusion lung scans because of suspected pulmonary embolism. The defects seen centrally in the lungs on the oblique views are due to prominent hila *(arrows)*, not embolism.

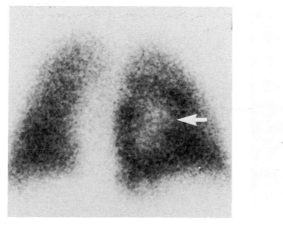
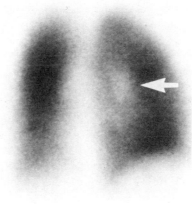

Ref.: Mettler FA, Guiberteau MJ. Essentials of Nuclear Medicine Imaging. New York: Grune & Stratton, 1983; p 147.

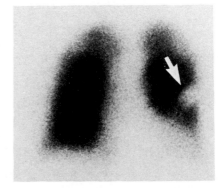

Figure 25–6. PHOTOPENIC DEFECT CAUSED BY PACEMAKER ON PERFUSION SCAN. Perfusion lung scan image demonstrates a photopenic defect caused by a pacemaker *(arrow)*. This should not be confused with embolism. Correlation with the chest x-ray will reveal the true nature of this defect.

Ref.: Wells LD, Berner DR. Radionuclide Imaging Artifacts. Chicago: Year Book Medical Publishers, 1982; p 109.

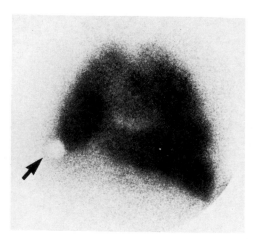

Figure 25–7. METALLIC ARTIFACT ON THE PER-FUSION SCAN. This patient had a pocketful of coins when the perfusion scan was performed, causing the photopenic defect seen on the oblique view *(view)*. All objects should be removed before imaging to prevent misinterpreting the defect as embolism.

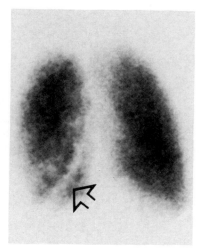

Figure 25–8. CHEST TUBE TRACT ON PERFU-SION SCAN. This patient had recently had a chest tube removed from the left lung. Correlation with the chest x-ray was necessary to identify the pleural thickening caused by the thoracostomy tube that resulted in the oblique defect *(arrow)* seen on the perfusion scan.

Figure 25–9. PLEURAL EFFUSION ON VENTILATION/PERFUSION SCAN. This patient underwent ventilation and perfusion imaging for suspected pulmonary embolism. The left lung demonstrates a rounded edge to the inferior portion of the lung on both the ventilation *(A)* and perfusion *(B)* scans *(arrows)*. Correlation with the chest x-ray revealed the pleural effusion that was causing the defect.

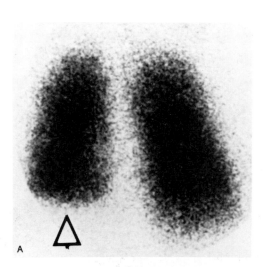

Figure 25–9A. Ventilation scan.

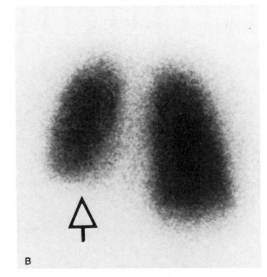

Figure 25–9B. Perfusion scan.

Ref.: Tow DE, Wagner HN. Effect of pleural fluid on the appearance of the lung scan. J Nucl Med 1970; 11:138–139.

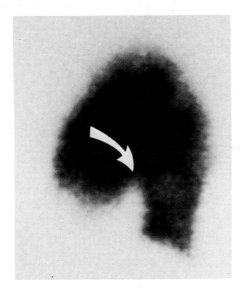

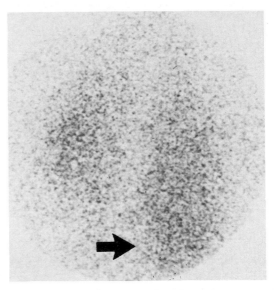

Figure 25–10. PLEURAL EFFUSION ON PERFU-SION SCAN. Perfusion scan image demonstrates a wedge-shaped peripheral defect *(arrow)*. Correlation with the chest x-ray revealed a focal accumulation of pleural fluid in the major fissure, which should not be misinterpreted as embolism.

Ref.: Tow DE, Wagner HN. Effect of pleural fluid on the appearance of the lung scan. J Nucl Med 1970; 11:138–139.

Figure 25–11. XENON ACCUMULATION WITHIN THE LIVER. Xenon accumulation *(arrow)* is present in the area beneath the right lung on this posterior image from a ventilation lung scan. The xenon is accumulating in the liver. Computed tomography demonstrated fatty infiltration.

Ref.: Carey JE, Purdy JM, Moses DC. Localization of 133Xe in the liver during ventilation studies. J Nucl Med 1974; 15:1178–1181.

Figure 25–12. XENON ACCUMULATION IN THE STOMACH. This infant underwent ventilation and perfusion lung scanning. The ventilation study reveals accumulation *(arrow)* in the left upper quadrant of the abdomen on the anterior view. This represents swallowed xenon. A crying infant will swallow large amounts of air, making a good ventilation study difficult to obtain without intubation of the trachea.

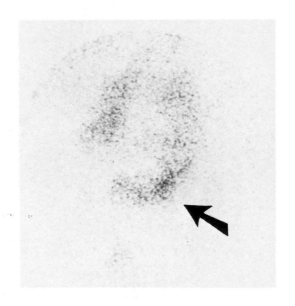

Brain Imaging

DONALD E. JACKSON, M.D.
CHARLES E. PETERSON, M.D.

Figure 26–1. EAR ARTIFACT.

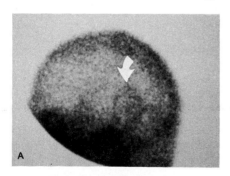

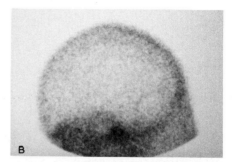

Figure 26–1A. Blood pool activity *(arrow)* in the pinna of the ear is seen on this lateral view from a technetium 99m-glucoheptonate brain scan.

Figure 26–1B. The defect is gone when a repeat image is obtained with the pinna taped down. Awareness of this potential defect, and re-imaging when necessary, will prevent the misdiagnosis of this finding as intracranial pathology.

Ref.: Patton DD, Brasfield DL. "EAR" artifact in brain scans. J Nucl Med 1976; 17:305–306.

Figure 26–2. COMPTON SCATTER ON BRAIN FLOW STUDY. The Compton scatter arising from the radioactivity of the bolus as it traverses the mediastinum may sometimes be visualized as an artifactual increase in the activity *(arrow)* in the patient's neck. This should not be mistaken for a hypervascular lesion in the neck. Its true nature can be determined by observing the fact that the activity is temporally related to the passage of the bolus through the subclavian vein. Cervical jugular reflux may also mimic this finding.

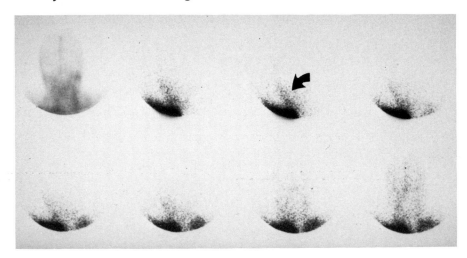

Ref.: Hayt DB, Perez LA. Cervical venous reflux in dynamic brain scintigraphy. J Nucl Med 1976; 17:9–12.

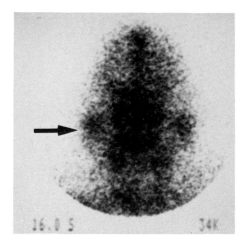

Figure 26–3. PAROTID BLUSH ON BRAIN FLOW STUDY. The parotid glands may demonstrate a prominent "blush" on the dynamic brain flow study *(arrow)*. In some cases, this has been related to parotitis and chronic alcoholism. It also occurs with obstruction of the internal carotid artery.

Ref.: Mishkin FS. Radionuclide salivary gland imaging. Semin Nucl Med 1981; 11:258–265.

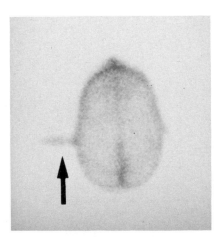

Figure 26–4. INADEQUATE SHIELDING ON THE VERTEX VIEW OF A BRAIN SCAN. The vertex view on a static brain image would be totally obscured by activity arising from the rest of the body if it were not for the use of lead shielding. When this shielding has gaps, some activity will "shine" through *(arrow)* and be a potential source of misinterpretation. Meticulous attention to detail by the technical staff will prevent this error.

Ref.: Holms RA. The central nervous system. In: Freeman LM, ed. Freeman and Johnson's Clinical Radionuclide Imaging. New York: Grune & Stratton, 1984; p 621.

CHAPTER 27

Venography and Gastrointestinal Bleeding

DONALD E. JACKSON, M.D.
CHARLES E. PETERSON, M.D.

Figure 27–1. VENOGRAM IN PREGNANCY. This pregnant patient had symptoms of acute deep vein thrombosis on the right side.

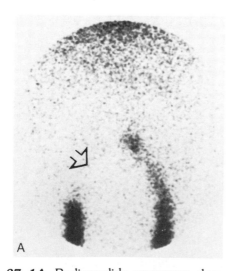

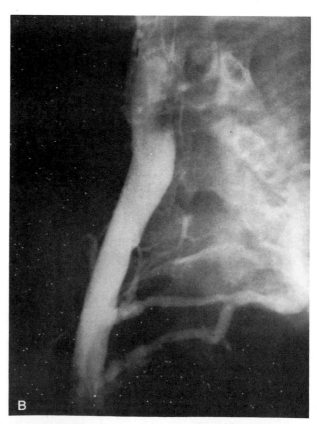

Figure 27–1A. Radionuclide venogram demonstrates absence of filling of the iliac vein on the right side *(arrow).*

Figure 27–1B. Contrast venography shows that the iliac vein and inferior vena cava are patent. The obstruction to flow was the result of the presence of the gravid uterus.

Ref.: Kerr MG, Scott DB, Samuel E. Studies of the inferior vena cava in late pregnancy. Brit Med J 1964; 1:532–533.

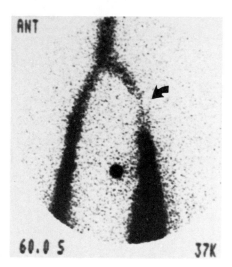

Figure 27–2. EXTRINSIC COMPRESSION OF THE ILIAC VEIN SIMULATING DEEP VEIN THROMBOSIS. This patient had symptoms of deep vein thrombosis on the left side. Radionuclide venogram demonstrates an area of decreased photon activity in the left iliac vein *(arrow)* and a build-up of activity distal to this area. Contrast venography revealed that the abnormality was due to extrinsic compression. Computed tomography showed enlarged lymph nodes from a lymphoma as the cause for the compression.

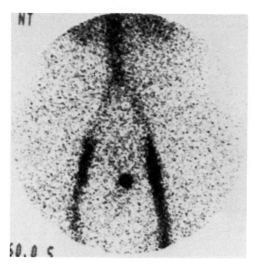

Figure 27–3. ATTENUATION BY PELVIC TISSUE. Venogram demonstrates a bilateral, symmetric decrease in the photon activity in the iliac veins. This is due to the normal attenuation of the photons by overlying pelvic tissues rather than venous occlusion. Note the lack of build-up of photon activity distal to the iliac veins.

Ref.: Dhekne RD, Moore WH, Long SE. Radionuclide venography in iliac and inferior vena caval obstruction. Radiology, 1982; 144:597–602.

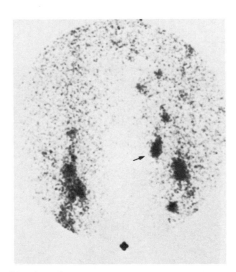

Figure 27–4. HOT SPOTS POST-VENOGRAPHY. Many areas of persistent radiopharmaceutical deposition *(arrow)* are present in the veins of the legs of this patient. Although these once were thought to indicate accumulation of the radiopharmaceutical on thrombus, they actually represent areas of pooling of pharmaceutical in varicosities and in the region of valves.

Ref.: Mettler FA, Guiberteau MJ. Essentials of Nuclear Medicine Imaging. New York: Grune & Stratton, 1983; p 177.

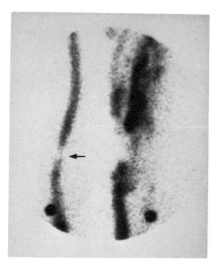

Figure 27–5. TOURNIQUET DEFECT. The venogram was performed with tight tourniquets about the ankles and knees of the patient. The defect shown *(arrow)* does not represent a luminal clot; rather, it is caused by the tight tourniquet above the knee.

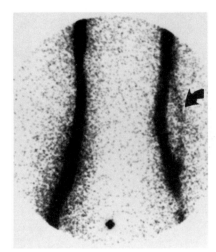

Figure 27–6. VARIANT VESSEL SIMULATING COLLATERALS. Venogram demonstrates a second channel in the deep system of the left thigh *(arrow).* This should not be interpreted as an indication of deep venous obstruction. Knowledge of the numerous variants that are common in the deep venous system of the thigh is necessary to prevent misinterpretation.

Ref.: Luzsa G. X-Ray Anatomy of the Vascular System. Philadelphia: J. B. Lippincott, 1974; p 306.

Figure 27–7. URINARY ACTIVITY SIMULATING LOWER GASTROINTESTINAL BLEEDING. This patient underwent a technetium-labeled red blood cell scan for a suspected lower gastrointestinal bleeding. The image shown in A demonstrates an area of tracer accumulation in the midline in the pelvis *(arrow).* Careful comparison of this image with an image obtained earlier in the study *(B)* reveals that the activity is accumulating in the area of the photopenic region caused by the bladder. Investigation of the tagging efficiency showed that only 80 per cent of the injected technetium was bound to the red blood cells. Free technetium was excreted via the urinary tract and was mistaken for sigmoid bleeding. Panendoscopy revealed no evidence of a colonic lesion and the bleeding was subsequently proved to be arising from another source. Excretion of technetium by the stomach and salivary glands and in the urinary tract are all potential sources for confusion on the labeled RBC scan. The tagging methodology must achieve a high percentage of technetium-labeled red blood cells.

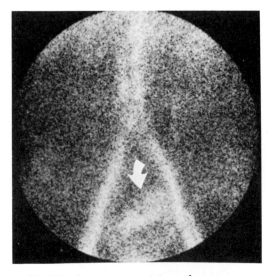

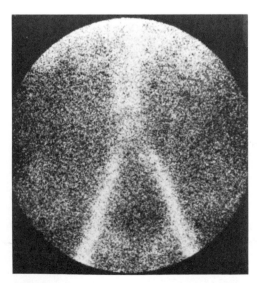

Figure 27–7A. An area suspicious for gastrointestinal bleeding *(arrow)* is seen on this image.

Figure 27–7B. This image, obtained earlier in the study, demonstrates the photopenic region of the bladder, which becomes the suspicious area seen in A.

Ref.: Haseman MK. Potential pitfalls in the interpretation of erythrocyte scintigraphy for gastrointestinal hemorrhage. Clin Nucl Med 1982; 7:309–310.

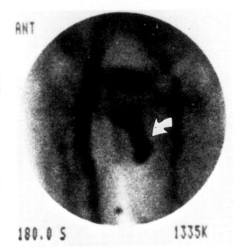

Figure 27–8. PENILE BLOOD POOL ON LABELED RED BLOOD CELL IMAGING. In a labeled red blood cell imaging study for suspected lower gastrointestinal bleeding, a spot image of the pelvis revealed an area of activity inferiorly in the pelvis. The patient's penis, which was positioned over his lower abdomen, was repositioned, and the repeat image (shown) demonstrates the intense blood pool activity seen in the penis *(arrow),* a potential source of confusion.

Ref.: Lisbona R, Leger J, Stern J, et al. Observations on Tc-99m-erythrocyte venography in normal subjects and in patients with deep vein thrombosis. Clin Nucl Med 1981; 6:305–309.

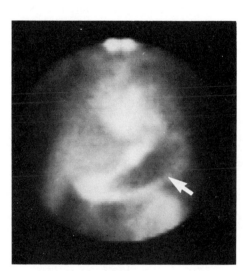

Figure 27–9. PHOTOPENIC DEFECT ON SCAN OF MECKEL'S DIVERTICULUM. This patient underwent a technetium pertechnetate scan to detect a suspected Meckel's diverticulum as the source of gastrointestinal bleeding. The photopenic defect *(arrow)* seen in the stomach is caused by coaptation of the stomach walls and should not be confused with a gastric mass. A repeat image in the upright position should reveal the true nature of the defect.

CHAPTER 28

Liver-Spleen Imaging

FREDERICK L. WEILAND, M.D.
FREDERIC A. CONTE, M.D.
JOSEPH A. ORZEL, M.D.
ALBERT S. HALE, M.D.

Figure 28–1. LIVER-SPLEEN SCINTIGRAPHY: ACQUISITION AND PROJECTIONS. Routine liver-spleen scintigraphy is performed using 3 to 5 mCi of Tc-99m sulfur colloid. The 0.3 to 1.0 micron colloidal particles are rapidly removed from the circulation by the reticuloendothelial system; the liver removes 80 to 90 per cent, the spleen 5 to 10 per cent, and bone marrow 3 to 5 per cent. Distribution of the radiopharmaceutical is dependent upon the integrity of the reticuloendothelial system, hepatic blood flow, particle size, opsonization, and colloidal charge (zeta potential). Plasma clearance of colloid approaches 95 per cent on each passage through the liver. Liver images are obtained in the following projections: anterior (ANT), posterior (POST), anterior with size marker, and right and left lateral (RT LAT, LT LAT). Oblique views may be obtained for further clarification. Imaging is usually performed 15 minutes after intravenous injection. A large field-of-view (LFOV) Anger scintillation detector with a low-energy all-purpose (LEAP) or high-resolution (High Res) collimator is the imaging system of choice.

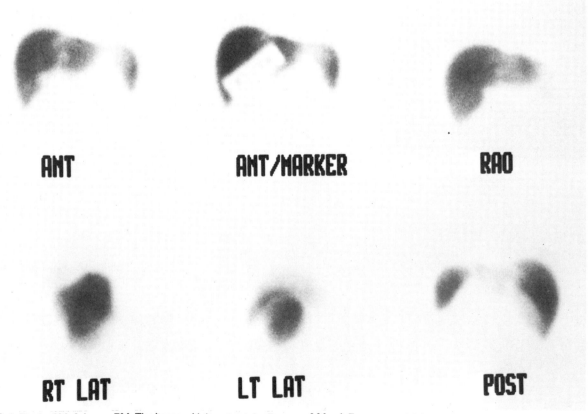

ANT   ANT/MARKER   RAO

RT LAT   LT LAT   POST

Ref.: Pinsky SM, Johnson PM. The liver and biliary tract. In: Freeman LM, ed. Freeman and Johnson's Clinical Radionuclide Imaging. Orlando: Grune & Stratton, 1984; pp 835–1049.

Figure 28–2. NORMAL HEPATIC ARCHITECTURE. Liver-spleen scintigrams are interpreted as to the size, shape, and position of the liver and spleen; the homogeneity of activity within the liver and spleen; the relative distribution of the radiopharmaceutical within the liver and spleen; and the presence of hepatic or splenic focal defects. The pliability of the liver creates a wide latitude in the normal shape. (Mould, in 1972, described 38 variations in liver shape in the anterior projection alone.) The liver is divided into four distinct lobes: the predominant right, the left, the quadrate lobe, which resides anteriorly, and the posterior caudate lobe. The predominant localization of the radiopharmaceutical is in the right hepatic lobe *(A).* There is typically a smooth reduction of intensity in the left hepatic lobe and the spleen. Visually the left lobe shows less tracer concentration due to its diminished hepatic mass, with attenuation and compression by the spine *(B* and C). The anterior quadrate lobe may be visualized, especially if hepatic enlargement has occurred *(F–H).* The spleen is normally ovoid or baseball glove–shaped, with the long axis oriented anterior to inferior *(D).* Increased splenic concentration of the isotope may be normal, especially in patients with a neoplasm receiving chemotherapeutic agents *(E).* The spleen is best visualized in the posterior and left lateral views. The caudate lobe usually is not identified on the normal liver-spleen scintigram.

Ref.: Mould RF. An investigation of the variations in normal liver shape. Br J Radiol 1972; 45:586–590.

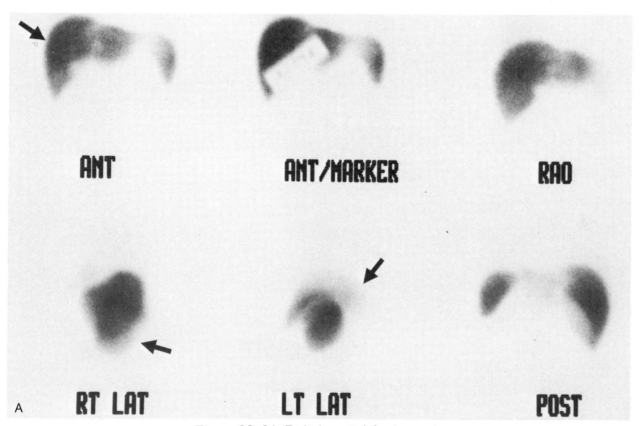

ANT   ANT/MARKER   RAO

RT LAT   LT LAT   POST

A

Figure 28–2A. Right hepatic lobe *(arrows).*

Illustration continued on following page

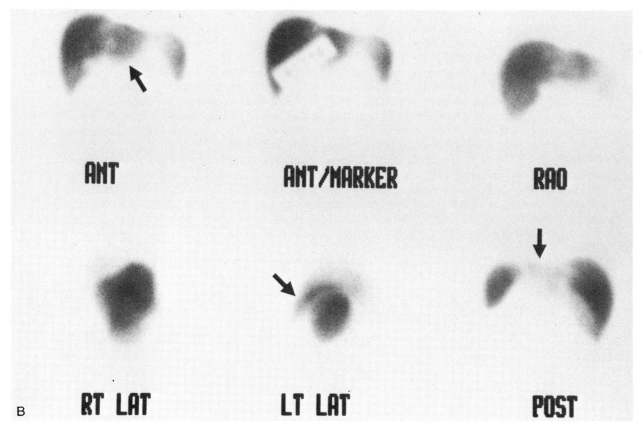

Figure 28–2B. Left hepatic lobe (*arrows*).

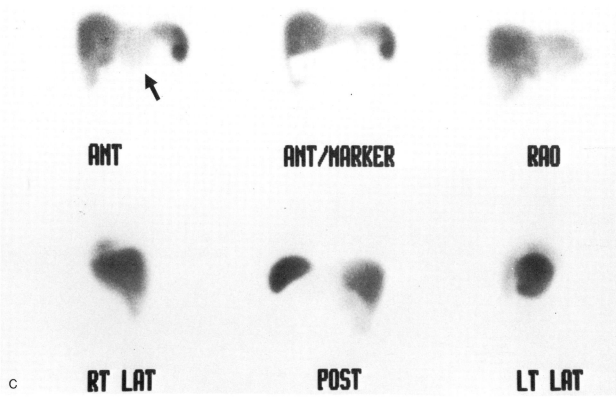

Figure 28–2C. Left hepatic lobe thinning (*arrows*).

Illustration continued on opposite page

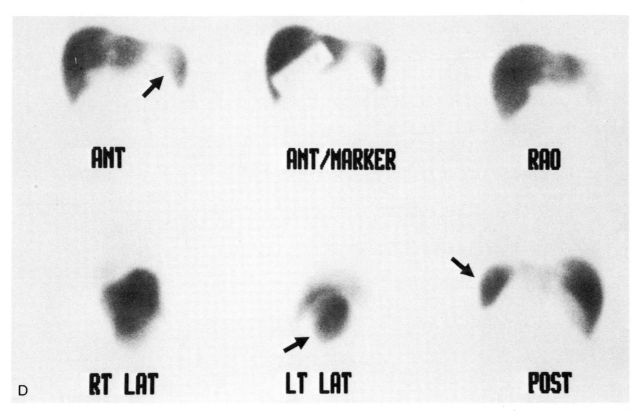

Figure 28–2D. Spleen (*arrows*).

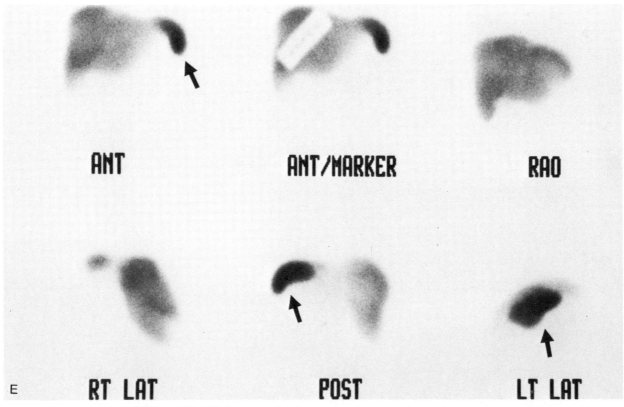

Figure 28–2E. Increased splenic tracer accumulation (*arrows*).

Illustration continued on following page

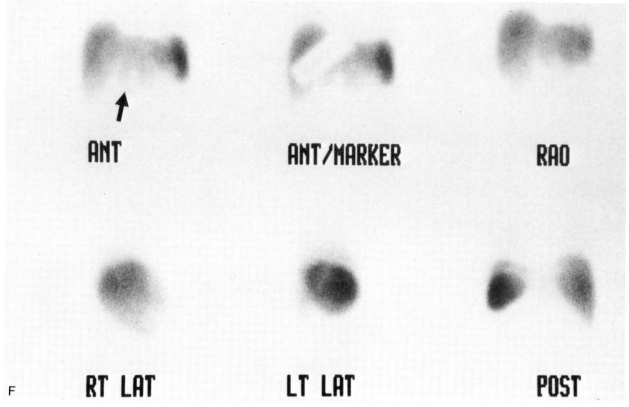

Figure 28–2F. Quadrate lobe (*arrow*).

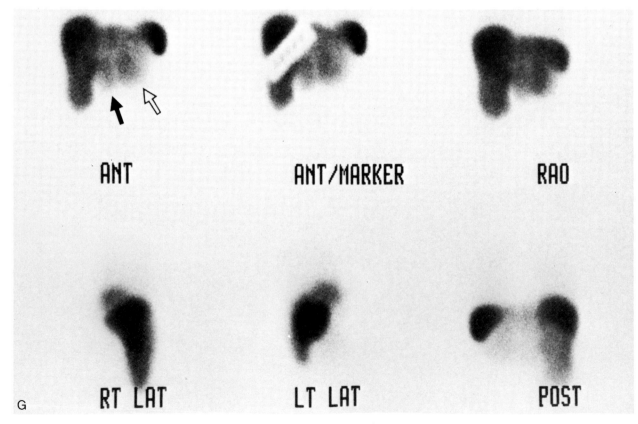

Figure 28–2G. Prominent left (*open arrow*) and quadrate lobes (*solid arrow*).

Illustration continued on opposite page

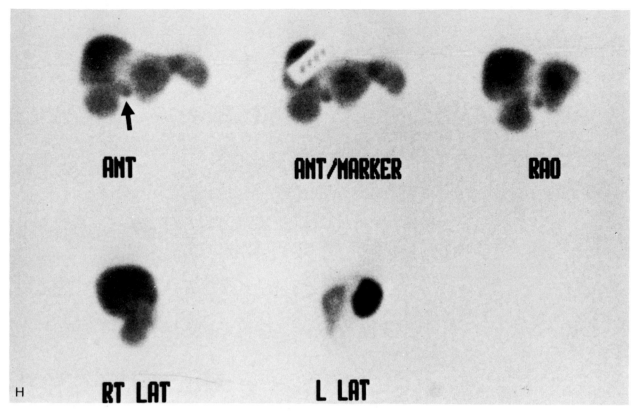

Figure 28–2H. "Cloverleaf" liver quadrate lobe (*arrow*).

Figure 28–3. RADIOPHARMACEUTICAL QUALITY CONTROL. Radiopharmaceutical quality control problems with Tc-99m sulfur colloid are infrequent. If images are obtained before complete extraction of the radiopharmaceutical by the liver, faint visualization of the blood pool may be observed *(A)*. The extraction half-life is about 2 to 6 minutes; however, hepatocellular dysfunction or congestive heart failure prolongs this circulation time. Free technetium results in visualization of the heart and renal parenchyma *(B)*. Macroaggregation of the radiopharmaceutical during intravenous injection results in focal hot spot artifacts in the pulmonary parenchyma. Aggregated colloid of greater than 10 microns in size will be trapped by the pulmonary capillary bed *(C and D)*. Injection of the radiopharmaceutical through intravenous tubing results in adherence of some of the colloidal particles to the tubing lumen due to charge attraction *(E)*.

Ref.: McAfee JG, Subramanian G. Radioactive agents for imaging. In: Freeman LM, ed. Freeman and Johnson's Clinical Radionuclide Imaging. Orlando: Grune & Stratton, 1984; pp 55–180.

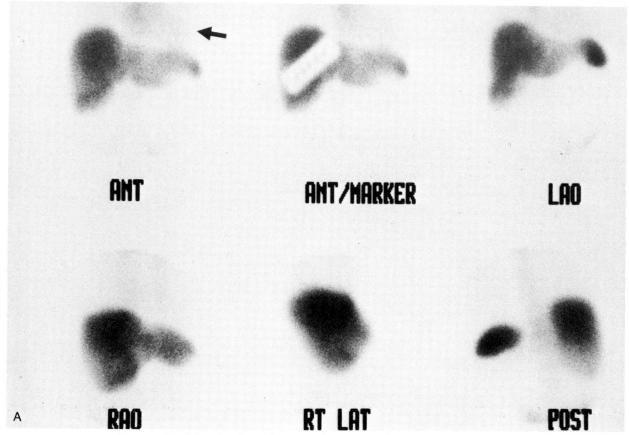

Figure 28–3A. Blood pool activity (*arrow,* cardiac chamber activity).

Illustration continued on opposite page

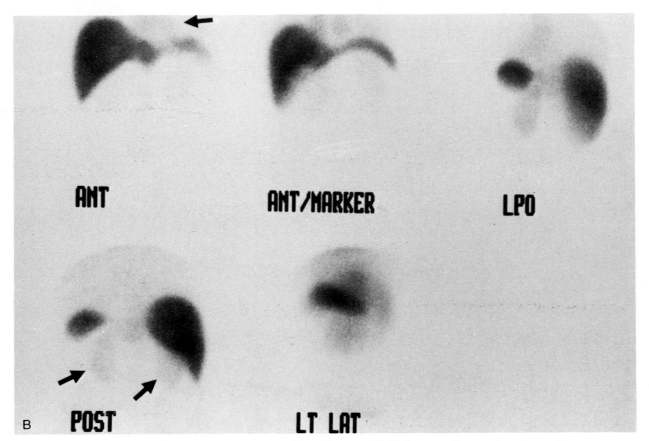

Figure 28–3B. Blood pool activity in the heart (*arrow*, ANT [anterior] image) and renal activity (*arrows*, POST [posterior] image).

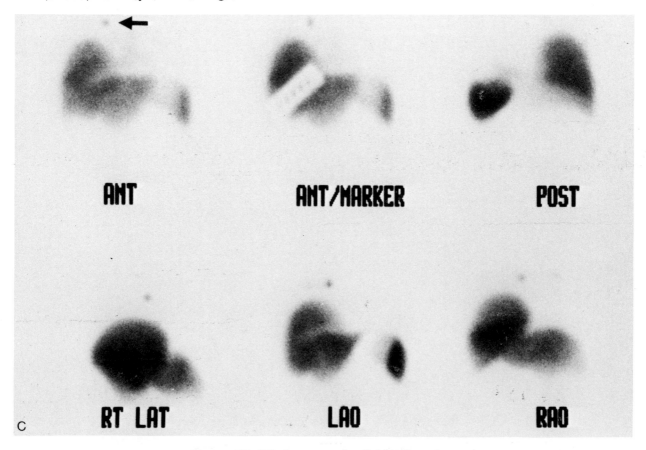

Figure 28–3C. Aggregated colloid in lung (*arrow*).

Illustration continued on following page

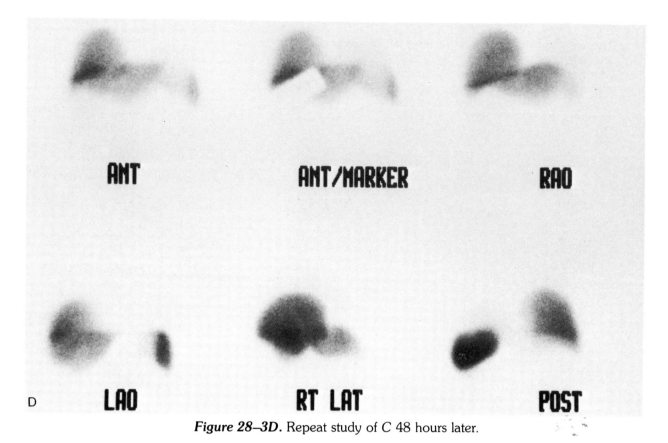

Figure 28–3D. Repeat study of C 48 hours later.

Figure 28–3E. Hickman catheter injection (*arrow*).

Figure 28–4. IMAGE QUALITY: SYMMETRIC AND ASYMMETRIC WINDOW SELECTION.
The 140-KeV photopeak of Tc-99m labeled radiopharmaceuticals is relatively symmetric with little scattering, permitting good pulse-height resolution. Routine liver-spleen scintigrams are obtained with a 140-KeV 20 per cent symmetric window. This combination allows good count rates during acquisition, while minimizing image degradation due to Compton scattering.

Asymmetric window placement above the 140-KeV photopeak provides adequate images but prolongs the acquisition time. Asymmetric window selection below the 140-KeV photopeak results in significant image degradation, reflecting the additive contribution by Compton scattering.

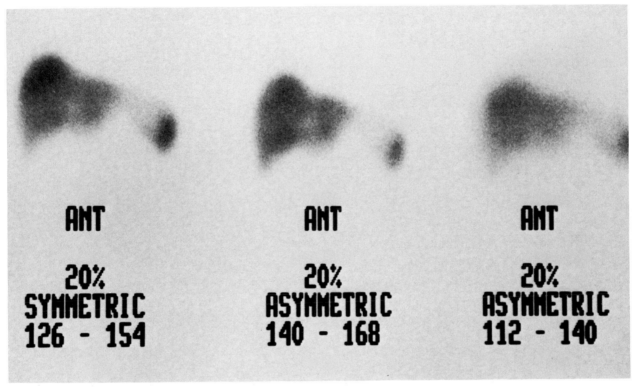

Ref.: Rollo FD, Harris CC. Factors affecting image formation. In: Rollo FD, ed. Nuclear Medicine Physics, Instrumentation, and Agents. St Louis: C V Mosby, 1977; pp 387–435.

Figure 28–5. IMAGE QUALITY: COUNT DENSITY. The number of counts required for an adequate liver scintigram is approximately 750,000 to one million counts per image. This number provides a count density of approximately 2000 to 3000 counts/cm². At this density, statistically adequate images that are clear and optimized for lesion detectability, are also acquired in an acceptable time of approximately 5 minutes per view. It is evident from the evaluation of both the liver-spleen scintigrams (*A*) and the corresponding bar phantoms (*B*) that information densities less than 2000 counts/cm² significantly compromise image quality.

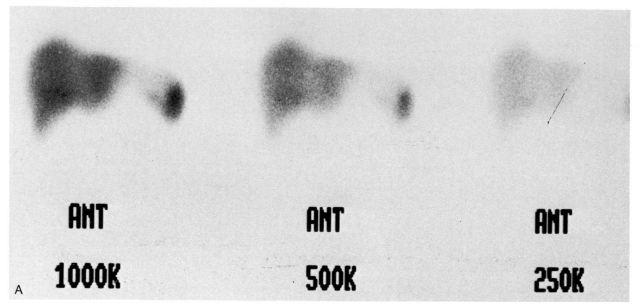

Figure 28–5A. Count acquisition of 1000 K, 500 K, and 250 K.

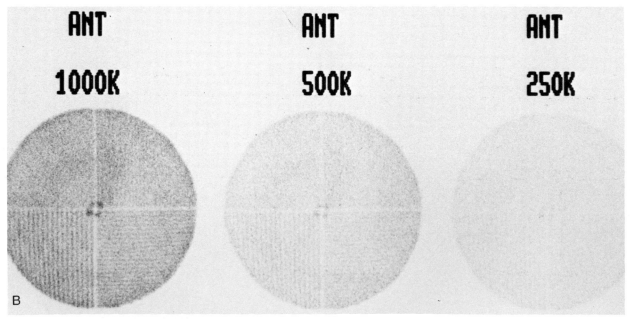

Figure 28–5B. Corresponding bar phantom to *A*.

Ref.: Rollo FD, Harris CC. Factors affecting image formation. In: Rollo FD, ed. Nuclear Medicine Physics, Instrumentation, and Agents. St Louis: C V Mosby, 1977; pp 387–435.

Figure 28–6. IMAGE QUALITY: COLLIMATOR SELECTION. The low-energy all-purpose (LEAP), high-resolution (High Res), and converging (CONV) collimators may be successfully used to perform liver-spleen scintigraphy. The LEAP collimator is used by most imaging laboratories; however, some physicians do prefer the High Res collimator because it provides slightly increased sensitivity. While sacrificing count density when imaging acquisition times are the same, this is not of practical importance, due to the high count rates available during liver-spleen scintigraphy. The CONV collimator by virtue of its magnification enhances resolution while sacrificing field of view. The entire normal liver and spleen, however, cannot be visualized in a single converging image. This is considered to be a distinct disadvantage.

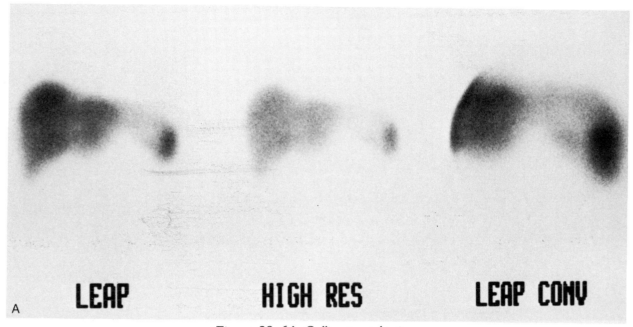

Figure 28–6A. Collimator selection.

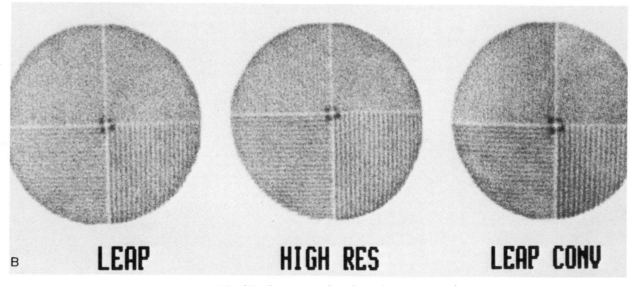

Figure 28–6B. Corresponding bar phantoms to *A*.

Ref.: Rollo FD, Harris CC. Factors affecting image formation. In: Rollo FD, ed. Nuclear Medicine Physics, Instrumentation, and Agents. St Louis: C V Mosby, 1977; pp 387–435.

Figure 28–7. HEPATIC MOTION CORRECTION. In routine liver-spleen scintigraphy, slight movement of the liver occurs as a result of respiration. Gross movement with double exposure of the liver as evident in *A and B* seldom occurs. Various techniques have been employed to minimize this hepatic movement and blurring of intrahepatic defects. They include breath holding; upright views; and, most recently, auto-motion correction devices *(C).* However, to date, these techniques and autocorrective devices have not been reported to substantially improve lesion detectability.

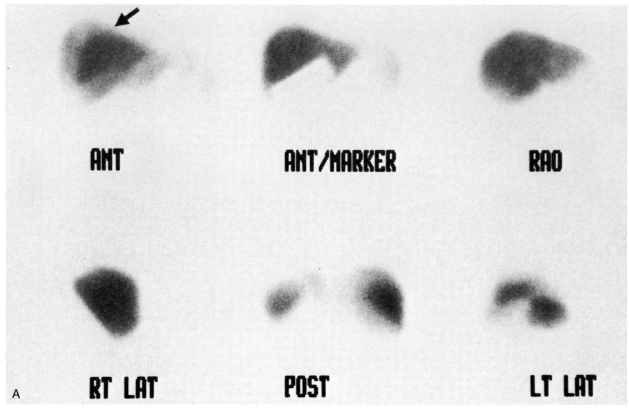

Figure 28–7A. Patient movement (*arrow*).

Illustration continued on opposite page

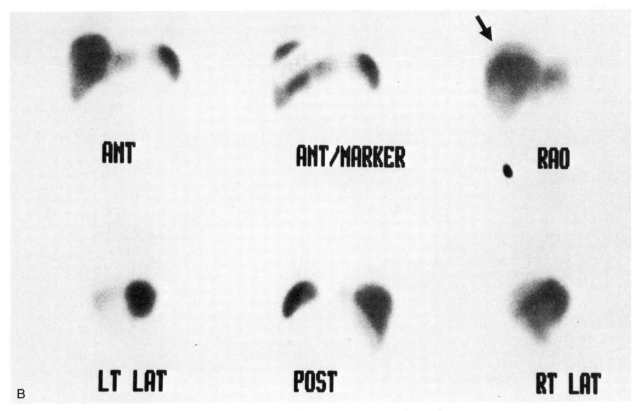

Figure 28–7B. Patient movement (*arrow*).

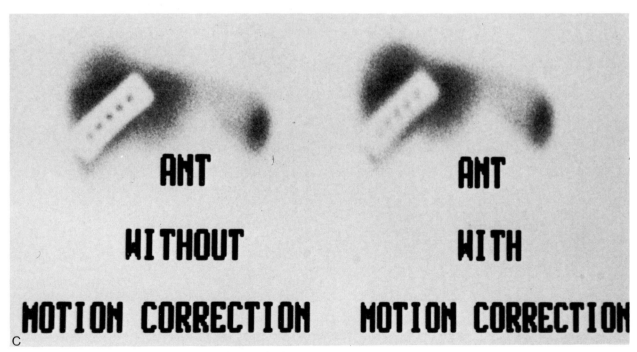

Figure 28–7C. Motion correction.

Ref.: Oppenheim BE. A method using a digital computer for reducing respiratory artifact on liver scans made with a camera. J Nucl Med 1971; 12:625–628.

Figure 28–8. RIEDEL'S LOBE. Riedel's lobe is an elongated, downward extension of the lateral portion of the right hepatic lobe. This variation occurs in approximately 4 per cent of normal individuals and is more frequent in females than males. First described by the German surgeon Bernhard Riedel (1846–1916), it is not a separate lobe but represents an anatomic inferior extension of the right lobe of the liver. The usual configuration is that of a long tongue-shaped extension; however, marked lobulation may occur. On physical examination, a hypertrophied Riedel's lobe may be misinterpreted as hepatomegaly or an abnormal abdominal mass.

Refs.: (1) McAfee JG, Ause RG, Wagner HN. Diagnostic value of scintillation scanning of the liver. Arch Intern Med 1965; 116:95–110. (2) Sham R, Sain A, Silver L. Hypertrophic Riedel's lobe of the liver. Clin Nuc Med 1978; 3:79–81.

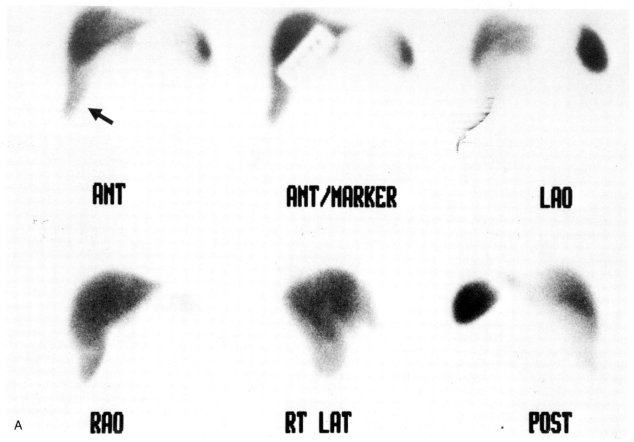

A

Figure 28–8A. Riedel's lobe (*arrow*).

Illustration continued on opposite page

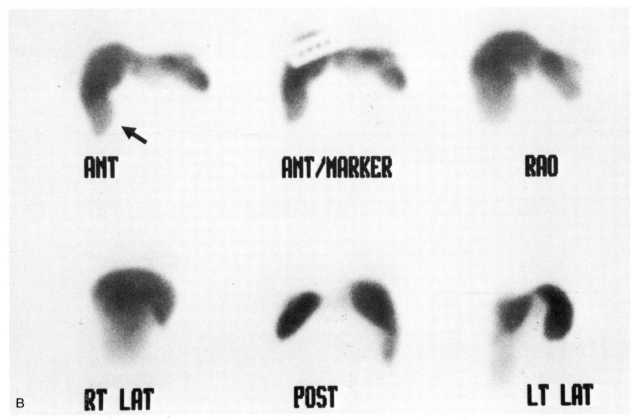

Figure 28–8B. Riedel's lobe (*arrow*).

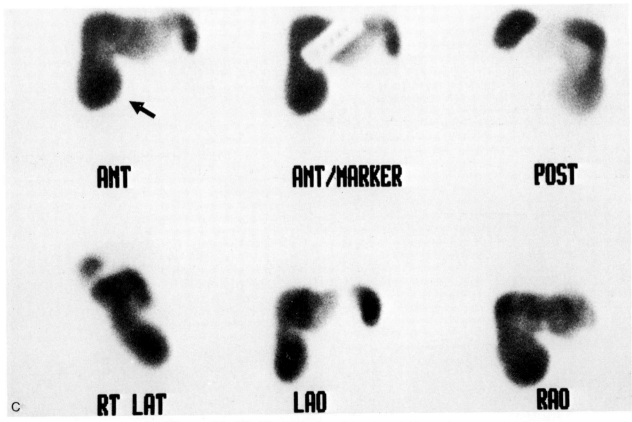

Figure 28–8C. Hypertrophy of Riedel's lobe (*arrow*).

Illustration continued on following page

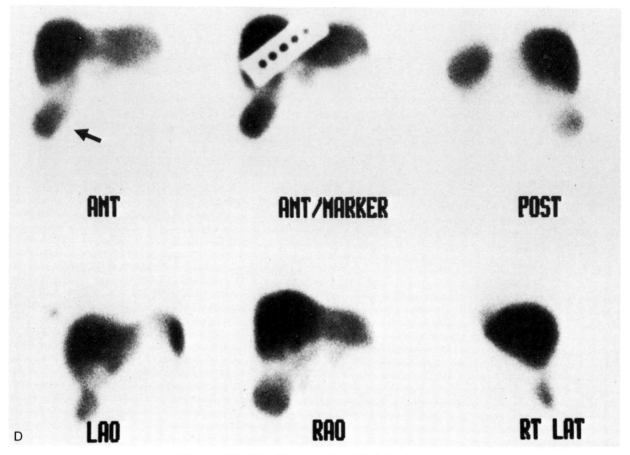

Figure 28–8D. Globular Riedel's lobe (*arrow*).

Figure 28–9. DIAPHRAGMATIC ALTERATIONS OF HEPATIC CONTOUR. The shape of the liver is highly variable in the anterior projection. As a pliable organ, the liver readily assumes the contour of any adjacent anatomic structures that impinge upon it. The superior aspect of the liver is normally convex on the diaphragmatic surface, proceeding to a concavity between the right and left hepatic lobes resulting from the crura of the diaphragm. Diaphragmatic changes often result in significant alterations of the superior hepatic contour. Eventration of the diaphragm (*A*) and partial or full right pneumonectomy produce a superior bulging of the right hepatic lobe. Chronic obstructive pulmonary disease results in the flattening of the superior aspect of the liver, due to hyperinflated lungs (*B*). Inferior displacement of the liver often results in the liver being palpable below the costal margin and in a clinical impression of hepatomegaly; the liver-spleen scintigram, however, reveals normal hepatic size. Flattening and inferior displacement may also occur with pleural effusions of any etiology (*C–E*). A liver-lung scintigram demonstrates the separation between the right lung and liver. Almost total absence of pulmonary activity in the right lung due to attenuation of photons by effusion is highly suggestive of a large pleural fluid collection. Radiographic correlation should be obtained to confirm the pulmonary process and exclude subphrenic abscess. Fibrothorax and pleural reaction result in marked straightening of the right hepatic border (*F* and *G*).

Ref.: Genant HK, Hoffer PB. False-positive liver scan due to lung abscess. J Nucl Med 1972; 13:945–946.

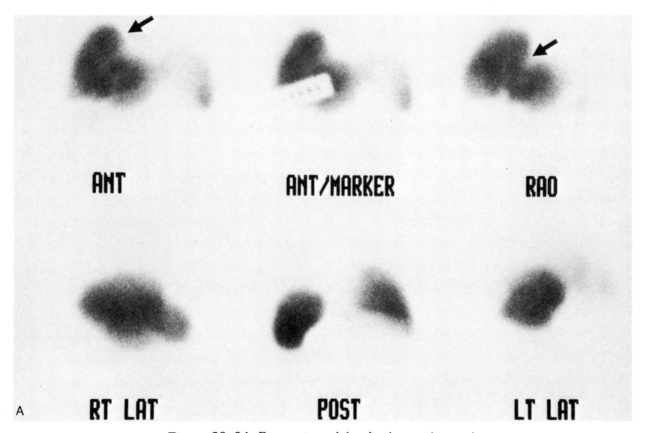

ANT   ANT/MARKER   RAO

RT LAT   POST   LT LAT

A

Figure 28–9A. Eventration of the diaphragm (*arrows*).

Illustration continued on following page

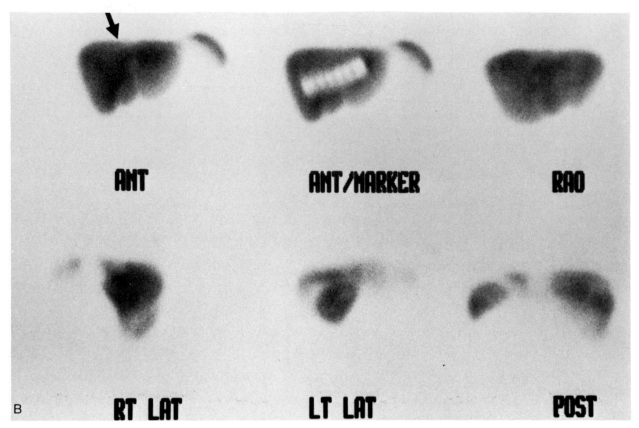

Figure 28–9B. Chronic obstructive pulmonary disease: Flattened hepatic dome (*arrow*).

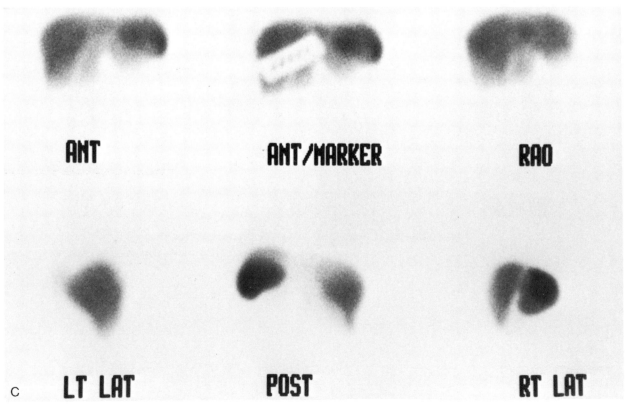

Figure 28–9C. Liver-spleen scintigram: Before pleural effusion.

Illustration continued on opposite page

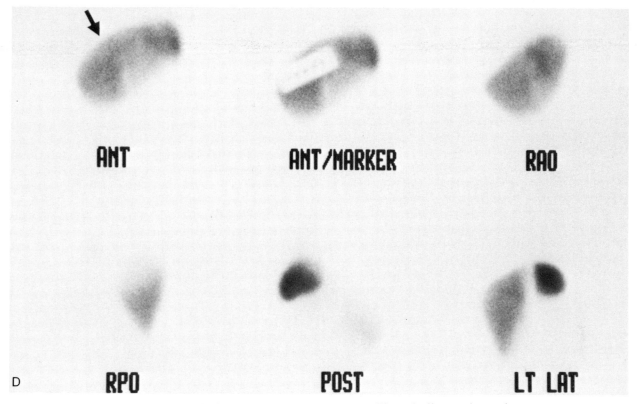

Figure 28–9D. Liver-spleen scintigram: Pleural effusion (*arrow*).

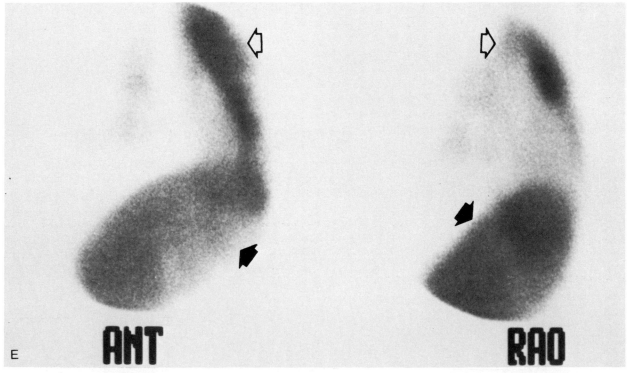

Figure 28–9E. Liver-lung scintigram: Pleural effusion (lung, *open arrows;* liver, *solid arrows*).

Illustration continued on following page

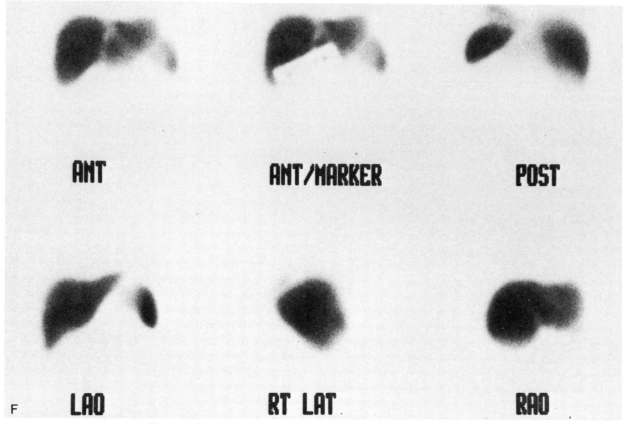

Figure 28–9F. Liver-spleen scintigram: Before fibrothorax.

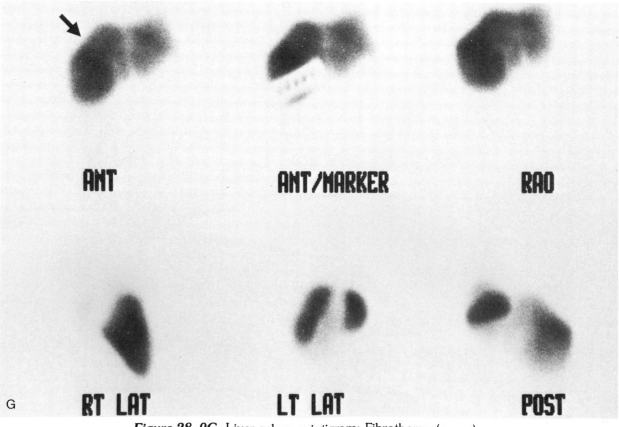

Figure 28–9G. Liver-spleen scintigram: Fibrothorax (*arrow*).

Figure 28–10. JUXTAHEPATIC IMPINGEMENT OF THE LIVER. The pliable nature of the liver allows extrinsic normal structures to alter either the shape of the liver or the distribution of the radiopharmaceutical. On occasion these pseudodefects may be misinterpreted as intrinsic liver masses *(A–E)*. The adrenal neoplasm illustrated in *F* demonstrates the extreme pliability of the liver. Anteriorly there is marked thinning of the right hepatic lobe, while the posterior scintigram reveals almost total absence of the right hepatic lobe due to attenuation. The right lateral projection verifies marked displacement. The hypernephroma *(G)* alters the normally smooth contour impression of the right kidney that is typically noted in the posterior view. The anterior view demonstrates a small photopenic area *(arrow)* in the superior aspect of the right hepatic lobe due to compression of normal hepatic tissue.

Refs.: (1) Covington EE. Pitfalls in liver photoscans. AJR 1970; 109:745–748. (2) Chaudhuri TK. Caution in interpreting liver scans in presence of hypernephroma. J Urol 1975; 114:481–482.

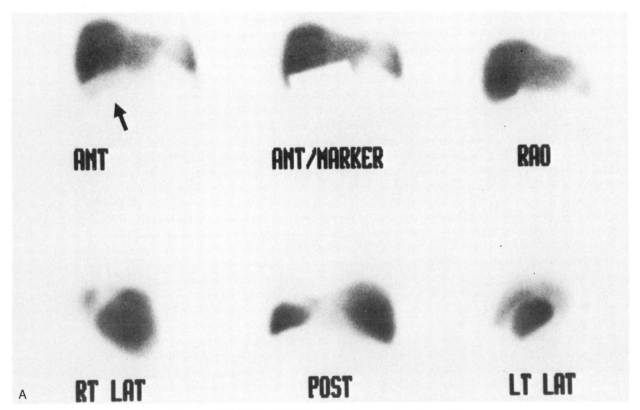

A

Figure 28–10A. Costal margin impression *(arrow)*.

Illustration continued on following page

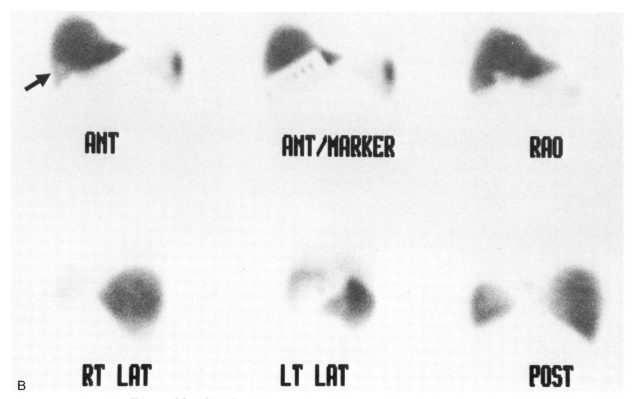

Figure 28–10B. Costal margin impression/rib impression (*arrow*).

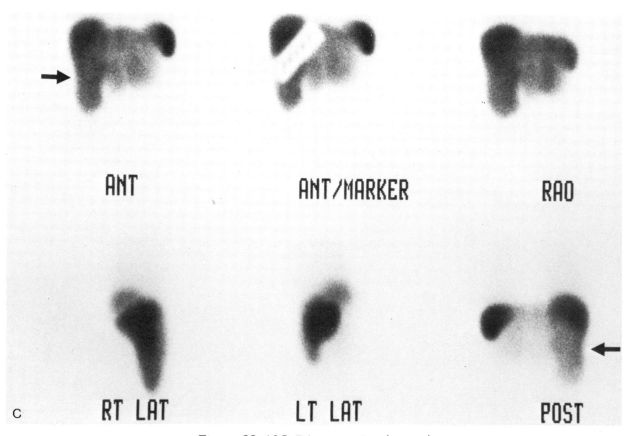

Figure 28–10C. Rib impression (*arrows*).

Illustration continued on opposite page

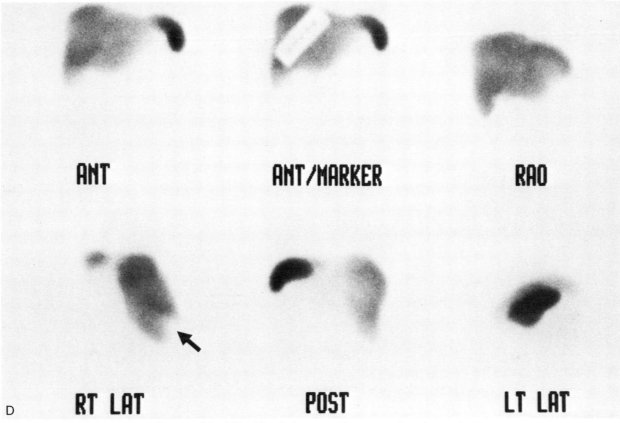

Figure 28–10D. Notch between hepatic lobes (*arrow*).

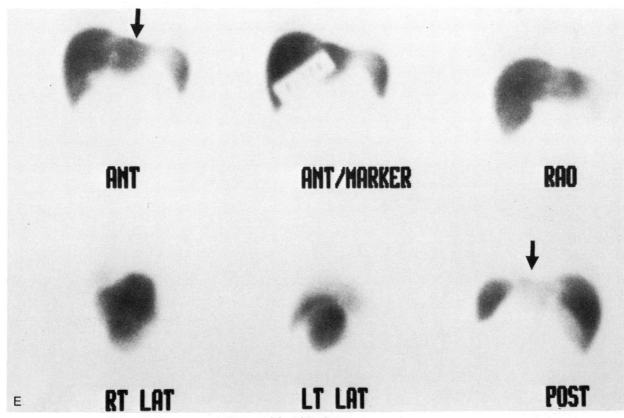

Figure 28–10E. Spine (*arrows*).

Illustration continued on following page

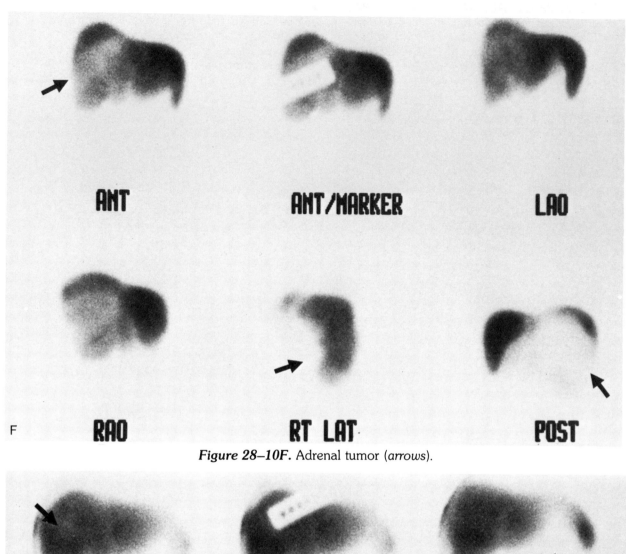

Figure 28–10F. Adrenal tumor (*arrows*).

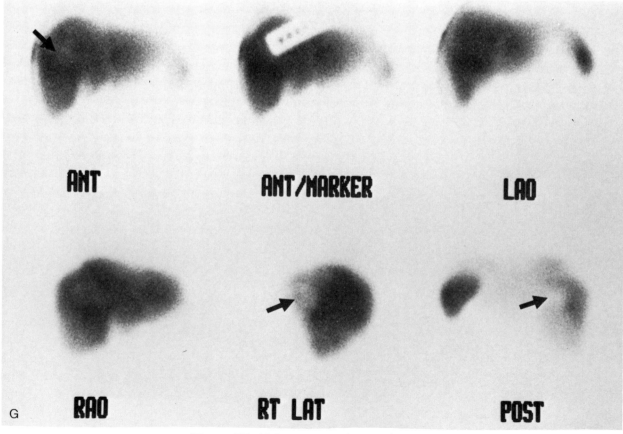

Figure 28–10G. Hypernephroma (*arrows*).

Figure 28–11. ALTERATION OF HEPATIC SHAPE. The liver-spleen scintigrams shown in A and B are from two patients who underwent subtotal right hepatic lobectomies for hepatoma. Compensatory hypertrophy of the left hepatic lobe is frequent after such surgery. The degree of compensatory hypertrophy is dependent on the total hepatic mass removed. In patients undergoing hepatectomy, the liver regenerates rapidly with a return to a normal hepatic mass in 1 to 3 months. Situs inversus may give a similar scintigraphic finding (C). The normally smaller left hepatic lobe artifactually appears as a surgically reduced right lobe of the liver.

Ref.: Samuels LD, Grosfeld JL. Serial scans of liver regeneration after hemihepatectomy in children. Surg Gynecol Obst 1970; 131:453–457.

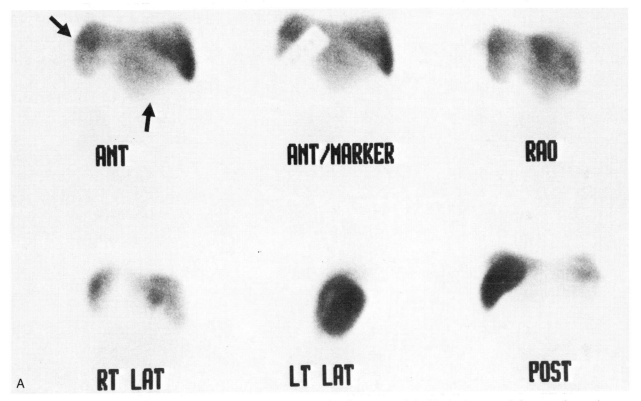

Figure 28–11A. Hepatectomy: Left lobe hypertrophy (*arrow, right*). (Right hepatic lobe is indicated by *arrow, left.*)

Illustration continued on following page

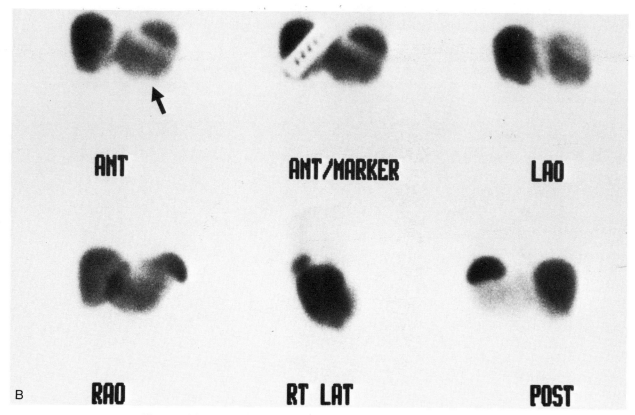

Figure 28–11B. Hepatectomy: Left lobe hypertrophy (*arrow*).

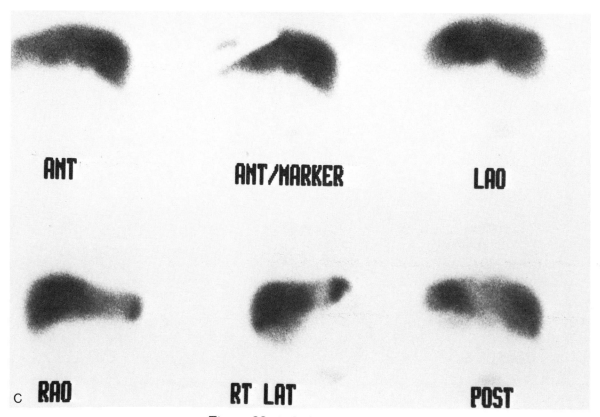

Figure 28–11C. Situs inversus.

Figure 28–12. HEPATIC MIGRATION SECONDARY TO SPLENECTOMY: "LIVER WALK."
Migration of the left hepatic lobe (B and C) following surgery is common. This migration is dependent upon the pliability of the liver, the patient's age, the size of the resected spleen, and whether the patient is obese. This hepatic movement results in the widening of the normal division between the left and right hepatic lobes. Scintigraphic confirmation of the absence of residual splenic tissue may be accomplished using heat-damaged red blood cells for a selective spleen scintigram.

Ref.: Custer JR, Shafer RB. Changes in liver scan following splenectomy. J Nucl Med 1975; 16:194–195.

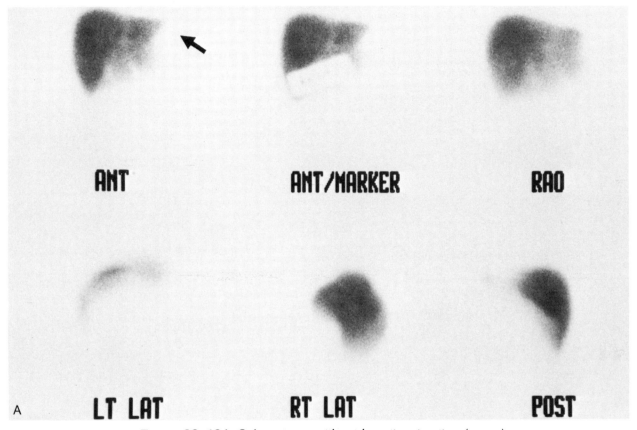

Figure 28–12A. Splenectomy without hepatic migration (*arrow*).

Illustration continued on following page

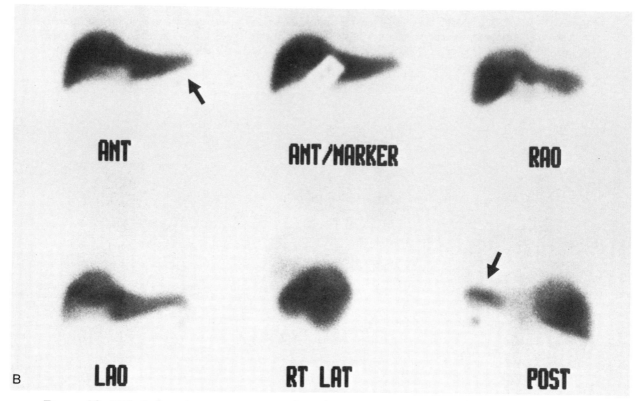

Figure 28–12B. Splenectomy, accessory spleen (seen on posterior image) with hepatic migration (*arrows*).

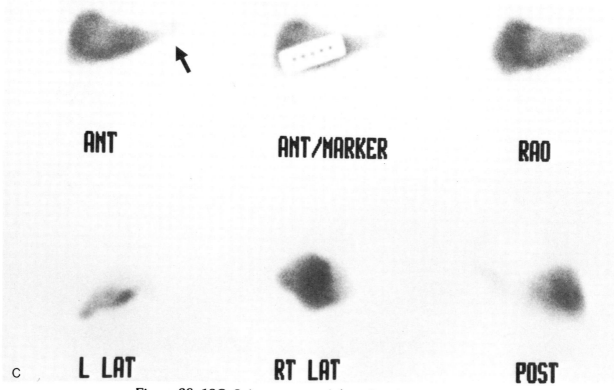

Figure 28–12C. Splenectomy with hepatic migration (*arrow*).

Figure 28–13. ANATOMIC STRUCTURES THAT MAY APPEAR AS FOCAL DEFECTS. The normal liver scintigram contains several anatomic structures that may be misinterpreted as focal hepatic defects (*A–F*). Familiarity with these normal anatomic variations should minimize confusion with space-occupying lesions.

Ref.: Covington EE. Pitfalls in liver photoscans. AJR 1970; 109:745–748.

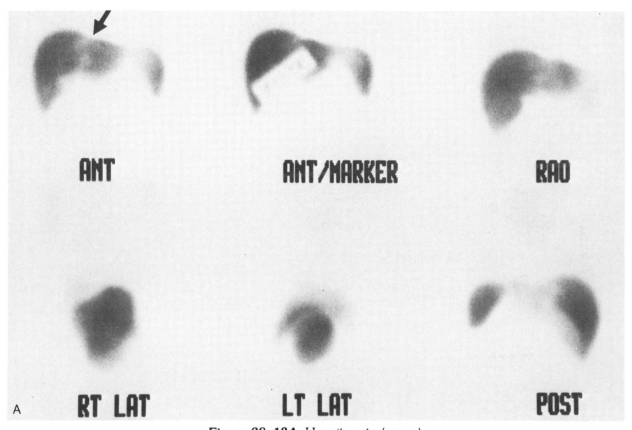

Figure 28–13A. Hepatic vein (*arrow*).

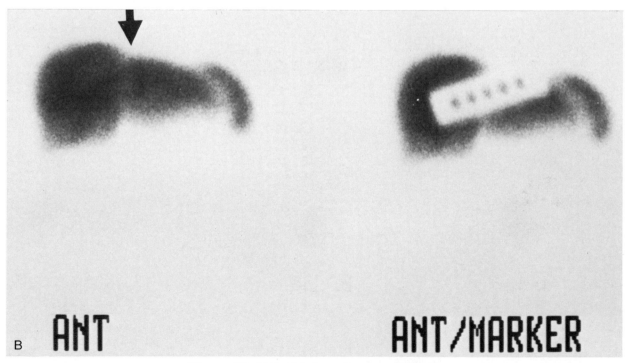

Figure 28–13B. Falciform ligament (*arrow*).

Illustration continued on following page

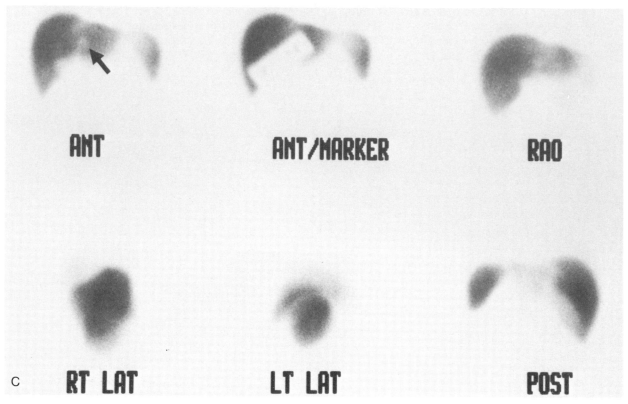

Figure 28–13C. Portal vein (*arrow*).

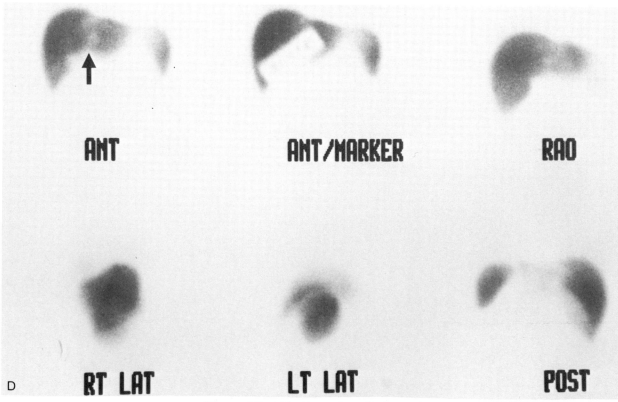

Figure 28–13D. Porta hepatis (*arrow*).

Illustration continued on opposite page

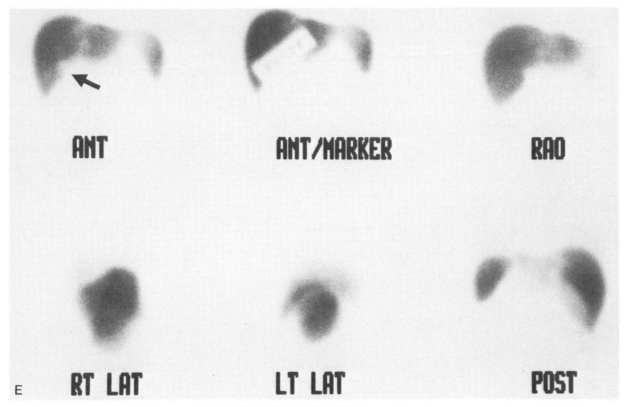

Figure 28–13E. Gallbladder fossa (*arrow*).

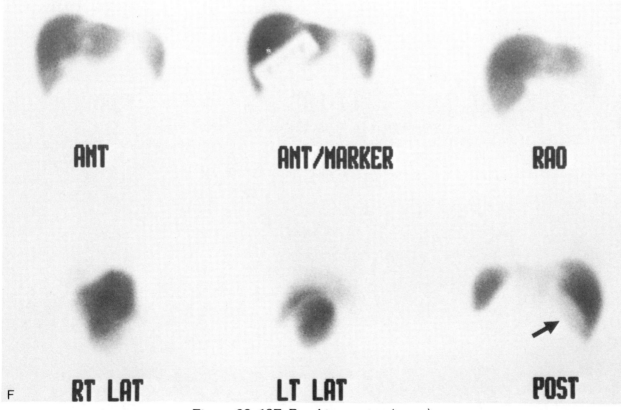

Figure 28–13F. Renal impression (*arrow*).

Figure 28–14. BREAST ATTENUATION. Tc-99m with a 140-KeV gamma energy has a tissue half-value layer of 4.6 cm. A pendulous breast or a breast prosthesis may result in a focal defect usually seen in the anterior and occasionally in the right anterior oblique projection. The defect is often easy to identify due to its uniform, smoothly demarcated appearance. Also, it is frequently associated with a stripe of relatively increased activity. This "stripe" sign is believed to result from small-angle scattering of photons emanating from the liver at the breast tissue/air interface. If this artifact is suspected, a repeat scintigram should be obtained with the breast retracted or prosthesis removed.

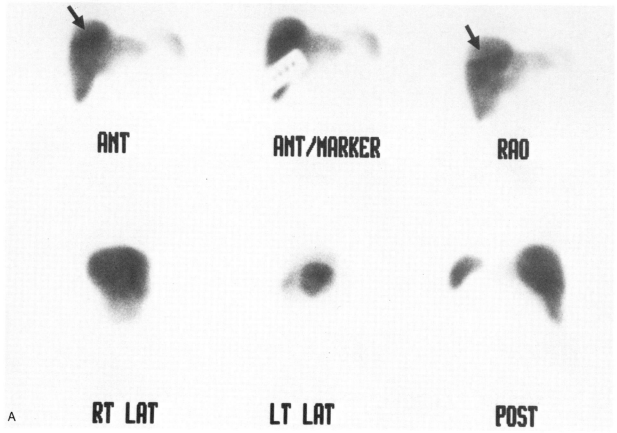

Figure 28–14A. Breast attenuation (*arrows*).

Illustration continued on opposite page

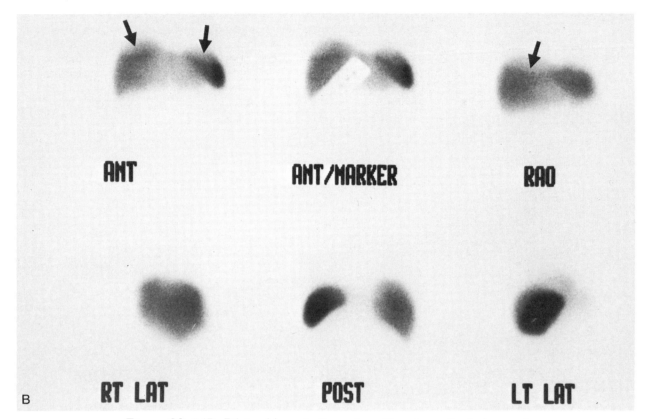

Figure 28–14B. Bilateral breast attenuation: Breast prosthesis (*arrows*).

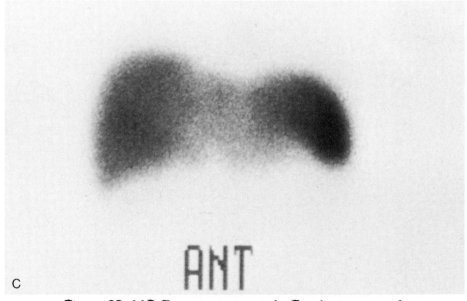

Figure 28–14C. Repeat anterior study: Prosthesis removed.

Refs.: (1) Milder MS, Larson SM, Swann SJ, et al. False-positive liver scan due to breast prosthesis. J Nucl Med 1973; 14:189. (2) Pinsky SM, Johnson PM. The liver and biliary tract. In: Freeman LM, ed. Freeman and Johnson's Clinical Radionuclide Imaging. Orlando: Grune & Stratton, 1984; pp 835–1049.

Figure 28–15. IATROGENIC-INDUCED HEPATIC DEFECTS. Residual barium in the hepatic flexure *(A)* may result in a pseudohepatic defect. This artifact is unusual due to the fact that the colon does not normally overlie the liver. Residual barium in the splenic flexure *(B)* results in a similar abnormality in the splenic views. An abdominal radiograph or repeat liver-spleen scintigram after evacuation of the barium *(C)* will confirm the artifactual cause of the abnormality. An abdominally located pacemaker *(D)* or coins *(E)* in a patient's shirt pocket results in significant photon attenuation. A typical coin of nickel and copper 2 mm thick results in a 30 per cent attenuation. Patients with paralysis or significant joint disease may be unable to move their arms from the camera's field of view *(F and G)*. All of these defects are usually well demarcated and appear in only one view.

Refs.: (1) Seymour EQ, Puckette SE Jr, Edwards J. Pseudoabnormal liver scans secondary to residual barium in the bowel. AJR 1969; 107:54–55. (2) Zwas ST, Braunstein P. Splenic focal defects produced by barium in the colon. Clin Nucl Med 1978; 3:202.

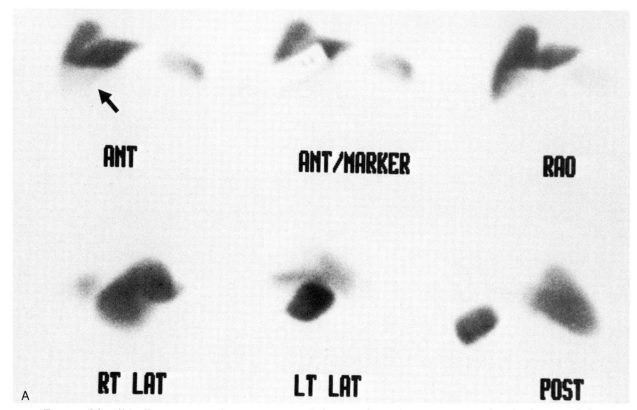

Figure 28–15A. Barium in colon causing a defect in the inferior portion of right hepatic lobe *(arrow)*.

Illustration continued on opposite page

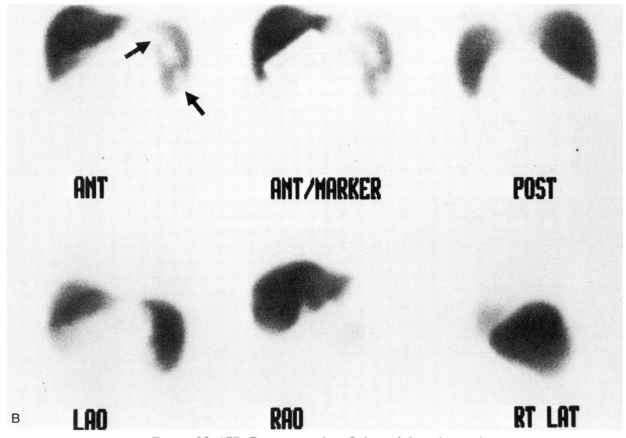

Figure 28–15B. Barium in colon: Splenic defects (*arrows*).

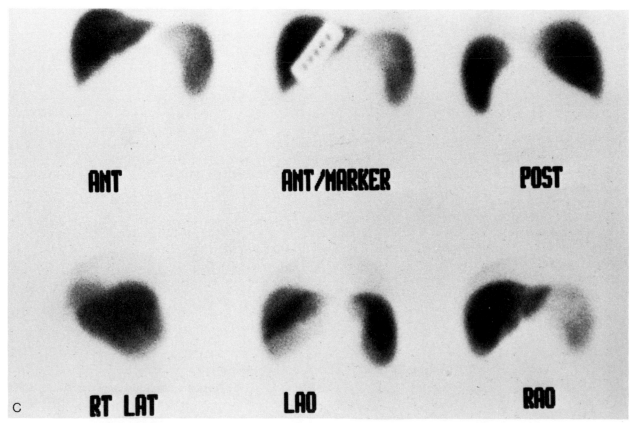

Figure 28–15C. Barium in colon: Repeat study after barium evacuation.

Illustration continued on following page

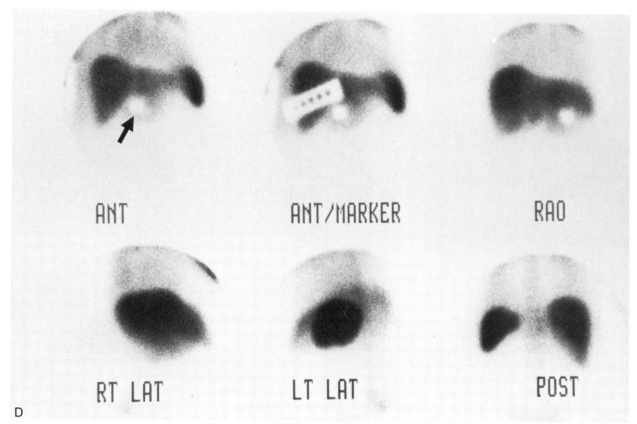

Figure 28–15D. Pacemaker artifact (*arrow*).

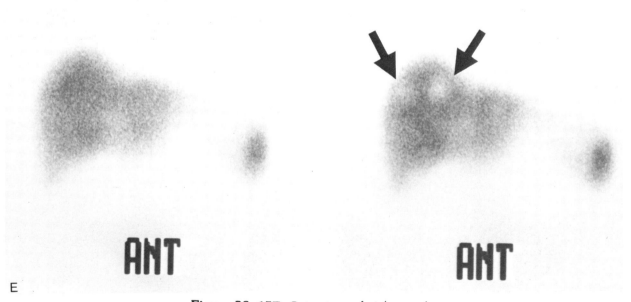

Figure 28–15E. Coins in pocket (*arrows*).

Illustration continued on opposite page

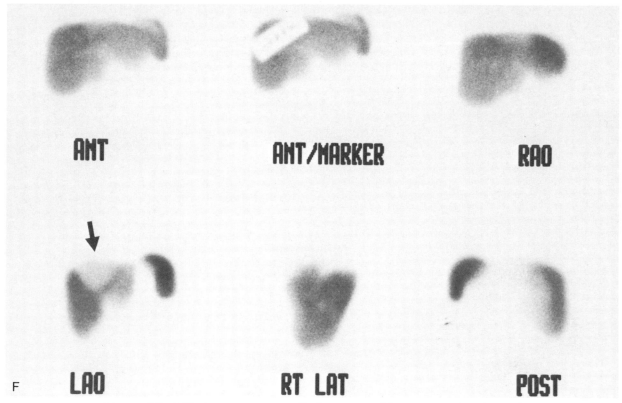

Figure 28–15F. Arm attenuation: Left anterior oblique projection (*arrow*).

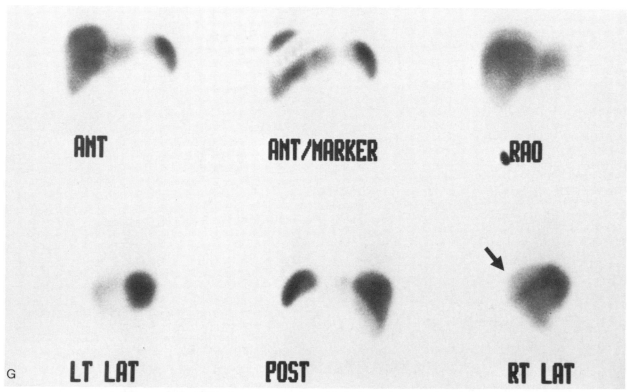

Figure 28–15G. Arm attenuation: Right lateral projection (*arrow*).

Figure 28–16. EXTRAHEPATIC BILIARY OBSTRUCTION WITH BILIARY DILATATION.
Significant obstruction and dilatation of the biliary tract may appear as an area of focally decreased Tc-99m sulfur colloid. The degree and shape of the abnormality reflects the amount of biliary dilatation and biliary ductal architecture. Often, the dilatation produces a stellate pattern or an enlarged porta hepatis when visualized in the anterior and right lateral views (arrows). Any suspected biliary dilatation can be confirmed by ultrasonography.

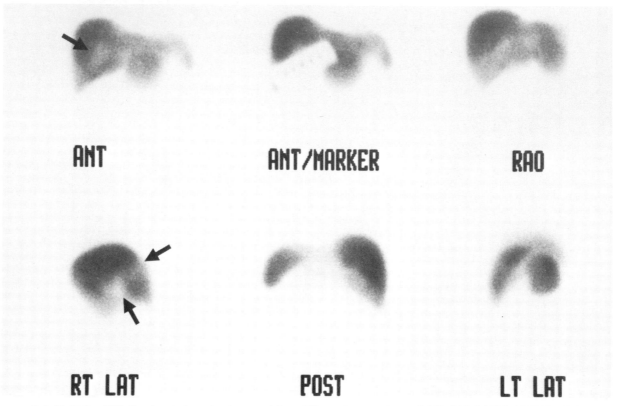

Ref.: McClelland RR. Focal porta hepatis scintiscan defects: What is their significance? J Nucl Med 1976; 16:1007–1012.

Figure 28–17. RADIATION-INDUCED RETICULOENDOTHELIAL CELL DYSFUNCTION.
If a radiation therapy port includes a portion of the liver, radiation-induced reticuloendothelial cell dysfunction may occur. This Kupffer cell dysfunction is often reversible and represents radiation hepatitis. The radiation threshold dose is in the range of approximately 3000 rads in 30 days or 3900 rads in 42 days. The area of radiation-induced hepatitis is often well demarcated on liver-spleen scintigraphy due to the precise collimation of the radiation port (A). This patient with cholangiocarcinoma and hepatic metastases received 3500 rads of irradiation to the liver. A follow-up liver-spleen scintigram obtained 8 months later (B) demonstrates the reversible nature of the hepatitis with the return of normal reticuloendothelial cell function.

Illustration on opposite page

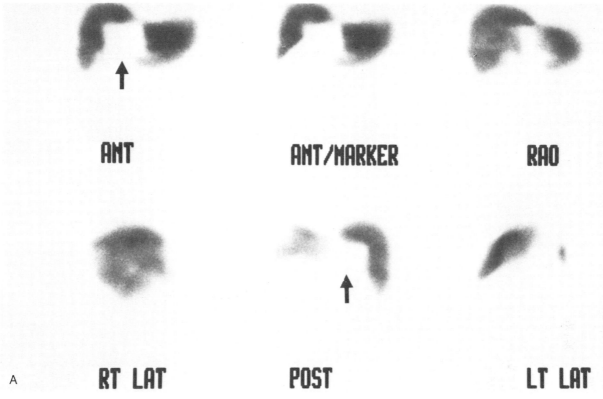

ANT　　　　**ANT/MARKER**　　　　**RAO**

RT LAT　　　　**POST**　　　　**LT LAT**

A

Figure 28–17A. Radiation hepatitis: Square radiation port (*arrows*).

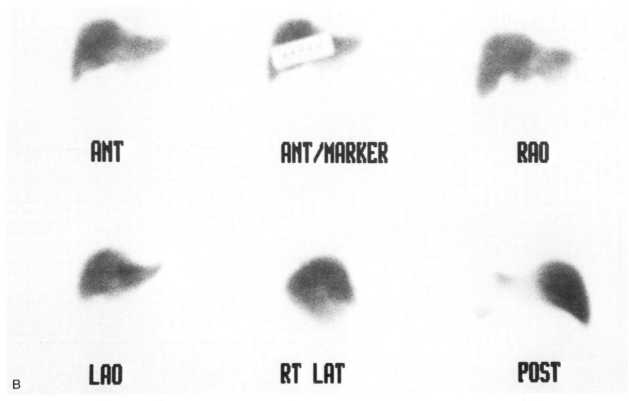

ANT　　　　**ANT/MARKER**　　　　**RAO**

LAO　　　　**RT LAT**　　　　**POST**

B

Figure 28–17B. Return of normal reticuloendothelial cell function 8 months later.

Refs.: (1) Kurohara SS, Swensson NL, Usselman JA, et al. Response and recovery of liver to radiation as demonstrated by photoscans. Radiology 1967; 89:129–135. (2) Johnson PM, Grossman FM, Atkins HL. Radiation-induced hepatic injury: Its detection by scintillation scanning. AJR 1967; 99:453–462.

Figure 28–18. FOCAL HOT SPOT: INJECTION SITE. Focal hepatic hot spots are an unusual finding during liver-spleen scintigraphy. The usual site of Tc-99m sulfur colloid injection is the antecubital fossa, and invariably there is extravasation of a small quantity of the radiopharmaceutical. If the site of injection is allowed to remain in the field of view, it will produce a focal hot spot.

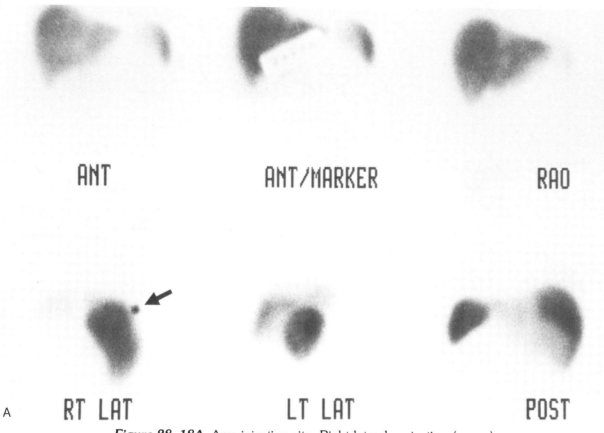

Figure 28–18A. Arm injection site: Right lateral projection (*arrow*).

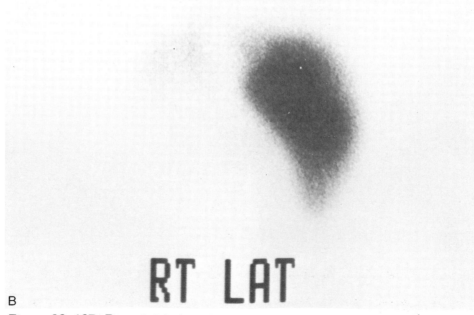

Figure 28–18B. Repeat right lateral projection; arm removed from field of view.

Illustration continued on opposite page

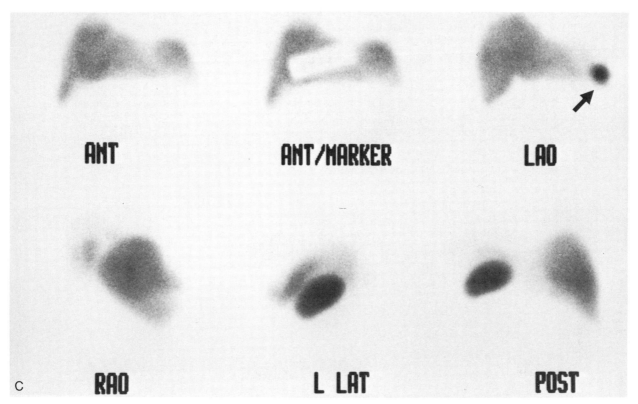

Figure 28–18C. Arm injection site: Left anterior oblique projection (*arrow*).

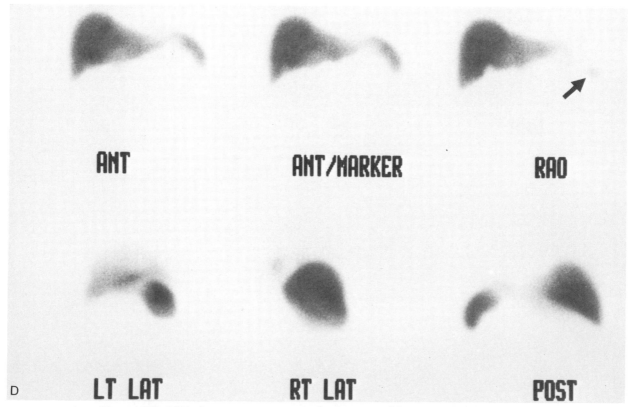

Figure 28–18D. Arm injection site: right anterior oblique projection (*arrow*).

Ref.: Stadalnik RC. "Hot spots"—liver imaging. Sem Nucl Med 1979; 9:220–221.

Figure 28–19. ALCOHOL-INDUCED LIVER DISEASE. The specificity of liver-spleen scintigraphy is poor. However, certain scintigraphic patterns have a strong correlation with alcohol-induced cirrhosis. These include hepatomegaly with heterogeneous uptake of the radiopharmaceutical in association with increased spleen and bone marrow tracer localization *(A).* Ascites may cause the liver to "float" away from the right lateral body wall due to the tendency of the liver to drift to the highest point within the ascites-filled abdominal cavity. Ascitic fluid containing no radioactivity surrounds the liver, resulting in the "halo" effect *(B* and *C).* Far-advanced cirrhosis may cause severe destruction of functional reticuloendothelial cells, resulting in virtual absence of colloid localization within the liver. This has been given the name "phantom" liver *(D).*

Refs.: (1) Drum DE, Beard JO. Liver scintigraphic features associated with alcoholism. J Nucl Med 1978; 19:154–160. (2) Alter AJ, Farrer PA. The perihepatic halo in liver scintiangiographic perfusion studies: A sign of ascites. J Nucl Med 1974; 15:396–398.

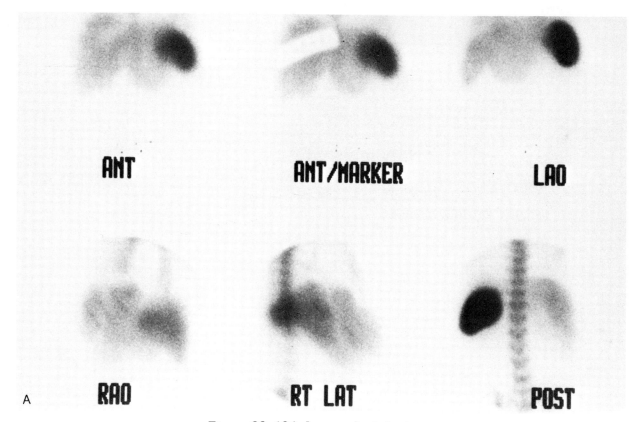

Figure 28–19A. Laennec's cirrhosis.

Illustration continued on opposite page

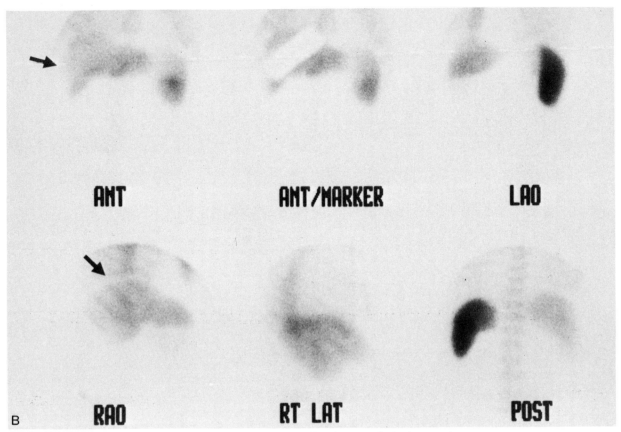

Figure 28–19B. Ascites: Perihepatic halo (*arrows*).

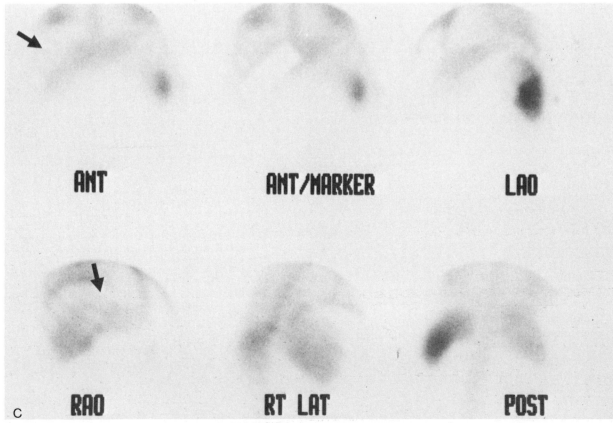

Figure 28–19C. Ascites: Perihepatic halo (*arrows*).

Illustration continued on following page

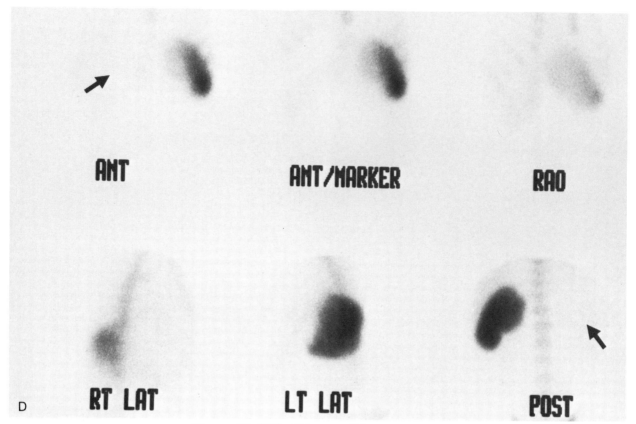

Figure 28–19D. "Phantom" liver (*arrows*).

Figure 28–20. DIFFUSE PULMONARY UPTAKE OF Tc-99m SULFUR COLLOID. The normal adult liver-spleen scintigram is devoid of any significant pulmonary accumulation of the tracer (A). The mechanism of lung colloidal uptake (B–D) is uncertain. It is hypothesized to originate from either in vivo aggregation with resultant pulmonary embolization or enhanced reticuloendothelial extraction in the pulmonary bed. Migration of macrophages from the liver, spleen, and marrow with trapping in the pulmonary capillary bed has been demonstrated during infection and neoplastic disease and under estrogen stimulation. In adults significant lung accumulation of Tc-99m sulfur colloid has been associated with a poor clinical prognosis.

Refs.: (1) Imarisio JJ. Liver scan showing intense lung uptake in neoplasia and infection. J Nucl Med 1975; 16:188–190.
(2) Keyes JW Jr, Wilson GA, Quinones JD. Evaluation of lung uptake of colloid during liver imaging. J Nucl Med 1973; 14:687–691.

Illustration on opposite page

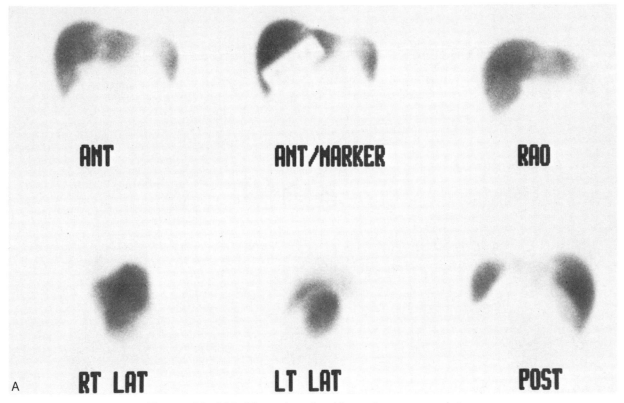

Figure 28–20A. Normal study: Absent lung accumulation.

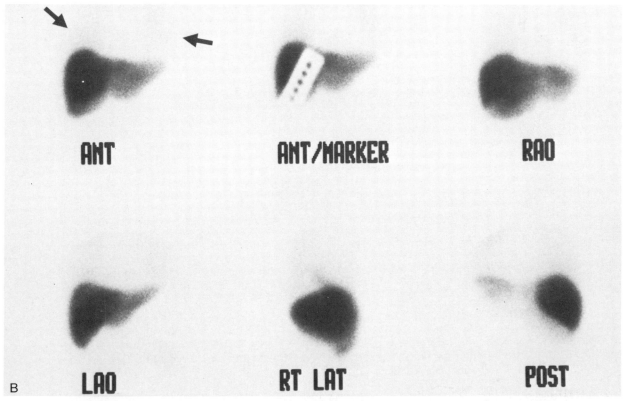

Figure 28–20B. Mild pulmonary accumulation of Tc-99m sulfur colloid (*arrows*).

Illustration continued on following page

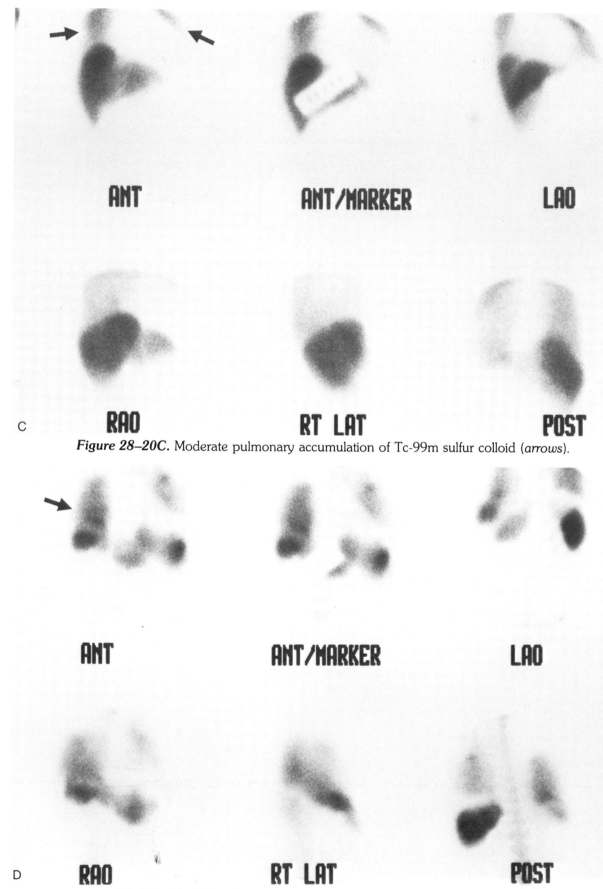

ANT   **ANT/MARKER**   **LAO**

RAO   **RT LAT**   **POST**

C

Figure 28–20C. Moderate pulmonary accumulation of Tc-99m sulfur colloid (*arrows*).

ANT   **ANT/MARKER**   **LAO**

RAO   **RT LAT**   **POST**

D

Figure 28–20D. Marked pulmonary accumulation of Tc-99m sulfur colloid (*arrow*).

Figure 28–21. ***ANATOMIC AND CONGENITAL VARIANTS OF THE SPLEEN.*** The normal spleen is an ovoid structure usually situated posteriorly and laterally in the left upper quadrant. Numerous variations in splenic orientation, shape, and location are possible. The spleen at birth is approximately 5 cm in length and grows in a linear fashion with age. In the adult, the normal range of splenic length is 7 to 13 cm. Normally the long axis of the spleen runs anteriorly and inferiorly; however, the splenic axis may be rotated in any position. The inverted spleen is an unusual variation that may mimic a mass (A). Normal lobulations or splenic notches occur and may be difficult to differentiate from infarcts, lacerations, or other pathological abnormalities (B–D and G). Accessory splenic tissue is rarely visualized in the presence of the major spleen, and is more commonly detected after splenectomy (E and F). Trauma or surgery may produce seeding of splenic tissue, resulting in splenosis (H and I).

Refs.: (1) Spencer RP, Wasserman I, Dhawan V, et al. Incidence of functional splenic tissue after surgical splenectomy. Clin Nucl Med 1977; 2:63. (2) Spencer RP, Johnson PM. The spleen. In: Freeman LM, ed. Freeman and Johnson's Clinical Radionuclide Imaging. Orlando: Grune & Stratton, 1984; pp 1241–1274.

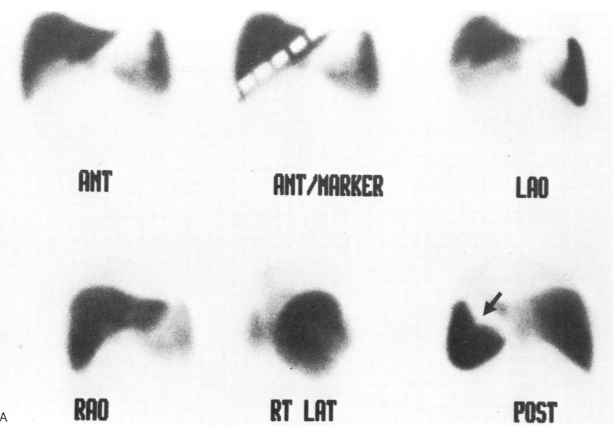

A

Figure 28–21A. Inverted splenic hilum (*arrow*).

Illustration continued on following page

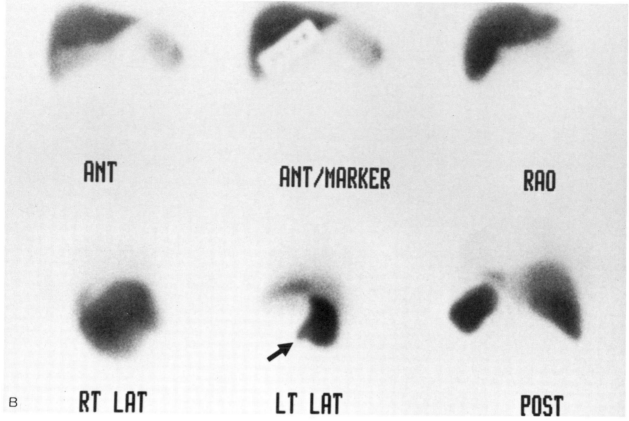

Figure 28–21B. Splenic lobulation (*arrow*).

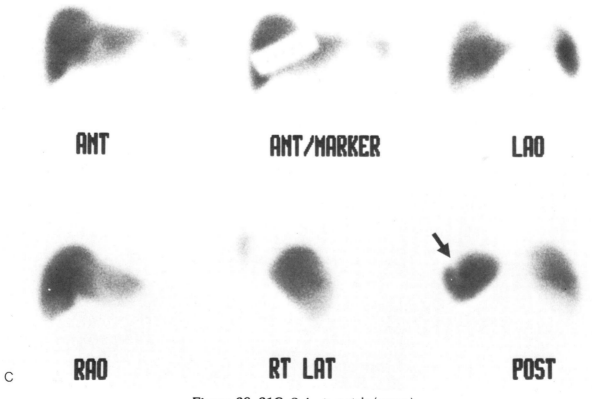

Figure 28–21C. Splenic notch (*arrow*).

Illustration continued on opposite page

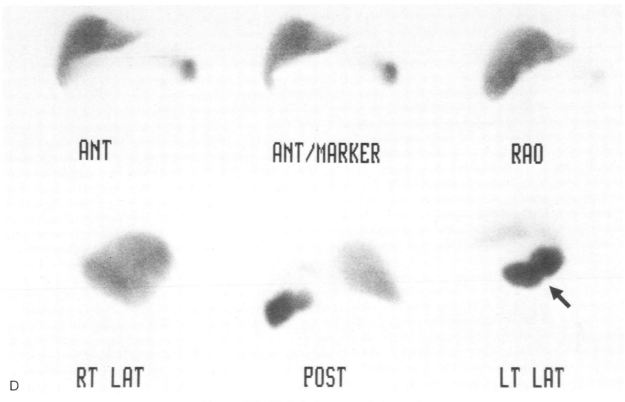

Figure 28–21D. Splenic notch (*arrow*).

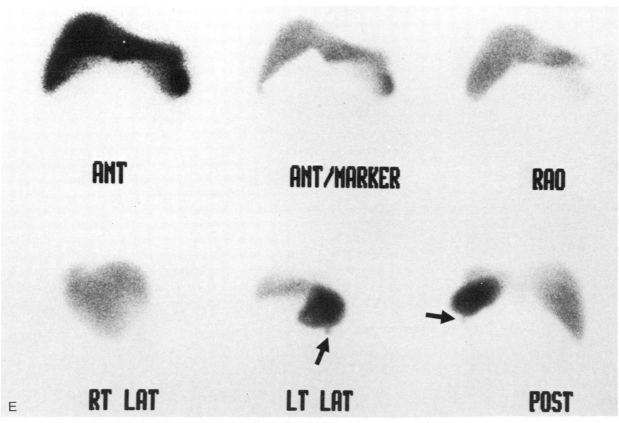

Figure 28–21E. Accessory spleen (*arrows*).

Illustration continued on following page

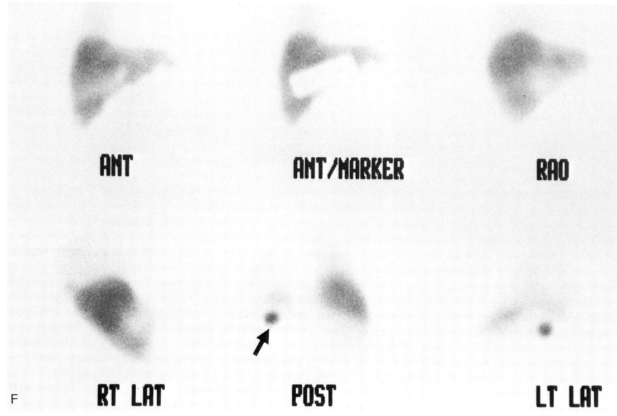

Figure 28–21F. Splenic bed remnant (*arrow*).

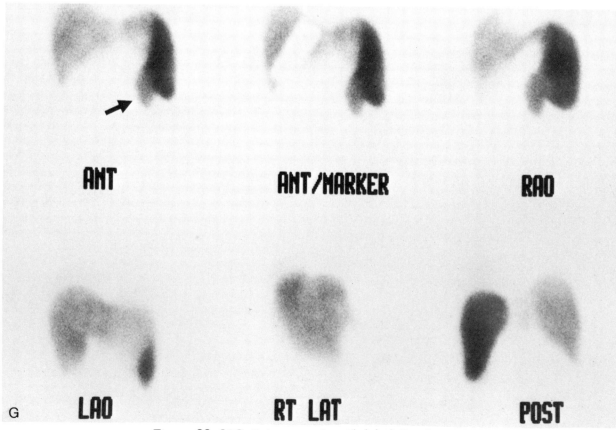

Figure 28–21G. Splenomegaly with lobulation (*arrow*).

Illustration continued on opposite page

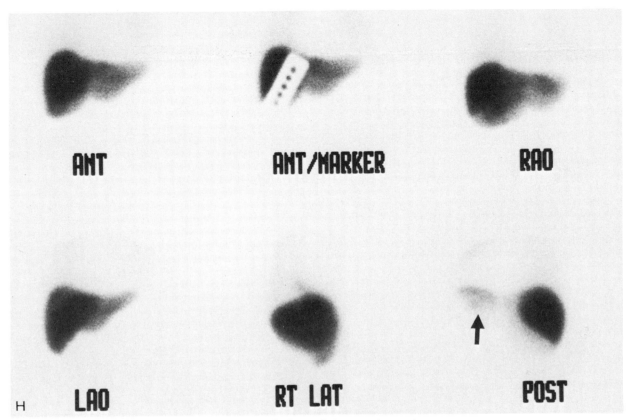

Figure 28–21H. Splenosis (*arrow*).

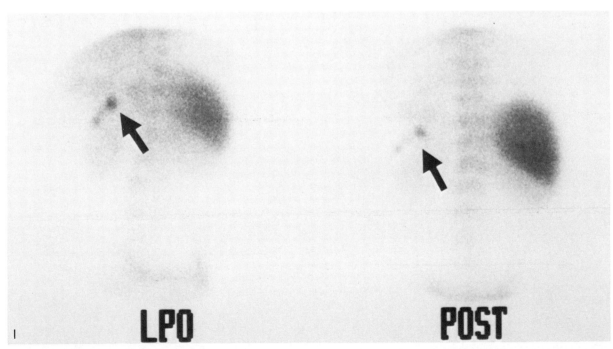

Figure 28–21I. Heat-damaged red blood cell spleen study of splenosis (*arrows*) (same patient as in *H*).

Illustration continued on following page

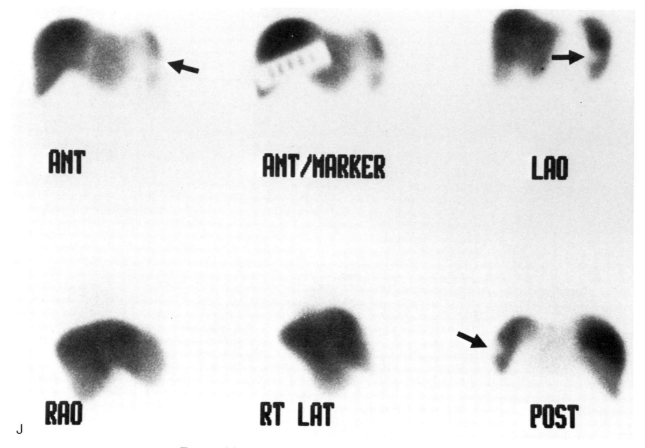

Figure 28–21J. Congenital splenic cyst (*arrows*).

Bone Imaging

FREDERICK L. WEILAND, M.D.
FREDERIC A. CONTE, M.D.
JOSEPH A. ORZEL, M.D.
ALBERT S. HALE, M.D.

Figure 29–1. A SPECTRUM OF NORMAL BONE SCINTIGRAMS. The sensitivity of bone scintigraphy for the detection of various benign and pathologic abnormalities is excellent; however, the specificity is modest. Thus it is imperative to recognize the numerous variations of normal scintigraphic bone images. The interpretation of the bone scintigram should not be limited to the evaluation of the osseous structures. It can supply valuable information regarding the soft tissues, including genitourinary abnormalities. The key to image interpretation is the comparison of contralateral regions for symmetry of tracer localization and intensity. Increased or decreased activity may be abnormal. Bone scintigrams are usually obtained using whole body imaging systems (A) with selected high-resolution spot images being reserved for clarification. An Anger tomographic imaging system may be employed if available (D and E). Younger patients show more avid bone accretion of the radiopharmaceutical in the entire skeleton, with intense activity in the metabolically active epiphyseal growth centers (B and C). Also, children are less likely to suffer from cardiac or renal diseases that might alter tracer transport to bone and clearance from the vascular spaces and soft tissues.

Ref.: O'Mara RE, Weber DA. The osseous system. In: Freeman LM, ed. Freeman and Johnson's Clinical Radionuclide Imaging. Orlando: Grune & Stratton, 1984, pp 1141–1239.

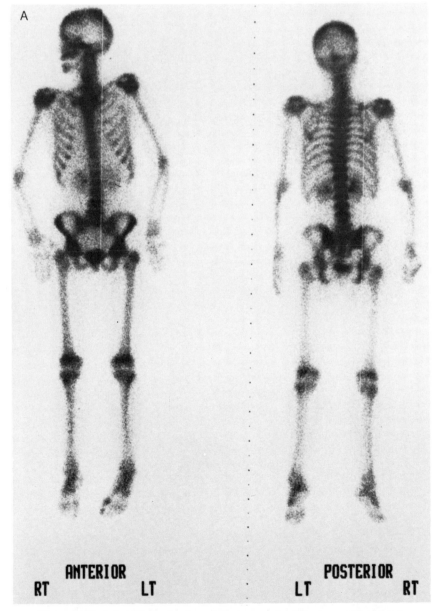

Figure 29–1A. Whole body scintigrams of a 30-year-old patient.

Illustration continued on following page

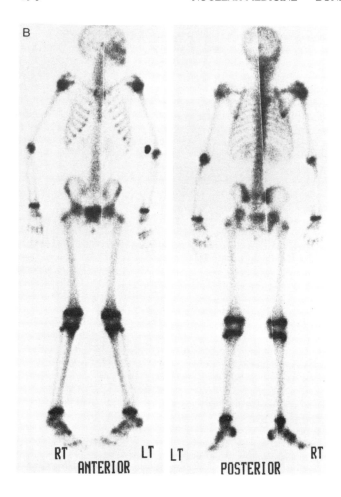

Figure 29–1B. Whole body scintigram of an 18-year-old patient.

Figure 29–1C. Whole body scintigram of a 9-year-old patient.
Illustration continued on opposite page

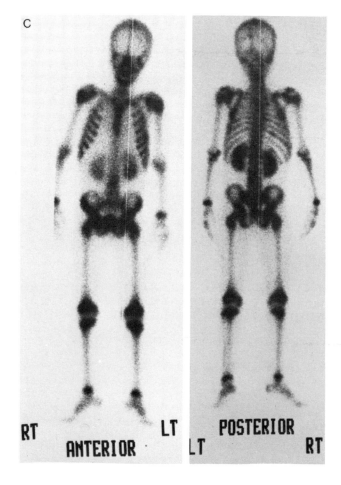

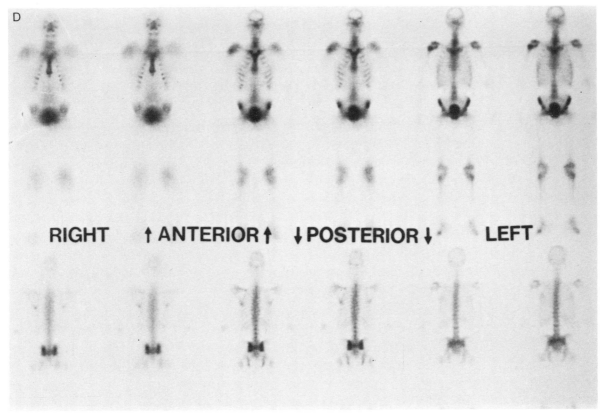

Figure 29–1D. Images made with a multiplane tomographic scanner of an adult male.

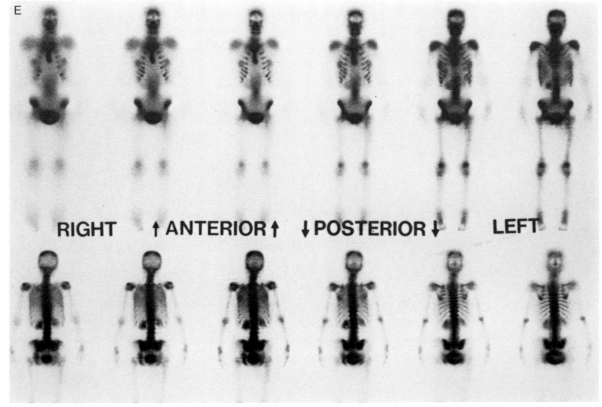

Figure 29–1E. Images made with a multiplane tomographic scanner of an adult female, showing physiologic breast accumulation.

Figure 29–2. RADIOPHARMACEUTICAL PREPARATION DIFFICULTIES. Bone scintigraphic radiopharmaceutical difficulties are increasingly rare due to the excellent kits available and the extreme stability of the radiopharmaceutical for many hours after tracer preparation. Artifacts attributable to poor bone radiopharmaceutical quality occur in three distinct scintigraphic patterns: (1) localization in the salivary gland, thyroid, and gastrointestinal tract due to free technetium *(A and B)*; (2) visualization of the reticuloendothelial system and kidneys resulting from colloid formation *(C)*; and (3) hepatic uptake and excretion of the radiopharmaceutical throughout the biliary system *(D)*.

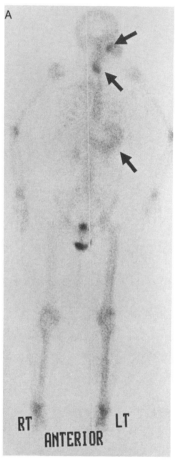

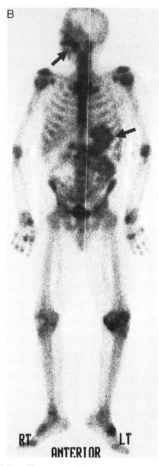

Figure 29–2A. Free technetium in salivary glands, thyroid, and stomach *(arrows)*.

Figure 29–2B. Free technetium in salivary glands *(upper arrow)*, thyroid, and stomach *(lower arrow)*.

Illustration continued on opposite page

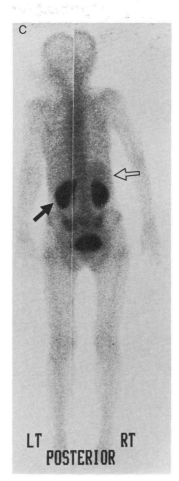

Figure 29–2C. Formation of colloids with reticuloendothelial (*open arrow*) and renal (*solid arrow*) activity.

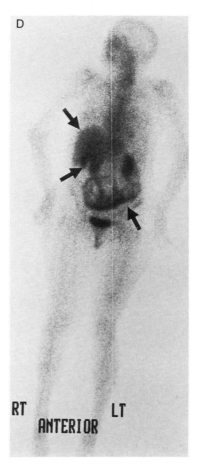

Figure 29–2D. Excretion of the radiopharmaceutical within the biliary system (*arrows*).

Ref.: McAfeè JG, Subramanian G. Radioactive agents for imaging. In: Freeman LM, ed. Freeman and Johnson's Clinical Radionuclide Imaging. Orlando: Grune & Stratton, 1984; pp 55–202.

*Figure 29–3. **EQUIPMENT AND TECHNICAL ARTIFACTS.*** Equipment and technical artifacts are often easy to identify by the bizarre nature of the scintigrams obtained. The current Anger scintillation detector systems are complex and rely extensively on integrated circuitry for their operation. These electronic circuits are extremely reliable but will occasionally malfunction *(A and B)*. The multiplane tomographic scanner utilizes a focusing collimator to obtain tomographic images. If the focal plane is not adjusted properly for each study, images will be constructed that do not represent adequate tomographic planes through the patient *(C)*. Significant image degradation occurs with improper photopeak selection. Image degradation *(D)* is a result of significant Compton scatter being included in the image. Low or high filters are employed depending on whether the study acquired is dynamic or static. The low filter allows additional light to strike the radiographic film to enhance image display when low count statistics are obtained in dynamic acquisition *(G)*.

Ref.: Rollo FD, Harris CC. Factors affecting image formation. In: Rollo FD, ed. Nuclear Medicine Physics, Instrumentation, and Agents. St. Louis: CV Mosby, 1977; pp 387–435.

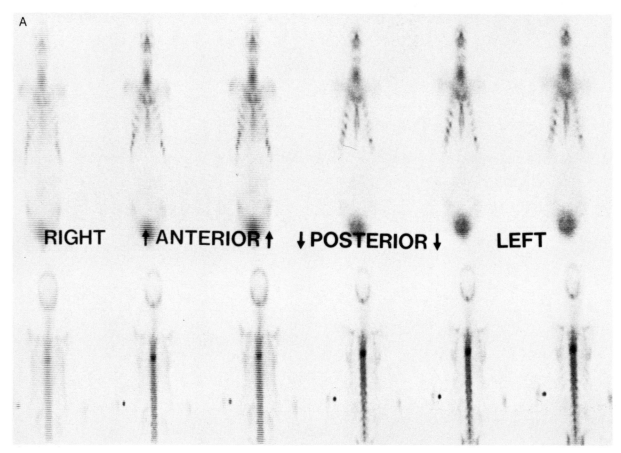

Figure 29–3A. XY coordinate circuitry malfunction.

Illustration continued on opposite page

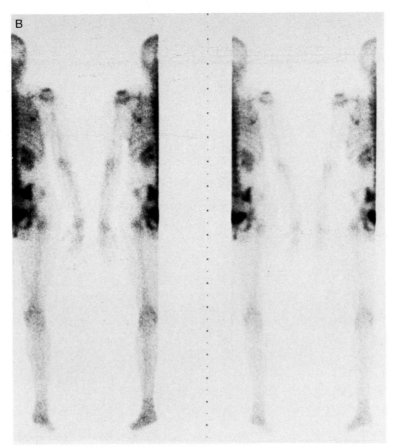

Figure 29–3B. Electronic malfunction in assembling two-pass whole body image.

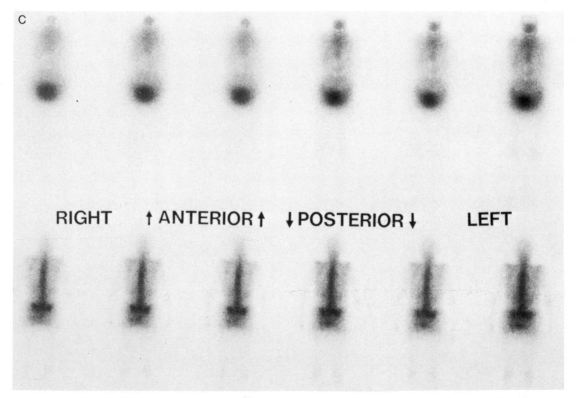

RIGHT   ↑ ANTERIOR ↑   ↓ POSTERIOR ↓   LEFT

Figure 29–3C. Multiplane tomographic scanner with collimator distance improperly set.

Illustration continued on following page

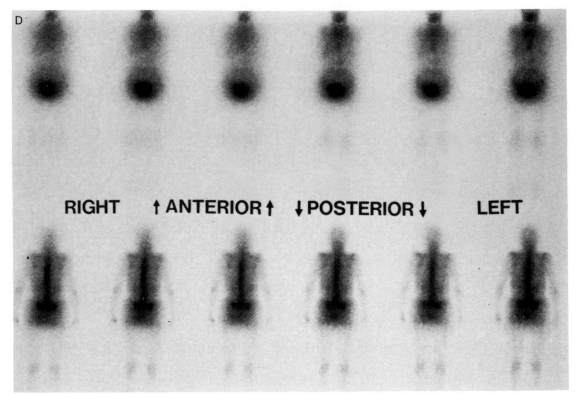

Figure 29–3D. Pulse height analyzer circuits set for Ga-67.

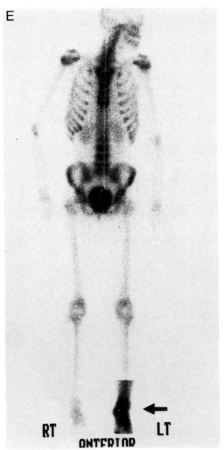

Figure 29–3E. Bone scintigraphic table stalled. Note region of prolonged imaging (*arrow*) as a result of table stalling.

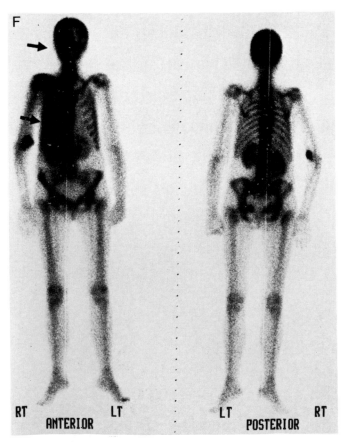

Figure 29–3F. Malfunctioning whole body table, with blur artifact (*arrows*).

Illustration continued on opposite page

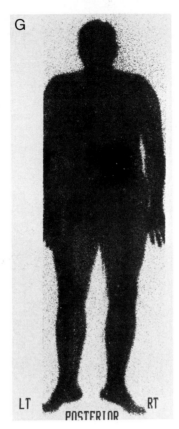

Figure 29–3G. Whole body image obtained with low filter.

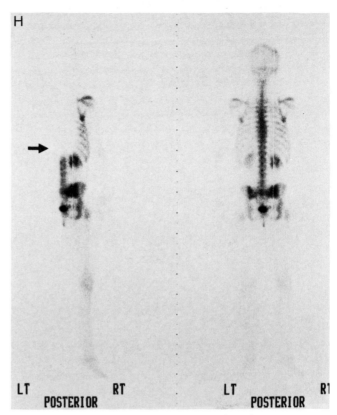

Figure 29–3H. Failure of photographic shutter to open properly, with resultant defect (*arrow*) in body scan.

Figure 29–4. PATIENT ARTIFACTS. Numerous artifacts are produced by the patient's body habitus, such as marked scoliosis *(A)*, amputations *(B)*, paralyzed extremities *(C)*, and, most commonly, patient movement *(D)*, especially when whole body reconstructed images are obtained. Patient movement and rotation occur frequently during the prolonged acquisition time necessary for whole body scintigrams and are augmented by the discomfort of whole body imaging tables. Patient rotation *(E)* is suggested when there is asymmetric localization of the radiopharmaceutical, with increased accumulation on the side of the patient that was closer to the detector. If a rotational artifact is suspected, repeat spot scintigrams should be taken after assuring that the patient's body is parallel to the camera. Due to the low-energy gamma photons of Tc-99m, poor bone visualization will occur in the obese individual from significant attenuation by the adipose tissue *(F)*.

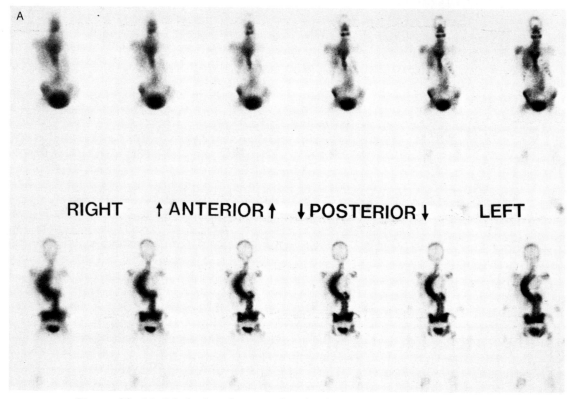

Figure 29–4A. Marked scoliosis artifact (multiplane tomographic scanner).

Illustration continued on opposite page

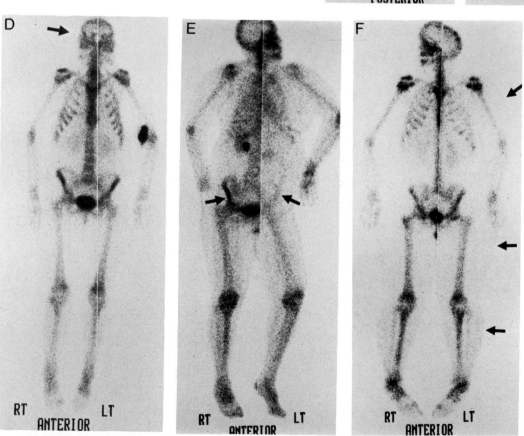

Figure 29–4B and C. *B,* Upper extremity amputation (*arrow*); *C,* paralyzed arm across the field of view (*arrow*).

Figure 29–4D, E, and F. *D,* Patient motion ("Janus" sign) (*arrow*); *E,* patient rotation (*arrows*); *F,* morbid obesity (photon attenuation) (*arrows*).

Ref.: O'Mara RE, Weber DA. The Osseous System. In: Freeman LM, ed. Freeman and Johnson's Clinical Radionuclide Imaging. Orlando: Grune & Stratton, 1984; pp 1141–1239.

Figure 29–5. BONE SCAN ABNORMALITIES IN DENTAL DISEASE. Focal increased concentration of bone scintigraphic agents in the maxilla or mandible is a common scintigraphic finding during routine bone imaging. Tow and coworkers demonstrated dental abnormalities in 14 of 25 patients with unsuspected dental disease. The underlying dental pathology included pulpitis and periodontitis, chronic irritations of the oral mucosa resulting from ill-fitting dentures, and healing bone following recent extractions or root canal treatments. The authors speculated that the etiology of the scintigraphic abnormalities represented bone reaction to chronic irritation.

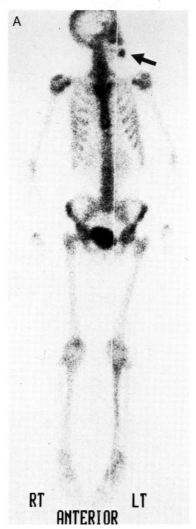

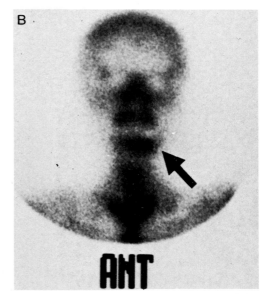

Figure 29–5A. Dental caries *(arrow).*

Figure 29–5B. Anterior spot scintigram of head of patient shown in *A.* Note dental caries *(arrow).*

Ref.: Tow DE, Garcia DA, Jansons D, Sullivan TM: Bone scans in dental diseases. J Nucl Med 1978; 19:845–847.

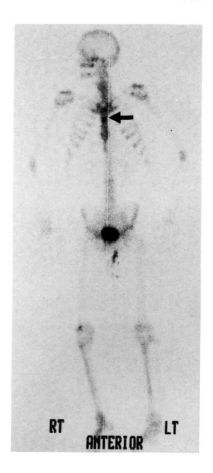

Figure 29–6. THE ANGLE OF LOUIS ("LOUIE'S HOT SPOT"). The angle of Louis is a palpable ridge along the anterior surface of the sternum *(arrow)*. It occurs at the fibrocartilaginous junction of the manubrium and body of the sternum. Fink-Bennett and Shapiro identified increased tracer concentration at this location in 36 of 100 consecutive bone scintigrams. All patients were asymptomatic, and 25 of 36 patients who had correlative radiographs were normal. The authors concluded that this finding was not a manifestation of an osseous abnormality but a normal scintigraphic finding.

Ref.: Fink-Bennett DM, Shapiro EE. The angle of Louis: A potential pitfall ("Louie's hot spot") in bone scan interpretation. Clin Nucl Med 1984; 9:352–354.

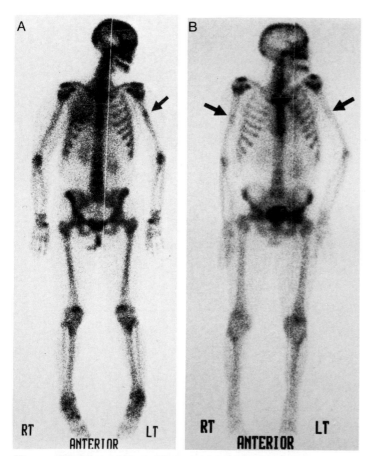

Figure 29–7. DELTOID TUBEROSITY: THE "DELTA" SIGN. The deltoid tuberosity is a bony prominence at the site of the distal insertion of the deltoid muscle. It is located on the lateral aspect of the proximal third of the humerus. Fink-Bennett and Vicuna-Rios identified this anatomic variant in 7 of 100 consecutive bone scintigrams. The characteristic appearance and location should be adequate to eliminate this as a potential source of bone-scintigraphic misinterpretation. If confusion does arise, a scintigram obtained with internal rotation of the humerus or a correlative radiograph should be diagnostic.

Ref.: Fink-Bennett DM, Vicuna-Rios J. The deltoid tuberosity—A potential pitfall (the "delta sign") in bone-scan interpretation: Concise communication. J Nucl Med 1980; 21:211–212.

Figure 29–7A and B. A, Unilateral deltoid tuberosity *(arrow)*; B, bilateral deltoid tuberosities *(arrows)*.

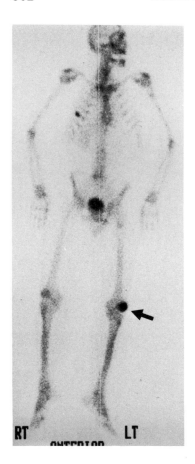

Figure 29–8. ASYMMETRIC INCREASED RADIOPHARMACEUTICAL UPTAKE IN THE PATELLA: THE "HOT PATELLA" SIGN. The incidence of either unilateral or bilateral increased uptake of bone radiopharmaceuticals in the patella *(arrow)* has been reported to be as high as 30 per cent by Fogelman and colleagues. Kipper and his co-authors reported this abnormality to be more frequent in patients with either malignant or metabolic bone disease. However, this finding has little diagnostic significance, being found in 20 per cent of patients without bone disease.

Refs.: (1) Fogelman I, McKillop H, Gray HW. The "hot patella" sign: Is it of any clinical significance? Concise communication. J Nucl Med 1983; 24:312–315. (2) Kipper Ms, Alazraki NP, Feiglin DH. The "hot" patella. Clin Nucl Med 1982; 7:28–32.

Figure 29–9. DEGENERATIVE ABNORMALITIES AS AN INCIDENTAL SCINTIGRAPHIC FINDING. Bone scintigraphy may be of use in evaluation of musculoskeletal pain if degenerative or arthritic causes are suspected. This is especially true if there are multiple symptomatic joints, as bone scintigraphy is more sensitive, easier to interpret, and less expensive than multiple radiographs. Asymptomatic degenerative changes are often incidentally found during bone scintigraphy performed for other purposes. Any joint may be involved; a few of the more common abnormalities are illustrated. Of particular interest is the scintigraphic finding of increased radiopharmaceutical disposition in the shoulder of the dominant hand *(B)*. This is believed to be due to increased articular utilization and repetitive mild trauma.

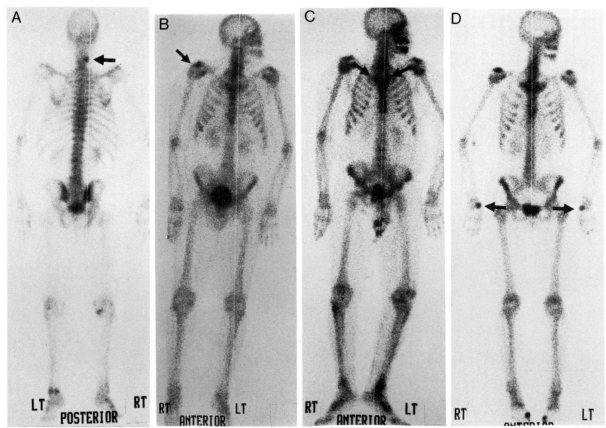

Figure 29–9A, B, C, and D. Degenerative abnormalities are indicated by *arrows* in these images. A, Cervical spine; B, right shoulder of a right-handed individual; C, sternoclavicular joint; D, primary osteoarthritis in wrists.

Ref.: Hoffer PB, Genant HK. Radionuclide joint imaging. Semin Nucl Med 1976; 6:121–137.

Figure 29–10. SCINTIGRAPHIC APPEARANCE OF TRAUMATIC RIB FRACTURES.
Trauma-induced rib fractures produce a characteristic scintigraphic pattern consisting of intense, focal, increased deposition in a linear fashion, as illustrated. In the vast majority of individuals, scintigraphic abnormalities will be apparent within 24 hours after acute injury, whereas in the elderly patient 3 to 4 days may need to elapse. The minimal time for rib fractures to return to normal scintigraphically is approximately 5 months, while 3 years may be required in certain individuals.

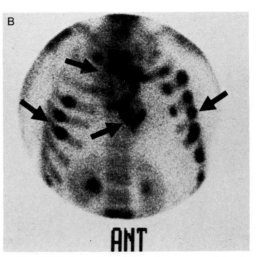

Figure 29–10B. Anterior spot scintigram of *A*, showing fractures *(arrows)*.

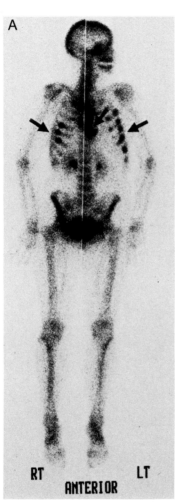

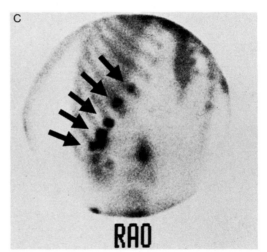

Figure 29–10A. Multiple rib fractures *(arrows)* as a result of cardiopulmonary resuscitation.

Figure 29–10C. Right anterior oblique view of multiple rib fractures *(arrows)* due to motor vehicle accident.

Ref.: Matin P. Bone scanning of trauma and benign conditions. In: Freeman LM, Weissmann HS, ed.: Nuclear Medicine Annual 1982. New York: Raven Press, 1982; pp 81–118.

Figure 29–11. SUPERSCAN. A superscan has been defined as homogeneous symmetrically increased uptake of tracer in bone relative to soft tissue *(A)*. Diffusely increased metabolic bone activity with accentuation of osseous tracer uptake results in less soft tissue and renal localization. This scintigraphic finding has been associated with various neoplastic, metabolic, and hematologic diseases. Heterogeneous increased distribution of radiopharmaceutical deposition may also result in a superscan *(B* and *C)*. Paget's disease of bone and fibrous dysplasia have also been associated with heterogeneous superscans.

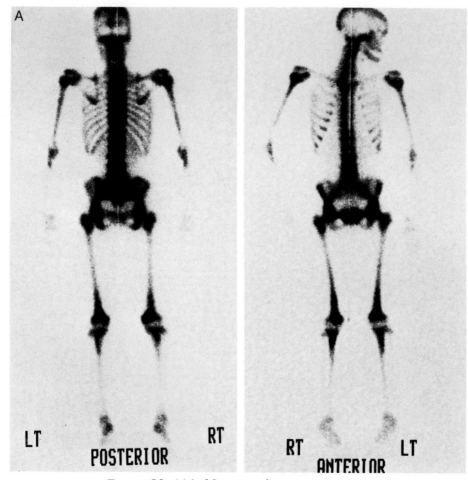

Figure 29–11A. Metastatic breast carcinoma.

Illustration continued on opposite page

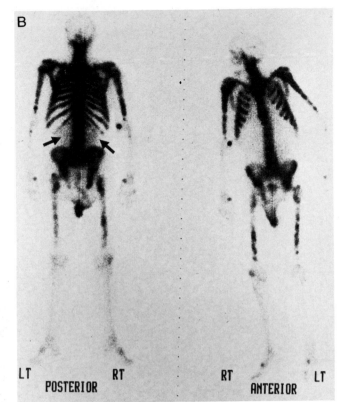

Figure 29–11B. Metastatic prostate carcinoma. Note poorly visualized kidneys (*arrows*).

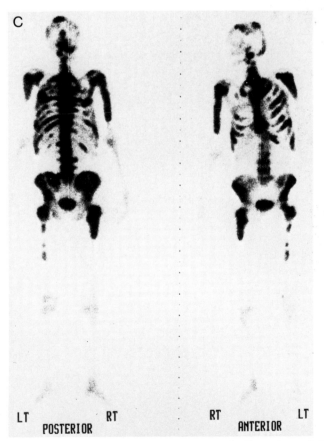

Figure 29–11C. Metastatic prostate carcinoma.

Refs.: (1) Constable AR, Cranage RW. Recognition of the superscan in prostate bone scintigraphy. Br J Radiol 1981; 54:122–125. (2) Sy WM, Patel D, Fauncie H. Significance of absent or faint kidney sign on bone scan. J Nucl Med 1975; 16:454–456.

Figure 29–12. HYPERTROPHIC PULMONARY OSTEOARTHROPATHY (HPO): "DOUBLE STRIPE" or "PARALLEL TRACK" SIGN. Hypertrophic osteoarthropathy is a humerally or neurally mediated syndrome that results in increased blood flow, edema of the periosteum, round cell infiltration, proliferation of connective tissue, and osteoid deposition with calcification. It is classified as primary when there is no known associated disease. Secondary osteoarthropathy has been associated with an extensive number of both benign and pathological conditions. Bone scintigraphy is more sensitive than conventional radiography for the detection of osteoarthropathy and often demonstrates more extensive involvement. The double stripe or parallel track sign is a common scintigraphic appearance *(arrows)*. With successful treatment of the underlying disorder, reversal of the periosteal abnormalities will occur, with bone scintigraphy returning to normal in 1 to 6 months.

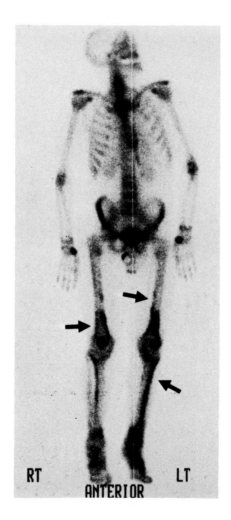

Ref.: Terry DW, Isitman AT, Holmes RA. Radionuclide bone images in hypertrophic pulmonary osteoarthropathy. AJR 1975; 124:571–576.

Figure 29–13. ATTENUATION ARTIFACTS. Tc-99m has a relatively low-energy gamma photon of 140 KeV with a tissue half-value layer of 4.6 cm. These low-energy photons are easily attenuated by metallic objects (*arrows A–F* and *H*) of any type and, as illustrated in *G* and *H* (*arrows*), by plastic breast prostheses. The appearance of the scintigraphic attenuation caused by these objects is often easy to identify. Most often the abnormality appears in only one projection and has a photon-deficient appearance. Misinterpretation can be avoided if all patients, prior to scintigraphy, completely disrobe and don hospital clothing. A sufficiently detailed history and physical examination should disclose the presence of pacemakers, implanted breast prostheses, orthopedic devices, and other objects.

Ref.: O'Mara RE, Weber DA. The osseous system. In: Freeman LM, ed. Freeman and Johnson's Clinical Radionuclide Imaging. Orlando: Grune & Stratton, 1984; pp 1141–1239.

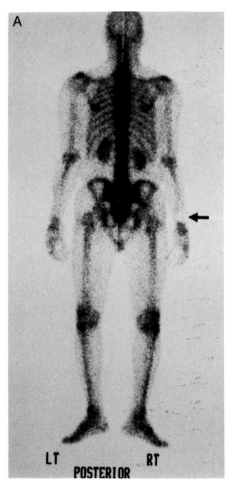

Figure 29–13A. Wrist watch.

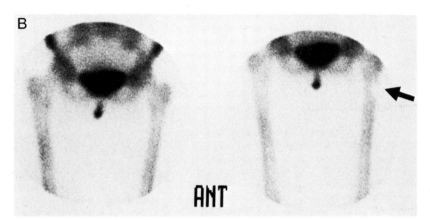

Figure 29–13B. Coins in pocket (*right*); repeat study with coins removed (*left*).

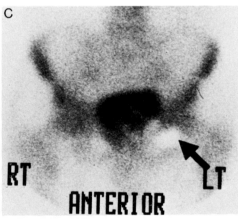

Figure 29–13C. Cigarette lighter.

Illustration continued on following page

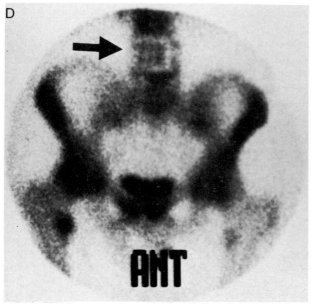

Figure 29–13D. Belt buckle.

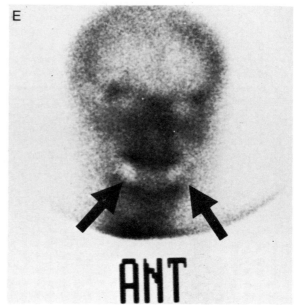

Figure 29–13E. Gold fillings.

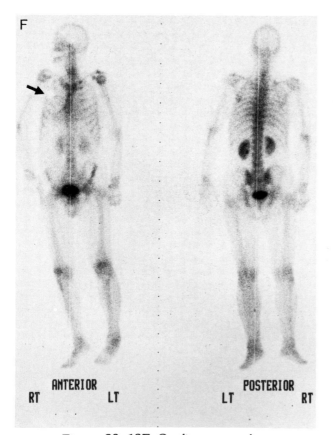

Figure 29–13F. Cardiac pacemaker.

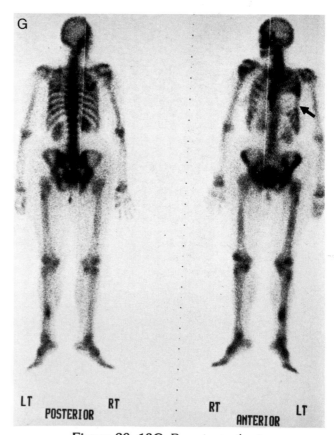

Figure 29–13G. Breast prosthesis.

Illustration continued on opposite page

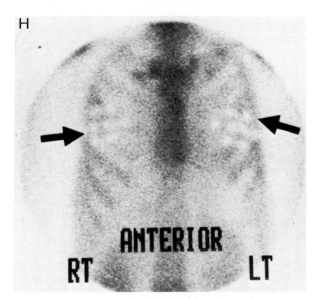

Figure 29–13H. Bilateral breast prostheses.

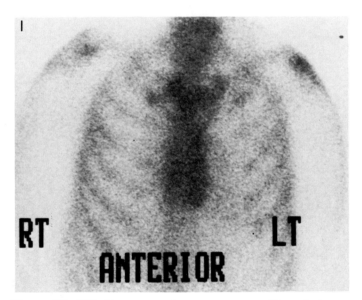

Figure 29–13I. Repeat study of patient in *H*, with breast prostheses removed.

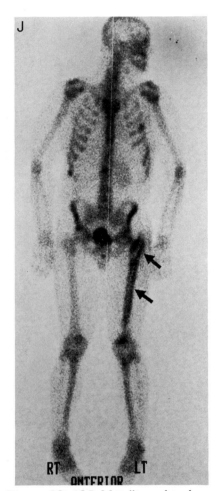

Figure 29–13J. Metallic rod in femur.

**Figure 29–14. PHOTON-DEFICIENT SCINTIGRAPHIC ABNORMALITIES OF THE AB-
DOMEN AND PELVIS DUE TO COLONIC RETENTION OF BARIUM.** *A* and *B* illustrate the
significant attenuation of the 140-KeV photons of Tc-99m by retained colonic barium *(arrows)*.
This classic artifact should be identified easily, usually by the patient's historical confirmation of a
recent radiographic gastrointestinal procedure, or, if needed, by a concurrent abdominal radiograph.
Repeat scintigraphic images should be obtained after complete evacuation of the retained barium.

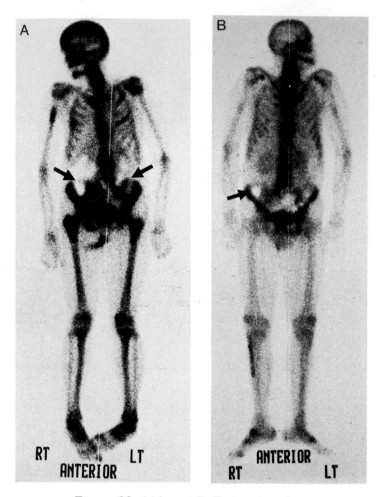

Figure 29–14A and B. Barium in colon.

Ref.: Karelitz JR, Richards JB. Pseudophotopenic defect due to barium in the colon. Clin Nucl Med 1978; 3:414.

Figure 29–15. RADIATION OSTEONECROSIS. Radiation damage to osseous tissue is believed to be secondary to alterations in the microvasculature resulting in partial or complete occlusion. This phenomenon occurs at doses exceeding 3000 rads in 3 weeks. The precise time course of radiation-induced osteonecrosis is not well defined. Initially, increased tracer concentration occurs due to radiation-induced hyperemia, followed by vessel occlusion and decreased radiopharmaceutical accumulation that may persist for years.

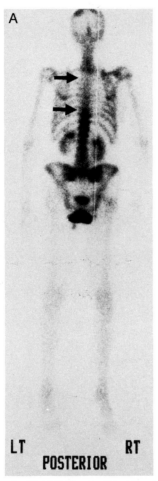

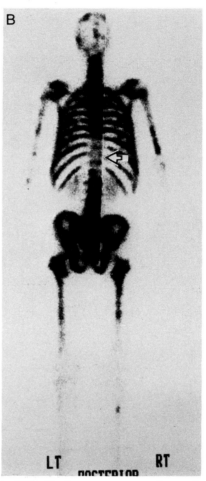

Figure 29–15A. Radiation osteonecrosis *(arrows)* at site of radiation therapy port.

Figure 29–15B. Radiation necrosis *(arrow)* at site of radiation therapy port (superscan).

Ref.: Bell EG, McAfee JG, Constable WC. Local radiation damage to bone and marrow demonstrated by radioisotope imaging. Radiology, 1969; 92:1083–1088.

Figure 29–16. INJECTION ARTIFACTS. Tc-99m methylene diphosphonate bone scintigrams are usually obtained 2 to 3 hours after the intravenous administration of the radiopharmaceutical. The usual site of injection is the antecubital fossa; however, the tracer may be injected wherever venous access may be obtained *(A–D, arrows)*. It is imperative that the injection site and the number of attempted injections be known prior to scintigraphic interpretation. This will prevent the misinterpretation of the injection site as a bone or soft-tissue abnormality. Extravasation of the radiopharmaceutical at the site of injection may obscure underlying osseous abnormalities *(E and G)*. If the photon flux is of sufficient intensity, penetration of the collimator lead septa may produce a star-like pattern *(F)*; this reflects the orthogonal geometry of the collimator holes.

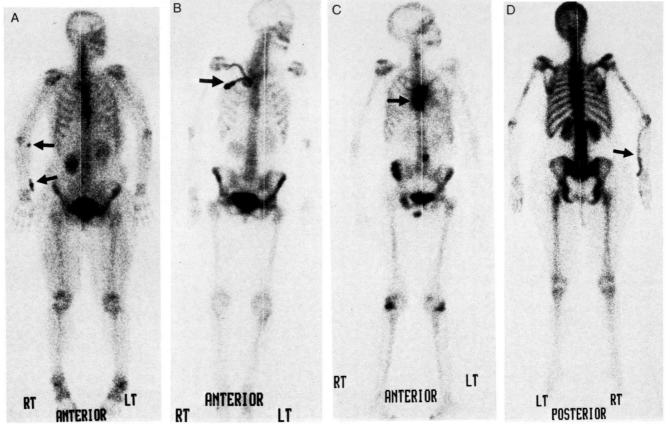

Figure 29–16A, B, C, and D. A, Multiple injection sites; B, injection through a subclavian catheter; C, injection through a Hickman catheter; D, injection through an intravenous line.

Illustration continued on opposite page

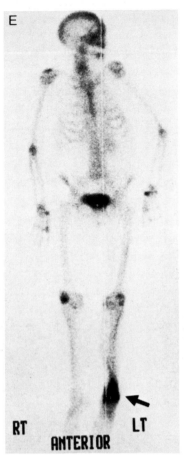

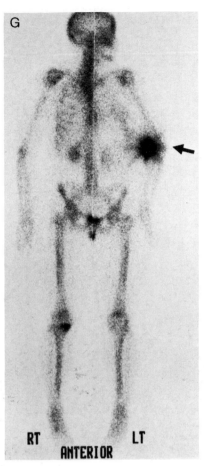

Figure 29–16E. Extravasation following injection through a dorsal vein in the foot.

Figure 29–16F. Extravasation of radiopharmaceutical, with star pattern *(arrow).*

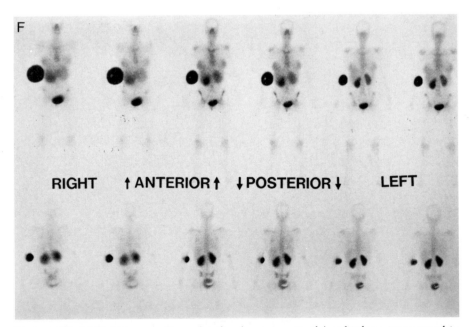

Figure 29–16G. Extravasation of radiopharmaceutical (multiplane tomographic scanner).

Ref.: O'Mara RE, Weber DA. The osseous system. In: Freeman LM, ed. Freeman and Johnson's Clinical Radionuclide Imaging. Orlando: Grune & Stratton, 1984; pp 1141–1239.

Figure 29–17. BREAST ACCUMULATION OF BONE RADIOPHARMACEUTICALS. Localization of phosphate bone radiopharmaceuticals *(A– J, arrows)* has been described in a variety of both benign and malignant breast lesions. Faint bilateral accumulation is not an unusual occurrence and is almost always benign. Unilateral deposition, however, should be investigated to exclude a malignant process. The precise mechanism of localization is not known. Calcium metabolism, alterations in pH, inflammatory reaction with hyperemia, deposition of immature collagen, and increased blood pool have all been proposed as mechanisms.

Refs.: (1) Burnett KR, Lyons KP, Brown WT. Uptake of osteotropic radionuclides in the breast. Semin Nucl Med 1984; 14:48–49. (2) Schmitt GH, Holmes RA, Isitman AT, Hensley GT, Lewis JD. Proposed mechanism for technetium-99 labeled polyphosphate and diphosphonate uptake by human breast tissue. Radiology 1974; 112:733–735.

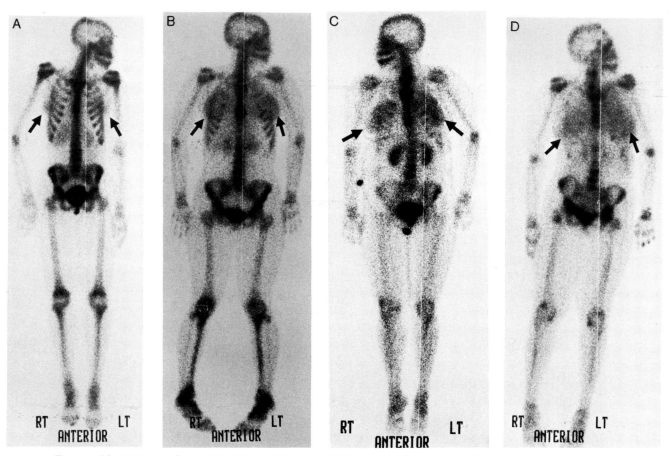

Figure 29–17A, B, C, and D. Bilateral symmetric breast uptake. *A* and *B,* Normal; *C,* lactation; *D,* drug-induced gynecomastia.

Illustration continued on opposite page

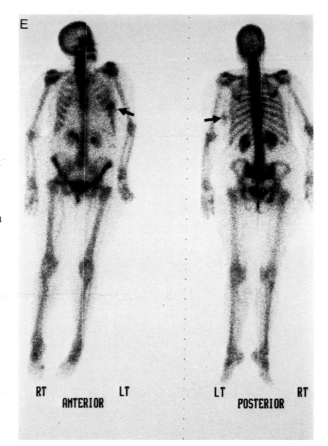

Figure 29–17E. Unilateral breast uptake: Adenocarcinoma of breast with metaplasia.

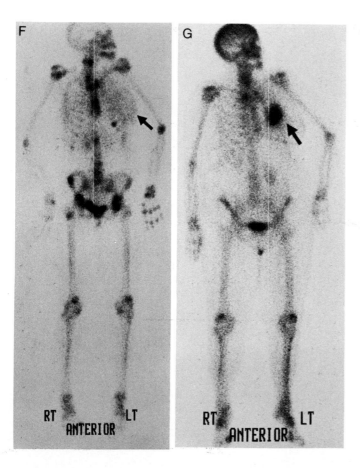

Figure 29–17F **and** *G.* Unilateral breast uptake: *F,* mastectomy contralateral breast; *G,* Chronic inflammation around prosthesis.

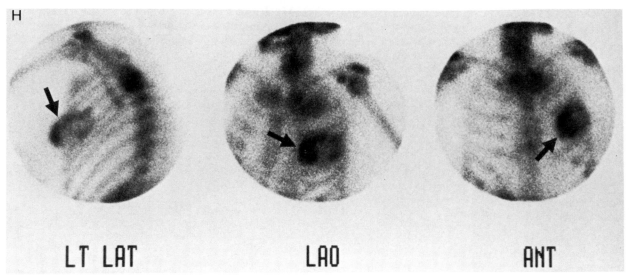

Figure 29–17H. Spot views of G.

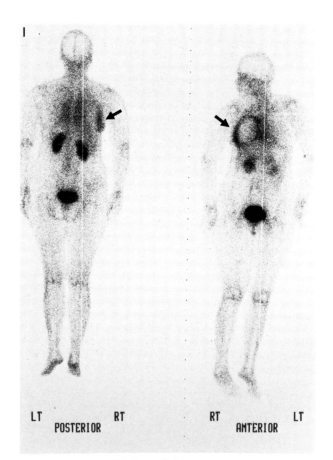

Figure 29–17I. Unilateral breast uptake: Rim sign; inflammation around prosthesis.

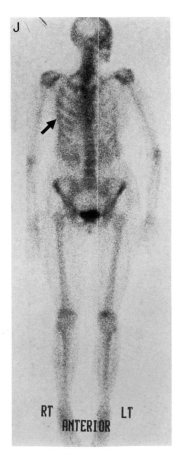

Figure 29–17J. Improved rib visualization due to mastectomy.

Figure 29–18. BONE SOFT-TISSUE SCINTIGRAPHIC CHANGES DUE TO LYMPHATIC OBSTRUCTION. Asymmetric distribution of the radiopharmaceutical *(arrows)* is noted in the extremities of the two patients shown in *A* and *B*. This increased soft-tissue deposition of tracer is the result of lymphatic obstruction, which causes soft-tissue swelling, increased fluid accumulation, altered blood flow, or extravascular protein binding.

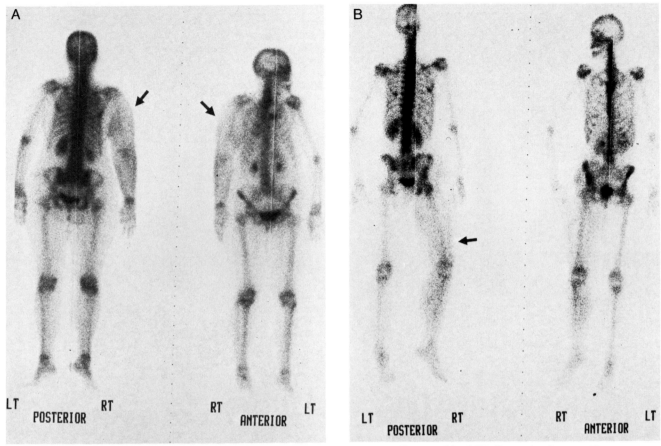

Figure 29–18A. Lymphedema of arm.   **Figure 29–18B.** Lymphedema of leg.

Ref.: Mandoli RS, Soin JS. Unilateral increased radioactivity in the lower extremities on routine 99mTc-pyrophosphate bone imaging. Clin Nucl Med 1978; 3:374–378.

Figure 29–19. EXTRA-OSSEOUS DEPOSITION OF PHOSPHATE BONE SCINTIGRAPHIC AGENTS. The visualization of extra-osseous localization of bone scintigraphic radiopharmaceuticals *(A–I, arrows)* is being identified with increasing frequency and over an increasing range of pathologic entities. The mechanism of soft-tissue deposition has not been precisely defined. Most pathologic processes are associated with either gross or microscopic calcification. Dystrophic areas of calcification may occur at sites of tissue injury, degeneration, or necrosis. Alteration in tissue pH or calcium/phosphorus metabolism may result in extra-osseous bone radiopharmaceutical deposition.

Ref.: Heck LL. Extra-osseous localization of phosphate bone agents. Semin Nucl Med 1980; 10:311–312.

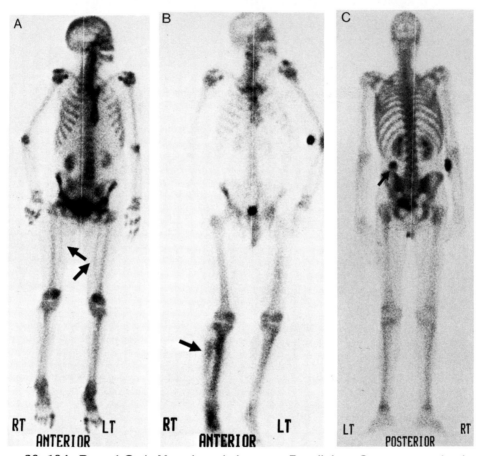

Figure 29–19A, B, and C. A, Vascular calcifications; *B,* cellulitis; *C,* psoas muscle abscess.

Illustration continued on opposite page

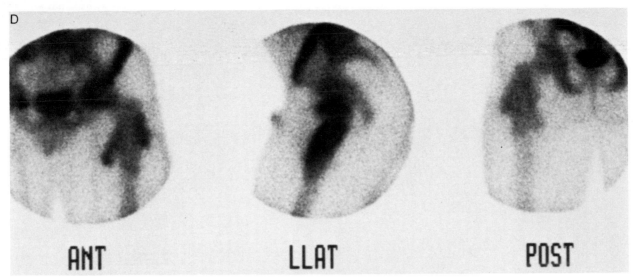

Figure 29–19D. Myositis ossificans.

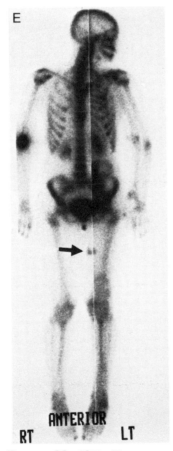

Figure 29–19E. Trauma-induced myositis ossificans.

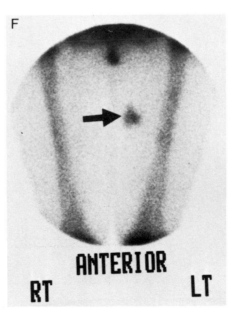

Figure 29–19F. Spot image of *E.*

Illustration continued on following page

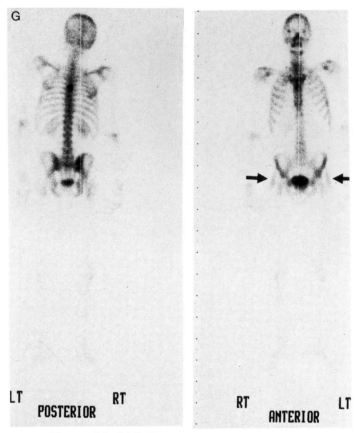

Figure 29–19G. Exertional rhabdomyolysis.

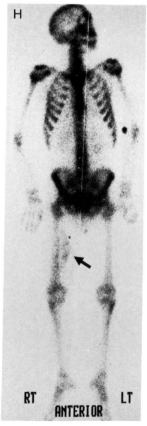

Figure 29–19H. Soft-tissue rhabdomyosarcoma.

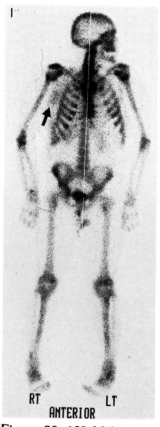

Figure 29–19I. Melanoma.

Figure 29–20. DIFFUSE PULMONARY ACCUMULATION OF BONE TRACER. The mechanism of soft-tissue localization of bone radiopharmaceuticals remains to be defined. Postulated mechanisms include adsorption onto hydroxyapatite crystal, immature collagen, extravascular diffusion secondary to altered capillary permeability, and adsorption onto intracellular calcium. Unilateral diffuse pulmonary concentration is frequently associated with malignant pleural effusion *(A, arrows)* and radiation therapy *(B, arrows)*.

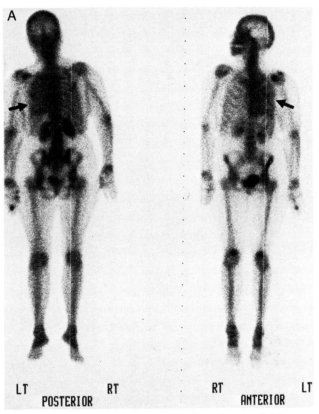

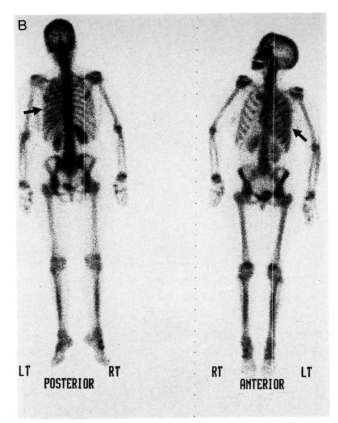

Figure 29–20A. Pulmonary accumulation: Malignant effusion; breast carcinoma.

Figure 29–20B. Pulmonary accumulation: Radiation.

Ref.: Sarreck R, Sham R, Alexander LL, Cortez EP. Increased 99mTc-pyrophosphate uptake with radiation pneumonitis. Clin Nucl Med 1979; 4:403–404.

Figure 29–21. HEPATIC VISUALIZATION DURING BONE SCINTIGRAPHY. Diffuse or focal accumulation of Tc-99m phosphate radiopharmaceuticals has been observed infrequently during bone scintigraphy. Focal uptake is most often associated with hepatic metastasis, such as those from oat cell carcinoma of the lung, malignant melanoma, squamous cell carcinoma of the esophagus, adenocarcinoma of the colon, and breast carcinoma (*B–D*). The precise mechanism of localization of bone radiopharmaceuticals remains unknown. Multiple factors are likely responsible, including tumor type, calcium deposition, phosphate binding, phosphate enzyme concentration, and altered calcium metabolism. The most frequent cause of diffuse hepatic visualization on bone scintigrams is a prior liver spleen study *(A)*. Faint hepatic visualization has been identified up to 48 hours after hepatic imaging. Faulty radiopharmaceutical preparation is an unusual but important cause and probably results from microcolloid formation of the phosphate compound. These microcolloids upon injection localize in the microvasculature of major organs such as kidneys, lung, and liver *(E)*.

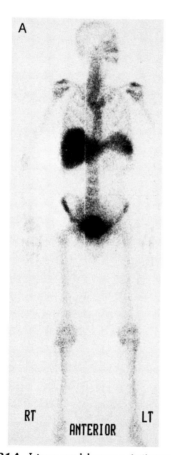

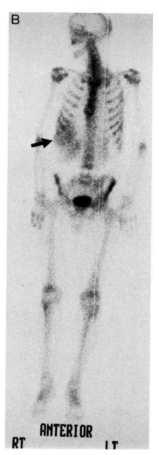

Figure 29–21A. Liver and bone scintigrams were performed on the same day.

Figure 29–21B. Colon carcinoma metastasis (*arrow*) to liver.

Illustration continued on opposite page

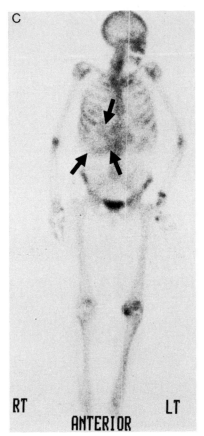

Figure 29–21C. Breast carcinoma metastasis (*arrows*) to liver.

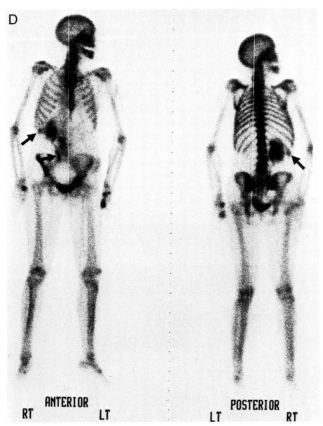

Figure 29–21D. Ovarian carcinoma metastasis (*arrows*) to liver and periaortic nodes; right hydronephrosis.

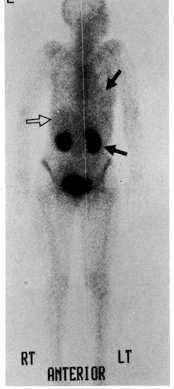

Figure 29–21E. Improper radiopharmaceutical preparation: Microcolloid formation (*open arrow,* liver; *solid arrow at upper right,* lung; *solid arrow at lower right,* kidney).

Refs.: (1) Hansen S, Stadalnik RC. Liver uptake of Tc-99m pyrophosphate. Semin Nucl Med 1982; 12:89–91. (2) Guiberteau MJ, Postaid MS, McKusick KA. Accumulation of Tc-99m diphosphonate in four patients with hepatic neoplasm: Case reports. J Nucl Med 1978; 3:355–358.

Figure 29–22. RENAL ABNORMALITIES IDENTIFIED DURING BONE SCINTIGRAPHY.
Renal excretion of Tc-99m methylene diphosphonate is approximately 30 to 50 per cent of the
injected dose during the imaging interval and tends to diminish with age. Due to this high extraction
rate by the kidneys, renal abnormalities are frequently identified as an incidental finding. Illustrated
are but a few of the renal abnormalities *(A–J, arrows)* that have been identified during routine
bone scintigraphy.

Ref.: Park CH, Glassman LM, Thompson NL, et al. Reliability of renal imaging obtained incidentally in 99m Tc-
polyphosphate bone scanning. J Nucl Med 1973; 14:534–536.

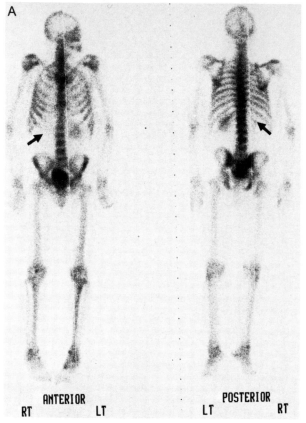

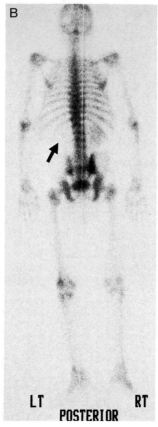

Figure 29–22A. Unilateral renal visualization: Nephrectomy.

Figure 29–22B. Unilateral renal visualization: Radiation damage.

Illustration continued on opposite page

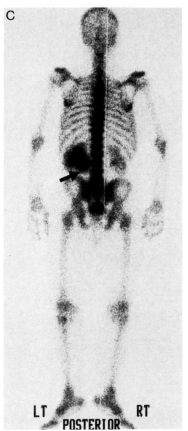

Figure 29–22C. Asymmetric renal visualization: Obstructed kidney.

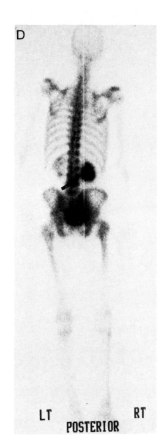

Figure 29–22D. Asymmetric renal visualization: Obstructed kidney.

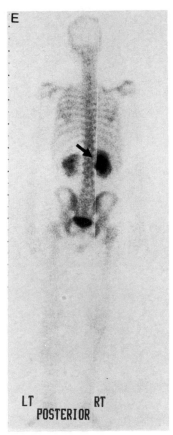

Figure 29–22E. Asymmetric renal visualization: Obstructed kidney.

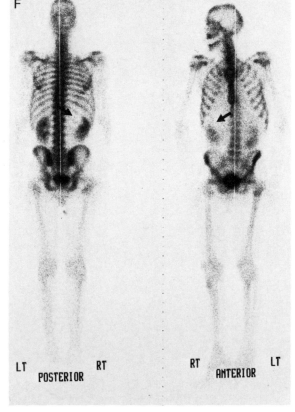

Figure 29–22F. Deviation of renal axis: Mass effect.
Illustration continued on following page

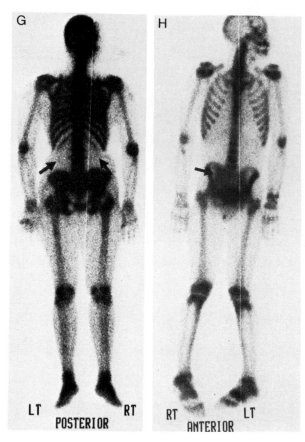

Figure 29–22G and H. G, Bilateral absent renal visualization (*arrow*): Renal failure. *H*, Renal transplant: Kidney in right pelvis (*arrow*).

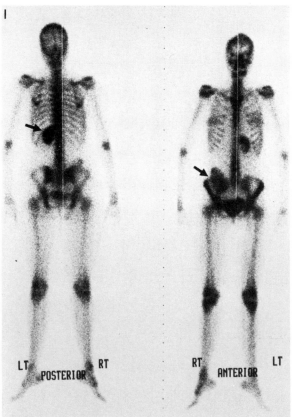

Figure 29–22I. Renal transplant (*arrow*, anterior view): Tracer localization in native kidney (*arrow*, posterior view).

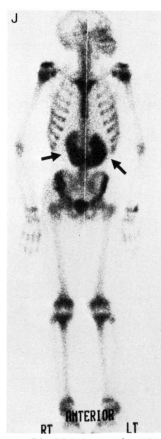

Figure 29–22J. Horseshoe kidney (*arrow*).

Figure 29–23. UROLOGIC ABNORMALITIES AND ARTIFACTS. Urologic abnormalities are frequently demonstrated during bone scintigraphy (*A–G, arrows*). Iatrogenic causes can also be identified (*H*, arrows). The ability to detect renal, ureteral, and bladder abnormalities is due to the high renal extraction of bone-seeking radiopharmaceuticals. Abnormalities identified during bone scintigraphy should be clinically correlated and radiographically evaluated when indicated.

Refs.: (1) Brill DR. Radionuclide imaging of nonneoplastic soft tissue disorders. Semin Nucl Med 1981; 11:277–288. (2) Park CH, Glassman LM, Thompson NL, et al. Reliability of renal imaging obtained incidentally in 99m Tc-polyphosphate bone scanning. J Nucl Med 1973; 14:534–536.

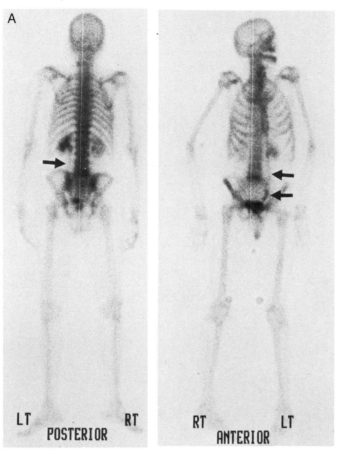

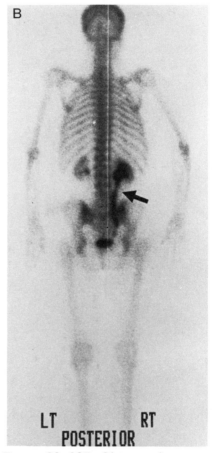

Figure 29–23A. Megaureter: Collimation of radiopharmaceutical in ureter.

Figure 29–23B. Obstructed ureter.

Illustration continued on following page

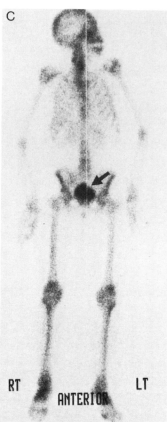

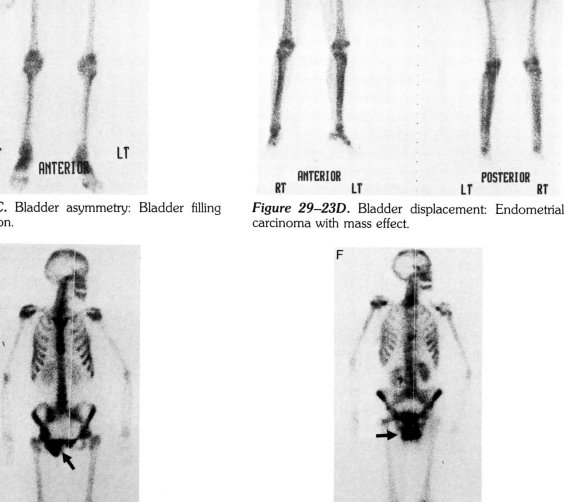

Figure 29–23C. Bladder asymmetry: Bladder filling during acquisition.

Figure 29–23D. Bladder displacement: Endometrial carcinoma with mass effect.

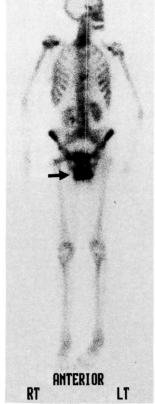

Figure 29–23E. Bladder prolapse: Postsurgery.

Figure 29–23F. Cystocele.

Illustration continued on opposite page

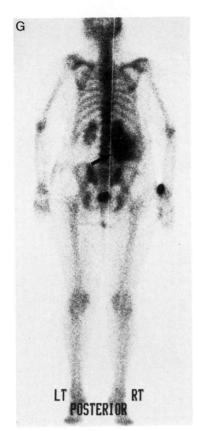

Figure 29–23G. Lacerated ureter with urine extravasation.

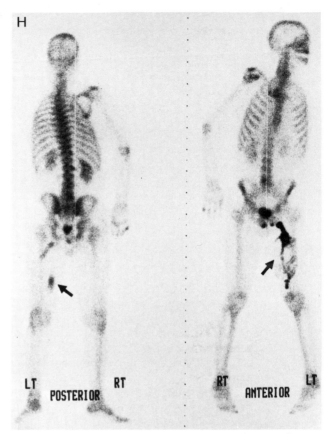

Figure 29–23H. Foley catheter and collecting bag.

Gallium-67 Imaging

FREDERICK L. WEILAND, M.D.
FREDERIC A. CONTE, M.D.
JOSEPH A. ORZEL, M.D.
ALBERT S. HALE, M.D.

Figure 30–1. NORMAL PATTERNS OF ADULT GALLIUM-67 CITRATE LOCALIZATION (MULTIPLANE TOMOGRAPHIC SCANNER). The normal gallium-67 scintigram is variable and depends upon the interval between injection of the radiopharmaceutical and imaging, in addition to the age of the patient and the patient's sex. Gallium-67 is cleared from the blood relatively slowly, with 20 per cent of the tracer remaining at 24 hours, which is reflected in the soft-tissue concentration noted at this time. Renal and bladder accumulation is often noted at 24 hours, due to the rapid renal clearance of gallium-67 citrate (A and B), whereas colonic activity is normally absent. Renal localization should be absent on subsequent images at 48 and 72 hours (E), and, if present, requires further evaluation. Colonic accumulation steadily increases as time elapses, due to bowel excretion of the radiopharmaceutical (C). Symmetric breast localization is a frequent scintigraphic finding in female patients (D). Uptake is usually noted in the nasal mucosa and, on occasion, faint visualization can be seen in the lacrimal and parotid glands. The images of the thorax may demonstrate the sternum, rib, and spine. Faint pulmonic visualization at 24 hours is due to blood pool activity and should be less than that of adjacent soft tissue at 48 hours. The liver is invariably visualized and increases in intensity over time; the spleen may or may not be identified. Colonic accumulation is unusual at 6 hours and has been associated with inflammatory bowel disease; however, colonic accumulation at 48 or 72 hours is considered normal.

Ref.: Larson SM, Hoffer PB. Normal patterns of localization. In: Hoffer PB, Bekerman C, Henkin RE, eds. Gallium-67 Imaging. New York: John Wiley and Sons, 1978; pp 23–38.

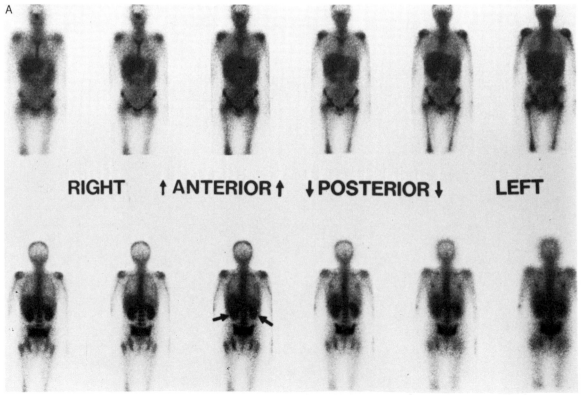

RIGHT ↑ **ANTERIOR** ↑ ↓ **POSTERIOR** ↓ **LEFT**

Figure 30–1A. 24-Hour study with renal visualization (*arrows*).

Illustration continued on opposite page

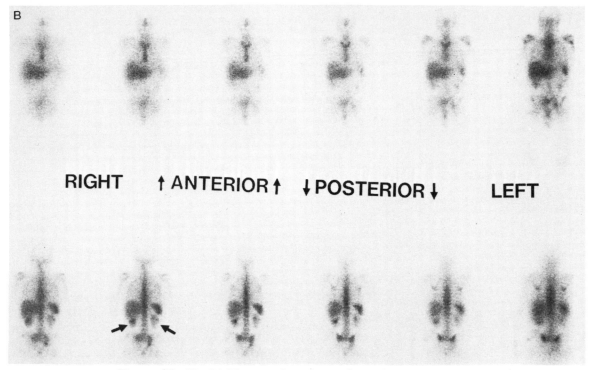

Figure 30–1B. 24-Hour study with renal visualization (*arrows*).

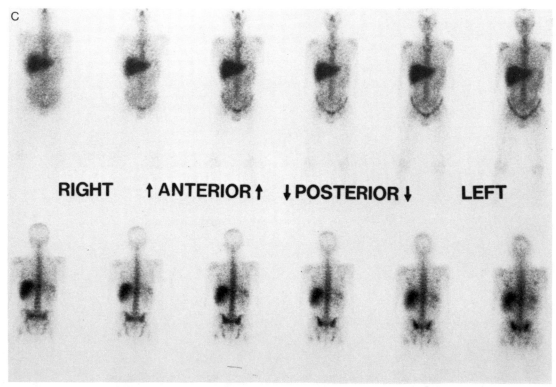

Figure 30–1C. 48-Hour study without bowel visualization.

Illustration continued on following page

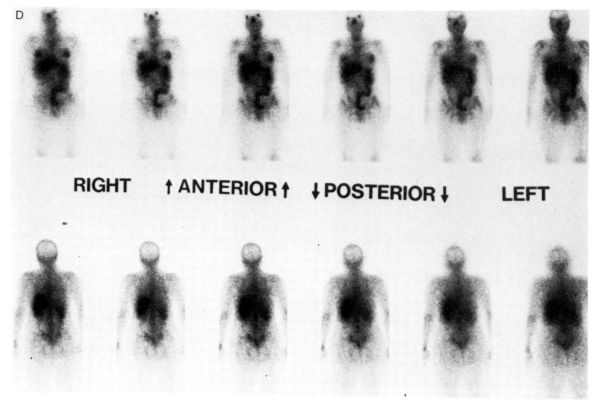

RIGHT   ↑ ANTERIOR ↑   ↓ POSTERIOR ↓   LEFT

Figure 30–1D. 48-Hour study: Breast and bowel accumulation.

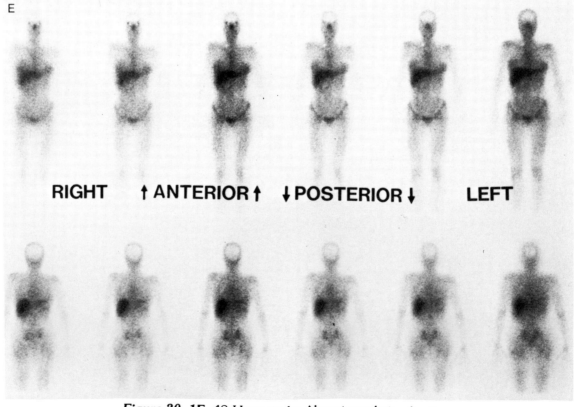

RIGHT   ↑ ANTERIOR ↑   ↓ POSTERIOR ↓   LEFT

Figure 30–1E. 48-Hour study: Absent renal visualization.

Figure 30–2. NORMAL PATTERNS OF PEDIATRIC GALLIUM-67 CITRATE LOCALIZATION. The pediatric gallium-67 scintigram differs somewhat from that of an adult. Increased activity may be found in the epiphyseal regions (*arrow,* posterior image). The precise location of gallium-67 deposition in the epiphysis remains unclear and may be in the bone matrix, cartilaginous structures, or adjacent marrow. The more active the growth, the more prominent the uptake. Normal thymic accumulation of gallium-67 may occur (*arrow,* anterior image). This increases interpretation difficulty if the mediastinum is being evaluated for a pathologic process. For unknown reasons, bowel accumulation of gallium-67 is less, rendering the abdomen easier to evaluate.

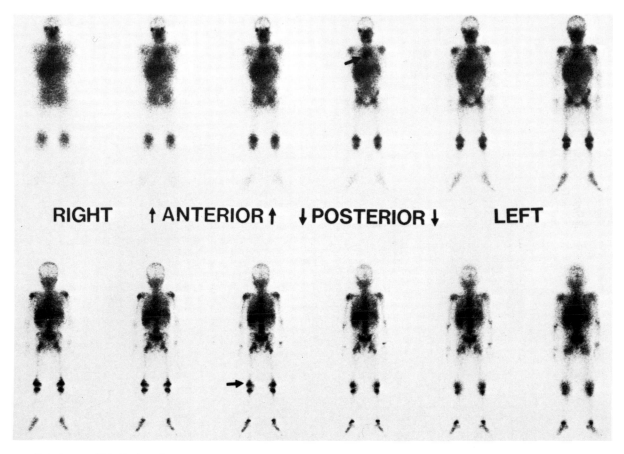

RIGHT   ↑ **ANTERIOR** ↑   ↓ **POSTERIOR** ↓   **LEFT**

Ref.: Larson SM, Hoffer PB. Normal patterns of localization. In: Hoffer PB, Bekerman C, Henkin RE, eds. Gallium-67 Imaging. New York: John Wiley and Sons, 1978; pp 23–38.

Figure 30–3. COLONIC ACCUMULATION AND MOVEMENT OF GALLIUM-67 CITRATE.
Colonic accumulation of gallium-67 is frequently present on scintigraphic images 48 *(A, arrows)*
and 72 *(B, arrows)* hours postinjection. This increases the difficulty in detecting abdominal lesions.
Bowel activity is variable from patient to patient and is generally less in the pediatric age group.
The use of a bowel preparation or cathartic preceding or during the examination remains
controversial. This results from reports that bowel preparation is ineffectual in eliminating colonic
activity. Our approach is to use a bowel preparation if colonic activity obscures a region of the
abdomen under evaluation or when confusion exists as to whether a focus of tracer localization is
within bowel. *A* and *B* demonstrate movement of colonic gallium after magnesia of citrate
administration.

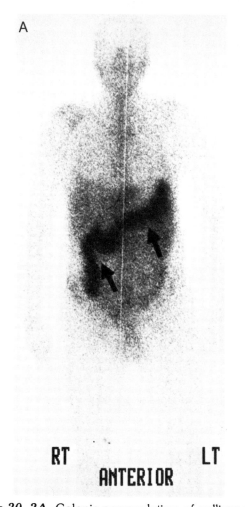

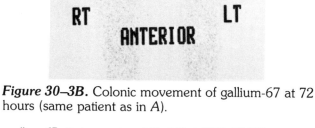

Figure 30–3A. Colonic accumulation of gallium-67 at 48 hours.

Figure 30–3B. Colonic movement of gallium-67 at 72 hours (same patient as in *A*).

Ref.: Zeman R, Reyerson T. The value of bowel preparation in gallium-67 citrate scanning. J Nucl Med 1976; 17:559 (Abstract).

Figure 30–4. BREAST DISTRIBUTION OF GALLIUM-67 CITRATE. Prominent gallium-67 citrate accumulation may occur normally in the breast. This finding is most frequently observed when the breasts are under the physiologic stimulus of cyclic estrogens or progestational agents such as oral contraceptives or during menarche *(A and B).* Kim and colleagues found gallium-67 localization in normal breast tissue in 12 per cent of female patients undergoing gallium-67 scintigraphy. Uptake in the normal breast is always symmetric. Gallium-67 citrate is excreted in breast milk as a result of gallium-67 binding to lactoferrin. The uptake of gallium-67 in the lactating female is extremely intense *(C).* Unilateral uptake of gallium in the breast may suggest a pathologic process and should always be investigated further; *D* demonstrates this unilateral gallium-67 citrate concentration in breast carcinoma and involved lymph nodes. The use of gallium-67 for the detection of primary or metastatic breast carcinoma has not been rewarding. The reported sensitivity for the detection of primary or metastatic disease is approximately 52 per cent.

Ref.: Kim Y, Brown M, and Thrall J. Scintigraphic patterns of gallium-67 uptake in the breast. Radiology 1977; 124:169–175.

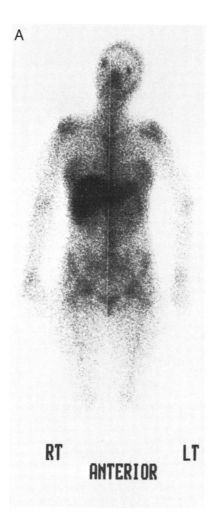

Figure 30–4A. Bilateral breast accumulation: Normal.

Illustration continued on following page

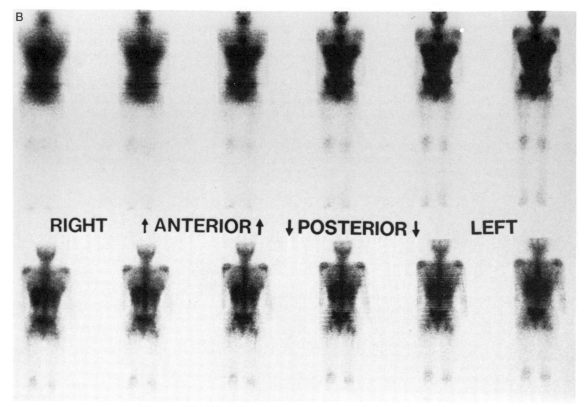

Figure 30–4B. Bilateral breast accumulation: Normal.

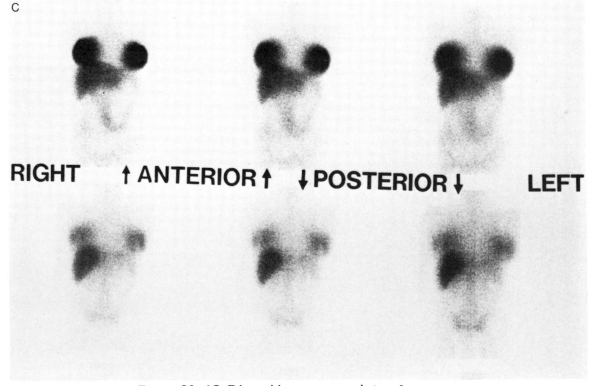

Figure 30–4C. Bilateral breast accumulation: Lactation.

Illustration continued on opposite page

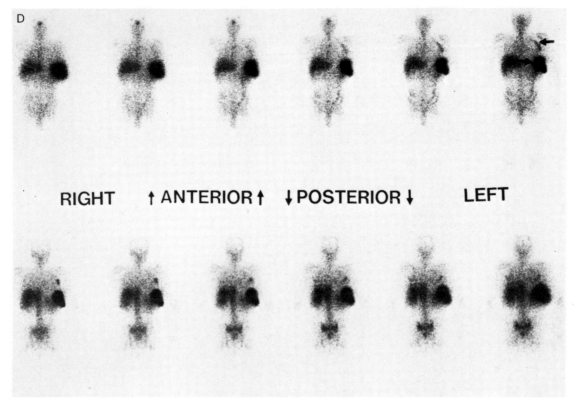

Figure 30–4D. Unilateral breast accumulation: Breast carcinoma.

Figure 30–5. GALLIUM-67 ACCUMULATION AT SURGICAL INCISION SITES. Gallium-67 will accumulate in areas of recent surgical incisions *(A and B, arrows).* This reflects localization of the radiopharmaceutical at sites of normal healing. Uptake in a surgical wound beyond the second or third operative week requires further investigation to exclude wound infection. Surgical incision sites are usually easy to identify due to their linear appearance. Oblique or lateral scintigraphic images may be obtained to demonstrate the superficial nature of tracer localization and to evaluate areas obscured by the incision site.

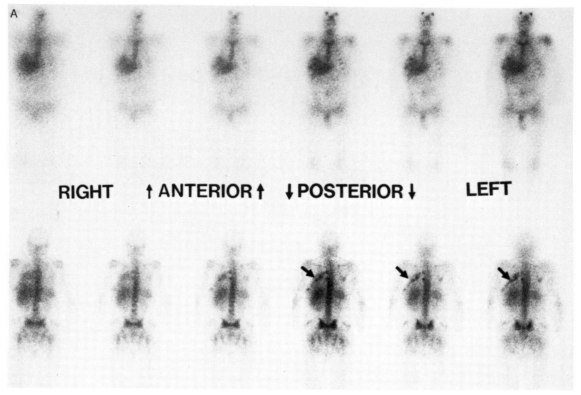

Figure 30–5A. Gallium-67 accumulation: Thoracotomy scar.

Illustration continued on opposite page

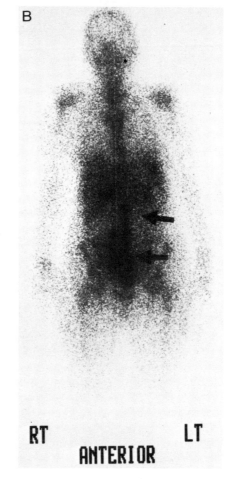

Figure 30–5B. Gallium-67 accumulation: Abdominal incision.

Ref.: Henkin RE. Gallium-67 in the diagnosis of inflammatory disease. In: Hoffer PB, Bekerman C, Henkin RE, eds. Gallium-67 Imaging. New York: John Wiley and Sons, 1978; pp 65–92.

Figure 30–6. IATROGENIC ALTERATIONS IN GALLIUM-67 BIODISTRIBUTION: INJECTION SITES. Gallium-67 is frequently noted in postoperative surgical incision sites for two to three weeks following surgery. On occasion, minimal tissue injury such as that which occurs following intramuscular injections (A and B, arrows), pressure abrasions (C, arrows), or cellulitis may localize gallium-67 citrate.

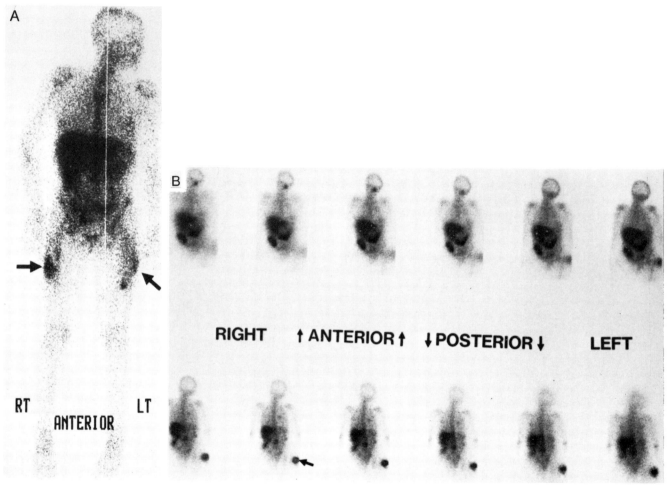

Figure 30–6A. Intramuscular injection sites.

Figure 30–6B. Intramuscular injection site: Abscess.

Illustration continued on opposite page

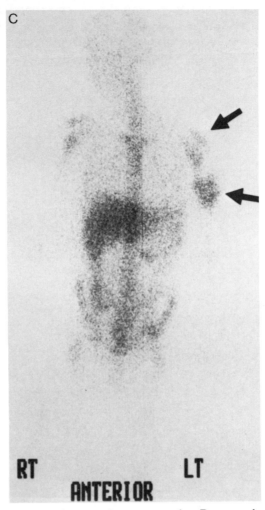

Figure 30–6C. Proximal arm soft tissue uptake: Pressure lesion from cast.

Ref.: Jackson FI, Dierich HC, Lentle BC. Gallium-67 citrate scintiscanning in testicular neoplasia. J Can Assoc Radiol 1976; 27:84–88.

Figure 30–7. RADIATION-INDUCED IATROGENIC ALTERATIONS IN GALLIUM-67 BIO-DISTRIBUTION. Radiation-induced sialadenitis has been associated with head and neck irradiation. It is characterized by intense localization of the radiopharmaceutical in the salivary glands *(A).* This sialadenitis has been reported to last up to 3 years. Irradiation for breast carcinoma, lung carcinoma or lymphoma may result in radiation pneumonitis and sialadenitis *(B).* Radiation-induced thyroiditis is an unusual complication in patients receiving irradiation for lymphoma. The patient shown in *C* had a repeat gallium-67 scintigram *(D)* on a follow-up study 11 months later, with absence of gallium localization in the thyroid. At this time, the patient had become hypothyroid. Of greater concern is the possibility of local irradiation decreasing the detectability of remote lesions. This occurs as a result of release of iron from irradiated tissue, which saturates transferrin, displacing gallium-67. The transferrin–galllium-67 transport mechanism is important in the delivery of circulating gallium-67 to sites of tumor or inflammation.

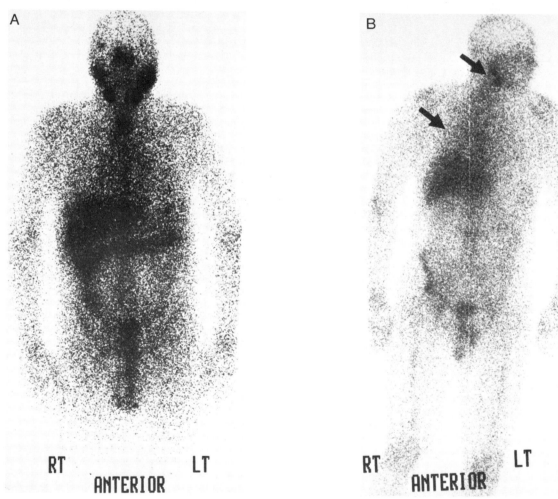

Figure 30–7A. Radiation-induced sialadenitis.

Figure 30–7B. Radiation-induced pneumonitis (*lower arrow*) and sialadenitis (*upper arrow*).

Illustration continued on opposite page

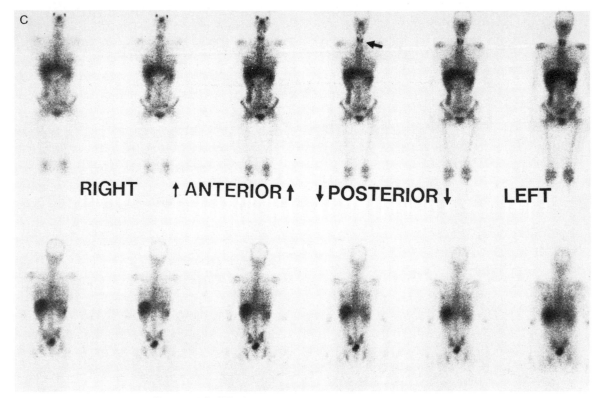

Figure 30–7C. Radiation-induced thyroiditis *(arrow)*.

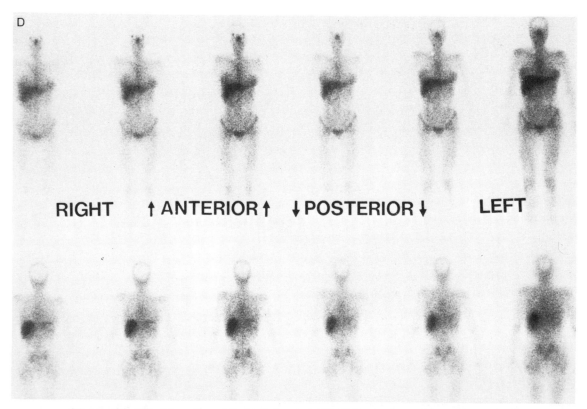

Figure 30–7D. Hypothyroidism eleven months later in the patient shown in C.

Refs.: (1) Van der Schoot JB, Groen AS, DeJong J. Gallium-67 scintigraphy in lung diseases. Thorax 1972; 27:543–546.
(2) Lentle BC, Jackson FI, McGowan DG. Localization of gallium-67 citrate in salivary glands following radiation therapy. J Can Assoc Radiol 1976; 27:89–91.

Figure 30–8. IATROGENIC ALTERATIONS IN GALLIUM-67 BIODISTRIBUTION: LYM-PHANGIOGRAPHIC CONTRAST AGENTS. Diffuse pulmonary accumulation of gallium-67 citrate has been reported in patients who had gallium-67 scintigrams within several days of lymphangiography. The oily contrast medium used results in a chemical pneumonitis, as demonstrated below, which is believed to be responsible for the gallium-67 deposition.

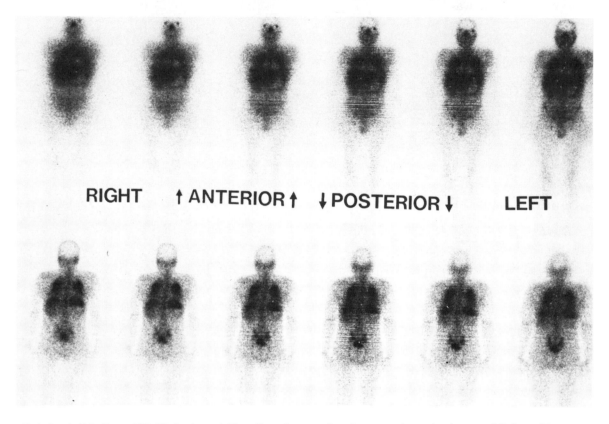

RIGHT ↑ ANTERIOR ↑ ↓ POSTERIOR ↓ LEFT

Ref.: Lentle BC, Castor WR, Khalig A, et al. The effect of contrast lymphangiography on localization of Gallium-67 citrate. J Nucl Med 1975; 16:374–376.

Figure 30–9. *IATROGENIC ALTERATIONS IN GALLIUM-67 BIODISTRIBUTION: CIS-PLATINUM.* Chemotherapeutic agents such as cis-platinum at a dosage of 20 mg/m² have been reported to result in unusual tracer biodistribution of gallium-67 up to two weeks post-administration. Scintigraphic findings include high blood tracer concentration with minimal or no radiopharmaceutical in the liver. Cis-platinum is nephrotoxic; however, 2 of 14 patients in which this abnormal gallium-67 pattern was reported had no clinical evidence of nephrotoxicity. The mechanism responsible for this tracer biodistribution has yet to be elucidated.

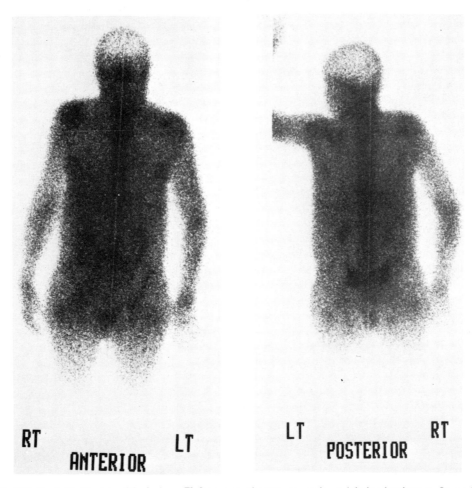

Ref.: Lentle BC, Scott JR, Noujaim AA, Jackson FI. Iatrogenic alterations in radionuclide biodistribution. Semin Nucl Med 1979; 9:131–143.

Figure 30–10. IATROGENIC ALTERATIONS IN GALLIUM-67 BIODISTRIBUTION: BLEO-MYCIN LUNG. Although numerous chemotherapeutic agents are suspected of producing pulmonary interstitial fibrosis, only bleomycin has been associated with pulmonary localization of gallium-67 citrate, as demonstrated below. The pulmonary toxicity of bleomycin is not strictly dose-related. It may be both a toxic reaction that develops into pulmonary interstitial fibrosis or an acute hypersensitivity reaction that is steroid responsive. It remains to be determined if the pulmonary accumulation of gallium-67 is a result of the toxic or hypersensitivity reaction or both.

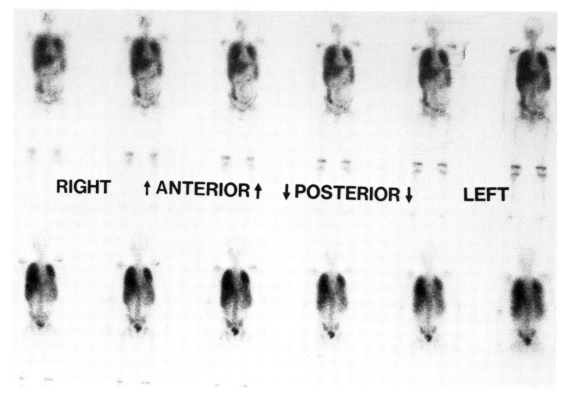

Ref.: Richman SD, Levenson SM, Bunn PA, et al. Gallium-67 accumulation in pulmonary lesions associated with bleomycin toxicity. Cancer 1975; 36:1966–1972.

Figure 30–11. IATROGENIC ALTERATIONS IN GALLIUM-67 BIODISTRIBUTION: BCG SYSTEMIC GRANULOMATOSIS. BCG has been administered orally and by scarification to induce a non-specific immune response in the treatment of melanoma patients. It has been reported that patients treated by scarification may develop a systemic bacteremia resulting in BCG granuloma and pneumonitis of the lung and cutaneous granulomatosis. Gallium-67 localization has been observed both diffusely in the lung and, as in this patient, in cutaneous granulomas.

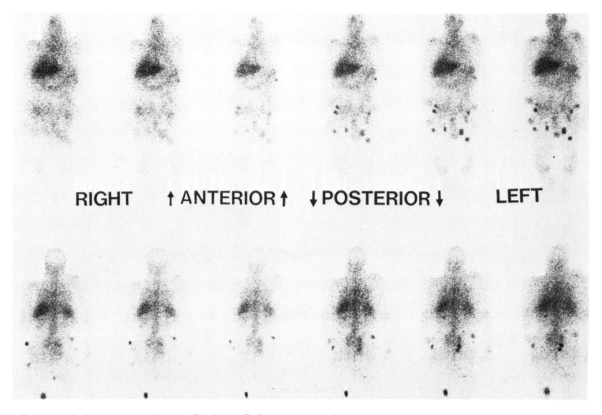

Ref.: Bilgi C, Brown NE, McPherson TA, Lentle B. Pulmonary manifestations in patients with malignant melanoma during BCG immunotherapy. A preliminary report. Chest 1979; 75:685–687.

Figure 30–12. EXTERNAL PHOTON-DEFICIENT ARTIFACTS ON GALLIUM-67 SCINTI-GRAMS. As with all nuclear medicine procedures, external objects markedly attenuate the photon flux of the radiopharmaceutical as illustrated in *A–C*. Photon-deficient lesions due to pathologic processes are extremely rare. Identification of a photon-deficient lesion on a gallium-67 scintigram is most likely artifactual. Clinical examination and history should readily clarify any artifactual abnormality.

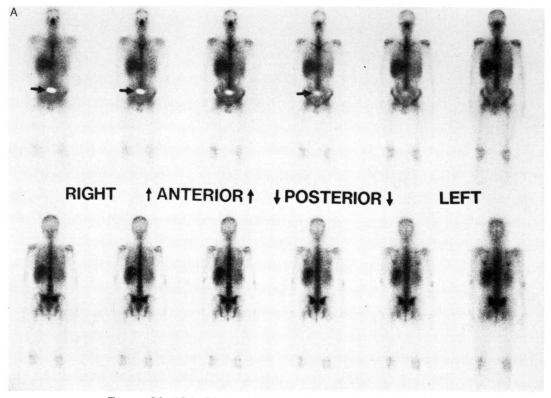

Figure 30–12A. Photon-deficient abnormality: Belt buckle.

Illustration continued on opposite page

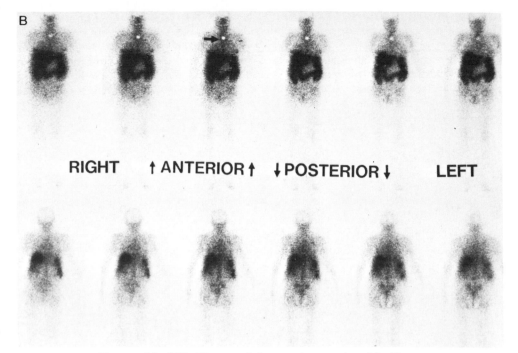

RIGHT   ↑ **ANTERIOR** ↑   ↓ **POSTERIOR** ↓   **LEFT**

Figure 30–12B. Photon-deficient abnormality: Necklace.

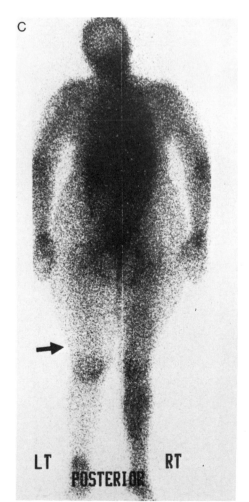

Figure 30–12C. Asymmetric lower extremity attenuation: Cast on leg.

Figure 30–13. MANIFESTATION OF GALLIUM-67 IN SARCOIDOSIS. Faint visualization of gallium-67 citrate in the lacrimal and parotid glands may be observed on normal gallium-67 images. A caveat of gallium-67 imaging is that in a patient who has not received irradiation, gallium-67 accumulation in both the parotids and lung indicates sarcoidosis until proven otherwise *(A and B).* Additionally, gallium-67 imaging offers the evaluation of unsuspected extrapulmonic involvement *(C, arrows).* Gallium-67 uptake in sarcoidosis correlates extremely well with histologic findings. Gallium-67 scintigraphy has been utilized successfully as a noninvasive method to evaluate the success of therapy.

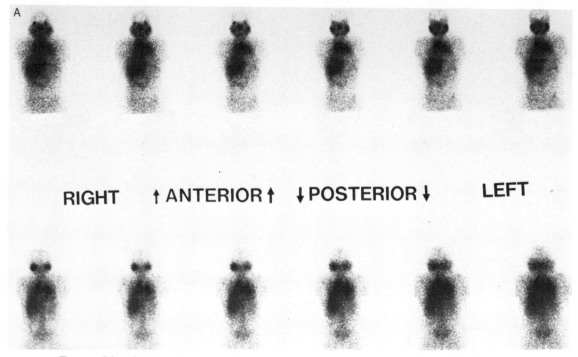

RIGHT ↑ ANTERIOR ↑ ↓ POSTERIOR ↓ LEFT

Figure 30–13A. Sarcoidosis: Parotid and pulmonary accumulation of gallium-67.

Illustration continued on opposite page

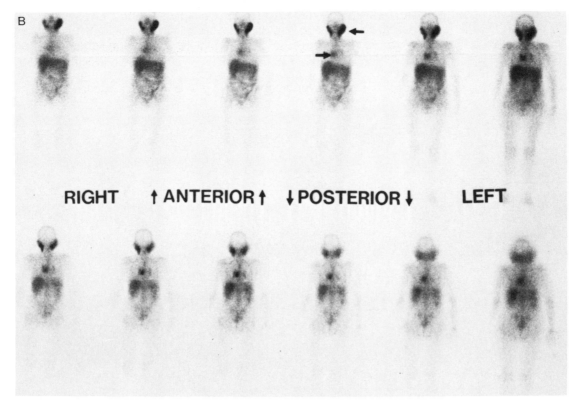

Figure 30–13B. Sarcoidosis: Parotid (*upper arrow*) and mediastinal (*lower arrow*) accumulation of gallium-67.

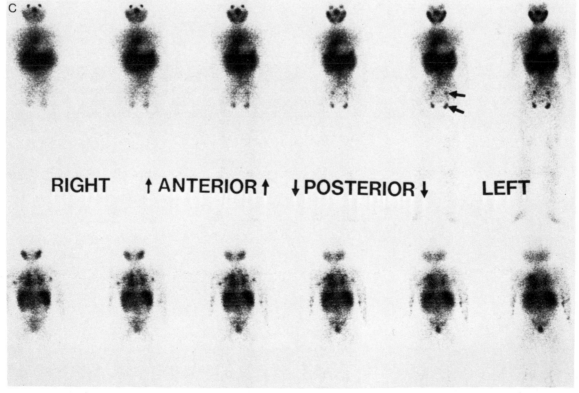

Figure 30–13C. Sarcoidosis: Accumulation in the parotid glands, lungs, lacrimal glands, and inguinal nodes (*arrows*).

Refs.: (1) Heshiki A, Schatz SL, McKusick KA, et al.: Galllium-67 scanning in patients with pulmonary sarcoidosis. Am J Roentgenol 1974; 122:744–749. (2) Niden AH, Mishkin FS, Khurana M. Use of Gallium-67 lung scan to assess pathologic activity of pulmonary sarcoidosis. Am Rev Resp Dis 1976; 113:164 (Abstract).

Figure 30–14. DIFFUSE ABDOMINAL DISTRIBUTION OF GALLIUM-67 CITRATE DUE TO PERITONITIS. Peritonitis is characterized by a diffuse abdominal distribution of gallium-67 citrate (*illustrated below*). In peritonitis, gallium-67 is often not limited by anatomic barriers of the abdominal cavity. Gallium-67 citrate has been found to be superior in the detection of peritonitis and phlegmons when compared to CT or ultrasound. However, CT and ultrasound are much more sensitive in detecting formed abscesses in the abdomen.

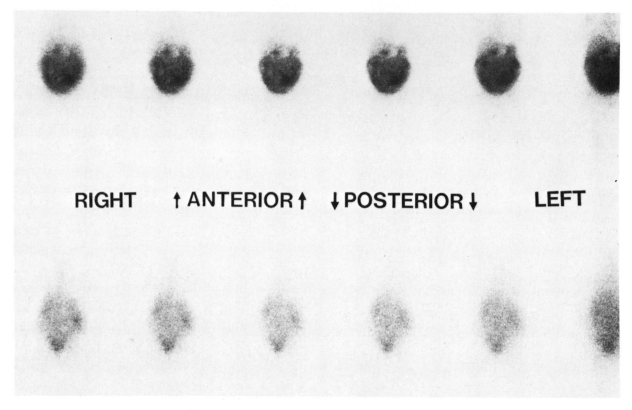

RIGHT   ↑ ANTERIOR ↑   ↓ POSTERIOR ↓   LEFT

Refs.: (1) Myerson PJ, Myerson D, Spencer RP. Anatomic patterns of gallium-67 distribution in localized and diffuse peritoneal inflammation. J Nucl Med 1977; 18:977–980. (2) Shimshak RR, Korobkin M, Hoffer PB, et al. The complementary role of gallium citrate imaging and computed tomography in the evaluation of suspected abdominal infection. J Nucl Med 1978; 19:262–269. (3) Korobkin M, Callen PW, Filly RA, et al. Comparison of computed tomography ultrasonography, and gallium-67 scanning in the evaluation of suspected abdominal abscess. Radiology 1978; 129:89–93.

IV

MAGNETIC RESONANCE IMAGING (MRI)

Head

WILLIAM M. KELLY, M.D.

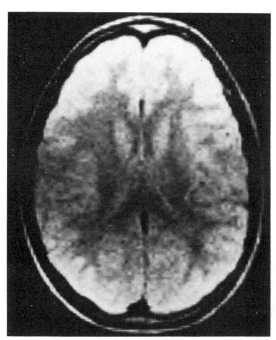

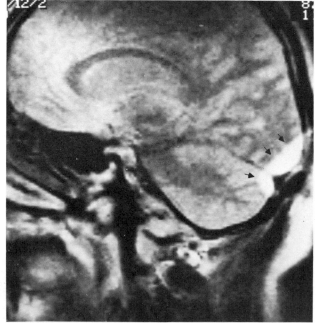

Figure 31–1. NONUNIFORM SIGNAL RECEPTION RELATED TO COIL DESIGN. Normal tissue in the frontal and occipital regions is displayed with greater signal intensity than at the lateral convexities. This is an artifact due to nonuniformity of signal reception by the RF antennae (cylindrical coil in this instance) and the proximity of the anterior and posterior tissues to the coil surface. Calculated T_1 and T_2 values for both gray matter and white matter were normal and varied little throughout the cerebrum.

Figure 31–2. "ROLLOVER" DISPLAY ARTIFACT. A well-demarcated region of bright signal *(arrows)* is superimposed over the occipital and cerebellar cortex on this sagittal image. Close inspection reveals that this unlikely pattern for any form of pathologic involvement conforms in contour to the anterior facial anatomy (nose). This artifact occurs when the planar dimensions of the tissue slice exceed the field of view (FOV) selected. Peripheral tissue is redisplayed or "rolled over" onto the opposite edge of the image.

Figure 31–3. ARTIFACT FROM FERROMAGNETIC DENTAL APPLIANCES. On transaxial images shown in A and B, increased signal in the left frontal region might confuse an inexperienced observer and lead to an erroneous suspicion of pathology. Clues to recognition of this type of artifact include unusual patterns of distortion of the architectural anatomy of the brain rather than discrete compartmental mass effect, and bizarre zones of signal "abnormality" that do not respect the usual anatomic boundaries. Suspicion regarding the type of artifact shown in A and B often can be confirmed merely by questioning the patient concerning the presence of metallic implants (mostly commonly dental hardware such as stainless steel bridges or braces). Alternatively, an additional pulse sequence obtained in a different plane (C) may reveal the source of signal distortion. Ferromagnetic artifact usually causes a zone of signal void corresponding to the location of the metallic implant (C) bordered by a perimeter of artifactually increased signal intensity. If needed, a CT scout view (D) or limited radiographic survey can be used to identify the precise location and nature of metallic implants.

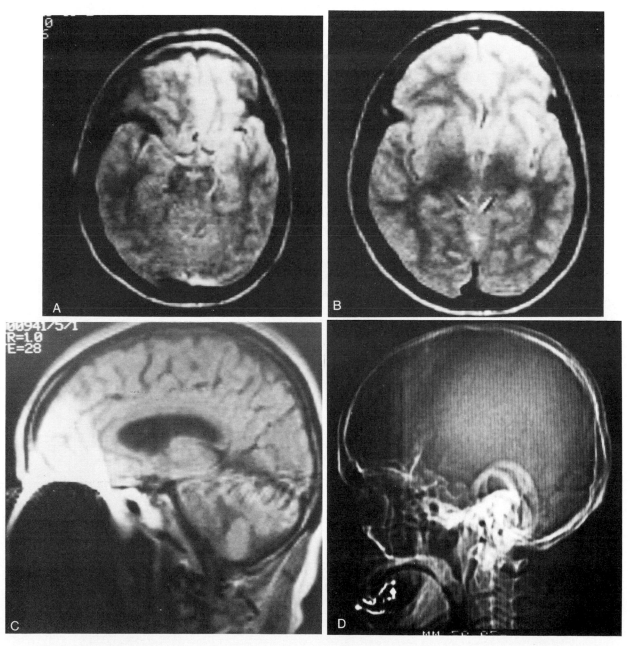

Ref.: New PFJ, Rosen BR, Brady TJ, et al. Potential hazards and artifacts of ferromagnetic and nonferromagnetic surgical and dental materials and devices in nuclear magnetic resonance imaging. Radiology 1983; 147:139–148.

Figure 31–4. MOTION ARTIFACT: HICCOUGHING. Repetitive episodes of reciprocating motion due to intractable hiccoughs resulted in multiple curvilinear artifacts *(A, arrows)* and anatomic blurring in an AIDS patient with mental status changes. Bihemispheric signal abnormalities due to herpes encephalitis remain visible on MRI *(A)* even though the right-sided involvement is not seen on a CT scan *(B)* that was not compromised by motion artifact. The crescents of increased signal demarcated by arrows actually represent partial reproductions of "ghost" images. This phenomenon of image harmonics is caused by the effects of motion on the acquisition and reconstruction methods utilized in the two-dimensional Fourier transform (2DFT) technique. The "ghosts" always appear in the phase encoding dimension (vertical, as in this instance) independent of the direction of motion. Cancellation and reinforcement of signal artifact results in partial copies of patient anatomy. The spacing between the partial copies (ghosts) is related both to instrument parameters (TR interval) and frequency of motion.

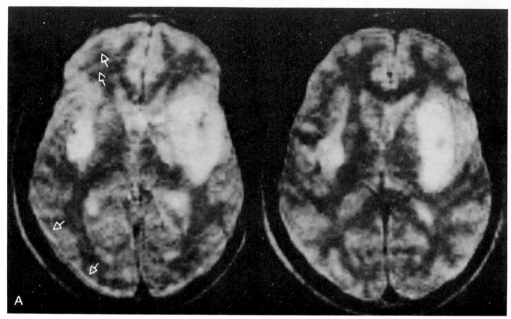

Figure 31–4A. MRI.

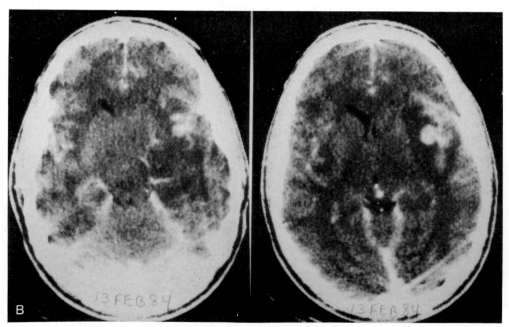

Figure 31–4B. CT scan.

Ref: Shultz CL, Alfidi RJ, Nelson AD, et al. The effect of motion on two-dimensional Fourier transformation magnetic resonance images. Radiology 1984; 152:117–121.

Figure 31–5. MOTION ARTIFACT: "PSEUDO–DOUBLE EXPOSURE." Slight movement of the neck occurred during the acquisition of this midsagittal image of a patient with a mixed solid/cystic cervical astrocytoma. The subject shifted once halfway through the pulse sequence and then maintained a slightly different position. Resulting displacement of anatomic interfaces along the upper vertebral body margins anteriorly creates the illusion of "double exposure." Also note multiple alternating bands of high and low signal intensity between the lower vertebral bodies, due to a component of axial motion at the endplate–disc margins. Blurring of edges or "pseudo–double exposure" assumes dominance over image harmonics (see Figure 31–4) as a manifestation of motion artifact when the underlying motion occurs only occasionally or especially as a single isolated event. Unlike "ghost images," this component of motion artifact is seen in the direction of motion, not necessarily the phase-encoding dimension.

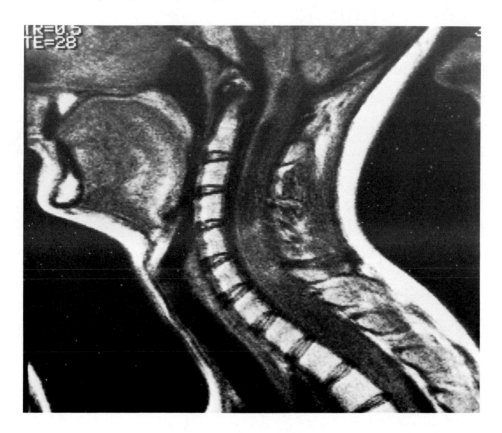

Figure 31–6. VENTROPERITONEAL SHUNT ARTIFACT SIMULATING CEREBROSPINAL FLUID SPREAD OF MEDULLOBLASTOMA. The patient is a 10-year-old child with recurrent medulloblastoma.

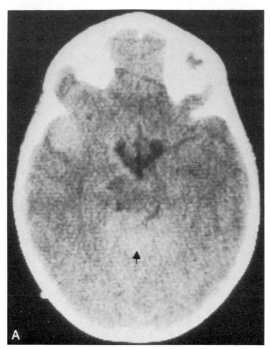

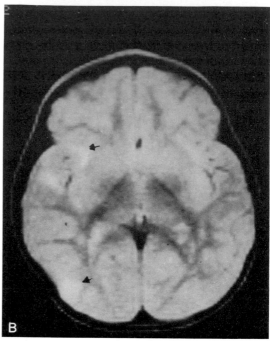

Figure 31–6A. The medulloblastoma *(arrow)* is visible on CT at its primary site near the superior vermis.

Figure 31–6B. On MRI, ferromagnetic artifact seen in the lower right parietal area is caused by the presence of metallic shunt tube hardware in the overlying scalp. The artifact produced closely resembles true signal abnormality due to cerebrospinal fluid spread of tumor *(arrows)* visible at the right sylvian fissure near the pterion.

From: Kucharczyk W, Brant-Zawadzki M, Sobel D, et al. Central nervous system tumors in children: detection by magnetic resonance imaging. Radiology 1985; 155:131–136. Reproduced with permission.

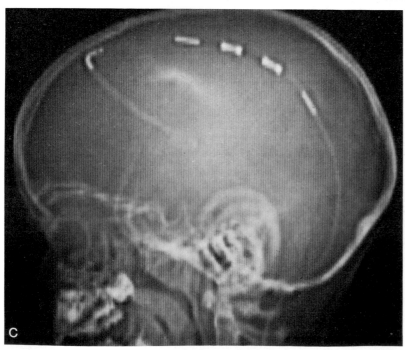

Figure 31–6C. Observer awareness of the presence and location of shunt tube hardware and, if needed, correlation with plain films, as shown here, may help avoid false-positive interpretations.

Figure 31–7. "CROSS-OVER" EFFECT LIMITING VISIBILITY OF ARACHNOID CYST. A potential pitfall related to the use of single echo T_2 weighted spin-echo imaging for screening purposes is the cancellation of contrast between a lesion and surrounding brain due to a cross-over effect of signal intensities. This problem is illustrated in A, in which a large, left retro-occipital arachnoid cyst is poorly seen on a 56-msec film of a 2-second repetition time (TR) spin-echo pulse sequence. However, it is well-visualized in B (arrow). Although the cerebrospinal fluid–containing lesion has markedly different T_1 and T_2 magnetic relaxation times when compared to adjacent neural tissue, the cyst as displayed is isotense because of the instrument parameters utilized—specifically, the TR and TE values. This problem may be alleviated by using a multi-echo technique that enables depiction of tissue with a greater spectrum of T_2 weighting (B). Alternatively, a supplementary pulse sequence obtained using a short TR value (e.g., 0.5 second) can be routinely employed with little reduction in patient throughput and perhaps more thorough tissue characterization.

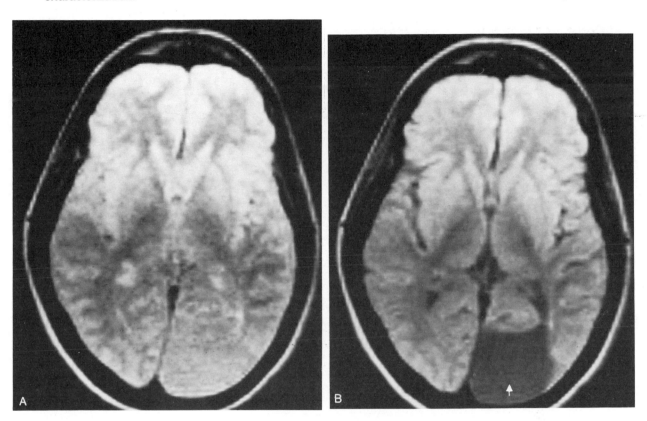

Ref.: Kelly WM, Brant-Zawadzki M, Norman D, Newton TH. Limitations and pitfalls of MRI in brain tumor diagnosis. Paper presented at the 23rd Annual Meeting of the American Society of Neuroradiology, Februrary 1985.

Figure 31–8. EVEN-ECHO REPHASING, SHRAPNEL ARTIFACT, AND SUBDURAL HY-GROMA. An even-echo rephasing phenomenon is apparent at three separate locations *(arrows)* when comparing the first *(A)* and second *(B)* echo images of this elderly patient with dementia and an incidental shrapnel injury from World War II. At the right side of the superior sagittal sinus adjacent to the left parietal convexity, and in the superficial scalp on the left, there are inversions of signal intensities when comparing *A* and *B*. These foci of signal change correspond in configuration to vascular structures. This is due to the effect of relatively slowly flowing blood in venous channels in combination with the even-echo rephasing phenomenon, which cause a slight absolute increase in signal intensity from these vascular structures on each even-numbered echo sample compared with the immediately preceding odd-numbered echo sample. Also of interest on this study is the presence of ferromagnetic artifact from retained shrapnel in the left frontal scalp. A right-sided subdural hygroma, which cannot be appreciated on *B* due to the so-called cross-over effect of signal intensities, is more thoroughly discussed in the legend for Figure 31–7.

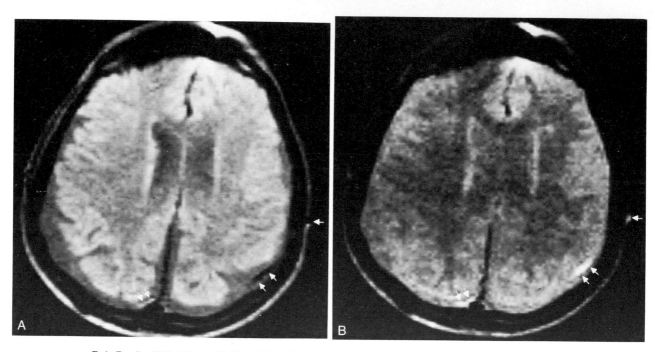

Ref.: Bradley WG, Waluch V. Blood flow: Magnetic resonance imaging. Radiology 1985; 154:443–450.

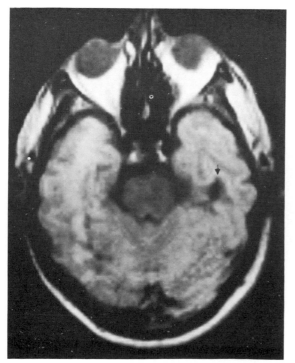

Figure 31–9. PARTIAL VOLUME AVERAGING: FALSE-POSITIVE. A focus of low intensity signal (signal void) *(arrow)* is visible in the vicinity of the mid left temporal lobe. This finding does not represent either a dilated temporal horn or a calcified intra-axial lesion. It is a partial volume averaging effect caused by incorporation of the arcuate eminence (petrous apex) into the imaged slice, in this case unilateral due to patient tilt.

Figure 31–10. PARTIAL VOLUME AVERAGING: FALSE-NEGATIVE. MR imaging techniques (characterized by relatively thick tissue sections and interslice gaps) are often inappropriate for accurate detection of small lesions, especially extra-axial tumors unaccompanied by cerebral edema. This patient has subtle widening of the left internal auditory canal, as shown on thin-section CT of the right *(A)* and left *(B)* temporal bones. Soft-tissue windows showed a small enhancing lesion *(arrow)* representing an eighth-nerve neurinoma on the left *(C)*. Direct coronal T$_2$ weighted MRI *(D)* failed to detect the lesion, due in part to partial volume averaging effects. This problem can often be alleviated with the use of newer techniques, including interleaved slices, thin contiguous sections, paramagnetic contrast agents, and specialized RF coils designed to improve signal reception.

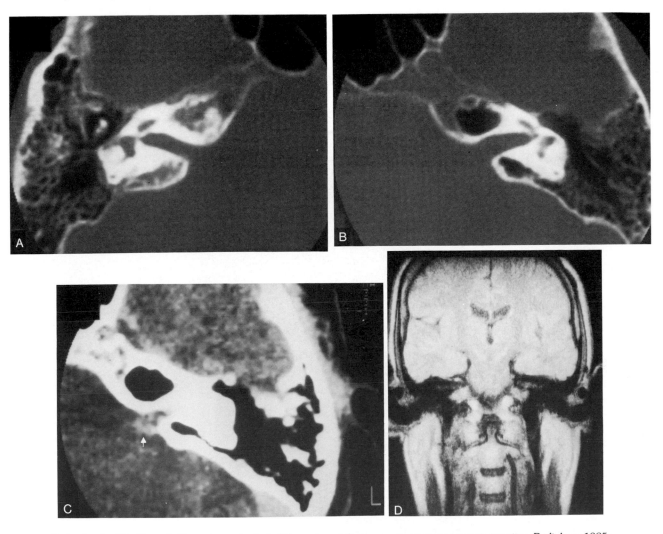

Ref.: Crooks LE, Watts J, Hoenninger J, et al. Thin-section definition in magnetic resonance imaging. Radiology 1985; 154:463–467.

Figure 31–11. CAVUM SEPTI PELLUCIDI/CAVUM VERGAE. Transaxial spin-echo images at the level of the frontal horns and bodies of the lateral ventricles show cerebrospinal fluid–like signal intensity within a cystic structure *(arrows)* situated in the midline. This collection is partitioned from the adjacent lateral ventricles on either margin by a thin rim of increased signal intensity representing the septum pellucidum and constituting the normal variant known as cavum septi pellucidi *(A)* with caudal extension into a cavum vergae *(B, arrow).* This pattern is not uncommon in infants and is often seen in premature neonates. The midline cerebrospinal fluid collection should not be confused with either a neuroepithelial cyst or superior extension of the third ventricle, as may occur in association with agenesis of the corpus callosum (see Figure 31–17).

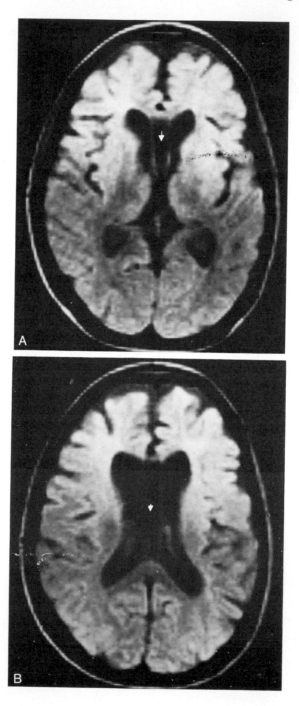

Figure 31–12. ASYMMETRY OF THE LATERAL VENTRICLES. Ventricular coarctation. On T$_2$ weighted spin-echo MRI (*A* and *B*), there is marked asymmetry of the lateral ventricles. The septum pellucidum is situated to the right of midline, a finding initially regarded as suspicious for pathologic enlargement of the left lateral ventricle. However, no obstructing mass lesion was visible at the foramen of Monro on MRI. Also, CT scans performed following injection of metrizamide into the left lateral ventricle (cerebrospinal fluid pressures were normal) were unrevealing. The absence of interstitial edema bordering the ependymal surfaces of the lateral ventricles militates against the presence of active obstructive hydrocephalus from an occult lesion. Nevertheless, because of the clinical history and degree of ventricular dilatation, the patient underwent craniotomy via a transcallosal approach, which failed to reveal either a small lesion or foraminal stenosis to account for the findings shown. This MRI appearance is believed to represent ventricular coarctation on the right.

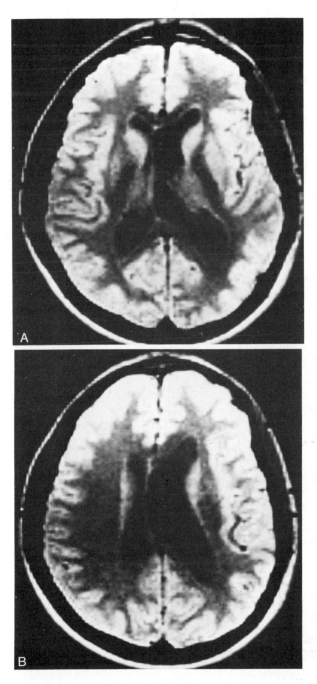

Figure 31–13. VENTRICULAR COARCTATION, MEGA CISTERNA MAGNA, AND CHIARI I MALFORMATION. The patient presented with cough-induced headache and down-beat nystagmus.

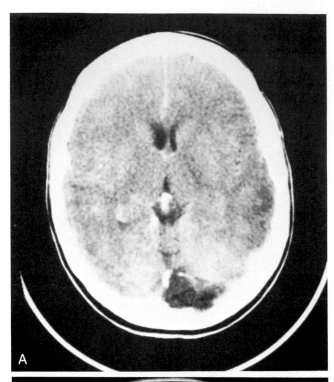

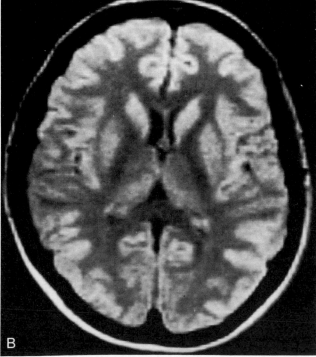

Figure 31–13A and B. An initial evaluation *(A)* demonstrated asymmetry of the lateral ventricles in addition to a cerebrospinal fluid attenuation region *(arrow)* in the left retro-occipital area. In *B*, transaxial T$_2$ weighted S/E MRI shows normal signal emanating from the periventricular neural tissue of each hemisphere, reducing the likelihood of either a parenchymal lesion on the left or an atrophic process on the right. The pattern shown is typical for normal variant ventricular asymmetry owing to coarctation of the left lateral ventricle.

Illustration continued on opposite page

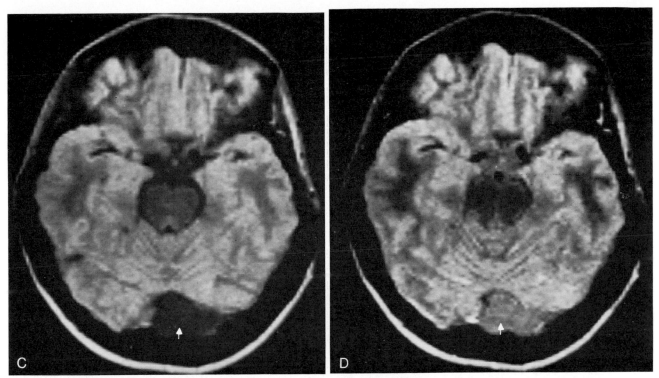

Figure 31–13 C and D. At the level of the torcula, first (E), and second (F) echo images document a cerebrospinal fluid–like signal, accounting for the circumscribed lesion *(arrows)* in the retro-occipital region on the left which abuts the straight sinus and torcula. This is characteristic of a mega cisterna magna.

Figure 31–13E. On a direct sagittal T$_1$ weighted spin-echo image, tonsillar ectopia *(double arrows)* is noted, indicating a Chiari I malformation. The cerebellar tonsils extend down to the level of C2 where the herniated cerebellar tissue abuts the "kinked" cervicomedullary junction anteriorly. Also note the large normal variant mega cisterna magna *(single arrow)* in the retro-occipital and retrocerebellar regions at the midline.

Ref.: Spinos E, Laster DW, Moody DM, et al. MR evaluations of Chiari I malformations at 0.15 T. AJNR 1985; 6:203–208.

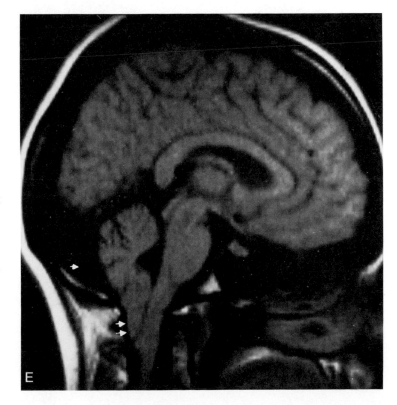

Figure 31–14. **VENTRICULAR ASYMMETRY SECONDARY TO MASS EFFECT FROM LOW-GRADE GLIOMA.** Contrast-enhanced CT *(A),* the initial imaging study in this adolescent patient with headaches and temporal lobe seizures, shows asymmetry of the lateral ventricles (right larger than left), with a slight midline shift but lack of attenuation abnormality in either hemisphere. In this patient, T$_2$ weighted spin-echo space MRI *(B)* was extremely useful in documenting a parenchymal abnormality diffusely involving much of the left hemisphere and exerting a mass effect that accounts for the subtle finding on CT. This signal abnormality is due to regional prolongation of the T$_2$ relaxation component involving the head of the left caudate nucleus, left basal ganglia, and lateral temporal convexity. A Grade II astrocytoma was diagnosed upon biopsy.

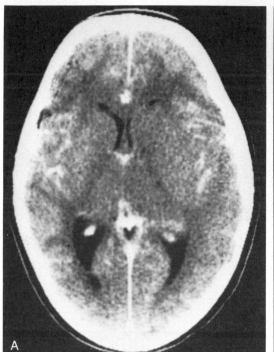
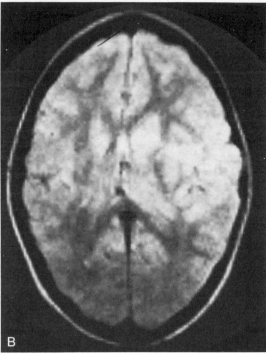

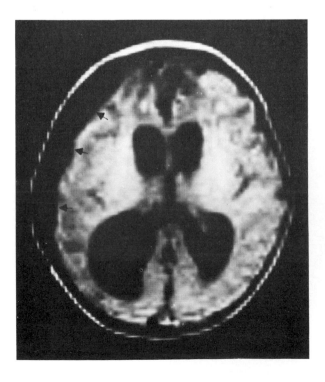

Figure 31–15. **ASYMMETRIC VENTRICLES AND SUBDURAL HYGROMA.** One week following initiation of treatment for bacterial meningitis, this infant demonstrated asymmetrically enlarged lateral ventricles in addition to a right extra-axial fluid collection *(arrows)* on MRI. In this instance, the ventricular asymmetry is caused by asymmetric ex vacuo dilatation of cerebrospinal fluid spaces as a result of an anoxic (hypotensive) episode which complicated the infant's early course. The absence of increased signal surrounding the ventricles (as would be expected from interstitial edema) and lack of midline shift in the face of a concomitant extra-axial fluid collection (subdural hygroma) on the right argue against the possibility of communicating hydrocephalus, a major clinical consideration in this child with treated meningitis. Similar patterns of atrophy may develop in response to in utero vascular accidents such as the Davidoff-Dyke-Masson syndrome that result in cerebral hemiatrophy with associated ex vacuo enlargement of the ipsilateral cerebrospinal fluid spaces.

Figure 31–16. MULTIPLE SCLEROSIS AND "LOOK-ALIKE" LESIONS. *B–J exhibit findings that, although similar to those seen in multiple sclerosis (A), are either normal or represent a variety of disease processes other than multiple sclerosis.*

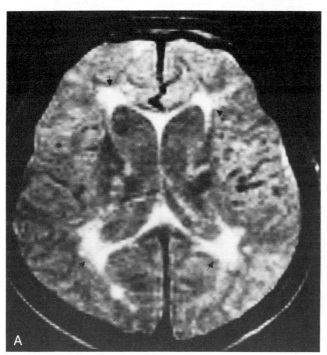

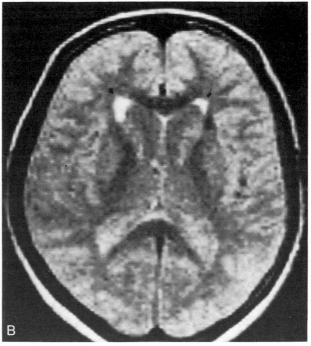

Figure 31–16A. Multiple sclerosis. On this T$_2$ weighted spin-echo MR image of a young adult with recurrent paresthesias, hyperreflexia, and spastic weakness, patchy foci of bright signal intensity *(arrows)* are distributed throughout the periventricular white matter, a pattern highly suggestive of demyelinating disease. In this instance the enlarged ventricles are due to central atrophy, a not uncommon association with chronic multiple sclerosis. However, the pattern of abnormalities demonstrated is not specific for multiple sclerosis and must be interpreted within the context of the patient's age, clinical findings, and available laboratory data.

Ref.: Jackson JA, Leake DR, Schneiders NJ, et al. Magnetic resonance imaging in multiple sclerosis: Results in 32 cases. AJNR 1985; 6:171–176.

Figure 31–16B. Normal. The subject is a 36-year-old man with increased periventricular signal intensity *(arrow)* bordering the frontal horns. This asymptomatic volunteer demonstrated symmetrically increased signal adjacent to the anterolateral fornices of the frontal horns. This pattern is not uncommonly observed as an incidental finding in otherwise normal patients, including young children. As a solitary finding, and in the absence of symptoms, it may be regarded as a normal finding. The focal T$_2$ prolongation that normally occurs at this location is related to edema from ependymitis fibrosa, a degenerative process that may begin in utero and can be identified in most adult patients at autopsy. It has been hypothesized that the proximity and perpendicular alignment of deep white matter fiber tracts to the frontal horns at this location predisposes the intervening ependymal surface to microscopic disruption and early degeneration, even in the absence of elevation in cerebrospinal fluid pressure.

Ref.: Sze G, DeArmond S, Brant-Zawadzki M, et al. "Abnormal" MRI foci anterior to the frontal horns: Pathologic correlations and relationship to normal maturation and aging. Paper presented at the 23rd Annual Meeting of the American Society of Neuroradiology, February 1985.

Illustration continued on following page

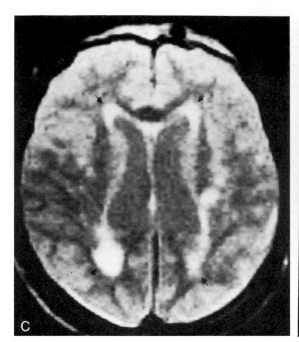 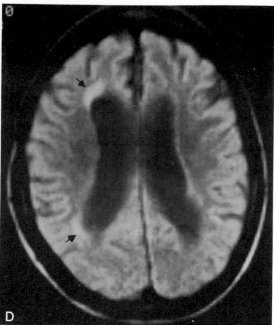

Figure 31–16C and D. C, Normal variant senescent change in an older patient. MRI in this 73-year-old individual without a history of demyelinating symptoms or a focal neurologic deficit demonstrates periventricular intensity *(arrows)* very similar in appearance to that of multiple sclerosis. This pattern is observed with increasing frequency in elderly patients (30 per cent of those over age 60) and may occur as an accelerated aging phenomenon in middle-aged persons. The topographical location of such lesions may at times correspond clinically to focal neurologic deficits attributable to cerebral vascular disease. More commonly, they are noted as an incidental finding in patients without either neurologic deficit or dementia. Presumably this pattern results from subclinical small vessel disease. The periventricular neural tissue is functionally a watershed vascular territory fed by small perforating arterioles that are vulnerable to early atherosclerotic change. Resulting atherosclerotic leukoencephalopathy may occur and lead to increased focal water concentration, yielding the foci of bright signal intensity shown on the T_2 weighted image. *D,* Periventricular encephalomalacia from shunt tube tracts. This patient has had multiple ventriculoperitoneal shunt tube revisions. The right frontal and trigonal periventricular white matter show foci of increased signal *(arrows)* caused by edema and encephalomalacic change as a result of shunt tube placements. The pattern shown is not unlike that of demyelinating disease.

Ref.: (Fig. 31–16C): Bradley WG, Waluch V, Brant-Zawadzki M, et al. Patchy periventricular white matter lesions in the elderly: A common observation during NMR imaging. Non-Invasive Medical Imaging 1984; 1:35–41.

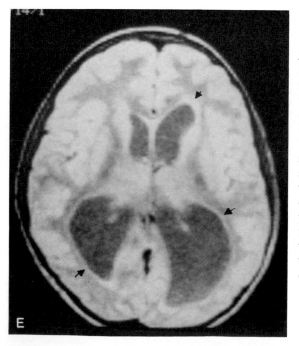

Figure 31–16E. Interstitial edema due to obstructive hydrocephalus. This adolescent patient with neurofibromatosis has a mid-brain lesion causing obstruction at the aqueduct of Sylvius. The lateral ventricles are dilated, and a thin rim of increased signal *(arrows)* bordering the ependymal surfaces is due to so-called "transependymal flow of cerebrospinal fluid," or interstitial edema. This process may also resemble multiple sclerosis. Ventricular enlargement and, certainly, direct visualization of an obstructing lesion would implicate obstructive hydrocephalus as the most likely cause of periventricular intensity. On the other hand, discrete non-confluent foci of increased signal within the centrum semiovale white matter (separate from a periventricular band), is a more characteristic manifestation of demyelinating disease.

Illustration continued on opposite page

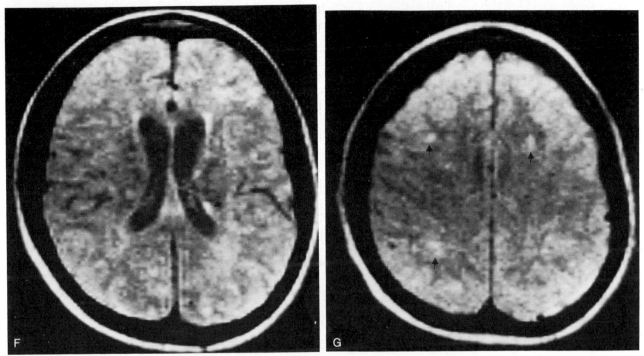

Figure 31–16F and G. Viral meningoencephalitis simulating multiple sclerosis. A 27-year-old woman rapidly developed an encephalopathic state following a viral upper respiratory infection. Cerebrospinal fluid studies revealed pleocytosis and elevated protein concentration (aseptic meningitis). MRI shows subtle periventricular *(F, arrows)* as well as centrum semiovale *(G, arrows)* foci of increased signal intensity similar to that seen in the early stages of multiple sclerosis.

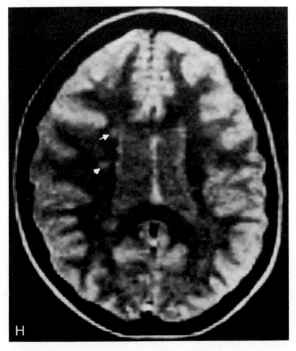

Figure 31–16H. Idiopathic retinocerebral angiitis (Susac's syndrome). Small rounded foci of increased signal intensity *(arrows)* are seen in the deep white matter adjacent to the ependymal surfaces of the lateral ventricles. In this instance the findings are due to a rare vasculitic syndrome in a young adult characteristically presenting with bilateral hearing loss. Funduscopic findings were considered pathognomonic of this disease entity and the patient did not have symptoms suggestive of demyelinating disease.

Illustration continued on following page

Figure 31–16I and J. Ependymal spread of tumor simulating periventricular intensity. A germinoma is situated in the pineal region at the posterior third ventricle. MRI *(I)* reveals increased signal intensity especially prominent at the ependymal margins of the frontal horns *(arrows)*. Without consideration of the CT findings, this abnormality could well be misinterpreted as indicative of interstitial edema, owing to the concomitant presence of obstructive hydrocephalus. The periventricular intensity is also not too dissimilar from that of MS. The CT scan *(J)* clearly shows linear deposits of enhancing tissue bordering the ependymal surfaces of the frontal horn representing spread of tumor rather than interstitial edema. The primary tumor (germinoma) is also visible at the posterior third ventricle on this slice.

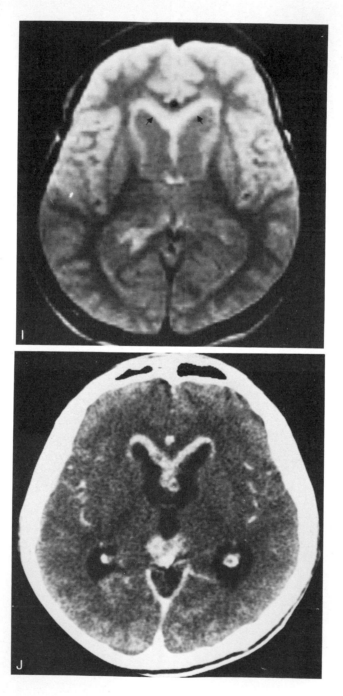

Figure 31–17. EPENDYMAL TUMOR SPREAD MASKED BY PERIVENTRICULAR EDEMA.
A 12-year-old boy presented with both systemic and central nervous system recurrence of non–Hodgkin's lymphoma. CT *(A)* clearly depicts an enhancing tumor mass in the septum pellucidum. The CT scan also demonstrates ventricular dilatation and interstitial edema due to concomitant obstructive hydrocephalus. Note that the presence of periventricular lucency due to the obstructive hydrocephalus serves to highlight the visibility of enhancing curvilinear ependymal deposits of tumor near the foramen of Monro on the right *(single arrow)* and at the left trigone *(triple arrows)*. A limitation of MRI in this setting relates to the relative prolongation of both T_1 and T_2 relaxation components of interstitial edema. These changes in relaxation times are similar to those of most forms of neoplastic disease (including ependymal tumor spread). Consequently, the periventricular edema is displayed in the same intensity range as ependymal tumor spread on either a T_1 or in this case a T_2 weighted image *(B)*. Thus, ependymal tumor deposits may be masked by edema (from either hydrocephalus or prior radiation treatment) and hence may escape detection if MRI is relied upon for screening purposes. In this instance, however, the large tumefactive deposit of tumor in the septum pellucidum is easily seen, owing to its size and protrusion into both dilated frontal horns.

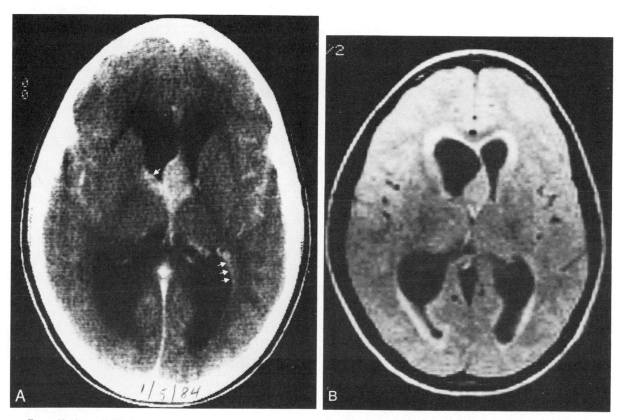

From: Kucharczyk W, Brant-Zawadzki M, Sobel D, et al. Central nervous system tumors in children: detection by magnetic resonance imaging. Radiology 1985; 155:131–136. Reproduced with permission.

Refs.: (1) Kelly WM, Brant-Zawadski M, Norman D, Newton TH. Limitations and pitfalls of MRI in brain tumor diagnosis. Paper presented at the 23rd Annual Meeting of the American Society of Neuroradiology, February 1985. (2). Brant-Zawadzki M, Kelly W, Kjos B, et al. Magnetic resonance imaging and characterization of normal and abnormal intracranial cerebrospinal fluid (CSF) spaces: Initial observations. Neuroradiology 1985; 27–38.

Figure 31–18. MISCELLANEOUS CAUSES OF CEREBROSPINAL FLUID INTENSITY WITHIN THE SELLA: "PRIMARY" EMPTY SELLA. On a midsagittal reformatted image *(A)*, contrast-enhanced CT shows predominantly low attenuation (in the range of cerebrospinal fluid density) within the sella. A vertically oriented linear density representing the infundibulum is visible immediately anterior to the dorsum sella, characteristic for this normal variant. On direct sagittal MRI *(B* and *C)*, T_2 weighted spin-echo images show high signal intensity near the floor of the sella, representing the pituitary gland *(B, arrow)*, bordered by cerebrospinal fluid intensity superiorly. Note the relative increase in signal intensity emitted from the intrasellar cerebrospinal fluid on the second echo image *(C)*, which corresponds in magnitude to other basal cerebrospinal fluid spaces such as the interpeduncular fossa or pontine cistern. Artifact from ferromagnetic dental hardware *(C, arrow)* is visible anteriorly at the alveolar ridge and soft palate.

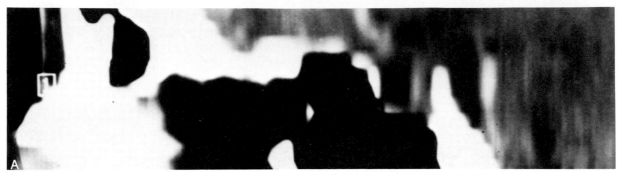

Figure 31–18A. Contrast-enhanced CT: Midsagittal reformatted image.

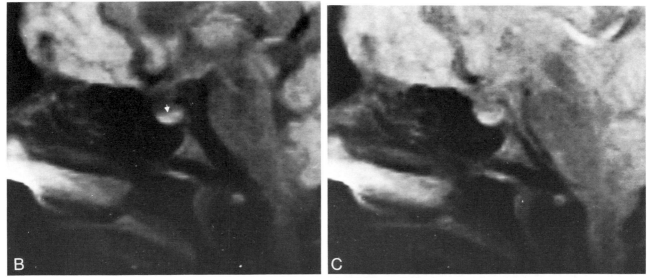

Figure 31–18 B and C. Direct sagittal MRI: T_2 weighted spin-echo images.

Figure 31–19. MISCELLANEOUS CAUSES OF CEREBROSPINAL FLUID INTENSITY WITHIN THE SELLA: "POST-THERAPEUTIC" EMPTY SELLA. Six months following initiation of bromocriptine therapy for a pituitary macroadenoma, direct coronal *(A)* and sagittally reformatted CT *(B)* showed an expanded sella with "cystic" appearance suggestive of cerebrospinal fluid–like contents. The dorsum sella is thinned. Differentiation of a tumor cyst from a secondary empty sella (following tumor regression) is hindered by the inability to visualize the infundibulum on CT. In this case, the availability of MRI obviated the need for a metrizamide CT study and enabled an accurate diagnosis.

On direct coronal MRI *(C)*, the infundibulum *(arrow)* is well visualized from its origin at the inferior aspect of the third ventricle where it extends inferiorly and obliquely, the left aspect of the sellar floor merging with a remnant of the pituitary. Compare the signal intensity of the remainder of the sellar contents to known cerebrospinal fluid spaces such as the sylvian cisterns or frontal horns. Note that the magnetic relaxation characteristics of these fluid compartments are qualitatively similar on the first *(C)* and second *(D)* echo samplings of this T_2 weighted pulse sequence, further securing the diagnosis of empty sella. A tumor cyst would tend to be associated with elevated protein concentration, causing a reduction in the T_1 relaxation time, yielding increased signal relative to cerebrospinal fluid on this type of pulse sequence.

From: Brant-Zawadzki M, Kelly W, Kjos B, et al. Magnetic resonance imaging and characterization of normal and abnormal intracranial cerebrospinal fluid (CSF) spaces: Initial observations. Neuroradiology 1985; 27:3–8. Copyright © 1985 by Springer-Verlag, New York and Heidelberg. Reproduced with permission.

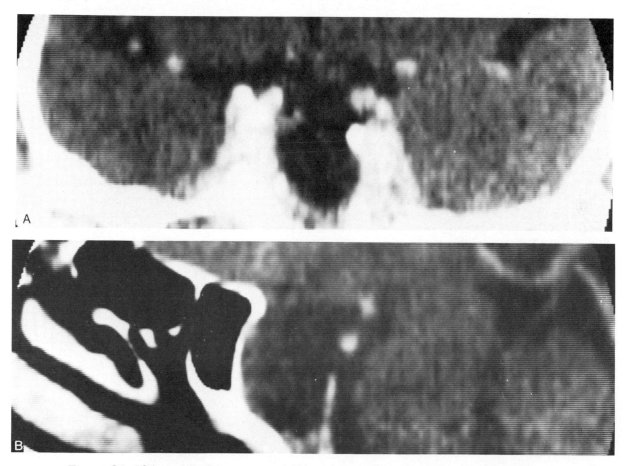

Figure 31–19A and B. Direct coronal *(A)* and sagittally reformatted *(B)* CT images.

Illustration continued on following page

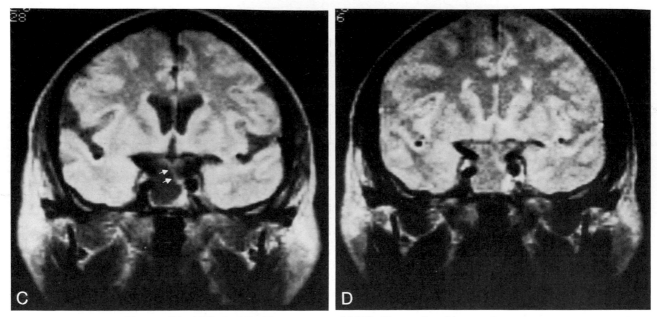

Figure 31–19C and D. Direct coronal MRI: T$_2$ weighted spin-echo images.

Figure 31–20. MISCELLANEOUS CAUSES OF CEREBROSPINAL FLUID INTENSITY WITHIN THE SELLA: HERNIATED THIRD VENTRICLE. This adolescent patient presented with progressive headaches. A transaxial CT scan *(A)* obtained at the level of the skull base shows cerebrospinal fluid density *(arrow)* within the sella, somewhat resembling the appearance of an "empty" sella. However, the sella is slightly enlarged and the dorsum is truncated. A sagittal reformation *(B)* shows a striking superior extension of the "cyst," which is contiguous with a mixed-density, partially calcified lesion (astrocytoma) posteriorly. Direct sagittal MRI *(D* and *E)* helps identify a herniated inferior third ventricle *(arrows)* as the inferior component of the abnormality. Note the proportional changes in signal intensity on the first *(D)* and second *(E)* echo images when comparing the dilated inferior third ventricle with the fourth ventricle or other cerebrospinal fluid spaces, mitigating the possibility of a proteinacious tumor cyst accounting for the lower portion of the abnormality. Other lesions that may account for cerebrospinal fluid–like signal within the sella might include neuroepithelial cysts of arachnoidal origin or benign cysts derived from Rathke pouch remnants.

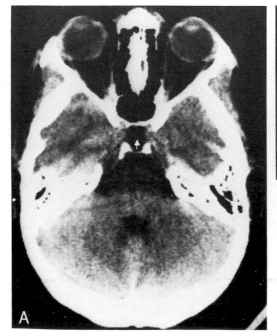

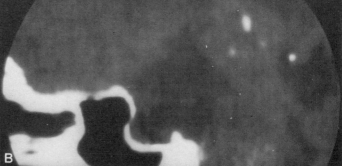

Figure 31–20A and B. Transaxial *(A)* and sagittally reformatted *(B)* CT images.

Illustration continued on opposite page

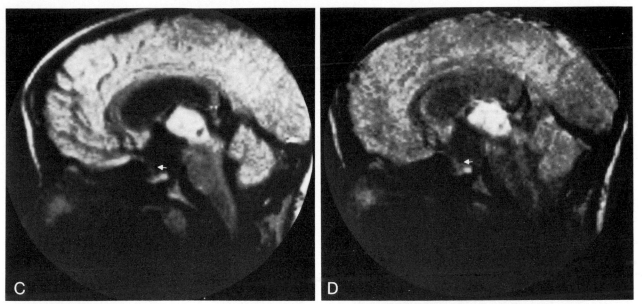

Figure 31–20C and D. Direct sagittal MRI: T_2 weighted spin-echo images.

Figure 31–21. AGENESIS OF THE CORPUS CALLOSUM. Agenesis of the corpus callosum may be a solitary structural anomaly of the brain or may occur in association with a variety of other entities including Chiari malformations, holoprosencephaly and midline lipoma. Agenesis of the corpus callosum may be partial or complete. The partial forms involve agenesis of the caudal portion (body and splenium), consistent with embryologic development of this structure in a cephalocaudad direction. In the isolated forms, mental retardation or developmental delay, although common, are by no means constant findings, as these patients may be functionally normal. The architectural derangements that are present are well suited for demonstration by MRI. On an axial section *(A)*, these findings include dilated lateral ventricles with preponderant enlargement of the trigones relative to the frontal horns, causing a so-called "race car" appearance wherein the elevated third ventricle (due to absence of the body of the corpus callosum) forms the body of the car and the enlarged trigones represent the rear wheels. On MRI, the serpiginous course of the pericallosal artery is also well demonstrated in *A*, due to both the absence of the pericallosal cistern and the presence of conspicuous signal void within the arterial lumina. The absence of commissural fibers bridging the midline can be directly visualized in the coronal plane *(B)*.

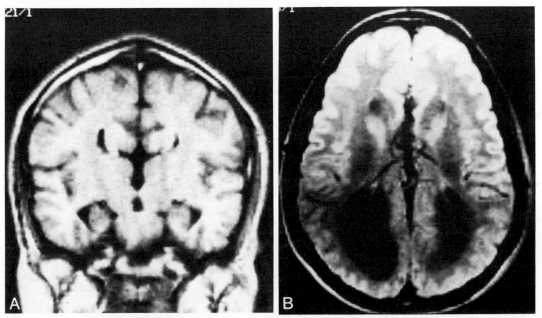

Figure 31–21A. MRI: Axial section. *Figure 31–21B.* Direct coronal MRI.

Figure 31–22. TUMOR CALCIFICATION NOT VISIBLE ON MRI. This patient has a "butterfly" glioma situated at the level of the genu of the corpus callosum. Thin crescentic arcs of calcification are clearly visible on CT (A). Some form of calcification—coarse, punctate, or curvilinear as shown in A—may be seen in 5 to 8 per cent of patients with astrocytomas. On MRI *(B)*, the calcification is not appreciated because the small crescents of signal void that they produce are "drowned out" by confluent zones of increased signal due to relative T_2 prolongation of both the tumor and associated vasogenic edema.

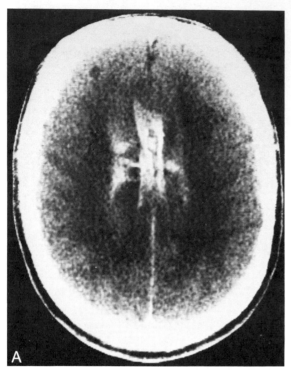

Figure 31–22A. Calcification is clearly visible on this CT image.

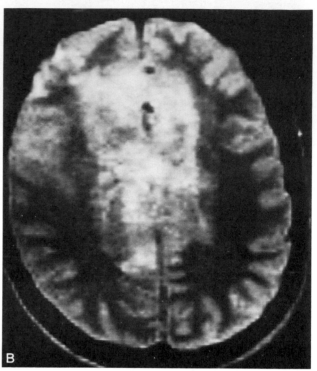

Figure 31–22B. On MRI, calcification cannot be seen, although the lesion is clearly demonstrated.

From: Brant-Zawadzki M, Norman D, Newton TH, et al. Magnetic resonance of the brain: The optimal screening technique. Radiology 1984; 152:71–77. Reproduced wth permission.

Figure 31–23. PINEAL SHIFT CAUSED BY A BENIGN ARACHNOID CYST. A skull series of a 35-year-old man with acromegalic features revealed an unsuspected shift of the calcified pineal gland from left to right. Follow-up contrast-enhanced CT *(A)* shows a low attenuation region *(arrow)* adjacent to the pineal gland, accounting for the midline shift. Mass effect is also evidenced by a convex impression on the pulvinar of the left thalamus. A metrizamide-enhanced CT cisternogram (MTTC) *(B)* shows no direct communication of the lesion with adjacent subarachnoid space. A malignant pineal region lesion with a cystic component, although unlikely, could not be excluded on the basis of CT alone. Dual echo images *(C* and *D)* of a T_2 weighted spin-echo MRI study help considerably in corroborating the diagnosis of arachnoid cyst. Note that the intensity characteristics of the lesion are identical to that of cerebrospinal fluid in the frontal horn, and a proportional degree of signal decay is evidenced by comparable changes in displayed signal intensity on the second echo sampling *(D)*.

Illustration on opposite page

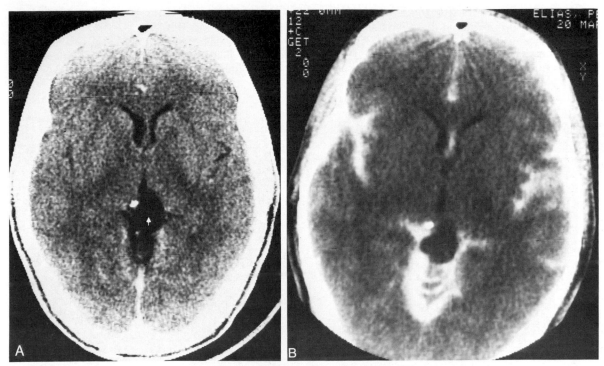

Figure 31–23A and B. Contrast-enhanced CT images.

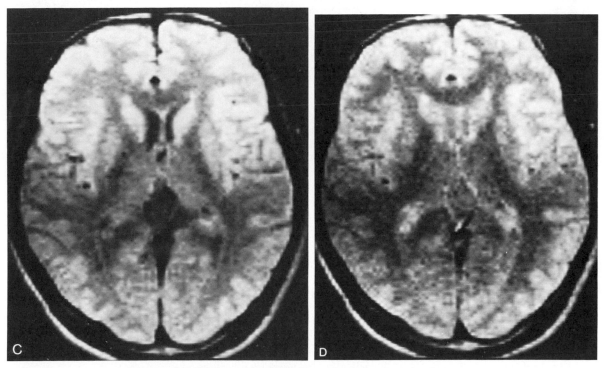

Figure 31–23C and D. MRI: T$_2$ weighted spin-echo images.

Ref.: Brant-Zawadzki M, Kelly W, Kjos B, et al. Magnetic resonance imaging and characterization of normal and abnormal intracranial cerebrospinal fluid (CSF) spaces: Initial observations. Neuroradiology 1985; 27:3–8.

Figure 31–24. CALCIFIED LESION NOT VISIBLE ON MRI. CT scan *(A)* reveals a densely calcified lesion *(arrow)* in the deep left hemisphere not associated with perifocal edema. This lesion is not apparent at the corresponding level on the T$_2$ weighted MRI screening study *(B)*. Failure to detect small foci of calcium, especially when punctate or curvilinear, is a known relative limitation of MRI when compared with CT. However, this shortcoming seldom accounts for failure to demonstrate active lesions, as there is usually some associated component of T$_2$ prolongation due to either soft tissue portions of the lesion or surrounding perifocal edema. In this instance, presumably the lesion contained an admixture of calcium and soft tissue, causing its magnetic relaxation properties to be very similar to that of adjacent neural tissue.

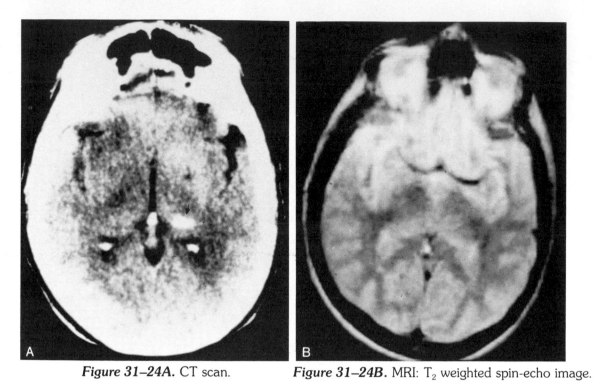

Figure 31–24A. CT scan.   ***Figure 31–24B.*** MRI: T$_2$ weighted spin-echo image.

Ref.: Brant-Zawadzki M, Norman D, Newton TH, et al. Magnetic resonance of the brain: The optimal screening technique. 1984; Radiology 152:71.

Chest

W. RICHARD WEBB, M.D.

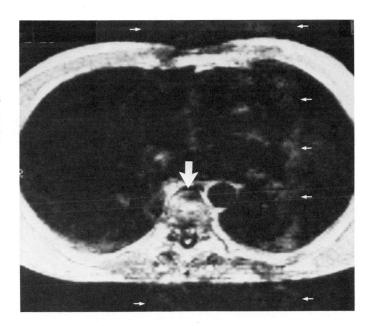

Figure 32–1. CARDIAC MOTION ARTIFACT. This spin-echo image (TR 2.0 sec, TE 28 msec) at the level of the heart shows a marked reduction in signal from the heart as a result of cardiac motion. A band of increased noise *(small arrows)* extending from anterior to posterior, and corresponding to the position of the heart is also a result of cardiac motion. The anterior vertebral cortex *(large arrow)* results in a crescentic area of low signal intensity and can be confused with air in the esophagus or the azygos vein.

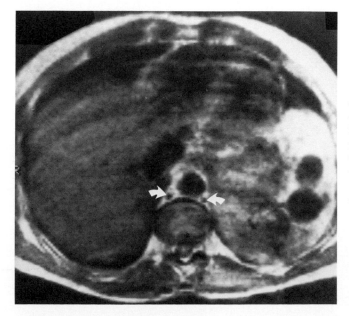

Figure 32–2. BREATHING ARTIFACT. Breathing results in a series of crescentic stripes overlapping the image and actually represents ghost images of the anterior chest wall. In this subject, the azygos and hemiazygos veins *(arrows)* are easily distinguished from the anterior vertebral cortex.

Ref.: Schultz CL, Alfidi RJ, Nelson AD, et al. The effect of motion on two-dimensional Fourier transformation magnetic resonance images. Radiology 1984; 52:117–121.

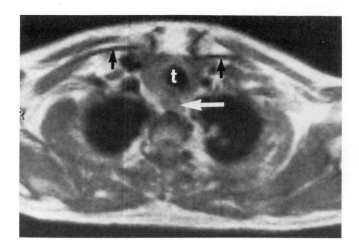

Figure 32–3. MEDIASTINAL THYROID. Thyroid gland extending into the mediastinum results in intermediate intensity signal surrounding the trachea (t). The esophagus *(white arrow)* also is intermediate in intensity. Cortices of the clavicles *(black arrows)* can simulate vascular structures.

Ref.: Stark DD, Moss AA, Gamsu G, et al. Magnetic resonance imaging of the neck. Part I: Normal anatomy. Radiology 1984; 150:447–454.

Figure 32–4. NORMAL MEDIASTINAL LYMPH NODES. Normal-sized mediastinal lymph nodes *(small arrows)* are occasionally visible on MR studies with short TR values (0.5 sec). In comparison with spin-echo images performed with a long TR value (2.0 sec, as in Fig. 32–3), mediastinal nodes as well as the esophagus (e) and chest wall muscles decrease in intensity relative to mediastinal fat and become more readily visible. The anterior vertebral cortex *(curved arrow)* is identified posterior to the esophagus.

Ref.: Webb WR, Gamsu G, Stark DD, et al. Evaluation of magnetic resonance sequences in imaging mediastinal tumors. AJR 1984; 143:723–727.

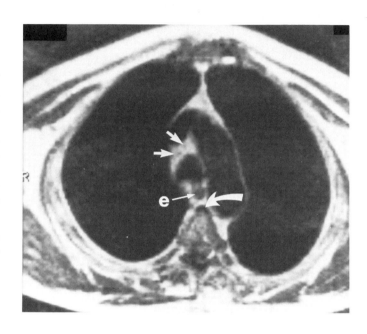

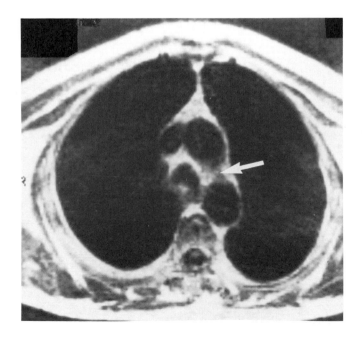

Figure 32–5. VOLUME AVERAGING SIMULATING A MEDIASTINAL NODE. At a lower level, volume averaging of the aortic arch produces an area of intermediate intensity *(arrow)* that can simulate a mediastinal node.

Figure 32–6. FLUID-FILLED ESOPHAGUS. Spin-echo images with TR values of 0.5 sec *(A)* and 2.0 sec *(B)* show the esophagus *(arrows)* as a circular low-intensity structure. Fluid in its lumen is higher in intensity. This characteristic appearance should not be mistaken for a pathologic process.

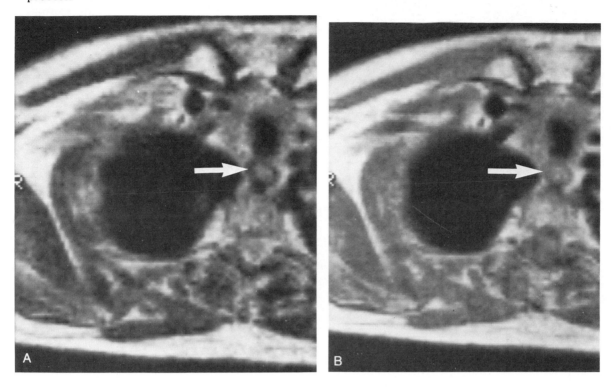

Figure 32–7. THYMUS GLAND. In a young patient, a gated spin-echo image (TR 0.75 sec) shows the thymus gland as an ill-defined area of low intensity *(arrow)* surrounded by mediastinal fat. This appearance is characteristic of the thymus and aids in differentiating it from other processes. The esophagus between the trachea and descending aorta is similar in intensity.

Ref.: Stark DD, Moss AA, Gamsu G, et al. Magnetic resonance imaging of the neck. Part I: Normal anatomy. Radiology 1984; 150:447–454.

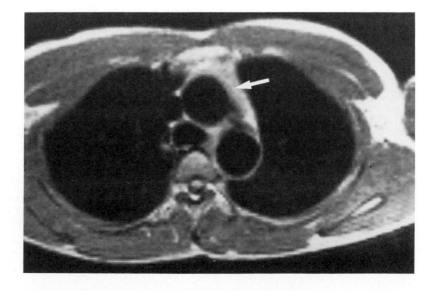

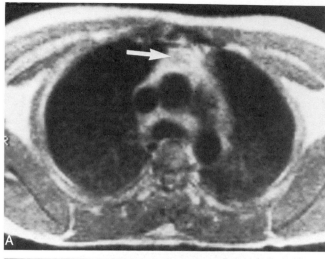

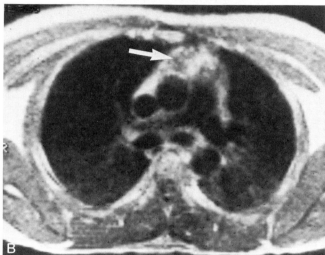

Figure 32–8. THYMUS GLAND. In another subject, the thymus is visible as an area of low intensity *(arrows)* surrounded by mediastinal fat but is more poorly seen than in Figure 32–7 because the scan is ungated.

Figure 32–9. NORMAL PERICARDIAL RECESSES.

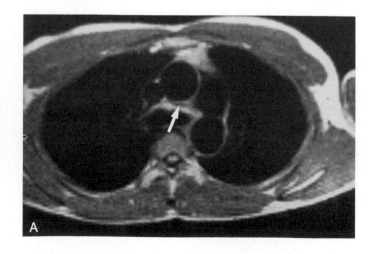

Figure 32–9A. As on CT, the superior pericardial recess is commonly visible as an area of low intensity *(arrow)* posterior to the aorta (see also Fig. 32–15A).

Illustration continued on opposite page

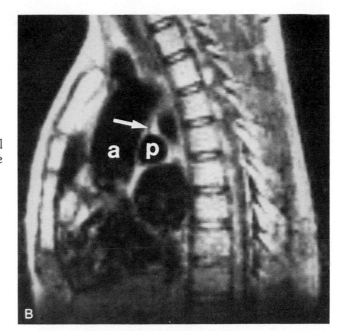

Figure 32–9B. On sagittal images the superior pericardial recess can be seen *(arrow)* behind the aorta (a) and above the right pulmonary artery (p).

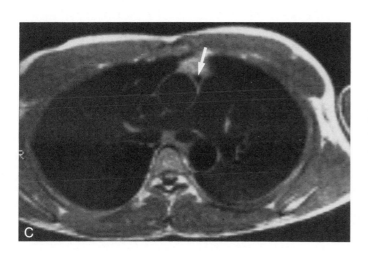

Figure 32–9C. In some patients the recess is also visible anteriorly *(arrow)* between the aorta and pulmonary artery. It should not be confused with a vessel or lymph node.

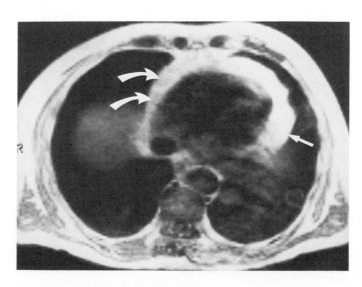

Figure 32–10. PARACARDIAC FAT. Paracardiac fat *(straight arrow)* is normally high in intensity. Near the level of the diaphragm, however, volume averaging can result in intermediate intensity areas *(curved arrows)* simulating lymphadenopathy.

Figure 32–11. FLOW ARTIFACTS.

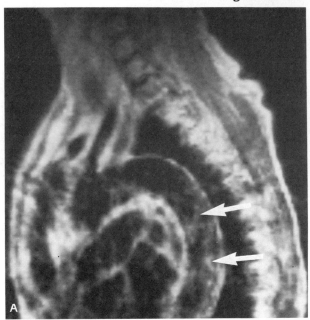

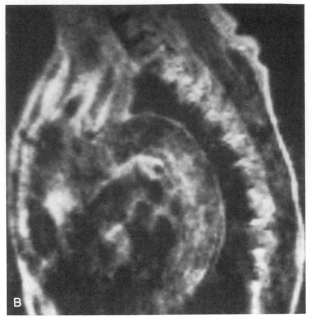

Figure 32–11A. Generally speaking, vessels with rapid flow, including all mediastinal arteries and veins, are devoid of signal on ungated magnetic resonance (see Figs. 32–4 and 32–5). However, in some cases higher intensity signals *(arrows)* from the lumen of large vessels are visible, as in the aorta of this patient.

Figure 32–11B. As shown in this image, flow-related signal generally increases on second echo (TE 56 msec) images.

Ref.: Higgins CB, Stark DD, McNamara M, et al. Multiplane magnetic resonance imaging of the heart and major vessels: Studies in normal volunteers. AJR 1984; 142:661–667.

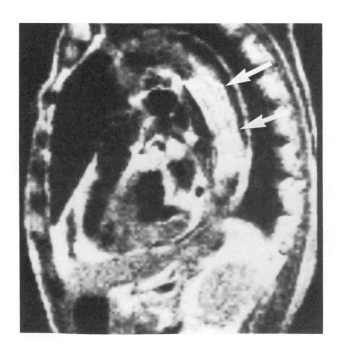

Figure 32–12. DIASTOLIC FLOW ARTIFACTS IN THE AORTA. On EKG gated images, scans obtained during systole (see Fig. 32–8A and B), show the vessels as devoid of signal as a result of rapid flow. However, as in this case, during diastole blood is flowing slowly and a strong signal can be seen from the vessel lumen *(arrows)*. This is also evident on second-echo images.

Figure 32–13. NORMAL HILAR TISSUE. In normal patients, soft tissue representing fat and normal lymph nodes is generally visible at three levels, illustrated in *A, B,* and *C.* Also note the left lung nodules in *C.*

Figure 32–13A. Hilar tissue is visible on the right, at the level of the bifurcation of the right pulmonary artery *(arrows).*

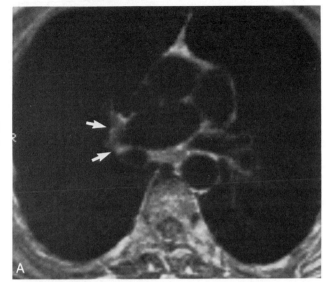

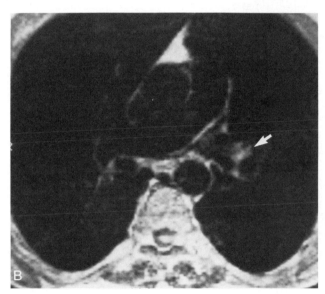

Figure 32–13B. Hilar tissue can be seen on the left, at the level of the upper lobe bronchus *(arrow).*

Figure 32–13C. Hilar tissue is visible on the right, at the level of the origin of the right middle lobe bronchus *(arrow).*

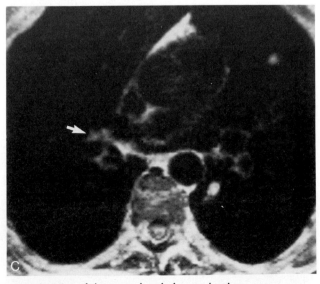

Ref.: Webb WR, Gamsu G, Stark DD, Moore EH. Magnetic resonance imaging of the normal and abnormal pulmonary hila. Radiology 1984; 152:89–94.

Figure 32–14. NORMAL HILAR TISSUE. As in Fig. 32–13, normal soft tissue *(arrows)* is visible in the pulmonary hila.

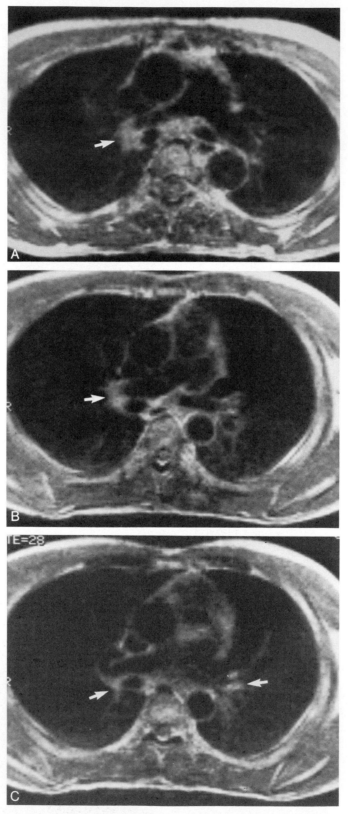

Figure 32–15. FLOW ARTIFACT SIMULATING HILAR MASS. In some patients, particularly those with pulmonary hypertension, flow signal not evident on first echo images *(A)* can be seen on second echo images *(B, arrow).* This should not be confused with a hilar mass.

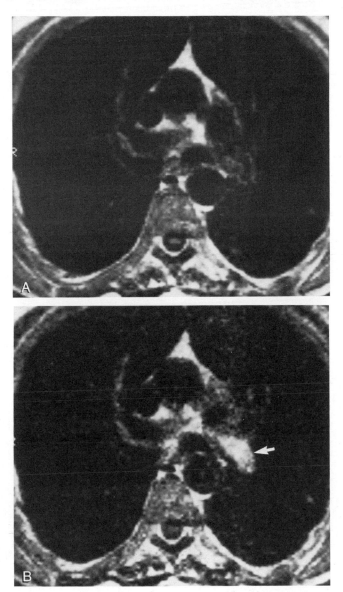

Figure 32–16. NORMAL LUNG MARKINGS. Although the lungs are largely devoid of signal, linear structures can sometimes be seen radiating from the hila on axial (*A* and *B*), sagittal (*C* and *D*), and coronal images. These may represent the walls of vessels or bronchi or both; however, by themselves they do not necessarily indicate parenchymal disease.

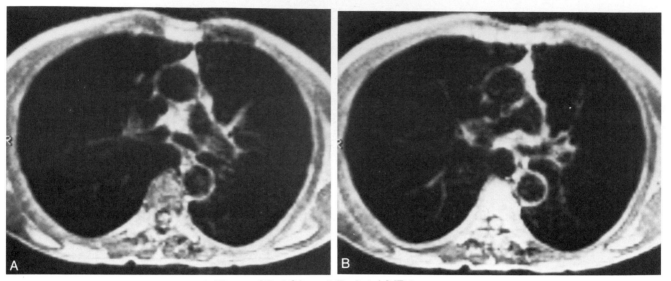

Figure 32–16A and B. Axial MR images.

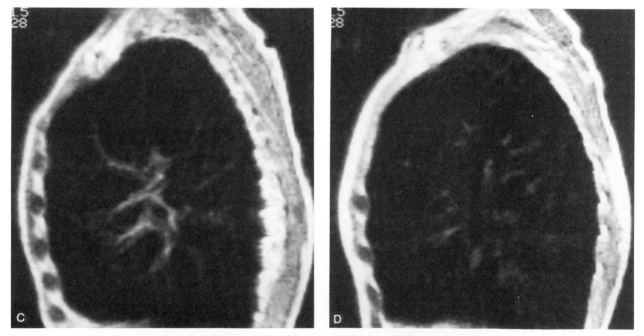

Figure 32–16C and D. Sagittal MR images.

Figure 32–17. VOLUME AVERAGING SIMULATING PARENCHYMAL LUNG DISEASE. At the level of the top of the aortic arch, the aortic lumen (a), due to its low signal intensity, can simulate lung, thus causing fat lateral to the aorta *(arrow)* to be misinterpreted as parenchymal lung disease.

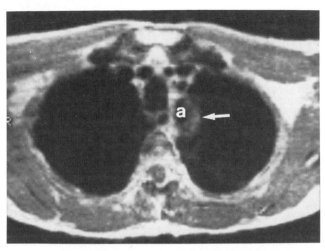

Figure 32–18. INCREASED SIGNAL IN NORMAL LUNG. As on CT, some increased signal may be encountered in dependent portions of the lungs. This is considered to reflect condensed lung parenchyma that is otherwise normal.

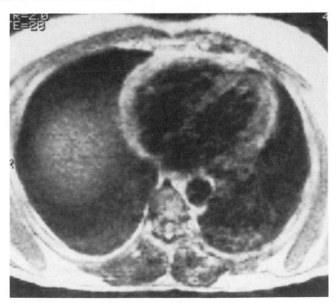

Abdomen and Pelvis

SUSAN D. WALL, M.D.
HEDVIG HRICAK, M.D.

Figure 33–1. "HERRINGBONE" ARTIFACT. A homogeneous pattern of signal intensity of the hepatic parenchyma can be seen in A. In B, an alternating pattern of high and low signal intensity is demonstrated. This "Herringbone" artifact is not present on the first echo image (A). It is due to the fact that the program sequence is out of calibration, causing a banding effect in the longer TE image only.

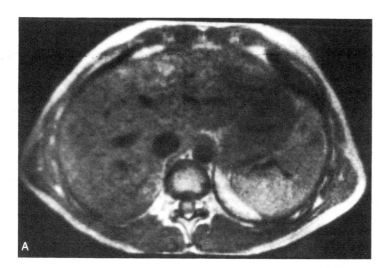

Figure 33–1A. First echo MR image (TE 28 msec).

Figure 33–1B. Second echo MR image (TE 56 msec).

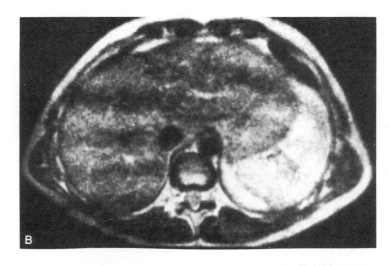

Figure 33–2. ARTIFACT: ARM TOUCHING RADIO FREQUENCY COIL.

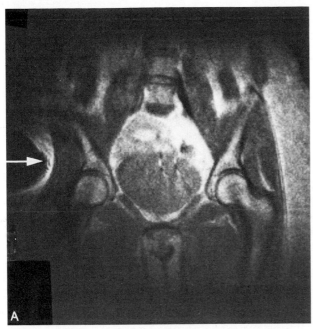

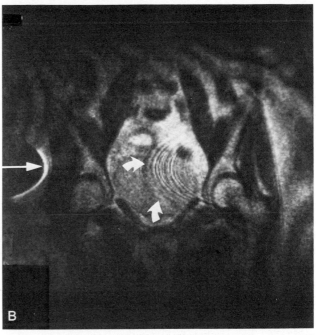

Figure 33–2A. Artifactual distortion *(arrow)* involving the right aspect of this coronal image (TR 2.0 sec, TR 28 msec) is caused by the touching of the subject's right arm to the radio frequency coil.

Figure 33–2B. In this second echo image (TE 56 msec), the same artifact *(straight arrow)* shown in *A* is seen. Also demonstrated is an additional artifact involving the left side of the image *(curved arrows)* that was not apparent on the shorter TE image *(A)*.

Figure 33–3. ARTIFACT: ARMS TOUCHING RADIO FREQUENCY COIL. Artifactual distortion *(arrows)* of a coronal image of the abdomen in a normal volunteer is caused by the touching of the upper extremities *(arrowheads)* to the radio frequency coil.

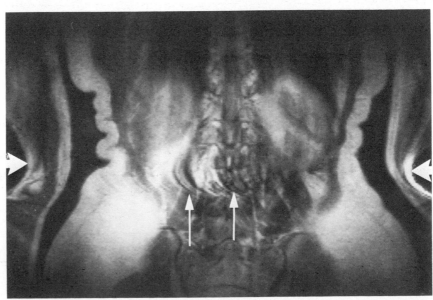

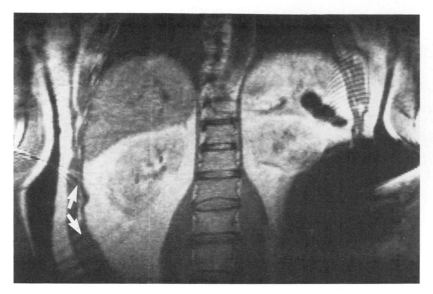

Figure 33–4. ARTIFACT: ARM TOUCHING RADIO FREQUENCY COIL. Artifactual distortion of the left side of this coronal image (TR 2.0 sec, TE 28 msec) is caused by touching of the patient's left arm to the radio frequency coil. Note that there is less distortion of the right side of the image *(arrows)*, owing to minimal touching of the radio frequency coil by the right arm.

Figure 33–5. METALLIC ARTIFACT.

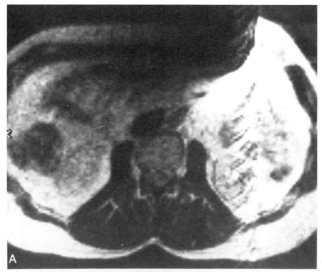

Figure 33–5A. This axial MR image (TR 1.5 sec, TE 56 msec) demonstrates marked artifact along the left side of this volunteer subject who did not remove the keys from his pants pocket.

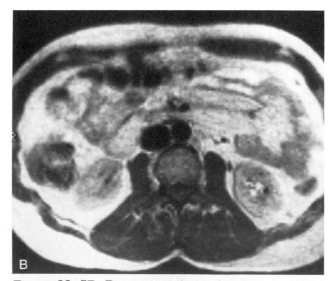

Figure 33–5B. Repeat imaging at the same level (TR 1.5 sec, TE 28 msec) demonstrates absence of the artifact after the keys were removed.

Figure 33–6. METALLIC ARTIFACT.

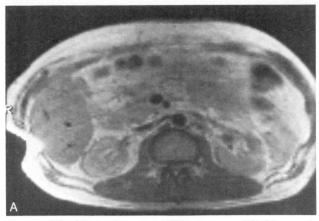

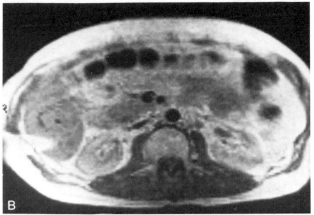

Figure 33–6A. In this image (TR 0.5 sec, TE 28 msec), there is distortion of the right lateral abdominal wall and the peripheral aspect of the right lobe of the liver, which was caused by the metallic connector of the patient's biliary drainage tubing that was on the abdominal wall at this level.

Figure 33–6B. In a repeat scan one cm caudal to A, the artifact distorts the abdominal wall to a less severe degree but still obscures the hepatic parenchyma by a streak of high-intensity artifact from the metallic connector.

Figure 33–7. INTENSITY CHANGES IN VESSELS.

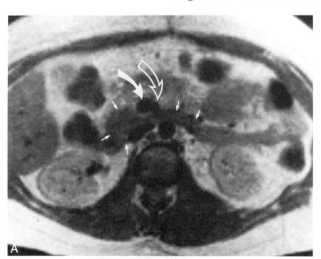

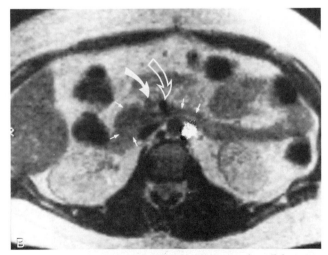

Figure 33–7A. In this MR image (TR 1.5 sec, TE 28 msec), there is absence of signal from both the superior mesenteric vein *(closed curved arrow)* and the superior mesenteric artery *(open curved arrow)*. The transverse duodenum is also identified *(straight arrows)*.

Figure 33–7B. When the TE is prolonged to 56 msec, due to slower flow in the superior mesenteric vein *(closed curved arrow)* than in the superior mesenteric artery *(open curved arrow)* the signal from the former is isointense relative to the transverse duodenum *(straight arrows)*, but the superior mesenteric artery remains signal-free.

Figure 33–8. SIGNAL WITHIN VESSELS.

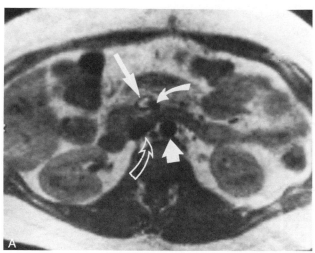

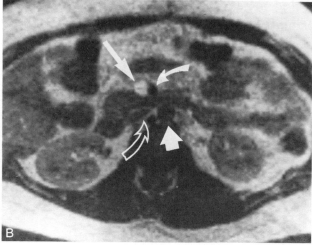

Figure 33–8A. In this MR image (TR 0.5 sec, TE 28 msec), the superior mesenteric vein *(straight arrow)* has high-intensity signal centrally and low-intensity signal peripherally. This is the result of velocity profile and does not indicate pathology. There is absence of signal from the superior mesenteric artery *(closed curved arrow).* The aorta *(arrowhead)* and inferior vena cava *(open curved arrow)* are also demonstrated.

Figure 33–8B. When the TE is 56 msec, the lumen of the superior mesenteric vein *(straight arrow)* is completely filled with high-intensity signal. This is due to the rephasing phenomenon. Similar to the superior mesenteric vein, the inferior vena cava *(open curved arrow)* exhibits some signal at this TE. There is absence of signal from the superior mesenteric artery *(closed curved arrow)* at this TE also. The aorta *(arrowhead)* is also identified.

Figure 33–9. REPHASING PHENOMENON.

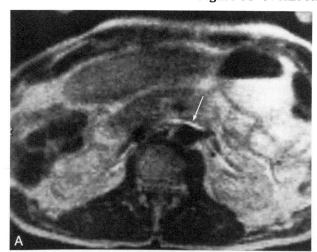

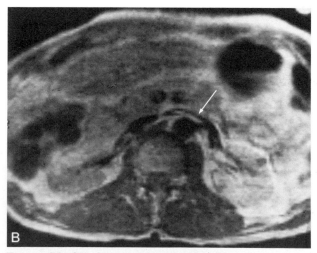

Figure 33–9A. High-intensity signal due to rephasing phenomenon is seen in the left renal vein *(straight arrow)* on this second echo image (TR 2.0 sec, TE 56 msec).

Figure 33–9B. The renal vein *(straight arrow)* is signal-free on the first echo image (TE 28 msec).

Figure 33–10. HIGH-INTENSITY ARTIFACT.

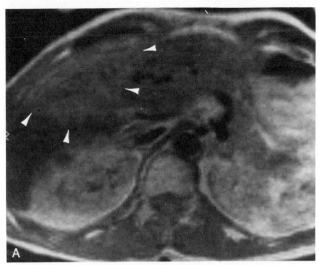

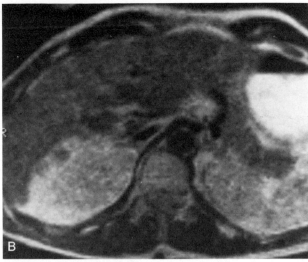

Figure 33–10A. On an MR image with a TR of 2.0 sec and a TE of 28 msec, there is a diffuse high-intensity signal artifact *(arrowheads)* in the medial segment of the left lobe of the liver of a normal volunteer.

Figure 33–10B. When the TE is 56 msec, the artifact is not evident. The origin of the artifact could not be determined.

Figure 33–11. INTERLOBAR FAT. This inversion recovery image (T1 210 msec, TE 56 msec) demonstrates an unusual (but normal) amount of fat (F) in the interlobar fissure. This was due to a small medial segment of the left lobe of the liver. Note the gastric wall *(straight arrow)* and air-fluid level *(curved arrow)* within the stomach. The lateral segment of the left lobe (L) and the right lobe of the liver (R) are indicated.

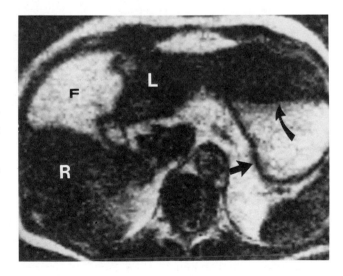

Figure 33–12. SMALL MEDIAL SEGMENT OF LEFT LOBE OF THE LIVER.

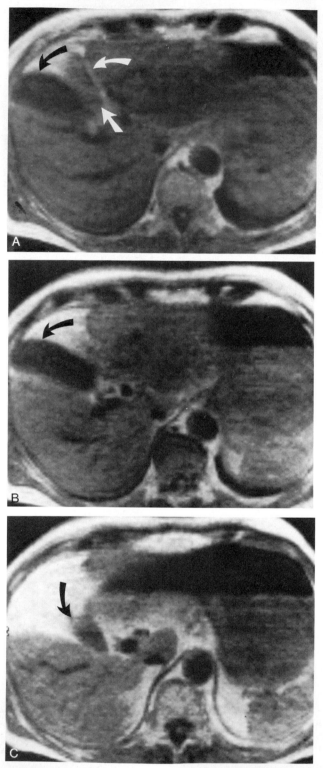

Figure 33–12A, B, and C. Consecutive images (TR 1.0 sec, TE 28 msec). *A* demonstrates a very small medial segment *(straight white arrow)* of the left lobe of the liver. High-intensity fat *(curved white arrow)* is seen in the left intersegmental fissure. An increasing amount of high-intensity fat abutting the gallbladder *(curved black arrows)* is seen on the more caudal images, *B* and *C*. Note that poorly concentrated gallbladder bile appears hypointense compared with the liver parenchyma.

Illustration continued on opposite page

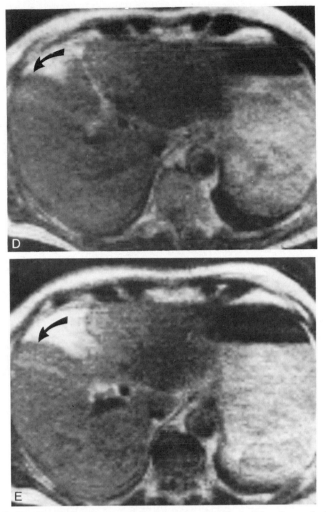

Figure 33–12D and E. D and *E* correspond anatomically with *A* and *B*, respectively, and demonstrate an isointense signal from the gallbladder (*curved arrow*) when the TR is 1.0 sec and the TE is prolonged to 56 msec. On these images, the gallbladder bile is isointense with surrounding tissue and cannot be differentiated from the liver.

Figure 33–13. LAYERING OF BILE. This MR image (TR 1.0 sec, TE 28 msec) demonstrates the normal layering of dependent, concentrated (high-intensity) bile *(open curved arrow)* and non-concentrated (low-intensity) bile *(arrowhead)* within the gallbladder. Note the fluid-fluid level *(straight arrow)*.

Ref.: Hricak H, Filly RA, Margulis AR, et al. Work in progress: Nuclear magnetic resonance imaging of the gallbladder. Radiology 1983; 147:481–484.

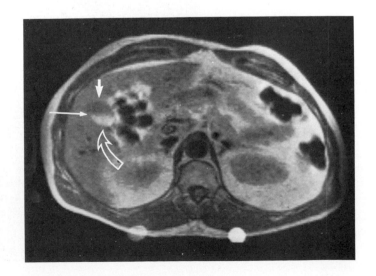

Figure 33–14. PARTIAL VOLUME AVERAGING OF THE GALLBLADDER. An ill-defined, high-intensity signal *(arrow)* simulates a lesion within the hepatic parenchyma in A. This was caused by partial volume averaging of the gallbladder, which is more clearly demonstrated *(arrow)* on the next caudal image, B. Note the absence of signal from the gallstone *(arrowhead, B)*, which has displaced the high-intensity, concentrated bile within the gallbladder. These MR images demonstrate that the gallbladder is still able to concentrate bile even though the patient has cholelithiasis. (TR 1.0 sec, TE 28 msec.)

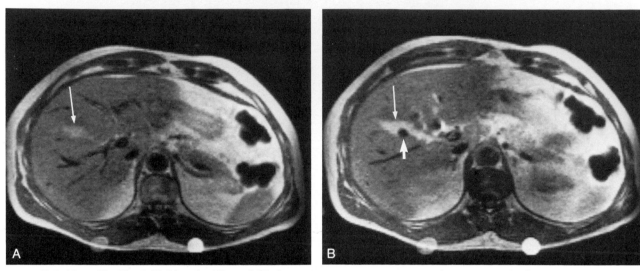

Ref.: Moon KL, Hricak H, Margulis AR, et al. Nuclear magnetic resonance imaging characteristics of gallstones in vitro. Radiology 1983; 148:753–756.

Figure 33–15. NECK OF THE GALLBLADDER. The stomach (S) and duodenal sweep *(straight arrows)* are filled with a dilute (1 mM) ferric ammonium citrate solution that emits a high-intensity signal on this image (TR 0.5 sec, TE 28 msec.), in addition to maintaining a relatively high-intensity signal on images with more prolonged TR (2.0 sec) and/or TE (56 msec) (not demonstrated). Note the ease of identification not only of the stomach and duodenum, but more importantly of the tail, body, and head of the pancreas (p). A focal area of high intensity *(open arrow)* is seen along the medial border of the liver near the contrast-filled duodenum *(straight arrows)*. Although sometimes mistaken for contrast agent in an ulcer or fistula, this high intensity represents concentrated bile in the neck of the gallbladder. Note the signal-free vascular structures, the left renal artery *(curved arrow)* as it takes off from the aorta, the left renal vein anterior to the aorta and behind the superior mesenteric artery, and the splenic vein, which is dorsal to the pancreas and anterior to the superior mesenteric artery, as it enters the splenoportal confluence.

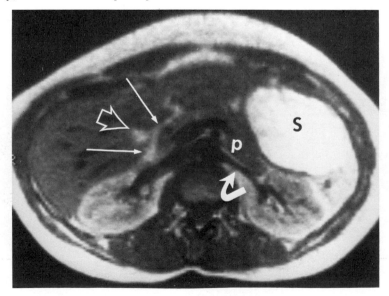

Figure 33–16. BILIARY STENT.

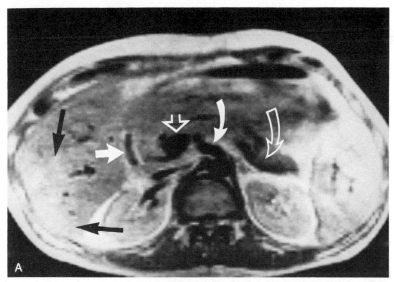

Figure 33–16A. A curvilinear signal-free biliary stent *(closed straight white arrow)* is seen in the second portion of the duodenum (TR 1.5 sec, TE 28 msec). Artifact of high-intensity signal *(black arrows)* is seen diffusely over the periphery of the right lobe of the liver and is caused by the metallic connector of the external drainage tube, which is attached to the patient's abdomen and is approximately 3 cm caudal to this image. Normal vascular structures are seen, including the splenic vein *(open curved arrow)*, the celiac axis *(closed curved arrow)*, and the portal vein *(open arrowhead)*.

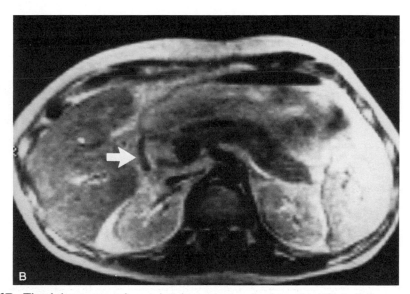

Figure 33–16B. The biliary stent *(arrow)* is less apparent when the TR is 2.0 sec and the TE is prolonged to 56 msec.

Figure 33–17. UPPER ABDOMEN WITH CONTRAST AGENT: NORMAL FINDINGS.

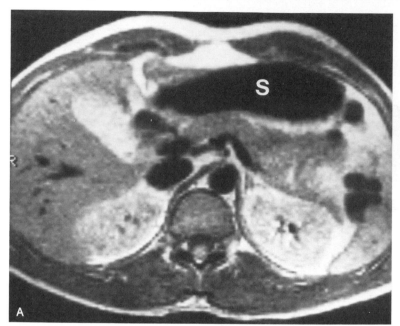

Figure 33–17A. A gas-distended stomach (S) is seen after the oral ingestion of effervescent granules along with 10 ml of water with simethicone. The CO_2 produced by this readily identifies the body and antrum of the anteriorly positioned stomach in this supine subject.

Figure 33–17B. The same normal volunteer as in A is imaged at a slightly more caudal level after the ingestion of a dilute (1 mM) solution of ferric ammonium citrate, which has produced a high-intensity signal within the stomach (S). The iron-filled stomach is clearly differentiated from the anterior wall of the body and tail of the pancreas (p), which can be assessed as normal. Note that the dorsal extent of the pancreas is delineated by the signal-free splenic vein (arrow).

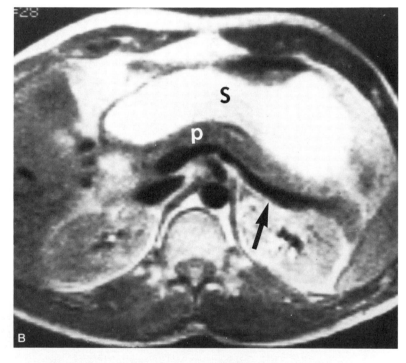

Figure 33–18. FULLNESS OF THE PANCREATIC TAIL/LIGAMENTUM TERES/CRUS OF THE RIGHT DIAPHRAGM.

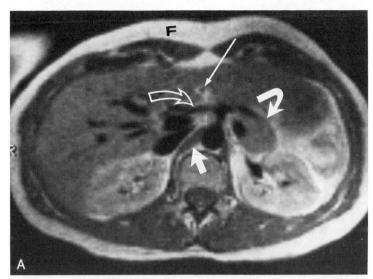

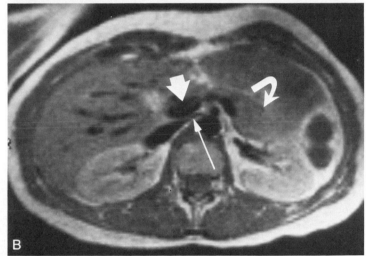

Figure 33–18A and B. (TR 1.5 sec, TE 28 msec.) This normal volunteer has a slight fullness in the tail of the pancreas *(curved closed arrow)*. In the absence of signal changes and when an isolated finding, this should not be mistaken for a mass. In *A*, the signal-free ligamentum teres *(long straight arrow)* is surrounded by high-intensity fat. This identifies the left intersegmental fissure and the division of the left lobe of the liver into its lateral and medial segments. The hepatic artery *(open curved arrow)* and the crus of the right diaphragm *(short straight arrow)* are seen in *A*. Note also the high-intensity fatty deposition (F) in the subcutaneous tissue in this woman, compared with intraperitoneal or retroperitoneal fatty deposition, which is more common in men. In *B*, the signal-free splenoportal confluence *(short straight arrow)* is demonstrated and the left renal vein *(long straight arrow)* can be seen.

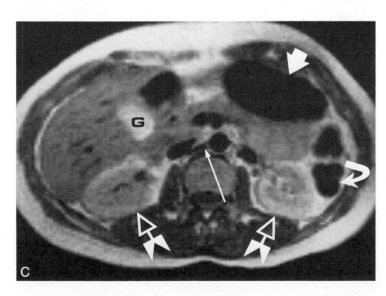

Figure 33–18C. High-intensity, concentrated bile is seen in this normal gallbladder (G) of the same individual as in *A* and *B*. Also identified are the right renal artery *(long straight arrow)*, right and left kidneys *(open arrows)*, air-filled stomach *(short straight arrow)*, and left colon *(curved arrow)*. (TR 1.5 sec, TE 28 msec.)

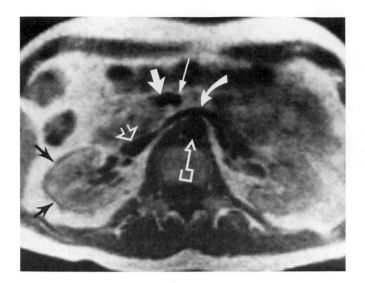

Figure 33–19. ABDOMINAL VASCULATURE/ PERIRENAL LOW-INTENSITY ARTIFACT. In this image (TR 1.0 sec, TE 28 msec), the superior mesenteric artery *(straight white arrow)* and the slightly fuller, more rightward superior mesenteric vein *(closed white arrowhead)* are seen to abut each other and simulate a signal-free dumbbell-shaped lesion. Note the left renal vein *(curved white arrow)* coursing anteriorly to the aorta *(boxed open arrow)* as it enters the inferior vena cava *(open white arrowhead)*. Note also the normal flattening of the inferior vena cava at the level of entrance of the left renal vein and the low-intensity line around the kidney *(black arrows)* representing chemical shift artifact.

Figure 33–20. SPLENOPORTAL CONFLUENCE.

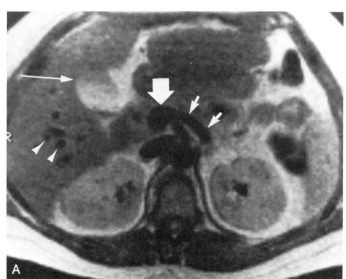

Figure 33–20A. This image (TR 1.5 sec, TE 28 msec) demonstrates a full but normal splenoportal confluence *(wide arrow)* and splenic vein *(small arrows)*. Note that when the TE is 28 msec, layering *(long arrow)* of non-concentrated and concentrated gallbladder bile can be seen. Intrahepatic vessels *(arrowheads)* appear hypointense at this TE.

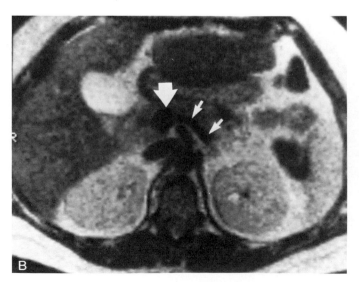

Figure 33–20B. This is the same axial image seen in A; however, the TE has been prolonged to 56 msec. At this TE setting, both concentrated and non-concentrated gallbladder bile are relatively more intense and the intrahepatic vessels have become isointense relative to the hepatic parenchyma. The normal splenoportal confluence *(wide arrow)* and splenic vein *(small arrows)* are again demonstrated.

Figure 33–21. **SPLENIC VESSELS.** The subject is a normal adult volunteer. (TR 0.5 sec, TE 28 msec.)

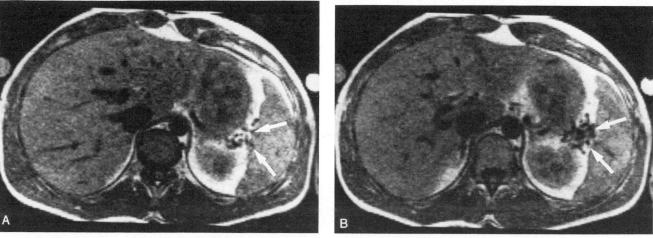

Figure 33–21A and B. Multiple signal-free, round and curvilinear structures in the area of the splenic hilum *(arrows)* represent splenic arteries and veins.

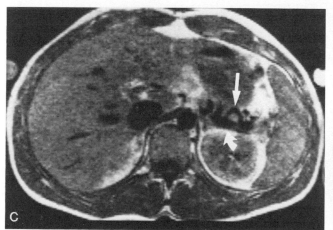

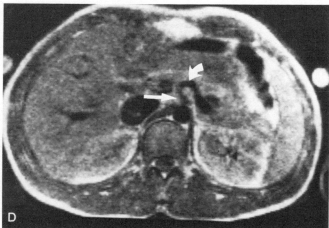

Figure 33–21C. This image, 1 cm caudal to *B,* demonstrates the more proximal, tortuous splenic artery *(straight arrow)* and the splenic vein *(curved arrow).*

Figure 33–21D. In this image, 1 cm caudal to *C,* the take-off of the splenic artery *(curved arrow)* from the celiac axis *(straight arrow)* is seen.

Figure 33–22. BOWEL IN HEPATORENAL FOSSA. (TR 2.0 sec, TE 28 msec.)

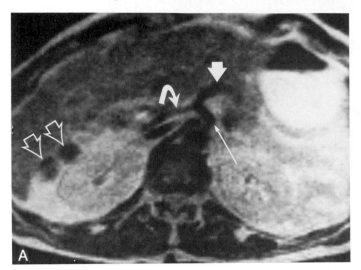

Figure 33–22A. Hypotense signal (round structures indicated by *open arrowheads*) originating from the hepatorenal fossa might be misinterpreted as abnormal in this postoperative patient clinically suspected of having an abscess. Note also the normal celiac axis *(straight arrow)*, hepatic artery *(curved arrow)*, and splenic artery *(closed arrowhead)*.

Figure 33–22B. This consecutive caudal image and other images confirmed that these structures *(open arrowheads)* represented bowel in the hepatorenal fossa. Also demonstrated are the superior mesenteric artery take-off *(curved arrow)* and the left renal vein *(double straight arrows)* as it enters the inferior vena cava.

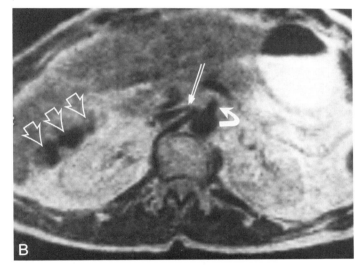

Figure 33–23. FLUID-FILLED SMALL BOWEL/MISREGISTRATION ARTIFACT. While bowel *(curved arrow, A and B)* may be difficult to detect on images with short TE, such as *A*, fluid content within the bowel increases the signal intensity on second echo (56 msec) images, as in *B*. Also note the air within the colon *(short arrows, A and B)*, which is signal-free on both the first and second echo images.

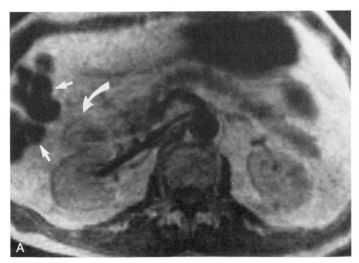

Figure 33–23A. This image was obtained with a TR of 0.2 sec and a TE of 28 msec.

Illustration continued on opposite page

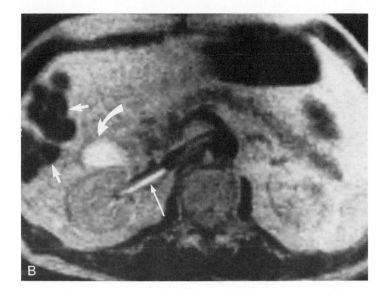

Figure 33–23B. When the TE is prolonged to 56 msec, there is high-intensity signal posterior to the right renal vein *(long straight arrow)*, which represents the artifact misregistration along the y axis.

Figure 33–24. FLUID-FILLED SMALL BOWEL/ASCENDING AND DESCENDING COLON. As in computed tomographic examinations of the abdomen, fluid-filled loops of small bowel on MRI may simulate intra-abdominal masses when no oral contrast agent has been administered.

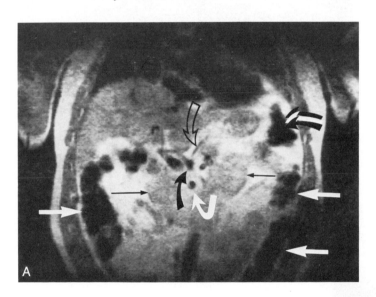

Figure 33–24A. A coronal image (TR 1.5 sec, TE 28 msec) demonstrates central "masses" *(straight black arrows)* that actually represent normal fluid-filled loops of small bowel. Air can be seen in the ascending and descending colon *(straight white arrows)*. Also identified are several vascular structures, including the celiac axis *(closed curved black arrow)*, the splenic artery *(open curved black arrow)* and the superior mesenteric artery *(curved white arrow)*.

Figure 33–24B. When the TE of the coronal image shown in A is prolonged to 56 msec, the contrast is increased but detail is decreased. Again are seen the fluid-filled loops of small bowel *(straight arrows)* and various vascular structures, including the hepatic artery *(open arrow)* and the portal vein *(boxed arrow)*.

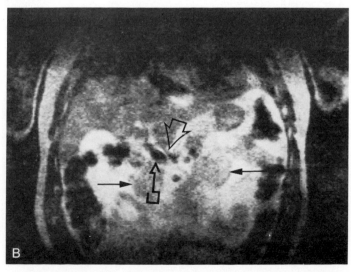

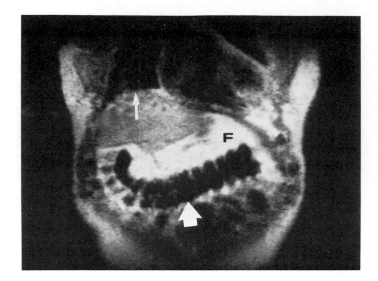

Figure 33–25. INTRAPERITONEAL FAT/ TRANSVERSE COLON. This coronal image (TR 1.5 sec, TE 28 msec) demonstrates high-intensity signal (F) situated superiorly to the transverse colon *(wide arrow)*. It represents normal intraperitoneal fat. Note the air-filled lung *(narrow arrow)*, which emits no signal in the right hemithorax.

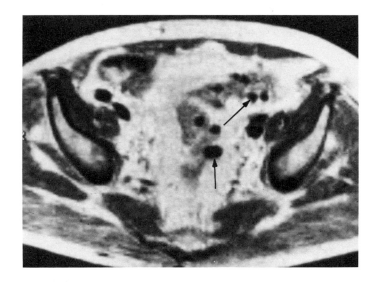

Figure 33–26. DIVERTICULOSIS. An axial image (TR 2.0 sec, TE 28 msec) of the pelvis demonstrates diverticulosis of the sigmoid colon. The air-filled diverticula *(arrows)* emit no signal and are easily differentiated from the high-intensity signal of the pelvic fat.

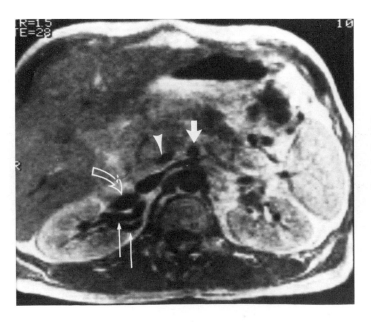

Figure 33–27. TWO RIGHT RENAL ARTERIES. Two right renal arteries *(long straight arrows)* are seen in this axial image (TR 1.5 sec, TE 28 msec) of the abdomen at the level of the renal hilum. The right renal vein *(curved arrow)* and the superior mesenteric artery *(short wide arrow)* and vein *(arrowhead)* are also demonstrated.

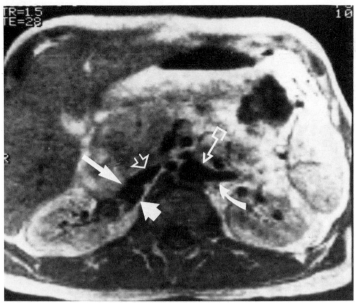

Figure 33–28. NORMAL RENAL VESSELS. Normal renal vascular structures are noted as follows: left renal artery *(curved arrow)*, right renal artery *(closed short arrow)*, right renal vein *(long straight arrow)*, inferior vena cava *(open short arrowhead)* and the aorta *(boxed arrow)*. (TR 1.5 sec, TE 28 msec.)

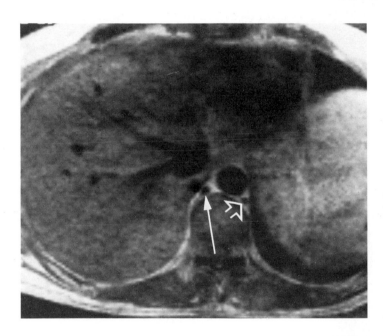

Figure 33–29. AZYGOUS AND HEMIAZYGOUS VEINS. Azygous *(arrow)* and hemiazygous *(arrowhead)* veins are demonstrated as small round structures that emit no signal and are seen to course parallel and adjacent to the aorta. (TR 2.0 sec, TE 28 msec.)

Figure 33–30. LEFT GONADAL VEIN. The left gonadal vein *(narrow straight arrow)* is seen before it enters the left renal vein *(wide arrow)*. Note the head of the pancreas (P) and the (normal) flattened inferior vena cava *(curved arrow)* posteriorly. The gonadal veins are easily recognized and differentiated from psoas muscle (M) on MRI. (TR 2.0 sec, TR 28 msec.)

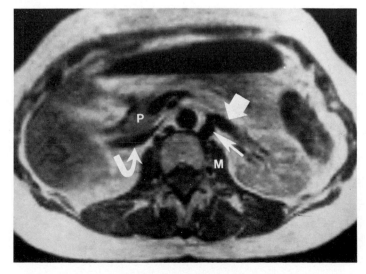

Figure 33–31. URETER AND GONADAL VEINS.

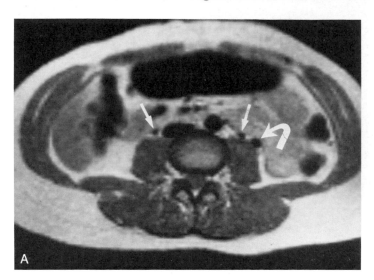

Figure 33–31A. In this image (TR 1.5 sec, TE 28 msec), the right and left gonadal veins *(straight arrows)* are demonstrated as round, tubular signal-free structures anterior to each psoas muscle. The ureter *(curved arrow)* is also identified.

Figure 33–31B. When the TE is prolonged to 56 msec, the gonadal veins exhibit high-intensity signal. Note that the left ureter *(curved arrow)* has low-intensity signal on both short and long TE images.

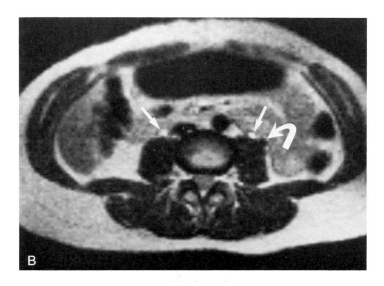

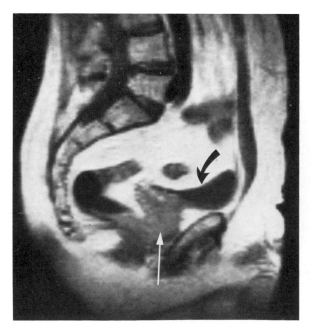

Figure 33–32. SAGITTAL PELVIS: NORMAL FINDINGS. A normal but incompletely distended urinary bladder *(curved arrow)* is seen. Note the air-filled rectum and high intensity fat within the presacral space and the medium-intensity signal of the prostate *(straight arrow)*.

Figure 33–33. PSEUDOMASS: PARTIAL VOLUME AVERAGING.

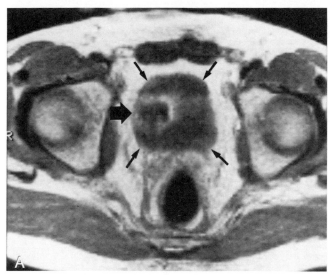

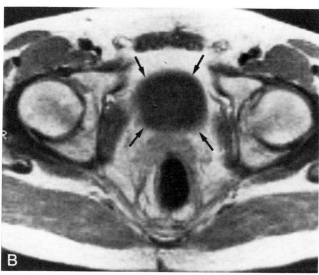

Figure 33–33A. In this image (TR 1.5 sec, TE 28 msec), the urinary bladder *(arrows)* appears to have a lesion *(wide arrow)* within it to the right of midline, but in fact this area of heterogeneity is an artifact of partial volume averaging of bowel and mesentery just superior to the urinary bladder.

Figure 33–33B. One cm caudal to *A,* this image demonstrates the urinary bladder *(arrows)* without partial volume averaging of bowel.

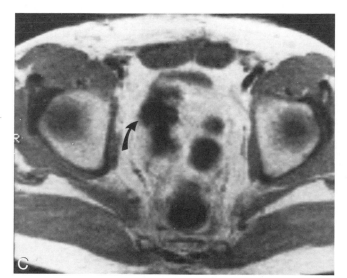

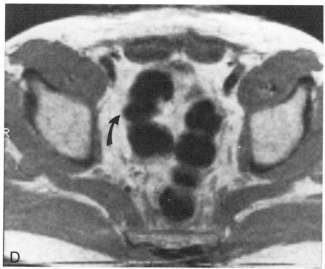

Figure 33–33C and D. Adjacent MRI images superior to the urinary bladder verify the artifactual findings on *A* and *B* as air-filled bowel *(curved arrows).*

Figure 33–34. PSEUDOMASS: MESENTERIC FAT. This MRI study includes sagittal (*A* and *B*) and transverse *(C)* images of the pelvis of a female patient with transitional cell carcinoma of the bladder.

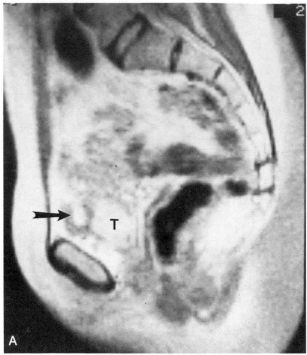

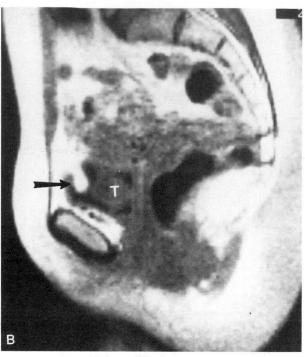

Figure 33–34A. In this sagittal image (TR 2 sec, TE 28 msec), the intensity of the transitional cell carcinoma (T) seen at the posterior aspect of the bladder is similar to that of the pseudomass seen anteriorly on the bladder dome *(arrow).* In this particular sequence, the etiology of the anterior mass is difficult to evaluate.

Figure 33–34B. When the study is repeated with a TR of 0.5 sec, it is clear that the anterior "mass" *(arrow)* is mesenteric fat indenting the non-distended urinary bladder. The tumor (T) is seen with medium-intensity signal.

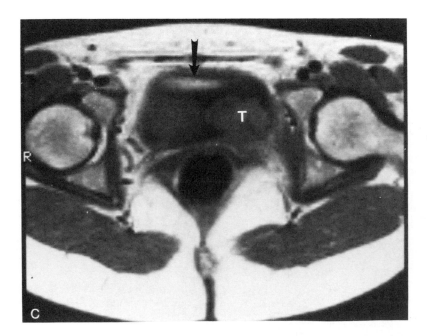

Figure 33–34C. The similar artifact of mesenteric fat *(arrow)* can be seen on the transverse image (TR 0.5 sec, TE 28 msec). Note, again, the papillary transitional cell carcinoma (T) of the left posterior bladder wall.

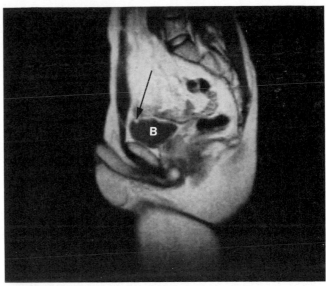

Figure 33–35. PSEUDOMASS: MESENTERIC FAT. A high-intensity pseudolesion *(arrow)* in the anterior dome of the bladder (B) is seen on a sagittal image (TR 2.0 sec, TE 28 msec) of the pelvis of a male patient. In reviewing consecutive scans, this was found to represent mesenteric fat indentation on an incompletely distended urinary bladder.

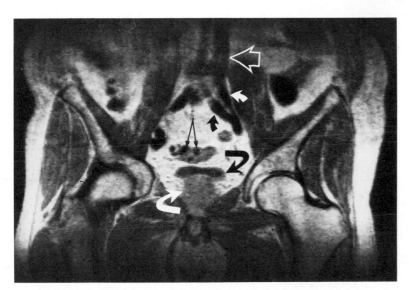

Figure 33–36. BENIGN PROSTATIC HYPERTROPHY/COLONIC DIVERTICULA. A nearly empty urinary bladder *(large curved black arrow)* is seen above a mildly enlarged prostate gland *(large curved white arrow)* (benign hypertrophy) on this coronal image. Note the air-filled, signal-free diverticula *(straight black arrows)* within the sigmoid colon. Normal pelvic vessels are seen as signal-free curvilinear structures and include the aorta *(open white arrow)*, the inferior vena cava (parallel to the aorta), the left common iliac artery *(small curved white arrow)*, and the left common iliac vein *(small curved black arrow)*. (TR 1.5 sec, TE 28 msec.)

Figure 33–37. PSEUDOMASS: SIGMOID COLON. A coronal image (TR 0.5 sec, TE 28 msec) of the pelvis of an adult man demonstrates a normal air-filled sigmoid colon *(curved black arrows)* in addition to a collapsed segment of sigmoid colon *(straight arrow)*, which should not be mistaken for a mass. Slight malpositioning accounts for the asymmetric appearance of iliac wings *(curved open arrows)* and of the pelvic muscles.

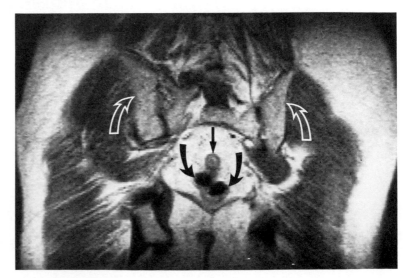

Figure 33–38. EFFECT OF DISTENDED URINARY BLADDER ON THE APPEARANCE OF THE CORPUS UTERI.

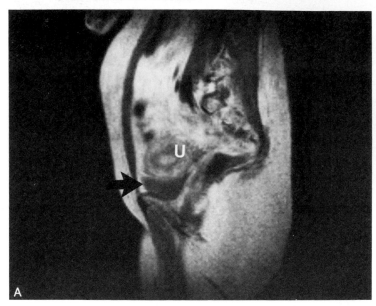

Figure 33–38A. In this sagittal image (TR 2.0 sec, TE 28 msec), the bladder *(arrow)* is nondistended and the corpus uteri (U) has a round configuration pressing on the bladder dome.

Figure 33–38B. A repeat scan of the same patient shown in A, with full bladder distention, demonstrates elevation of and change in the shape of the corpus uteri (U).

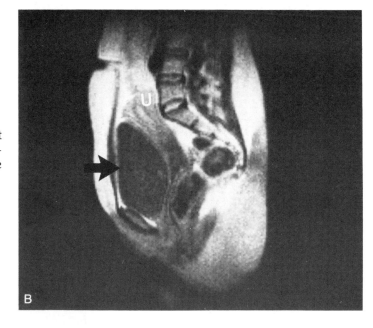

Figure 33–39. PSEUDOMASS: CERVIX.

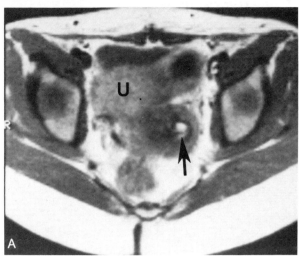

Figure 33–39A. In this transverse image (TR 1.5 sec, TE 28 msec), the corpus uteri (U) is seen to the right of the midline. There appears to be separate mass with high intensity in the center *(arrow).*

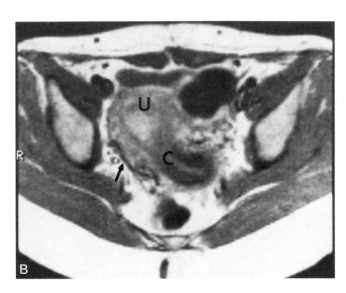

Figure 33–39B. One centimeter cephalad to A, the continuation between the corpus uteri (U) and the cervix (C) is apparent, confirming that the pseudomass seen in A represents the cervix. The uterine artery *(arrow)* is also demonstrated.

CHAPTER 34

Musculoskeletal System

CLYDE A. HELMS, M.D.
MICHAEL L. RICHARDSON, M.D.

Figure 34–1. METALLIC ARTIFACT: PROSTHESIS.

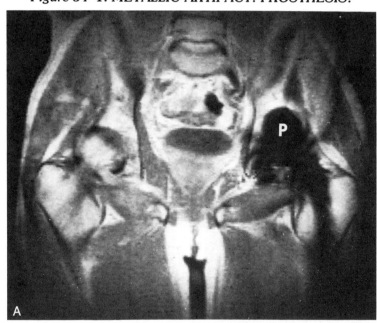

Figure 34–1A. A coronal scan through the pelvis in a patient with a left hip prosthesis (P) shows virtually no signal emanating from the prosthesis.

Illustration continued on opposite page

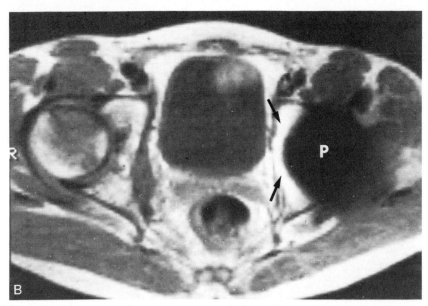

Figure 34–1B. An axial scan in the same patient shows a large area that is devoid of signal and represents the prosthesis (P). Note that the size of the low-intensity area does not correspond to the actual size of the prosthesis as seen on the coronal scan. A large, curvilinear high-intensity signal is seen medial to the prosthesis *(arrows)*, which represents an artifact occasionally seen with metallic prostheses.

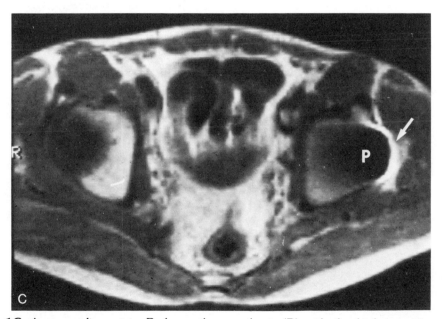

Figure 34–1C. A scan adjacent to *B* shows the prosthesis (P) with the high-intensity curvilinear artifact lateral to the prosthesis *(arrow)*.

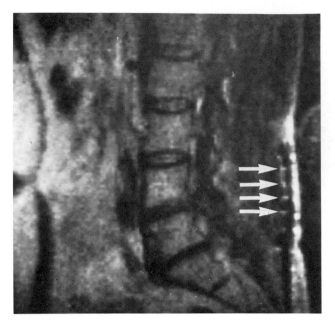

Figure 34–2. METALLIC ARTIFACT: WIRE SUTURES. A sagittal scan through the lumbar spine shows some high-intensity streaks in the posterior soft tissue *(arrows)* that are artifacts due to wire sutures.

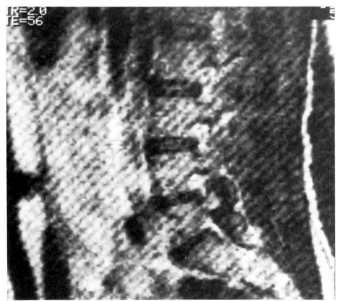

Figure 34–3. RADIO FREQUENCY ARTIFACT. A "herringbone pattern" is occasionally seen as a manifestation of radio frequency interference.

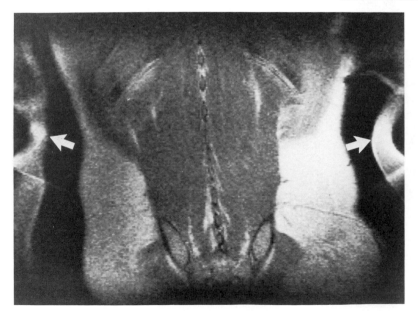

Figure 34–4. INTENSITY ARTIFACT. A coronal scan through the back has a frequently seen artifact, with one side of the image being darker than the opposite. Note the high-intensity signal from the muscles on the left compared with the muscles on the right. The exact cause of this is undetermined to date. Notice also the distortion to the arms *(arrows)*, which is due to patient contact with the coils.

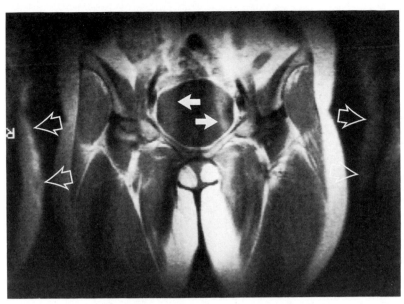

Figure 34–5. "WRAP AROUND" AR- TIFACT. A coronal image of the pelvis demonstrates a "wrap around" artifact *(open arrows)* seen as signal arising outside of the body. It is caused by the body part filling too much of the coil. It has also caused the streak artifacts *(solid arrows)* noted over the bladder.

Figure 34–6. MOTION ARTIFACT.

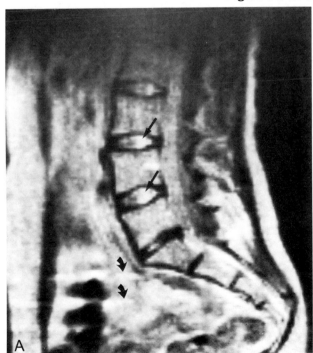

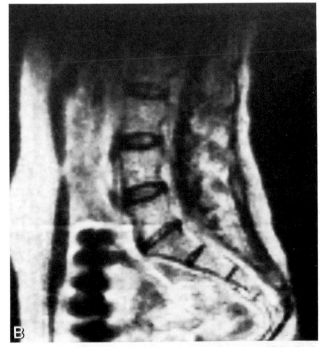

Figure 34–6A. A midline sagittal scan through the lumbar spine shows high-intensity streak-like artifacts parallel to the haustra in the colon *(curved arrows)*. These probably result from peristaltic motion of the bowel gas. Note the high-intensity signal from the nucleus pulposus *(straight arrows)* compared with the parasagittal scan in B. This probably results from partial volume averaging of annulus with the nucleus pulposus.

Figure 34–6B. Streak artifacts associated with bowel gas in the haustra of the colon are again seen. Note the low-intensity signal of the nucleus pulposus compared with the midline cut on A. A similar appearance of low-intensity signal of the nucleus can be seen in degenerative disc disease; however, this case illustrates how apparent degenerative disc disease can be mistakenly diagnosed if the midline scan is not obtained.

Figure 34–7. AREA OF LOW SIGNAL INTENSITY IN NUCLEUS PULPOSUS. Sagittal scans of the lumbar spine are shown.

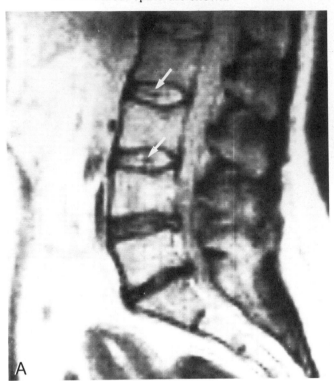

Figure 34–7A. The nucleus pulposus generates a high-intensity signal at L3-4 and L4-5 with a linear low-intensity area *(arrows)* in the center of each disc. This is occasionally seen in normal subjects; the cause is unknown. It has been called the intranuclear cleft.

Ref.: (1) Modic MT, Pavlicek W, Weinstein MA, et al. Magnetic resonance imaging of intervertebral disk disease. Clinical and pulse sequence consideration. Radiology 1984; 152:103–111. (2) Aguila LA, Piraino DW, Modic MT. Magnetic resonance imaging of the intranuclear cleft. Radiology 1985; 155:155–158.

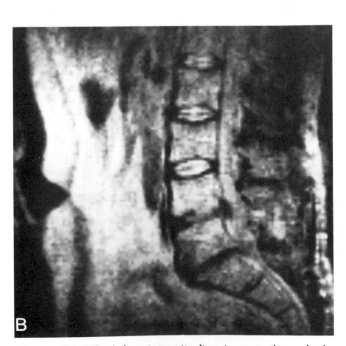

Figure 34–7B. A low-intensity line is seen through the center of each nucleus pulposus, similar to A. These are best seen above the level of L4.

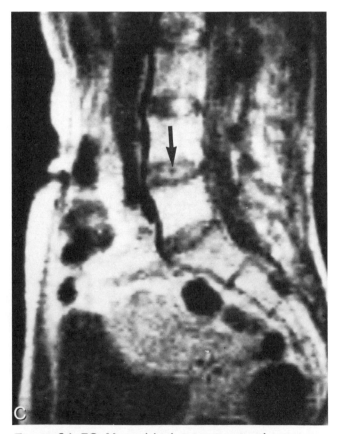

Figure 34–7C. Normal high-intensity signal originates from each nucleus pulposus, with the L4-5 nucleus demonstrating a focal area of low intensity *(arrow).* The etiology of this finding is not known; however, it is often seen in the lumbar spine.

Figure 34–8. LOSS OF DISC SIGNAL FROM PARTIAL VOLUME AVERAGING.

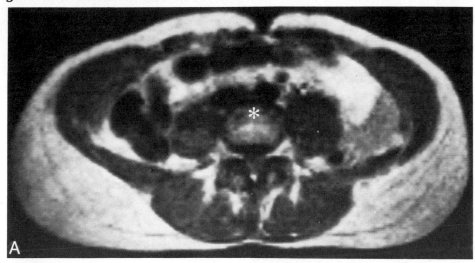

Figure 34–8A. An axial image of the lumbar spine at the level of the disc shows a low-intensity signal from the nucleus pulposus *(asterisk)*, suggesting degenerative disease. Because of partial volume averaging, definite degenerative disc disease should not be diagnosed on axial images alone. (See the normal-appearing disc in *B*.)

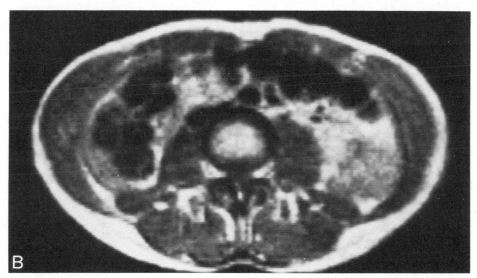

Figure 34–8B. The image adjacent to *A* shows the normal high-intensity signal from the nucleus. Not all normal discs show this high-intensity image on axial scans; occasionally the thickness of the slices and partial volume averaging will make the nucleus appear artificially low in intensity as on the prior slice.

Figure 34–9. LOSS OF DISC SIGNAL FROM PARTIAL VOLUME AVERAGING.

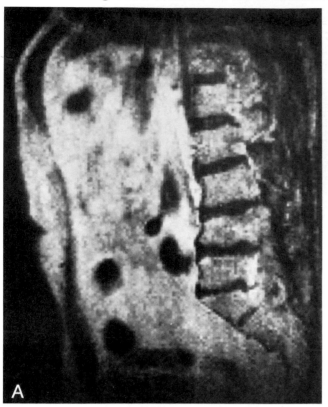

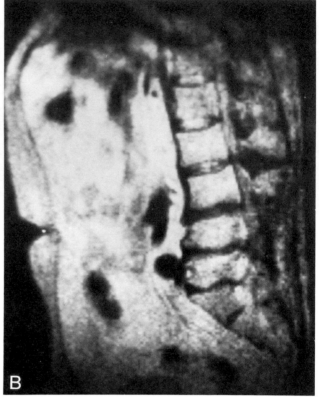

Figure 34–9A. A parasagittal scan shows low-intensity signal from all of the discs in the lumbar region, suggesting degenerative disease.

Figure 34–9B. A true sagittal scan in the same patient with the same scanning parameters demonstrates degenerative disc disease at the lumbar levels below L3 but normal-intensity signal from the nucleus pulposus in the lumbar discs above this level. The prior scan was done off midline, resulting in partial volume averaging of the annulus fibrosis with the nucleus giving the suggestion of degenerative disc disease. Care must be taken to evaluate the true midline scan before diagnosing degenerative disc disease.

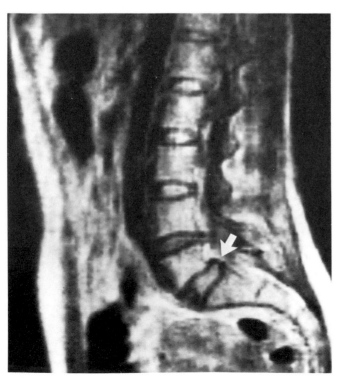

Figure 34–10. SPONDYLOLISTHESIS PRODUCING APPARENT DISC PROTRUSION. A parasagittal scan of the lumbar spine shows an apparent disc protrusion *(arrow)* extending into the L5–S1 neural foramen. This apparent protrusion, however, is the result of a grade one spondylolisthesis of L5 on S1 with the disc material staying with the S1 segment. It is important to evaluate the disc material in relation to the posterior endplate of S1 rather than the posterior endplate of L5 in order to avoid an erroneous diagnosis of a protruded disc in this setting.

Figure 34–11. KLIPPEL-FEIL DEFORMITY.

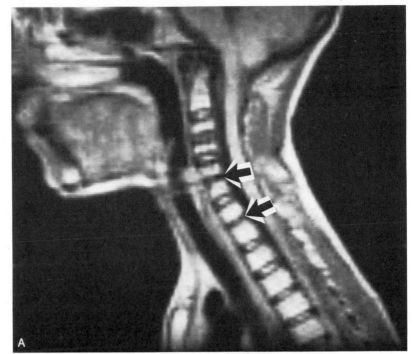

Figure 34–11A. A sagittal image through the cervical spine in this patient with Klippel-Feil deformity shows a narrow intervertebral disc space at C5-6 and at C7–T1 with loss of the high-intensity signal normally seen in the nucleus pulposus *(arrows)*. This indicates fusion of these vertebral bodies.

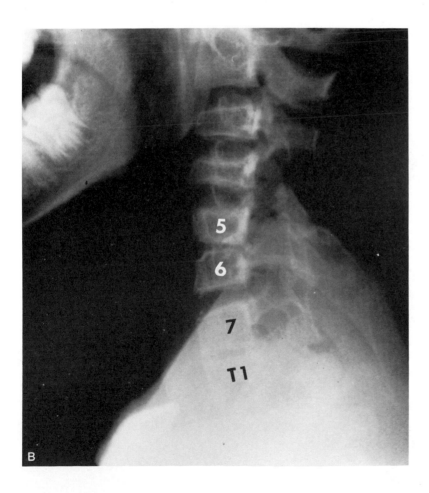

Figure 34–11B. The corresponding lateral C-spine plain film shows fusion of C5-6 and C7–T1 vertebral bodies.

Figure 34–12. BASIVERTEBRAL PLEXUS. In these axial MRI scans of the lumbar spine, a low-intensity signal *(arrows)* is seen in the region of the midvertebral body. The location and appearance of this structure are characteristic of the basivertebral plexus.

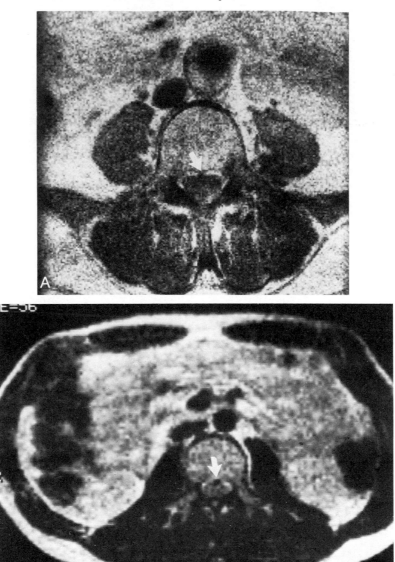

Figure 34–13. SCHMORL'S NODE AND BASIVERTEBRAL PLEXUS.

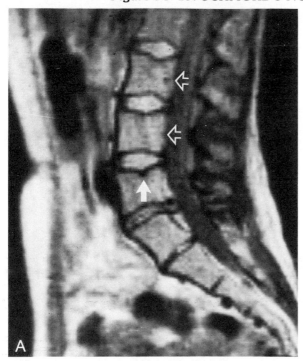

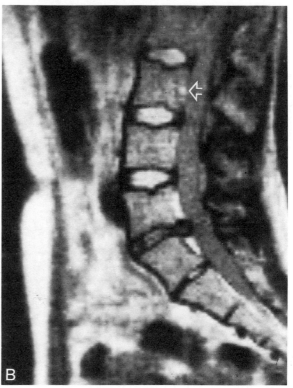

Figure 34–13A. A Schmorl's node *(arrow)* having a characteristic appearance is seen at the superior endplate of L5. Also note the low-intensity signal from the basivertebral plexus *(open arrows)* in the midvertebral bodies of L3 and L4 in this example. Note that the posterior cortex of all the vertebral bodies, particularly at L3 and L4, is not well seen. Poor visualization of posterior cortical margins of vertebral bodies on MRI scans is not uncommon and should not be misconstrued as indicative of pathology.

Figure 34–13B. A second echo image of the same scan as in *A* demonstrates the basivertebral plexus *(arrow)* to have a high-intensity signal. This probably represents even-echo rephasing in slow blood flow through the plexus.

Ref. Waluch V, Bradley WG. NMR even echo rephasing in slow laminar flow. J Comput Assist Tomogr 1984; 8:594–598.

Figure 34–13C. A sagittal second echo scan through the lumbar spine shows the basivertebral plexus at L2 and L3 in this patient to have a high-intensity signal *(arrows)*.

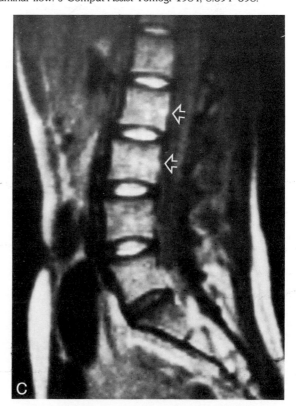

Figure 34–14. SCHMORL'S NODE.

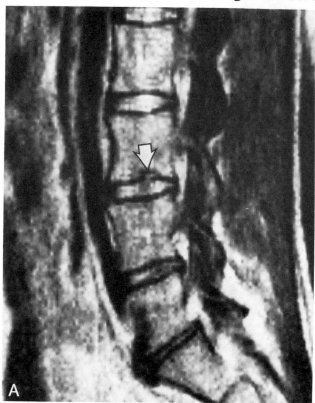

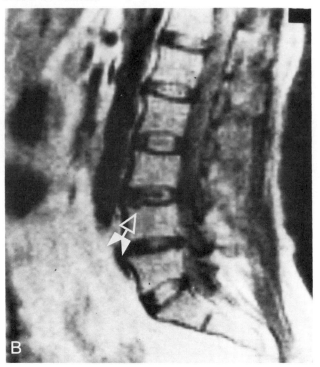

Figure 34–14B. A parasagittal scan of the lumbar spine demonstrates a typical Schmorl's node *(arrow)* in the superior endplate of the L4 vertebral body.

Figure 34–14A. A parasagittal scan through the lumbar spine shows herniation of disc material *(arrow)* through a defect in the inferior endplate of the L3 body. This appearance is characteristic of a Schmorl's node.

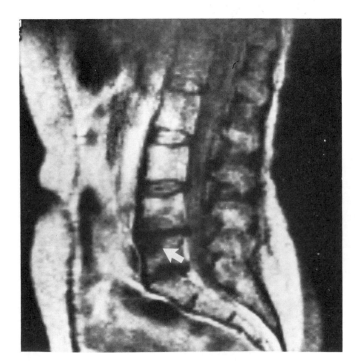

Figure 34–15. DISCOGENIC VERTEBRAL DIS-EASE. A sagittal scan of the lumbar spine shows an area of low-intensity signal *(arrow)* involving the L5 vertebral body anteriorly. This could be confused with metastatic disease (see Fig. 34–32B). In this example, however, the appearance is characteristic for discogenic vertebral disease that occurs with long-standing degenerative disc disease and is always associated with adjacent disc space narrowing, osteophytosis, and sclerosis. This entity is analogous to a Schmorl's node.

Ref.: Martel W, Seeger JF, Wicks JD, et al. Traumatic lesions of the discovertebral junction in the lumbar spine. AJR 1976; 127:457–464.

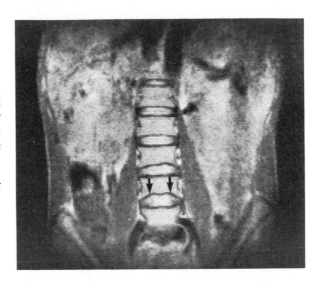

Figure 34–16. ***CUPID'S BOW DEFORMITY.*** A coronal image of the lumbar spine demonstrates a Cupid's bow deformity *(arrows)* at the inferior endplate of L4. This is often seen in the lower lumbar vertebral bodies. A milder example is seen at the inferior border of L3 in this patient.

Ref.: Dietz GW, Christensen EE. Normal "cupid's bow" contour of the lower lumbar vertebrae. Radiology 1976; 121:577.

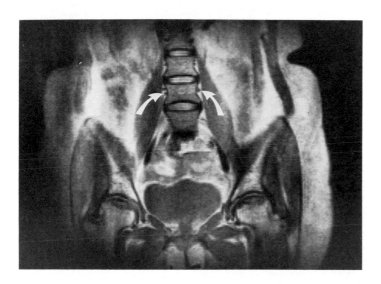

Figure 34–17. ***SEGMENTAL LUMBAR VEINS.*** A coronal image of the lumbar spine and pelvis in a patient with bilateral avascular necrosis of the hips shows a low-intensity signal from the segmental lumbar veins *(arrows).*

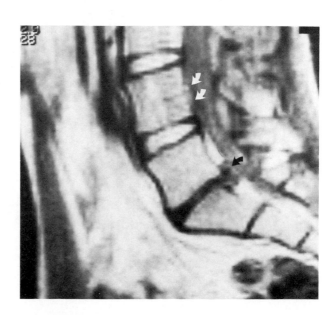

Figure 34–18. ***EPIDURAL FAT WITH PARTIAL VOLUME AVERAGING.*** A sagittal scan of the lumbar spine shows an intermediate-intensity signal *(white arrows)* adjacent to the posterior L4 vertebral body, which represents epidural fat. This should not be mistaken for a bony projection or free disc fragment, both of which should have a low-intensity MRI signal. Note the abundance of higher-intensity epidural fat posterior to the L5 vertebral body. The intermediate-intensity signal of epidural fat at L4 is, perhaps, due to partial volume averaging. In addition, this patient has a large herniated disc *(black arrow)* at the L5-S1 level.

Figure 34–19. HIGH-INTENSITY SIGNAL IN VERTEBRAL BODIES. Parasagittal scans through the lumbar and thoracic spine show several areas of increased-intensity signal *(arrows, A)*, which are of undetermined etiology. These are occasionally seen throughout the spine and the source remains unidentified.

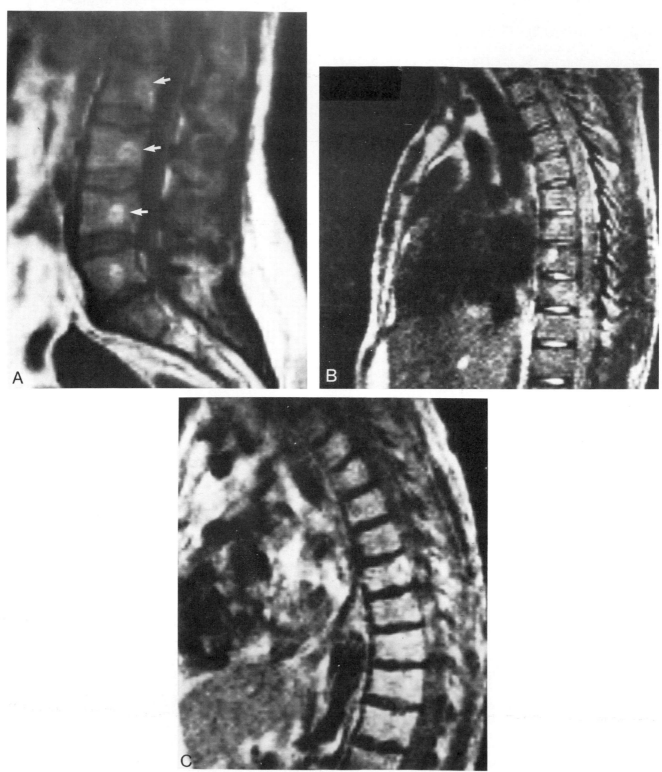

Figure 34–20. SACRAL NEURAL FORAMINA.

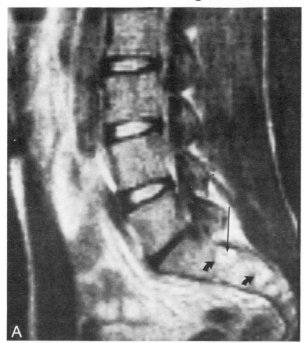

Figure 34–20A. A parasagittal scan through the lumbar spine and sacrum shows multiple high-intensity defects *(curved arrows)* in the sacrum, which can occasionally mimic a destructive process at this location. These are the normal sacral neural foramina. Note the low-intensity signal *(straight arrow)* representing the nerve root in the most superior sacral neural foramen.

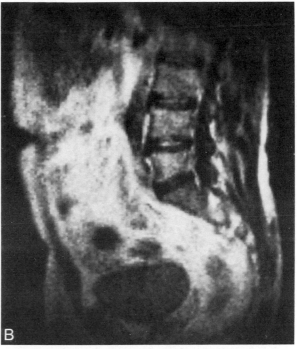

Figure 34–20B. A parasagittal scan of the lumbar spine and sacrum in another patient again demonstrates the high-intensity nature of the normal sacral neuroforamina. These structures are most evident in off-midline scans.

Figure 34–21. SCOLIOSIS.

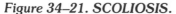

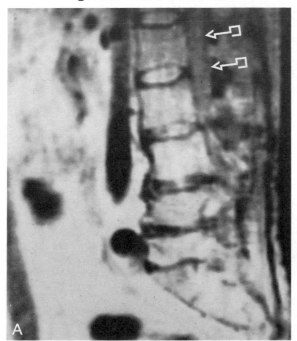

Figure 34–21A. A parasagittal scan of the lumbar spine shows a normal-appearing spinal cord and thecal sac *(arrows)* in the upper lumbar spine (above L3). Below this level, however, the thecal sac and nerve roots are not seen, suggesting possible impingement.

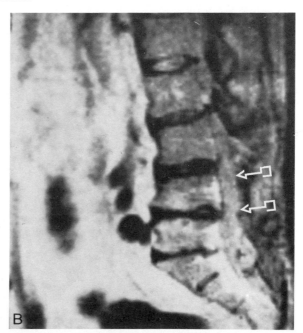

Figure 34–21B. An adjacent parasagittal scan shows the thecal sac *(arrows)* in the lower lumbar regions; however, now the cord and thecal sac in the upper spinal canal are not seen. The reason for this apparent disappearance of the central canal and cord in this patient is scoliosis. When scoliosis is present it should be identified on an anteroposterior examination in order to avoid mistakenly interpreting central canal abnormalities on parasagittal scans when the canal is only partially included in the section.

Figure 34–22. PARTIAL VOLUME AVERAGING OF THE HAMATE, SIMULATING A FRACTURE.

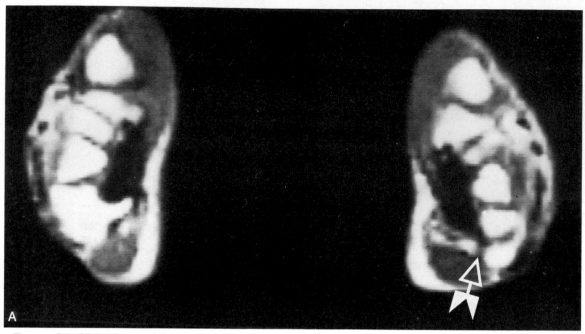

Figure 34–22A. An axial MRI scan of the wrists shows an apparent fracture *(arrow)* of the hook of the hamate on the right side. Compare this to the normal left side.

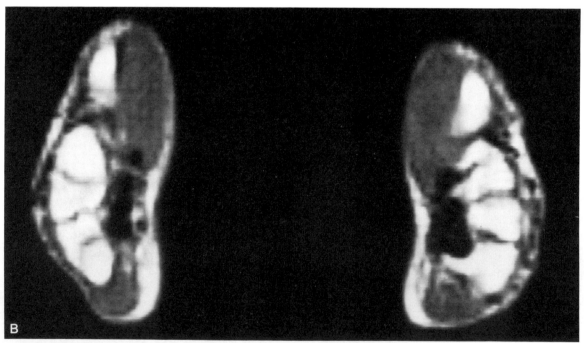

Figure 34–22B. A slightly more distal scan shows that the hook of the hamate is not fractured. The apparent fracture on the prior scan was due to partial volume averaging.

Figure 34–23. VASCULAR GROOVE—SCAPULA.

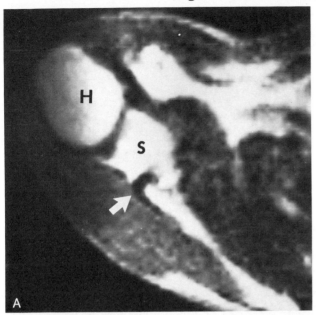

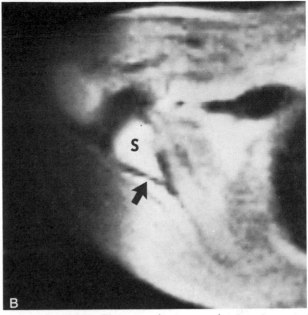

Figure 34–23A. An axial scan of the right shoulder demonstrates a low-intensity serpiginous structure *(arrow)* representing a normal vessel coursing through the scapula (S). The humerus (H) is also identified.

Figure 34–23B. The vessel seen in *A* is again noted *(arrow)* coursing through the scapula (S).

Figure 34–24. S1 JOINT SCLEROSIS. A coronal scan through the S1 joints shows low-intensity signal in the anterior portion of the right S1 joint, involving both the sacral and iliac sides. This is the typical, but not specific, appearance of degenerative disease involving the S1 joint. A spondyloarthropathy such as Reiter's psoriasis, or even infection, could certainly present with this appearance; however, it would be atypical for this to represent metastatic disease, since both sides of the joint are involved.

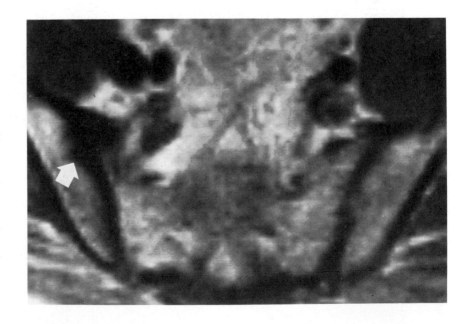

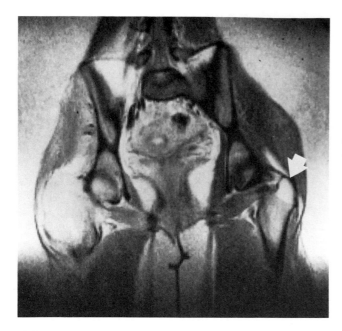

Figure 34–25. HIGH-INTENSITY SIGNAL FROM NORMAL APOPHYSES. This MR image of a 28-year-old woman with a giant cell tumor of the right hip illustrates the high-intensity signal often seen in normal epiphyses and apophyses *(arrow)* in young adults and children.

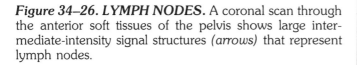

Figure 34–26. LYMPH NODES. A coronal scan through the anterior soft tissues of the pelvis shows large intermediate-intensity signal structures *(arrows)* that represent lymph nodes.

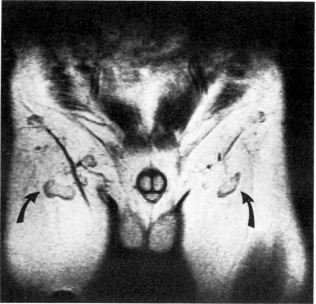

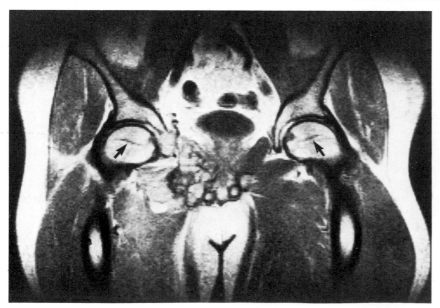

Figure 34–27. EPIPHYSEAL LINES. A coronal scan through the pelvis demonstrates a linear area of low-intensity signal in both femoral heads *(arrows)*. These are the normal physeal lines and should not be confused with fractures.

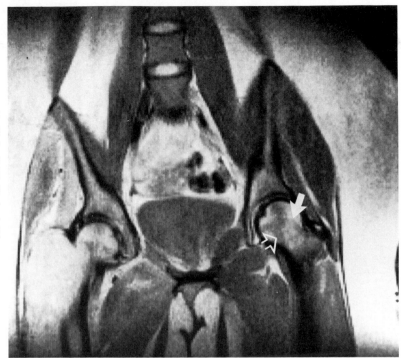

Figure 34–28. TRABECULAR PATTERNS IN THE HIP. In this coronal scan of the hips and pelvis of a patient with a giant cell tumor of the right hip, two areas of low-intensity signal *(arrows)* are seen in the left femoral head. These correspond to the primary tensile trabeculae *(solid arrow)* and the primary compressive trabeculae *(open arrow)*. These inhomogeneous areas should not be confused with avascular necrosis.

Figure 34–29. ACETABULAR NOTCH AND FOVEA CAPITIS.

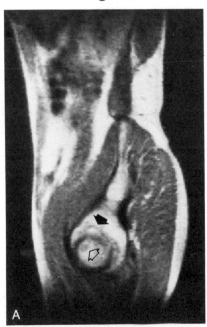

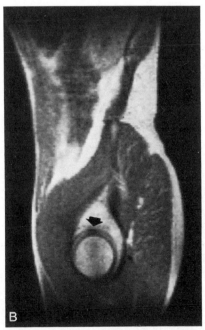

Figure 34–29A. A parasagittal scan through the acetabulum and femoral head shows a low-intensity signal *(black arrow)* in the acetabular region that represents the normal acetabular notch. Also note the low-intensity signal *(open arrow)* in the femoral head representing the normal fovea. Neither of these should be mistaken for degenerative disease or subchondral cysts.

Figure 34–29B. A more lateral parasagittal scan in the same patient as in *A* shows extension of the acetabular notch as rarefaction of the articular cartilage, yielding a low-intensity signal *(arrow)*.

Figure 34–30. FOVEA CAPITIS.

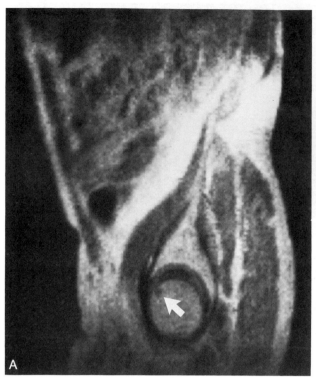

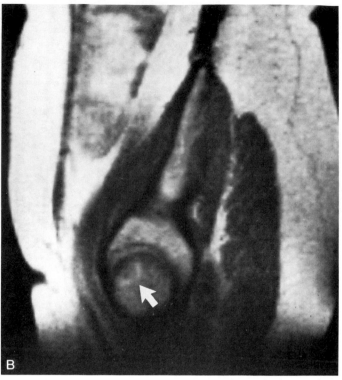

Figure 34–30A. A parasagittal scan through the medial portion of the femoral head shows an area of low intensity *(arrow)* located along the superoanterior articular surface. This represents the normal fovea and should not be mistaken for a geode or an area of avascular necrosis.

Figure 34–30B. A parasagittal scan through the medial portion of the femoral head in another patient shows a normal fovea *(arrow)*. Again, this should not be mistaken for a geode or an area of avascular necrosis.

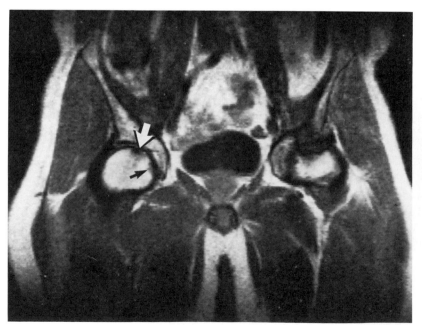

Figure 34–31. AVASCULAR NECRO-SIS OF THE HIPS VS. FOVEA CAPI-TIS. A coronal scan through the hips of a patient with bilateral avascular necrosis shows a small area of necrotic bone *(white arrow)* in the superior portion of the right femoral head. The location of necrosis is distinctly different from the normal fovea capitis *(black arrow)*, allowing differentiation of these entities.

Figure 34–32. HERNIATION PITS OF THE FEMORAL NECK.

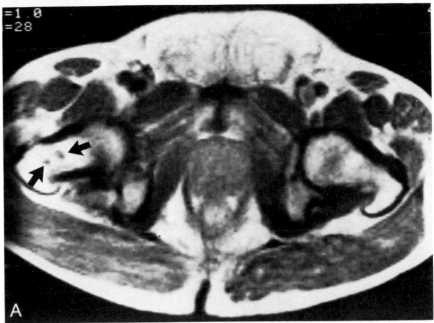

Figure 34–32A. An axial image through the hips shows two areas of low intensity *(arrows)* of a focal nature in the right femoral neck, which represent benign herniation pits of the femoral neck. These are not uncommonly seen and could be confused with metastatic disease (see *B*).

Ref.: Pitt MJ, et al. Herniation pit of the femoral neck. AJR 1982; 138:1115.

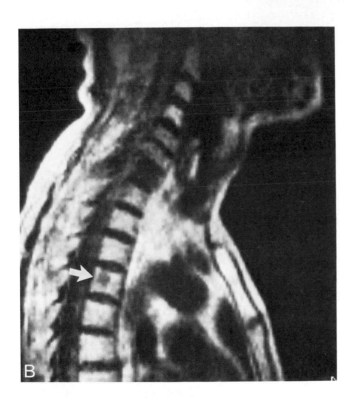

Figure 34–32B. A sagittal scan of the spine shows a focal low-intensity signal *(arrow)* in the body of T4 and a diffuse low-intensity signal from an ivory vertebra at the C7 level. These represent blastic prostatic metastases. The benign herniation pit defects in *A* can be differentiated from metastatic disease primarily by the clinical setting and the plain film appearance.

Figure 34–33. **PARTIAL VOLUME AVERAGING IN THE KNEE SIMULATING CORTICAL DESTRUCTION.**

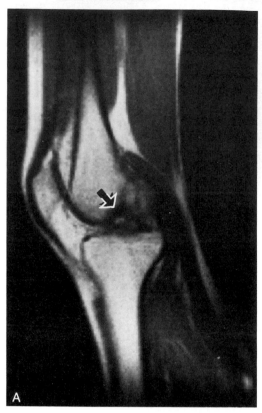

Figure 34–33A. A sagittal scan through the knee in a normal subject shows an apparent cortical defect posteriorly in the femur *(arrow).* This is due to partial volume averaging in the intercondylar notch.

Figure 34–33B. In the same patient as in *A*, an off-midline scan shows the normal posterior femoral cortex with no defect.

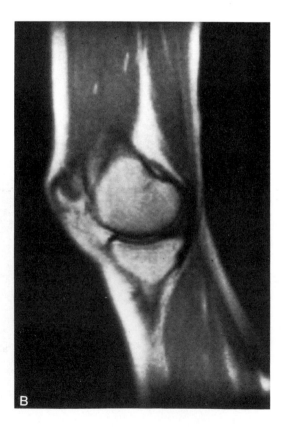

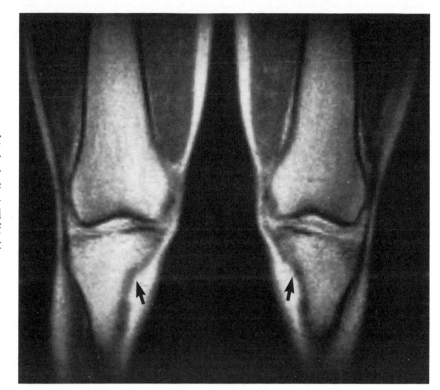

Figure 34–34. **PARTIAL VOLUME AVERAGING IN THE TIBIA SIMULATING CORTICAL DESTRUCTION.** A coronal scan through the knees of a normal subject shows apparent defects *(arrows)* in the proximal tibiae medially. These are the result of partial volume averaging and are not true cortical defects.

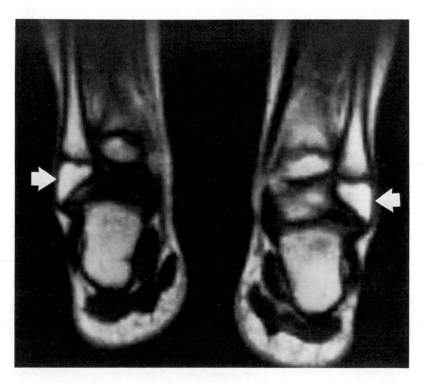

Figure 34–35. **HIGH-INTENSITY SIGNAL FROM NORMAL EPIPHYSES.** In this coronal view of the ankles of a child, a higher-intensity signal is noted in the epiphyses *(arrows)* than in the corresponding bony structures. This is normal in children and young adults.

CHAPTER 35

Pediatrics

HANS RINGERTZ, M.D.

Figure 35–1. MOTION ARTIFACT. In this transaxial MRI section through the upper abdomen of a 1-year-old boy with recurrent hepatoblastoma, repeated motion has degraded the image severely. Alternating lines of increased and decreased intensity parallel the anterior contour of the body. This motion artifact is caused by sobbing or crying and by pushing the lower thorax and upper abdomen upward while hyperextending the body. High-intensity areas such as subcutaneous fat imaged in multiple resonating positions produce these artifacts.

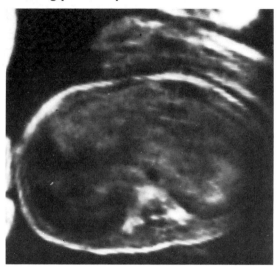

Figure 35–2. RF COIL ARTIFACT. Shown are two transaxial midabdominal MRI sections in a 2-year-old girl with renal failure due to bilateral renal vein thrombosis.

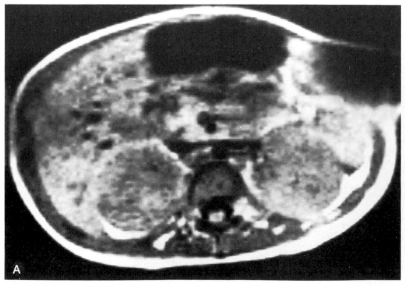

Figure 35–2A. Outward contour distortion and low intensity artifact are seen along the left side.

Illustration continued on opposite page

Figure 35–2B. Inward contour defect and high-intensity artifact of the same anatomic part as in *A* are evident on an adjacent section. The child held her hand in a firm grip around the edge of the RF coil during the study, producing these different artifacts. The hand and distal arm became capacitated and coupled to the coil, which distorted the RF field. The different anatomic details of the hand cause the difference in artifact appearance in neighboring sections.

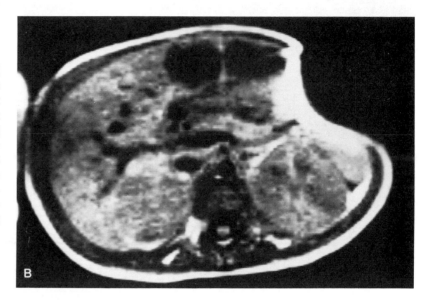

Figure 35–3. METALLIC ARTIFACT. Shown is a transaxial mid-chest MRI section in a 3-year-old boy with transposition of the great vessels. His congenital cardiac malformation has been corrected with a Senning operation. The MR image was made with ECG triggering. A dark, ring-shaped defect is seen in the sternum, with areas of higher intensity *(arrows)* to the right. This artifact is caused by a metallic sternal suture. The low-intensity ring represents the intermediate ferrous material with a very short T_2. The asymmetric high intensity is caused by deformity of the magnetic field gradient produced by the presence of the intrinsic magnetic field of the metal. The linear relationship between signal and mass is distorted so that the signal from a unit of mass is compressed on one side of the metal, producing a high-intensity area, while the opposite effect occurs on the other side.

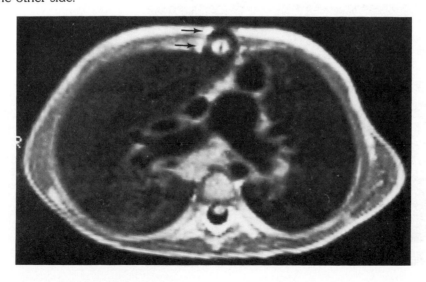

Figure 35–4. METALLIC ARTIFACT. Illustrated are transaxial upper abdominal MRI studies of a 4-month-old boy with a hemangioendothelioma of the pancreas.

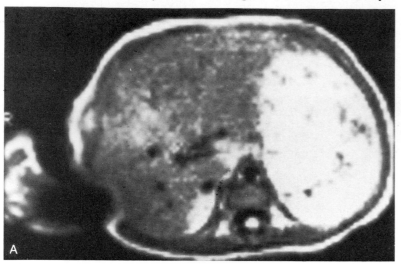

Figure 35–4A. In this section, diluted oral iron solution for positive contrast enhancement of the gastrointestinal tract is seen in the stomach. A low-intensity artifact in right arm and flank areas distorts the contours of both these structures. The artifact is caused by a metallic stopcock on an intravenous line to the patient's right arm.

Figure 35–4B. In this section the artifact is high in intensity, with outward distortion of the arm and inward distortion of the body.

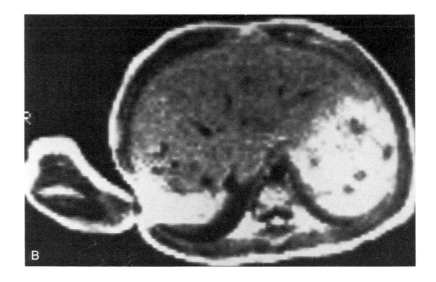

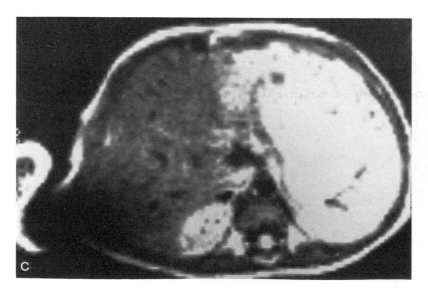

Figure 35–4C. In another section, the artifact is low in intensity with outward distortion of the body and inward distortion of the arm. Artifacts from single metallic objects can result in different appearances in neighboring sections.

Figure 35–5. MULTIPLE METALLIC ARTIFACTS. Shown are MRI studies of the abdomen of a 6-year-old boy with right renal agenesis and left renal hydronephrosis and pelvoureteric obstruction.

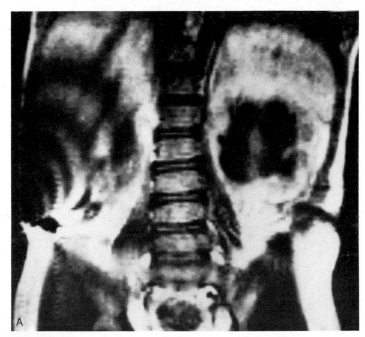

Figure 35–5A. In this coronal image, fan-shaped and diverging zones of alternating low and high intensity radiate from two separate sites. This artifact is caused by two metallic objects (iron eyes of a teddy bear lying on the patient's abdomen). The distortion close to the plane of the two metallic objects shows the artifactual magnetic field superimposed on the linear magnetic gradient as well as the effect of each single metallic object.

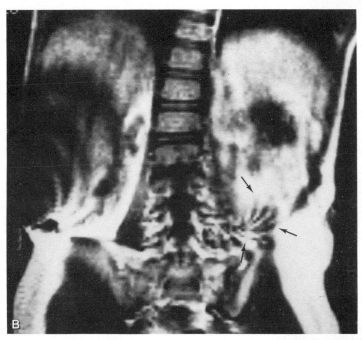

Figure 35–5B. In a coronal section adjacent to *A*, the fan-shaped artifact *(arrows)* to the left of the patient is seen more clearly; the right-sided artifacts are the same. No obvious distortion of the body or organ contours are seen (compare *C*).

Figure 35–5C. In this transaxial midabdominal image, severe body contour distortion and low-intensity artifact are evident along the right side of the body. Again, this artifact is caused by the presence of two metallic objects; however, only distortion of the magnetic gradient such as would be seen with one metallic object is present. The reason for this probably relates to the fact that the plane of the two objects is further away from the image plane than in *A* and *B*.

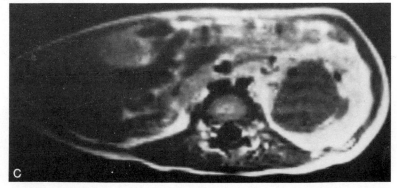

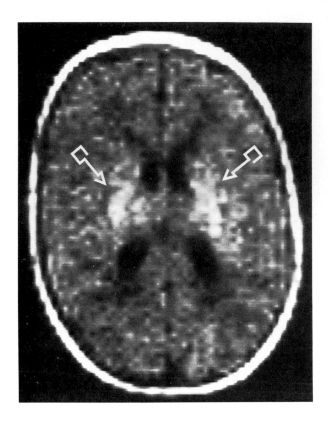

Figure 35–6. NORMAL MYELINIZATION. This transaxial cranial MRI section of a 4-month-old girl born 3 months prematurely is normal. The low-intensity areas of the lateral ventricles are surrounded by symmetric high-intensity areas *(arrows)*. These represent early myelinization of the thalamic region and are not to be misinterpreted as hemorrhage.

Figure 35–7. ARACHNOID CYST. The patient is a 10-year-old girl with minor motor symptoms. In this transaxial MRI section immediately superior to the quadrigeminal cistern, a small, probably congenital, parapineal arachnoid cyst *(arrows)* is seen within the cisternal space. The cyst does not result in obstructive hydrocephalus but is seen to minimally displace adjacent low-intensity, midline venous structures.

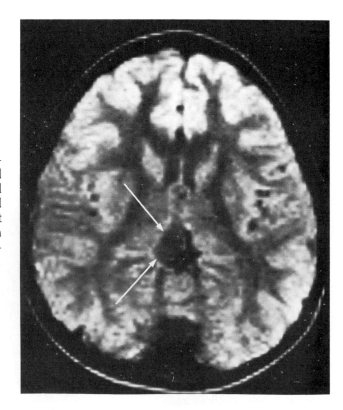

Figure 35–8. INTENSITY VARIATIONS IN VERTEBRAL BODIES. Two transaxial MRI sections of the lower abdomen of a 4-year-old girl are demonstrated. The variable normal appearance of the vertebral column is illustrated.

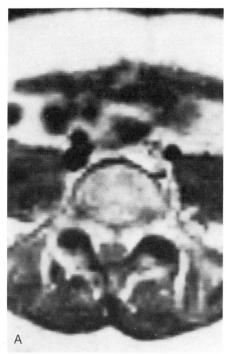

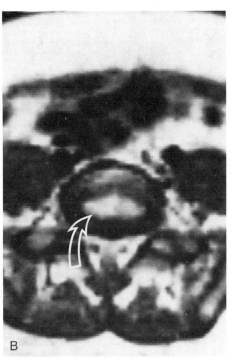

Figure 35–8A. This section through the center of a vertebral body demonstrates a relatively homogeneous area of average high intensity, due to the large quantity of fat in the bone marrow.

Figure 35–8B. A section through the region of the endplate demonstrates the low-intensity nature of cortical bone at this site. The focus of high intensity posteriorly *(arrow)* represents disc material seen in a Schmorl's node. A small area of high-intensity signal anterior to this is the result of partial volume averaging of part of the marrow of the vertebral body.

Figure 35–9. POSTOPERATIVE CHANGES IN THE HEART. Illustrated are two transaxial ECG-triggered MR images of the heart of a 2-year-old boy with a recent surgically corrected stenosis of the right ventricular outflow tract.

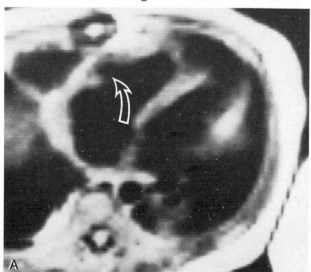

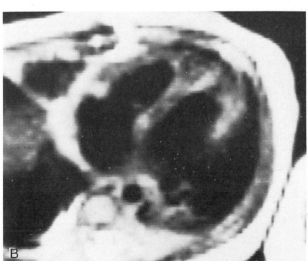

Figure 35–9A. A first echo image demonstrates a low-intensity myocardial area *(arrow)* at the bottom of the right ventricular outflow tract.

Figure 35–9B. The higher mixed intensity on this second echo image identifies the lesion as postoperative edema and hematoma. The findings seen in *A* should not be misinterpreted as a congenital malformation.

Figure 35–10. UMBILICUS. In a transaxial MRI section of the lower abdomen of a 4-year-old girl, the normal appearance of the umbilicus *(arrow)* is illustrated. This image also illustrates the variable intensity that can be seen in pediatric vertebral bodies on MRI. The section is close to the endplate and shows partial volume averaging of the cortical bone, creating a low-intensity ring around the higher-intensity marrow of the vertebral body.

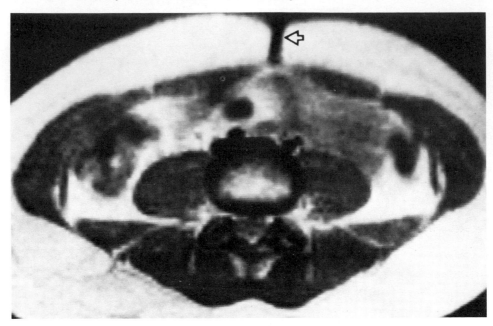

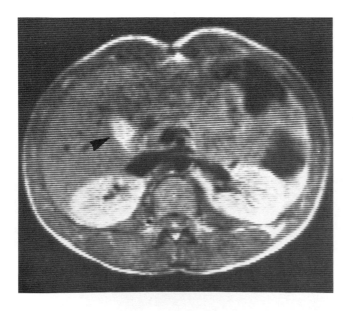

Figure 35–11. NORMAL GALLBLADDER. In this transaxial MRI section through the upper abdomen of a 15-year-old boy with suspected recurrent pheochromo-cytoma, the high-intensity area *(arrowhead)* near the liver hilum is the normal gallbladder and should not be mistaken for abnormal (chromaffin) tissue within the liver.

Figure 35–12. RADIATION CHANGES IN THE LIVER. Shown are two transaxial MR images of the upper abdomen of a 5-month-old boy who had his left kidney removed due to a Wilms tumor. He has received radiation therapy of approximately 1000 Rads to the left renal fossa. The radiation port included portions of the middle and left lobes of the liver.

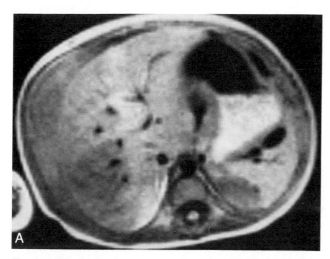

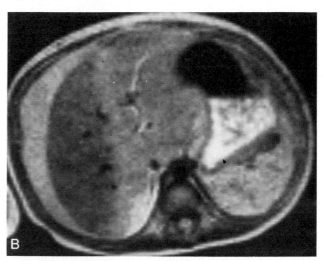

Figure 35–12A. On a first echo image, there is subtle higher intensity of the irradiated liver tissue.

Figure 35–12B. On a second echo image, the higher-intensity irradiated liver tissue is more evident. The increased intensity of irradiated tissue is believed in part to represent edema from the therapy. Ascites (as well as diluted, orally given iron solution for positive contrast enhancement of the stomach) is also visible.

Figure 35–13. THROMBOSIS IN AN ANEURYSM. A and B are first and second echo images of a transaxial MRI section of the lower abdomen of a 4-month-old girl with an acquired aortic aneurysm.

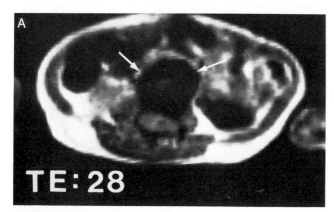

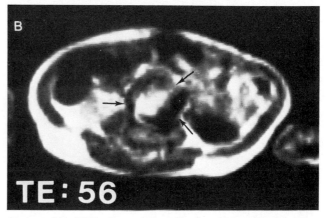

Figure 35–13A. On the first echo image the aortic aneurysm *(arrows)* appears to be of relative uniform low intensity, suggesting normal blood flow.

Figure 35–13B. On a second echo image, high-intensity areas *(arrows)* are identified within the lumen of the aortic aneurysm. These represent areas of slow-flowing blood and thrombosis. As in this case, second echo images are often necessary to diagnose vascular flow abnormalities. The lack of intensity seen on the first echo image should not be interpreted as freely flowing blood of normal velocity.

Figure 35–14. PROXIMAL HUMERAL PHYSIS. Shown is a transaxial upper thoracic MRI section of a 14-year-old boy with Hodgkin's lymphoma and upper mediastinal involvement. The dark line *(arrows)* through the right humerus represents an epiphyseal line. No such line is seen on the left side because of slightly asymmetric positioning, with the plane of the scan below the level of the left humeral epiphysis.

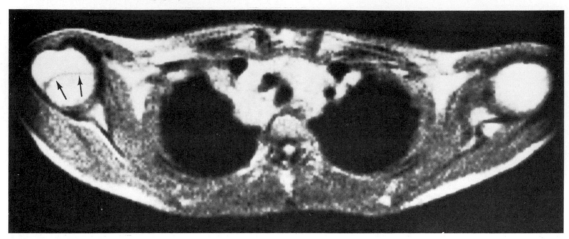

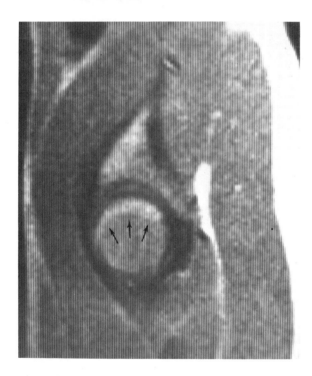

Figure 35–15. FEMORAL EPIPHYSIS. Parasagittal MRI section through the hip of a 15-year-old boy. The epiphyseal line of the femoral head is fused *(arrows)*, but the epiphysis can be seen as higher signal intensity than the metaphysis and the rest of the femoral head. This is a normal finding.

V

MAMMOGRAPHY

Mammography

EDWARD A. SICKLES, M.D.

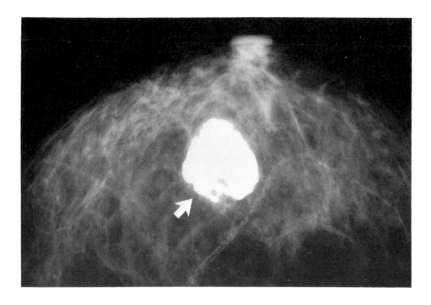

Figure 36–1. DENSELY CALCIFIED FIBROADENOMA. When densely calcified, a fibroadenoma presents on physical examination as a firm, dominant mass that often is thought to be suspicious for malignancy. However, its characteristic mammographic appearance is unequivocally benign *(arrow)*, with confluent calcific densities completely or almost completely obscuring the underlying mass. Biopsy can be averted if the mammographer can verify, by examining the patient, that the mammographic and palpable lesions are the same (see also Figures 36–16 and 36–26). Hematomas and areas of fat necrosis also undergo extensive calcification, similar to fibroadenomas.

Ref.: Sickles EA. Use of breast imaging procedures to avert the biopsy of benign lesions. In: Margulis AR, Gooding CA, eds. Diagnostic Radiology 1983. San Francisco: University of California Press, 1983; pp 423–426.

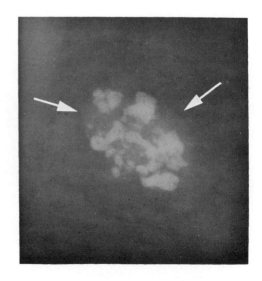

Figure 36–2. FIBROADENOMA: "POPCORN" CALCIFICATION. Partially calcified fibroadenomas can take on a wide variety of mammographic appearances. When calcification occupies only about half the volume of the mass, it often demonstrates this characteristic pattern, resembling that of a piece of popcorn. Portions of the noncalcified margins of the mass usually can also be identified *(arrows)*.

Ref.: Wolfe JN. Xeroradiography of the Breast, 2nd ed. Springfield: Charles C Thomas, 1983; pp 214–255.

Figure 36–3. FIBROADENOMA: EARLY CALCIFICATION. When a fibroadenoma first begins to calcify, most or all of its margins will still be visible, unless obscured by adjacent dense fibroglandular tissues. Calcific particles typically are large (> 0.5 mm) and display a variety of amorphous, often bizarre shapes. Frequently, some of the calcifications are located at the periphery of the mass *(arrows)*, a useful identifying feature. Fibroadenomas undergoing the earliest stages of calcification occasionally are mistaken for carcinoma if their calcifications are so small that they do not yet demonstrate the characteristic features shown here.

Ref.: Hoeffken W, Lanyi M. Mammography: Technique, Diagnosis, Differential Diagnosis, Results. Philadelphia: WB Saunders, 1977; pp 106–112.

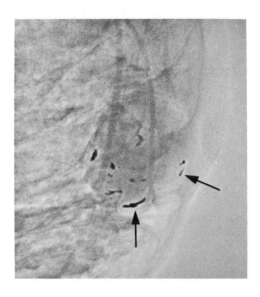

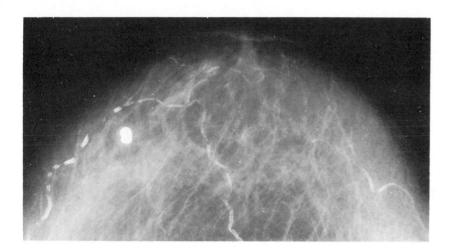

Figure 36–4. EXTENSIVE ARTERIAL CALCIFICATION. Arterial calcification is readily identified when it is extensive, presenting as parallel tracks of calcific density, often in discontinuous segments. The presence of arterial calcification correlates strongly with advancing age and to a lesser extent with coexistent diabetes mellitus. However, its association with diabetes is too weak to be useful clinically, and the only significance that mammographers should ascribe to arterial calcification is that it is unequivocally benign.

Also note the densely calcified fibroadenoma, similar in appearance to but considerably smaller than the lesion shown in Figure 36–1.

Ref.: Sickles EA, Galvin HB. Breast arterial calcification in association with diabetes mellitus: too weak a correlation to have clinical utility. Radiology 1985; 155:577–579.

Figure 36–5. EARLY ARTERIAL CALCIFICATION. In its earliest stages, arterial calcification presents as single discontinuous lines of faint calcific density *(arrows)*, at one edge of an otherwise visible vascular structure. Most examples of arterial calcification are intermediate between early (this example) and extensive (Fig. 36–4) involvement. A typical example of moderate arterial calcification is shown in Figure 36–1.

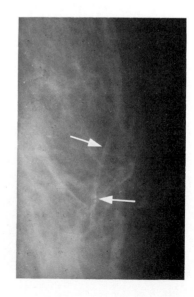

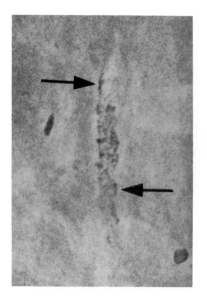

Figure 36–6. ARTERIAL CALCIFICATION SIMULATING CLUSTERED PARENCHYMAL MICROCALCIFICATIONS. Occasionally only one small segment of arterial calcification is visible. This may simulate the mammographic appearance of clustered microcalcifications, suspicious for malignancy, especially when the extent of arterial calcification is very slight (i.e., the tangentially imaged part of the artery does not present with a "line" of calcification) and also when adjacent dense fibroglandular tissues obscure the noncalcified margins of the artery. In such a case, fine-detail magnification mammograms may more clearly indicate the benign vascular nature of the calcification by emphasizing the linear features shown tangentially in the arterial walls *(arrows)*.

Ref.: Wolfe JN. Xeroradiography of the Breast, 2nd ed. Springfield: Charles C Thomas, 1983; pp 457–461.

Figure 36–7. SKIN CALCIFICATION: TYPICAL APPEARANCE. Skin calcifications invariably are benign and usually are somewhat larger than malignant microcalcifications. They are found most commonly along the medial aspects of both breasts, and characteristically are round or oval in shape, with relatively lucent centers. In this example, six skin calcifications are imaged tangentially in the parasternal part of the breast *(curved arrow)*, and another skin calcification projects over the subcutaneous tissues more anteriorly *(wide arrow)*. One more skin calcification, having a lucent center *(thin arrow)*, projects over a cluster of malignant microcalcifications.

Ref.: Wolfe JN. Xeroradiography of the Breast, 2nd ed. Springfield: Charles C Thomas, 1983; pp 386–393.

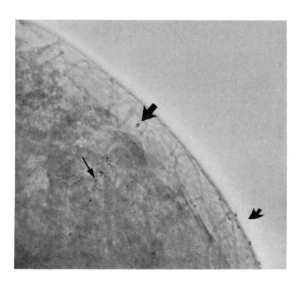

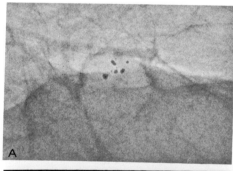

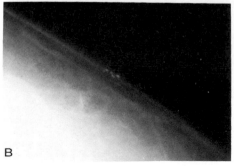

Figure 36–8. SKIN CALCIFICATION: NEED FOR TANGENTIAL VIEW. Occasionally skin calcifications are clustered only in one small area of one breast. In this circumstance they may be mistaken for malignant microcalcifications, especially if they are unusually small, do not show relatively lucent centers, and are projected over areas of breast parenchyma on standard mammographic views *(A)*. Such clusters of calcification will be considered suspicious for malignancy unless an additional mammogram is taken, tangential to the calcific particles, to demonstrate their benign nature by virtue of their dermal location *(B)*.

Ref.: Kopans DB, Meyer JE, Homer MJ, Grabbe J. Dermal deposits mistaken for breast calcifications. Radiology 1983; 149:592–594.

Figure 36–9. AXILLARY DEODORANT PARTICLES SIMULATING CLUSTERED PAREN-CHYMAL MICROCALCIFICATIONS. Zinc and aluminum salts in many underarm deodorants can closely mimic the clustered calcifications of breast carcinoma. This can lead to errors in interpretation, especially if only a small number of deodorant particles are seen, and if they are located so low in the axilla as to overlie the uppermost portions of breast parenchyma *(arrows, A)*. The concavity of the axilla precludes obtaining tangential views to demonstrate the superficial location of the simulated microcalcifications. However, whenever clustered calcific particles are seen in the axillary tail of the breast, one should take a repeat mammogram after the patient has vigorously washed the axilla with soap and water. Some or all deodorant particles will no longer be seen *(B)*, but intramammary calcifications will persist entirely unchanged.

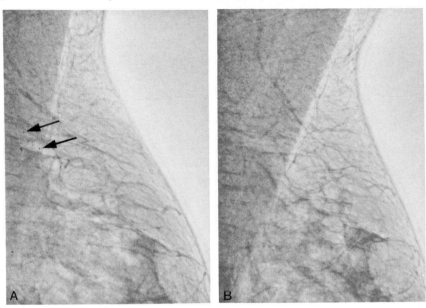

Ref.: Wolfe JN. Xeroradiography of the Breast, 2nd ed. Springfield: Charles C Thomas, 1983; pp 386, 394–397.

Figure 36–10. PARTICLES IN AREOLAR SKIN CREAM, SIMULATING CLUSTERED MICROCALCIFICATIONS. Patients occasionally apply skin creams to the areolar regions of the breast, and metallic particles within the creams may simulate clustered malignant microcalcifications on mammograms, as with axillary deodorants. Note the small size, clustering, and linear, curvilinear, and branching shapes of these skin cream particles, all of which are mammographic features suggesting the presence of carcinoma. The clue to proper diagnosis in this case is the areolar distribution of the simulated calcifications. A repeat mammogram after the areola was washed showed no residual particles of calcific density.

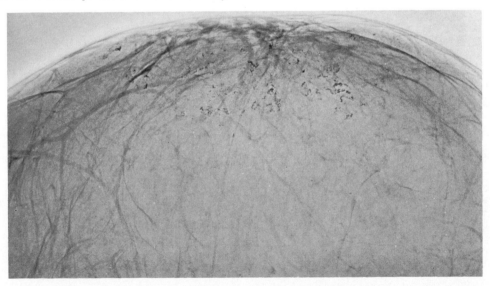

Figure 36–11. MILK OF CALCIUM WITHIN CYSTS: TYPICAL APPEARANCE. Small amounts of milk of calcium settling to the bottom of multiple tiny benign cysts produce the mammographic picture of clustered linear and curvilinear calcifications when imaged in lateral projection with a horizontal x-ray beam. These calcifications, although benign, may be confused with the microcalcifications of carcinoma. However, all of the linear and curvilinear shapes seen with milk of calcium are oriented parallel to the transverse body plane (perpendicular to the lines of gravitational force) on horizontal-beam lateral projection mammograms *(arrows, A)*, but they appear only as poorly defined smudges on vertical-beam craniocaudal projection images *(arrows, B)*: these features are useful in differentiation. Demonstration of calcification shape is crucial to the confident diagnosis of milk of calcium cysts. Magnification mammography usually is needed to provide sufficient image detail.

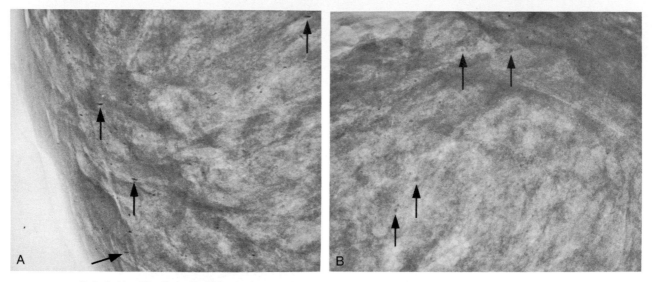

Ref.: Sickles EA, Abele JS. Milk of calcium within tiny benign breast cysts. Radiology 1981; 141:655–658.

Figure 36–12. MILK OF CALCIUM CYSTS: UNUSUAL APPEARANCE. Occasionally milk of calcium will be seen within large benign cysts. Its mammographic appearance is identical to that of tiny cysts, with horizontally oriented, sharply defined linear or curvilinear calcification on the horizontal-beam lateral projection mammogram *(large arrow, A)* and poorly defined smudges of increased density on the vertical-beam craniocaudal projection image *(large arrow, B)*. However, in addition, some or all of the margins of the cyst are seen *(small arrows, A and B)*, with the calcification sedimented at the bottom of the cyst on the horizontal-beam film. Other, more typical, tiny milk of calcium cysts also can be seen *(arrowheads, A and B)*.

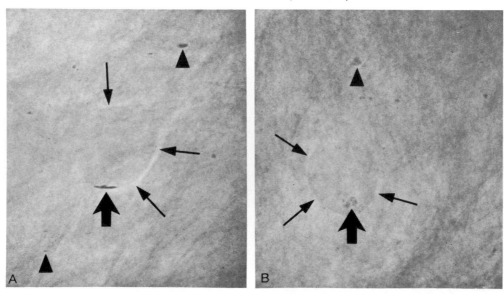

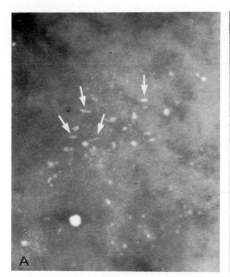 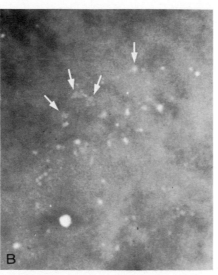

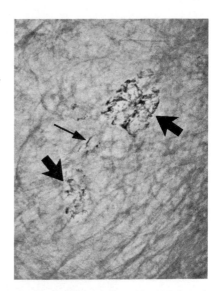

Figure 36–13. MILK OF CALCIUM WITHIN CYSTS, IN ADDITION TO CLUSTERED MICROCALCIFICATIONS. Not infrequently, tiny milk of calcium cysts coexist with clustered parenchymal microcalcifications. Although the milk of calcium collections present characteristic changing mammographic features on lateral *(A)* and craniocaudal *(B)* projection images *(arrows)*, the shapes of the stromal microcalcifications do *not* change with the orientation of the x-ray beam. Despite the presence of typically benign milk of calcium cysts, these lesions should be biopsied to obtain tissue diagnosis for the other, potentially malignant calcifications.

From: Sickles EA, Abele JS. Milk of calcium within tiny benign breast cysts. Radiology, 1983; 141:655–658. Reprinted with permission of the publisher.

Figure 36–15. BENIGN DUCT CALCIFICATION. Benign duct calcifications, otherwise known as secretory calcifications, characteristically are scattered throughout both breasts, demonstrating linear and occasionally branching shapes of wide caliber, indicative of the inspissated secretory debris from which they form. These calcifications usually are 5 to 10 times larger than those associated with malignancy, following the anatomic pattern of the ducts, with their long axes oriented primarily toward the nipple. Some may demonstrate relatively lucent centers. Patients usually are perimenopausal or postmenopausal, and often are found to have plasma cell mastitis if biopsy is done for non-mammographic indications. Only when the calcifications are unilateral, clustered, and unusually small in size will they resemble those of carcinoma, a circumstance encountered very rarely indeed.

Figure 36–14. DYSTROPHIC CALCIFICATION. Following trauma or infection, "dystrophic" calcification may occur within breast tissues. Characteristically, this appears as amorphous sheets of calcification *(wide arrows)*, with relatively large streaks or strands of discrete calcific particles, often associated with focal architectural distortion. When dystrophic calcification forms at a site of previous biopsy, the calcific sheets, streaks, and strands usually follow the plane of surgical incision. Only occasionally may discrete linear dystrophic calcifications simulate those of malignancy *(thin arrow)*, and even then the overall appearance of the lesion usually is clearly benign, because of the typical features of the associated sheets of calcification that almost always are present.

Ref.: Sickles EA, Herzog KA. Mammography of the postsurgical breast. AJR 1981; 136:585–588.

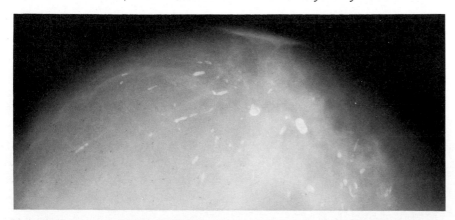

Ref.: Martin JE. Atlas of Mammography: Histologic and Mammographic Correlations. Baltimore: Williams & Wilkins, 1982; pp 196–202.

Figure 36–16. SUPERIMPOSITION OF CALCIFIC PARTICLES, SIMULATING CLUSTERED MICROCALCIFICATIONS. On a lateral projection mammogram *(A)*, a solitary cluster of calcifications was seen in the lower aspect of this patient's breast, an appearance usually considered suspicious for malignancy. However, on craniocaudal projection *(B)*, the calcific particles *(arrowheads)* were non-clustered in distribution, spread out in a track along the medial-lateral axis of the breast. The explanation of this case is that the "calcifications" represented tiny metallic fragments from a previous gunshot injury, the lateral projection mammogram by chance having been taken directly along the path of the wound, thereby causing the bullet fragments to be superimposed onto what seemed to be a cluster of calcifications.

As with Figure 36–25, it is necessary to identify a mammographic lesion on images taken in more than one projection before establishing the presence of a significant abnormality. Unassociated calcifications, like islands of normal fibroglandular tissue, can superimpose on a single image to simulate the presence of a suspicious lesion.

One final note: the large S-shaped calcification *(arrow)* in the central region of the craniocaudal projection image *(B)* represents a bizarre dystrophic calcification (see Figure 36–14) in the upper aspect of the breast, fortuitously superimposed over the track of bullet fragments but unrelated to the gunshot injury.

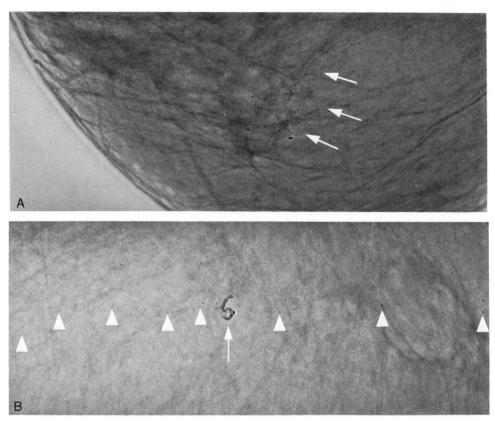

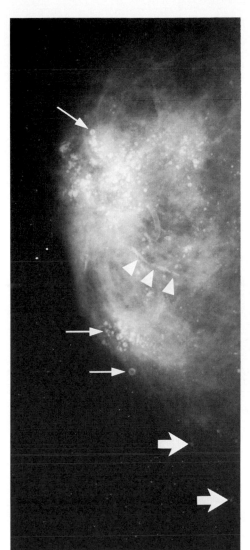

Figure 36–17. MULTIPLE PARAFFIN CALCIFICATIONS/NOD- ULES. Injection of paraffin into the breasts is an augmentation procedure occasionally done in the Far East in Oriental women. Injected paraffin forms smaller nodules than silicone, but induces a much more brisk calcific reaction, producing the characteristic mammographic appearance of bilateral round calcifications, many with relatively lucent centers, distributed throughout the breast tissue *(thin arrows)*. Because of the tendency of paraffinomas to migrate out of the breast to more dependent locations, some of the paraffin calcifications usually are seen in the anterior abdominal wall *(wide arrows)*.

Benign duct calcification *(arrowheads)* also is seen in this patient, similar to that shown in Figure 36–15. It is intriguing to speculate that some of the paraffin was inadvertently injected directly into a duct, producing the calcified ductal cast that now is so clearly seen.

Ref.: Koide T, Katayama H. Calcification in augmentation mammoplasty. Radiology 1979; 130:337–340.

Figure 36–18. FATTY MASS: TYPICAL APPEARANCE. Breast masses that are fatty in composition invariably are benign. A fatty mass surrounded by fatty tissues will be identified mammographi- cally only by its thin fibrous capsule *(arrows)*, even, as in this case, if superimposed over areas of dense fibroglandular tissue. Fatty masses surrounded by dense tissue will appear identical to the numerous fatty lobules seen to varying degrees on most normal mammograms, and will stand out only if considerably larger in size than fatty lobules. The differential diagnosis of fatty masses includes lipoma, fat necrosis, and galactocele, with a history of recent lactation suggesting galactocele and a history of prior trauma suggesting fat necrosis. However, biopsy is not needed to make a specific tissue diagnosis, since all these lesions are benign.

One must remember that areas of fat necrosis, such as the one illustrated, often are palpated as firm masses considered to be suspicious for malignancy. In such cases the mammographer must verify by examining the patient that the mammographic and palpable lesions are the same. Only under such circumstances can mammography be used to avert the biopsy of clearly benign lesions. (Also see Figures 36–1 and 36–26.)

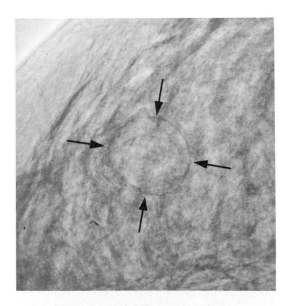

Ref.: Martin JE. Atlas of Mammography: Histologic and Mammographic Correlations. Baltimore: Williams & Wilkins, 1982; pp 251–256.

*Figure 36–19. **INTRAMAMMARY LYMPH NODE: TYPICAL APPEARANCE.*** Intramammary lymph nodes are very common lesions, usually located in the upper outer quadrants of the breasts. Typically, they appear as noncalcified masses up to 8 mm in greatest diameter, round or oval in shape, with smooth and well-defined margins. Although these mammographic features all suggest benign etiology, the intramammary lymph node is identified with certainty only when it demonstrates a radiolucent notch *(arrow)*, representing an area of fatty replacement around the hilus of the node. Occasionally the hilus is imaged en face instead of tangentially, producing a central radiolucent defect.

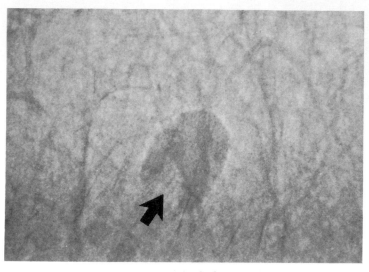

Ref.: Wolfe JN. Xeroradiography of the Breast, 2nd ed. Springfield: Charles C Thomas, 1983; pp 335–342.

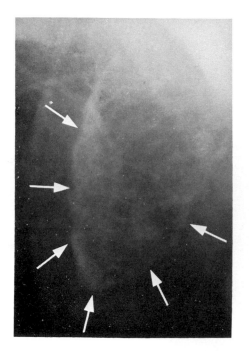

*Figure 36–20. **LYMPH NODE WITH MASSIVE FATTY REPLACEMENT.*** Occasionally a lymph node undergoes massive fatty replacement, usually in response to chronic or repeated episodes of acute infection or inflammation. This is seen most commonly in the axilla but rarely may occur in an intramammary node as well. Such a node is considerably enlarged, typically to more than 2 cm in greatest diameter. Because the node is almost completely replaced by fat, it presents mammographically as a thin crescent of nodal tissue *(arrows)* surrounding a large central fatty zone. This is an unequivocally benign radiographic appearance.

Ref.: Martin JE. Atlas of Mammography: Histologic and Mammographic Correlations. Baltimore: Williams & Wilkins, 1982; p 321.

Figure 36–21. RAISED SKIN MOLE SIMULATING INTRAMAMMARY MASS. Any raised skin lesion, most commonly a benign nevus, will simulate an intramammary mass when it overlies the breast, because air surrounding the margins of the lesion will provide sufficient contrast to indicate its presence (*arrows, A*). The best way to prove the benign nature of such a lesion is by imaging it tangentially and demonstrating its dermal location *(arrow, B)*, since primary breast carcinoma does not originate in the skin. Frequently, standard mammographic projections are not angled so fortuitously as to produce tangential images of a given skin lesion. Under these circumstances the mammographer must either obtain additional specially positioned tangential views or verify by physical examination that the location of the mammographic mass corresponds to that of the skin lesion.

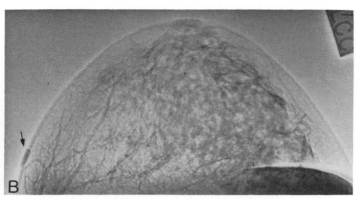

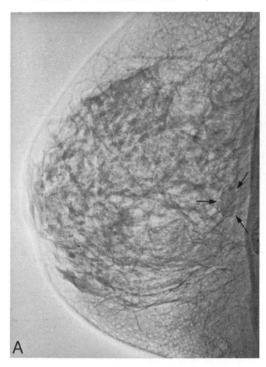

Ref.: Martin JE. Atlas of Mammography: Histologic and Mammographic Correlations. Baltimore: Williams & Wilkins, 1982; pp 301–305.

Figure 36–22. IRREGULAR SKIN LESION SIMULATING INTRA-MAMMARY MASS. If a raised skin lesion is irregular in contour, the mass that it projects over the breast on mammography will be correspondingly irregular in shape. This occurs frequently in women having keloids from prior burns or surgical scars. An even more characteristic appearance is that of raised verrucous lesions, such as the seborrheic (senile) keratosis. Although the finely lobulated, knobby borders of such a mass might be confused with carcinoma, small quantities of air trapped in the interstices between the tiny projections of the skin lesion produce typical mammographic lucencies overlying the mass itself.

Ref.: Wolfe JN. Xeroradiography of the Breast, 2nd ed. Springfield: Charles C Thomas, 1983; pp 367–369.

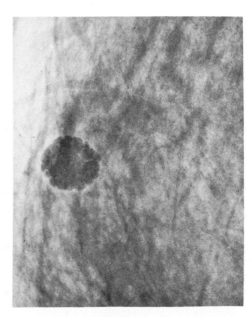

Figure 36–23. NON-RAISED SKIN LESION SIMULATING INTRAMAMMARY MASS. Sebaceous (epidermal inclusion) cysts are cutaneous lesions that do not usually produce externally raised outgrowths. When uncomplicated, such a cyst presents an identical mammographic appearance to the mass shown in Figure 36–21, but with a tangential view showing the mass arising in the skin but bulging into the subcutaneous fat rather than out externally. Occasionally one of these cysts may become infected, in which case there will be an adjacent inflammatory reaction that will make the cyst margins indistinct. Such a lesion may be interpreted as being suspicious for malignancy if it is not imaged tangentially *(arrow, A)* on standard mammographic projections. The clue to proper diagnosis in such a case is the superficial location of the mass on physical examination, since it will be fixed to the skin. Obtaining an additional tangential view *(B)* will demonstrate its true benign nature by demonstrating that it arises in the skin rather than in the breast parenchyma *(arrows)*.

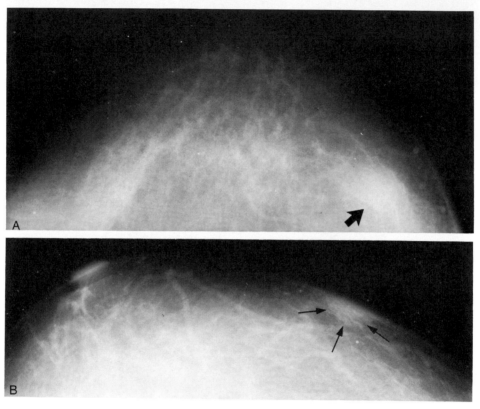

Ref.: Wolfe JN. Xeroradiography of the Breast, 2nd ed. Springfield: Charles C Thomas, 1982; pp 367, 372–381.

Figure 36–24. MULTIPLE SILICONE NODULES. Injection of silicone into the breasts is one type of cosmetic procedure done to augment breast size. Injected silicone collects in multiple small nodules, each of which is surrounded by a foreign-body granulomatous reaction. The resultant mammographic appearance is one of multiple, round, dense masses (silicone is more dense than fibroglandular breast tissue), some of which may demonstrate partial rim calcification *(small arrows)*. Dense confluent areas of injected silicone also may be seen, usually immediately anterior to the chest wall *(large, wide arrows)*. These features do not mimic those of malignancy; rather, they impair mammographic identification of small noncalcified carcinomas, just as the palpable silicone nodules themselves render quite difficult the detection of cancer by physical examination.

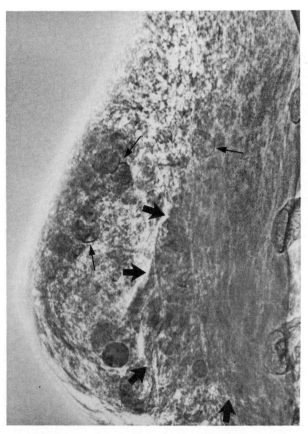

Ref.: Martin JE. Atlas of Mammography: Histologic and Mammographic Correlations. Baltimore: Williams & Wilkins, 1982; pp 330–333.

Figure 36–25. **ASYMMETRIC DENSITY DUE TO SUPERIMPOSITION OF NORMAL STRUCTURES.** On lateral projection mammograms of the left *(A)* and right *(B)* breasts, a vague asymmetric density was seen in the upper aspect of this patient's right breast *(arrow, B)*. No palpable masses were found nor was there any abnormality on either craniocaudal or oblique projection mammograms. The asymmetric "lesion" seen on the lateral projection image resulted from superimposition of islands of normal fibroglandular tissue, a fairly frequent occurrence.

To establish the true presence of an asymmetric mass by mammography, it is necessary first to identify the lesion on images taken in more than one projection; this may well require additional films for clarification. Failure to demonstrate a lesion on more than one projection not only effectively precludes localization for biopsy, but also strongly suggests that the "lesion" represents a summation shadow from superimposed normal breast structures.

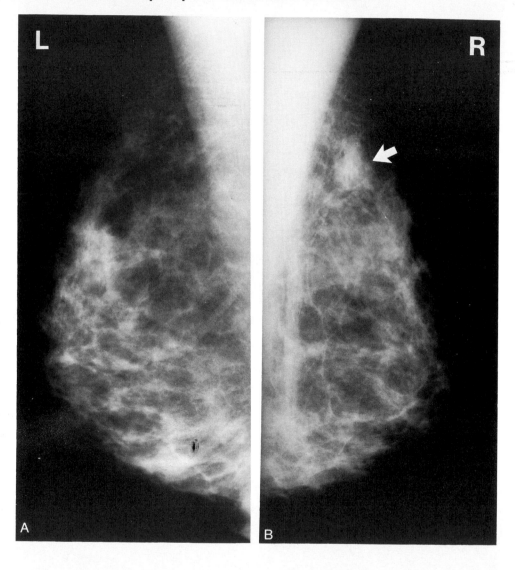

Figure 36–26. MAMMOGRAPHIC LESION IN A LOCATION DIFFERENT FROM THAT OF A PALPABLE MASS. This patient presented with a palpable upper outer quadrant mass but her mammograms demonstrated clustered microcalcifications suspicious for malignancy in a somewhat different location, deep in the central portion of the breast, slightly above and medial to nipple level *(arrows, A and B)*. By carefully examining the patient, the mammographer verified that the palpable and mammographic lesions were *not* the same, prompting biopsy of the suspicious clustered calcifications with the aid of mammographic needle localization. Had this correlative physical examination been omitted, biopsy probably would have been limited to excision of the palpable mass, which turned out to be benign fibroglandular tissue. The suspicious mammographic lesion (intraductal carcinoma) might thus have gone untreated until it grew large enough to become palpable.

Because the shape of the breast is vastly different during physical examination and mammography, the identity or non-identity of palpable and mammographic lesions must not be inferred simply by comparing descriptions of their respective locations. A correlative physical examination is necessary, with mammograms in hand, to plan properly for subsequent treatment. (Also see Figures 36–1 and 36–18.)

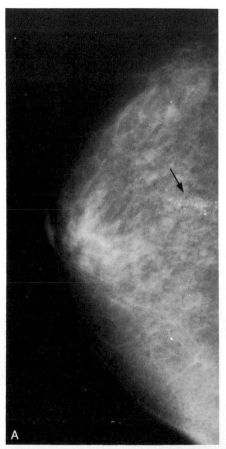

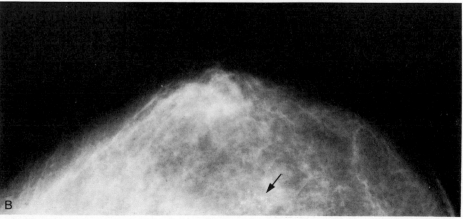

Figure 36–27. NEED FOR COMPRESSION DURING SPECIMEN RADIOGRAPHY. Mammographic visualization of a small spiculated mass, nonpalpable even in retrospect, prompted biopsy of the lesion immediately after mammographic needle localization. A radiograph *(A)* of the uncompressed biopsy specimen failed to indicate clearly whether the mammographic lesion had been removed, but a repeat radiograph *(B),* taken with the specimen flattened out by a standard mammography compression device, verified complete excision of the spiculated mass *(arrow).*

Breast biopsy specimens often have numerous irregular projections extending out in many directions. These projections may obscure visualization of a mammographic lesion, especially a noncalcified mass, by superimposing their own x-ray shadows onto those of the intrinsic lesion. To overcome this potential problem, one should routinely compress all breast specimens to uniform thickness with the same compression device used for mammography, thereby flattening out any confounding contour projections.

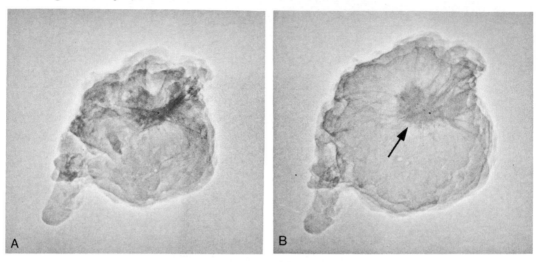

Ref.: Frankl G. Compression in specimen xeromammography. AJR 1978; 130:377–378.

Figure 36–28. GENERALIZED SKIN THICKENING. Generalized skin thickening is readily displayed on mammograms, usually accompanied by coarsening and increased prominence of trabecular markings (Cooper's ligaments). These findings are more apparent when unilateral, seen in comparison with the normal contralateral breast. The differential diagnosis is extensive, ranging from a variety of infectious and inflammatory conditions to congestive heart failure, chronic renal failure, scleroderma, recent prior radiation therapy, lymphoma, leukemia, and of course, locally advanced breast carcinoma. One of the more unusual causes of generalized skin thickening, illustrated, is prior axillary lymph node dissection, which was done in this patient as treatment for an upper extremity malignant melanoma. While it is impossible to make a specific diagnosis among the various possibilities on the basis of mammographic criteria alone, the appropriate past medical history may strongly suggest the correct choice.

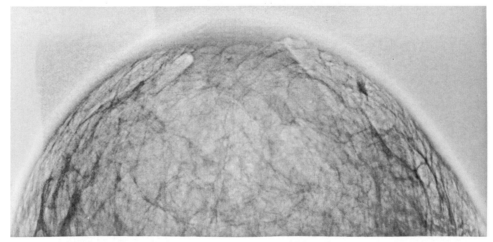

Ref.: Tabár L, Dean PB. Teaching Atlas of Mammography. New York: Thieme-Stratton, 1983; pp 211–215.

Figure 36–29. FOCAL SKIN THICKENING. Focal skin thickening is a nonspecific mammographic sign, usually associated with benign conditions but which occasionally may be seen due to contiguous invasion of the dermis by an underlying primary breast cancer or cross-lymphatic metastasis (medially) from a contralateral carcinoma. The differential diagnosis of benign lesions is not so extensive as for generalized skin thickening but includes localized infection, inflammation, and prior scarring from breast biopsy or blunt trauma. The correct diagnosis often is evident when correlating mammographic findings with those of history and physical examination, as in the case illustrated, in which lateral *(A)* and craniocaudal *(B)* views demonstrate focal skin thickening in the lower inner aspect of the breast *(arrows),* due to a patch of psoriasis in that location.

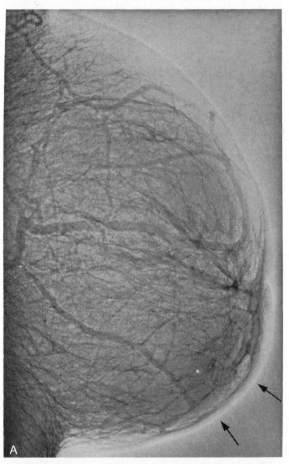

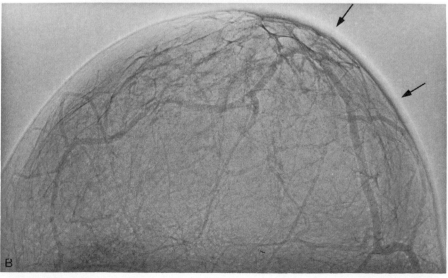

*Figure 36–30. **UNILATERAL VENOUS ENLARGEMENT.*** Asymmetric dilated veins may serve as an indirect indicator of a breast cancer, if locally advanced, by virtue of increased blood flow. However, in such cases the underlying tumor almost always is readily apparent mammographically, so that isolated unilateral venous enlargement usually is considered to be an innocuous finding. Not only do many normal breasts demonstrate such venous asymmetry, but so do breasts with a wide variety of infectious, inflammatory, post-traumatic, and benign neoplastic processes. In the case illustrated, the prominent draining veins *(arrows, A)* represent a normal variant in the breast contralateral to the breast that harbors a large palpable carcinoma *(arrow, B)*.

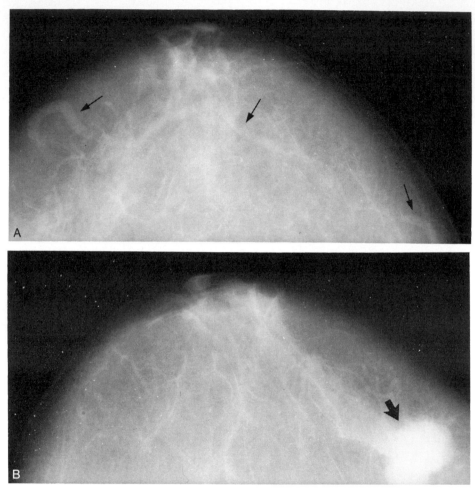

Ref: Martin JE. Atlas of Mammography: Histology and Mammographic Correlations. Baltimore: Williams & Wilkins, 1982; pp 29–31.

VI

DIGITAL
SUBTRACTION
ANGIOGRAPHY
(DSA)

Digital Subtraction Angiography (DSA)

WILLIAM M. KELLY, M.D.

Digital subtraction angiography (DSA) represents the product of relatively recent technologic innovation, even when compared with nuclear medicine, ultrasound, and computed tomography. Yet, somewhat ironically, the "hard-copy" result of a DSA study is an image long familiar to angiographers—a 2-dimensional projection of complex 3-dimensional vascular anatomy. In the past few decades, the general topic of diagnostic angiography relating to interpretation and recognition of normal variants and diagnostic pitfalls has been reviewed extensively in several texts and is beyond the intended scope of this section. Rather, the focus of this chapter is to emphasize the methodologic pitfalls and resulting artifacts intrinsic to DSA that most often compromise subtraction image quality. By necessity, the organization of this chapter differs from the format used in other portions of this book. Herein, the most troublesome aspects of DSA—problems relating to patient preparation, procedural techniques, and post-processing utilization—are emphasized in text form. A variety of techniques are presented that provide the radiologist with methods of avoiding, minimizing, or retrospectively compensating for the adverse effect these problems may have on image quality. Explanatory schemes and practical examples are illustrated to demonstrate limitations and convey specific strategies for optimal execution of different DSA examinations.

GENERAL CONSIDERATIONS

Mask mode (temporal subtraction) DSA has been clinically verified as a convenient, quick, and safe technique for obtaining reliable angiographic results.[1-3] Although early reports emphasized applications in conjunction with intravenous injections of contrast material (IVDSA), more recent experience suggests that this technology will become increasingly pervasive as intra-arterial DSA (IADSA) continues to replace conventional screen-film angiography at many centers.[4-5] At the same time, sophisticated design innovations, including both conventional fluoroscopic components as well as digital devices and computer software, have allowed extension of this modality to an increasing variety of angiographic procedures.

These same technologic advances permit the depiction of much finer spatial detail with state-of-the-art DSA systems, meeting user demands for improved spatial resolution. Moreover, the clinical utility of high-resolution conventional screen-film angiography for both diagnosis and surgical planning for many categories of disease has diminished considerably with the advent of computed tomography (CT) and magnetic resonance imaging (MRI). The availability of these newer modalities has further fueled support for the argument that in many instances DSA is a satisfactory and often desirable alternative to screen-film technique when angiographic evaluation is needed. Furthermore, for interventional procedures such as transcatheter embolization, DSA offers an expedient method of monitoring the progress of a procedure by providing virtually real-time feedback of angiographic results.[6]

Currently, the frequency with which diagnostic DSA results are achieved is seldom limited by inadequate contrast or spatial resolving ability. Instead, a variety of artifacts are usually responsible for suboptimal results. Their presence may obscure diagnostically important vascular detail or even simulate pathology. Major impediments which need to be addressed include (1) image degradation due to patient motion and (2) artifacts related to equipment limitations, particularly video saturation or "bright spots" produced by overstimulation of the television camera.

ARTIFACTS RELATED TO PATIENT MOTION

Many undesirable types of patient motion may occur during a pulsed exposure sequence. The movement of anatomic interfaces of tissues with different radiographic densities (such as bone abutting soft tissue or soft tissue abutting air) may adversely affect DSA image quality. Such motion often becomes patently obvious in the form of image-degrading misregistration artifact when a subtraction image is derived from a selected mask and contrast-laden image pair.

A variety of methods are available for dealing with undesirable effects of motion on DSA image quality. Procedural techniques intended to prevent or limit the occurrence of different types of motion include the use of restraining devices (head/mandibular taping, immobilization devices), abdominal compression, incorporation of a C-arm into the DSA system (thereby minimizing the need for awkward and unsteady patient positioning), psychological reinforcement, and even pharmacologic aids. Still other types of motion may be best dealt with by modification of the image acquisition technique (ECG-synchronized x-ray exposure control, dual energy/hybrid DSA, or temporal bandpass DSA). Finally, a variety of post-processing computer algorithms provides the option of retrospectively attempting to reduce motion artifact by further computer manipulation of the digitized images. These latter techniques, which include remasking and reregistration, may allow the salvaging of diagnostic results from an otherwise unsatisfactory study.

Sensible and effective employment of the maneuvers and techniques mentioned above is predicated on familiarity with the expected type or types of motion likely to impact upon image quality in any given study. Appropriate procedural modifications will, of course, vary with the anatomic region being evaluated. For the purposes of this chapter, it is useful to consider the various types of motion that may occur in terms of their origin and temporal evolution as listed in Table 37–1.

Patient motion can be subdivided into two major types: oscillatory and random (or non-oscillatory). In the case of oscillatory motion, the body or component substructure has a baseline or neutral position (e.g., diastole or expiration), from which it

Table 37–1. Patient Motion Affecting DSA

Oscillatory
Aperiodic
Swallowing
Periodic
Pulsatile vascular activity
Breathing
Non-Oscillatory (Random)
Peristalsis
Alimentary
Ureteric
Skeletal muscle activity
Minor reflex movements
Uncooperative patient/combativeness

undergoes a cyclic excursion. These types of motion are typically initiated by involuntary muscle contraction such as cardiac systole, inspiration, or swallowing and may be further categorized as periodic or aperiodic. Pulsatile vascular activity and breathing are periodic events in that the motion occurs with predictable timing or frequency while the oscillatory motion of swallowing is an isolated and usually unpredictable occurrence. Random or non-oscillatory motion that may interfere with DSA studies includes peristalsis (both alimentary and ureteric) as well as varying degrees of sudden gross skeletal muscle motion.

Oscillatory Motion

Swallowing

Optimal DSA image quality of the extracranial carotid arteries is often denied because of swallowing. Although swallowing artifact may obscure or simulate pathology on selective IADSA studies (Figure 37–1), this impediment poses an even greater challenge when the IVDSA technique is utilized. The sudden delivery of a large bolus (30 to 50 cc) of ionic contrast solution into a central vein followed by a 4 to 6 second exposure delay allows a startled and often unprepared patient ample time to respond predictably with a big "gulp" just as the contrast material is circulating through the cervical arteries.

Simultaneous opacification of all arterial structures in the case of the IVDSA technique requires the use of a steep oblique projection (60 to 70 degrees) in order to avoid superimposition of the vessels of interest. Therefore, if swallowing motion occurs in the time interval between the mask and peak opacified image, it is the carotid artery overlying the larynx which often fails to be visualized adequately because of swallowing artifact. The carotid bifurcation which overlies the cervical spine is generally depicted in profile free of artifact (Figure 37–2).

Prior to any IVDSA study, the patient should be both mentally and physically prepared for the sensations and impulses that will be experienced. Adequate psychological preparation includes emphatically communicating to the patient the overrid-

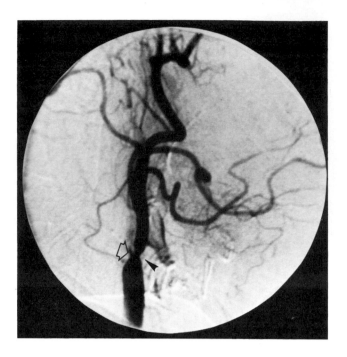

Figure 37–1. MOTION ARTIFACT: SWALLOWING. Lateral cervical view of an arterial injection common carotid DSA. Motion artifact *(arrowhead)* immediately anterior to the carotid bifurcation simulates the appearance of the ulcerative plaque *(open arrow)* present posteriorly.

ing importance of avoidance of swallowing as the single most important *controllable* factor of the entire examination. The importance of this step is supported by the anecdotal observation that the second and any subsequent runs of a DSA examination typically produce superior image quality when compared with the first run. This is due in part to the patient's rapidly acquired familiarity with the procedure and a reduction in apprehension and related motion with further injections.

Various physical maneuvers may also help reduce swallowing motion. Repetitive swallowing 4

Figure 37–2. REMASKING. Oblique IVDSA of neck.

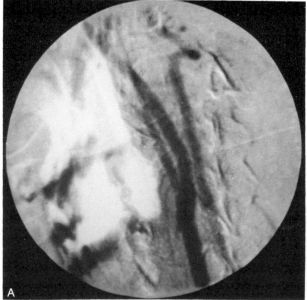

Figure 37–2A. The left carotid and vertebral arteries, superimposed over the stationary spine in this projection, are clearly seen, even though the right-sided vessels are obliterated by swallowing artifact.

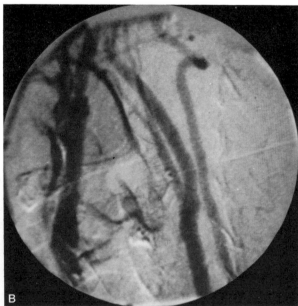

Figure 37–2B. Remasking of same DSA run shown in A. Rather than using the first exposure of the run as a mask, a late phase image, acquired after washout of the contrast material, was substituted. Because the larynx is now in the same anatomic orientation as on the contrast laden image, artifact is dramatically reduced.

or 5 times just prior to each DSA run may significantly reduce this type of artifact by temporarily fatiguing the patient's physiologic ability to initiate the contraction of the hypopharynx which precedes swallowing. In other patients, simple clenching of the teeth on a tongue blade or bite block is useful.

Pharmacologic agents such as viscous lidocaine (2 per cent) dripped over the oropharyngeal mucosa may also be effective in preventing swallowing.[7] If topical anesthesia is used, care must be taken to ensure that the patient fasts completely (no food or liquid by mouth) for several hours before and after the procedure in order to avoid the risk of aspiration.

It is obviously desirable to avoid awkward and uncomfortable patient positioning when performing a DSA study. Unfortunately, the oblique projections required for diagnostic cervical IVDSA results do not permit the patient to remain in a supine, neutral position when single-angle (x-ray tube stationary, beneath the table surface) systems are utilized. Many manufacturers now offer DSA units that feature a flexible C-arm, U-arm, or L/U-arm. These modifications permit rotation of the image axis into an increasing variety of angulations without moving the patient. Additional flexibility is provided by a fully movable table top, which also enables simple adjustment of projectional magnification without changing the image intensifier mode. Most importantly, these newer systems permit the patient to remain in a neutral, comfortable position and thus more likely to cooperate and remain motionless during an exposure sequence (Figure 37–3). Although the multi-angle capability increases equipment costs as well as space requirements, the additional expense can be justified by both improved image quality and reduced examination times.

While considerable effort may be expended in directing patients to avoid swallowing (as well as other types of motion), at least some degree of misregistration is visible on most IVDSA subtraction images. This problem is particularly commonplace in the elderly and seriously ill patients whose IVDSA studies may be further compromised by altered physiology such as low cardiac output, which may lead to reduced contrast resolution. Although little can be done to compensate for problems related to patient physiology, minor degrees of anatomic misregistration can often be retrospectively eliminated by computer manipulation. The two computer operations that have proved most useful for this purpose are known as remasking and reregistration.

Remasking is a post-processing function that allows the operator to select an alternate image pair upon which the computer performs the subtraction process. For many systems, the computer is programmed to automatically designate the image corresponding to the first x-ray exposure pulse as the "non-contrast" image. A series of subtraction images are then generated by subtracting this initial mask image from contrast-laden images acquired during the passage of the contrast bolus through vessels within the radiographic field. This procedure is inappropriate, however, for the relatively common situation wherein motion such as swallowing occurs during the beginning of the exposure series yet terminates just prior to arrival of the contrast bolus. Under these circumstances, remasking (designating a late phase post-washout image as the mask) will often reduce motion artifact in the reprocessed subtraction image (see Figure 37–2).

Reregistration, or pixel shifting, is another technique that involves computer-assisted manipulation of two separate digital images. The goal is to electronically restore the anatomic orientation of tissue that was disturbed because of intervening motion. Either automatically or under operator control, X and Y axis shifts (or translations) between the two images are made in subpixel increments until the desired subtraction effect is achieved. For minor degrees of misregistration, this method is easily implemented and consistently delivers improved image quality.

Unfortunately, ensemble reregistration often fails to salvage diagnostic quality results when dealing with DSA examinations marred by gross swallowing artifact. This is due in part to the complex three-dimensional movements associated with swallowing. X and Y axis reregistration of a two-dimensional projection is often inadequate in restoring anatomic alignment. Furthermore, the motion of swallowing is confined to the soft tissues (and laryngeal air column) of the anterior neck, and compensatory reregistration is ideally restricted to this area. The latter problem can be addressed by region-of-interest (ROI) algorithms that effectively limit pixel shifting to an operator-designated area (Figure 37–4).

Breathing

The undesirable effect of respiratory motion on DSA image quality can of course be avoided when a cooperative patient is able to stop breathing during a typical 10 to 15 second exposure sequence. Respiration should be consistently suspended in the mid-expiratory phase in order to provide reproducible results for "repeat" runs. The patient should be reminded not to perform a Valsalva maneuver, especially preceding an IVDSA, as this may adversely affect the bolus dynamics of contrast injections and thus reduce contrast resolution.

Some patients, especially children and elderly subjects, may not follow instructions or may find the situation anxiety-provoking and fail to restrict ventilation. Still other patients may be physically incapable of interrupting ventilatory effort for more than a few seconds due to either acute or chronic pulmonary disease. For such patients, rapid expo-

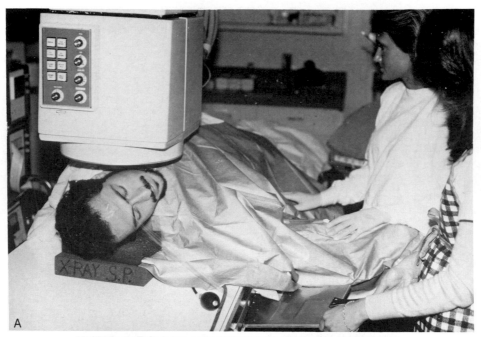

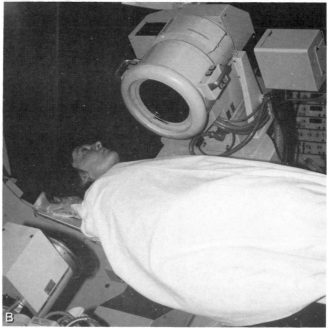

Figure 37–3. EQUIPMENT. Comparison of single angle *(A)* and more flexible C-arm *(B)* image axes. One of the many advantages of the more expensive configuration shown in *B* is the ability to avoid time-consuming delays due to repositioning and stabilizing the patient for different projections. A comfortable patient in a neutral position is considerably less likely to move during a DSA run.

sure rates (4 or more per second) improve the likelihood of a satisfactory result by increasing the selection of raw images available for remasking. Subsequent selection of an image pair in phase with the oscillatory motion of breathing may produce a more satisfactory subtraction. In patients who happen to be intubated for general anesthesia or other reasons, mechanical ventilation may usually be safely interrupted during the exposure series.

Pulsatile Vascular Activity

Misregistration artifact related to cardiovascular activity occurs when the mask and contrast-laden images happen to be exposed during different phases of the cardiac cycle. A large gradient of tissue density at the interface of the pulsatile structure and bordering tissues serves to enhance the visibility of such misregistration. These conditions

Figure 37–4. REREGISTRATION.

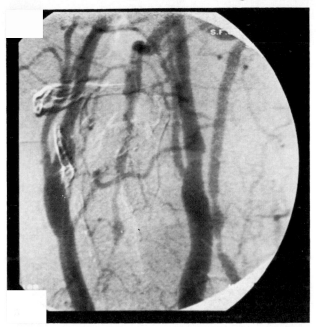

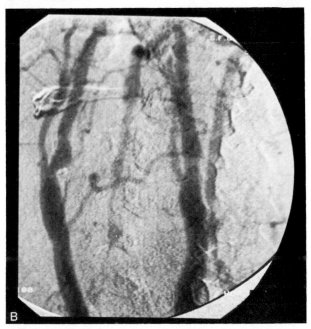

Figure 37–4A. Mask mode IVDSA image of cervical vessels shows diagnostic clips and vascular detail; motion artifact obscures the right internal carotid artery origin.

Figure 37–4B. Reregistration by ensemble pixel shifting eradicates the motion artifact visible in A but causes blurred misregistration of other vessels.

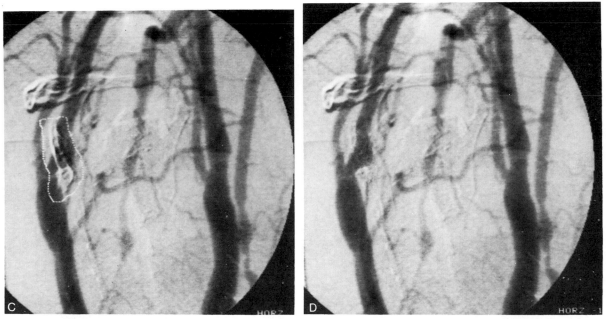

Figure 37–4C and D. Region-of-interest reregistration may be limited to the area enclosed by the oval *(C)*, resulting in improved visibility of all vessels in the field on a single image *(D)*.

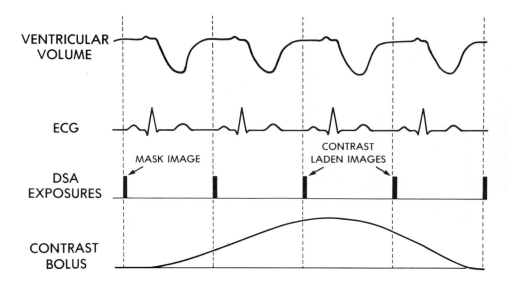

VENTRICULAR VOLUME

ECG

DSA EXPOSURES — MASK IMAGE — CONTRAST LADEN IMAGES

CONTRAST BOLUS

Figure 37–5. ECG-SYN-CHRONIZED DSA. Exposure pulses are under computer control and keyed by the R-wave of a patient's ECG. A trigger delay places each exposure in late diastole, capturing the heart and large arteries at their moment of least activity, thereby ensuring acquisition registration of pulsatile structures.

are most prevalent in the thorax (large pulsatile vessels bordering aerated lungs) but may also be significant in other fields such as the neck, where pulsating carotid plaques may contain calcium bordering the less dense soft tissues. In any case, the degree of artifact that may be produced is worsened by a greater amplitude of oscillatory motion. Hence, physiologic factors such as hypertension or aortic regurgitation may further aggravate this problem.

A teleologically appealing way to avoid or minimize motion artifact caused by pulsatile vascular activity is through the use of ECG-synchronized DSA exposure control. This method involves inter-

facing the patient's ECG signal to a computer-controlled x-ray generator. A software program calculates the average time interval between cardiac contractions and allows each x-ray exposure pulse to be "keyed" on the patient's R-wave. Ideally, at least one exposure is made in late diastole (the period of least cardiac motion) of each cardiac cycle (Figure 37–5). Thus each exposure is obtained "in phase" with the patient's cardiac cycle, allowing acquisition registration of pulsatile structures.

ECG-synchronized DSA may be used to help avoid the poor edge definition and vessel blurring that are often apparent on non-ECG gated subtrac-

Figure 37–6. ECG SYNCHRONIZATION FOR VASCULAR PULSATIONS.

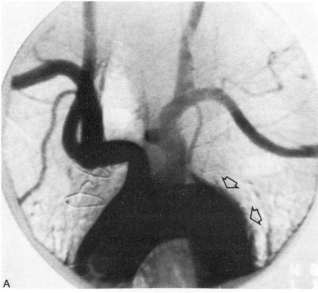

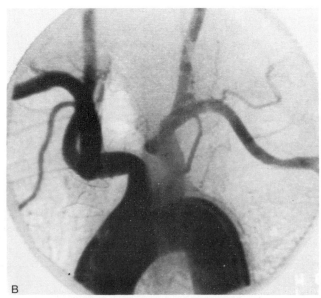

Figure 37–6A. DSA image was obtained without benefit of ECG synchronization. Note motion artifact at the aortic margin *(arrows)* and in lung fields due to pulsatile vascular activity.

Figure 37–6B. Improved image, in the same patient, was obtained with ECG-synchronized acquisition. Note the sharp edge definition at the aortic margin and the absence of vessel misregistration in lung fields.

tion images of the aortic arch (Figure 37–6).[10] This technique may also dramatically improve the quality of pulmonary angiograms that are otherwise difficult to perform satisfactorily using DSA equipment.

The pulsatile motion of calcified carotid plaques may hinder accurate quantitation of stenotic lesions or diminish the visibility of an associated intimal ulceration. Either of these problems can be substantially reduced with the aid of ECG-synchronized image acquisition (Figure 37–7).

Random Motion

Peristalsis

A number of factors can reduce the diagnostic quality of abdominal IVDSA studies. These include an often inadequate field of view, poor opacification of small vessels, limited spatial resolution, and motion artifacts. The use of IADSA technique in combination with a wide field-of-view image intensifier can help circumvent many of these problems

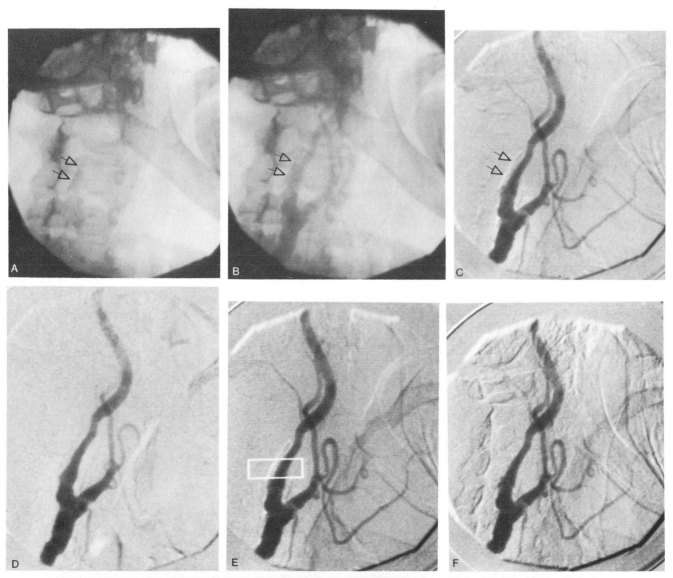

Figure 37–7. ECG GATING FOR IMPROVED REGISTRATION. Series of DSA images illustrates advantages of ECG-gated exposures for improved registration of calcified carotid plaque. Raw mask image *(A)* and contrast-laden image *(B)* show the location of calcium within the plaque and its relation to the vessel lumen *(arrows).* "Ungated" subtraction *(C)* shows misregistration of plaque *(arrows)* due to pulsatile motion occurring between the mask and raw image. *D* is an artifact-free "gated" subtraction image of the same lesion. In *E* and *F*, selective reregistration of ungated DSA (indicated by the rectangle in *E*) results in introduction of undesired misregistration along nonvascular interfaces.

From: Kelly W, Gould R, Norman D, et al. ECG-synchronized DSA exposure control: Improved cervicothoracic image quality. AJNR 1984; 5:429–432. Reproduced with permission.

and thereby extend the diagnostic utility of this modality for visceral angiography. However, peristaltic activity, the major source of motion artifact in the abdomen, may continue to obscure vascular detail. Although peristalsis of the urinary tract is by no means insignificant, alimentary contractions usually prove to be more troublesome. The following techniques have proved useful for dealing with bowel gas motion.

1. *Binding*: A cloth binder is strapped across the patient's abdomen and tightened so as to displace air-containing bowel to the periphery of the field. Thus, peristaltic activity may continue to occur, but away from and not overlapping the major vascular structures of interest. This method should be avoided in patients suspected of having an abdominal aortic aneurysm for obvious reasons.

2. *Prone Positioning*: Turning the patient into a prone position is functionally similar to binding in that aerated bowel is again displaced away from the center of the abdomen. In addition, gas within the transverse colon is reduced by the effect of gravity.[8] This maneuver is somewhat inconvenient and is feasible only when vascular access is gained from the upper extremity.

3. *Pharmacologic Intervention*: 1 mg of glucagon injected intravenously renders the bowel as well as ureters hypotonic within minutes. Clinical studies have documented the efficacy of this drug for reducing bowel gas motion on abdominal DSA studies.[9] Although the use of glucagon for this purpose generally appears safe, caution should be exercised to avoid the use of this drug in patients with a possible pheochromocytoma or insulinoma.

Skeletal Motion

Prior to each DSA run, it is worthwhile to spend a few moments reiterating to the patient the need to remain motionless during the exposure series. Small degrees of body motion related to minor or unintentional movements may be further diminished by ensuring that the patient is in a comfortable position. As mentioned earlier, a flexible C-arm–mounted image axis helps achieve this goal. A head cushion and table pad should also be used to help reduce patient discomfort, particularly when lengthy procedures are involved.

Additional benefit can be realized by the application of adhesive tape, Velcro strips, or other immobilization devices designed to help restrict patient motion.[11] Such techniques are especially useful for cervical or cerebral studies in which slight motion of the jaw, spine, or cranium may result in annoying artifacts. This step may help avert the need for reregistration following these commonly performed studies.

For persistent minor degrees of misregistration, pixel shifting may at times help confirm or rule out the presence of an otherwise equivocal finding

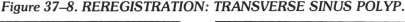

Figure 37–8. REREGISTRATION: TRANSVERSE SINUS POLYP.

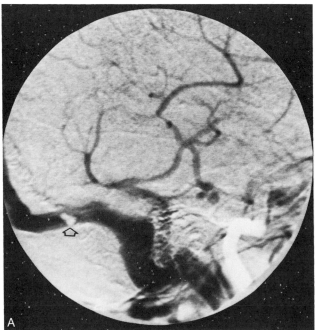

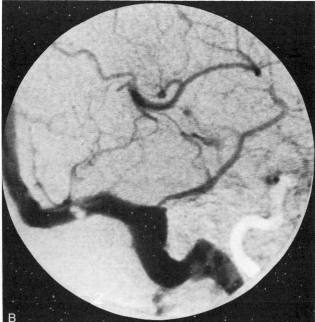

Figure 37–8A. Venous phase lateral cerebral DSA. The apparent filling defect *(arrow)* within the transverse sinus cannot be clearly separated from overlying misregistration of the lambdoidal suture, caused by patient motion.

Figure 37–8B. Reregistration of a remasked subtraction image eradicates all motion artifact, enabling confirmation of the normal variant polyp within the transverse sinus.

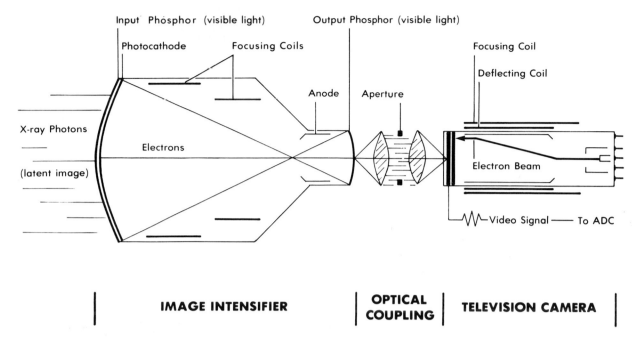

Figure 37–9. DSA INSTRUMENTATION. This is a diagrammatic illustration of the photoelectronic instrumentation responsible for signal transfer in the "front-end" of a typical DSA system. The television camera usually has less dynamic range compared with other components of the imaging chain and may produce annoying and sometimes confusing artifacts known as video saturation and cutoff. (ADC = analog-to-digital convertor.)

(Figure 37–8). More commonly, this maneuver serves to merely improve the esthetic appearance (and hopefully, diagnostic quality) of a subtraction image. The objection that reregistration may help elucidate findings obscured by motion artifact in one portion of an image and yet introduce potentially confusing misregistration artifact in other portions of an image is tenable under two conditions: (1) the motion at fault is a local phenomenon (including swallowing and blood vessel pulsations) confined to only a portion of the image, and (2) ensemble pixel shifting is used. Utilization of newer techniques such as ECG gating or region-of-interest reregistration (see Figures 37–4 and 37–5) may help circumvent these problems.

Patients who are extremely uncooperative may not be suitable candidates for DSA. Some of these patients are better studied with screen-film technique. Exceptions might include situations such as an aneurysm search in an intubated, struggling patient. In that clinical setting, we have used paralytic agents such as Pavulon (administered by an anesthesiologist) to induce a transient period of inactivity, enabling artifact-free diagnostic results.

ARTIFACTS RELATED TO EQUIPMENT LIMITATIONS

Conventional angiographic images are obtained in a direct and relatively simple fashion using a screen-film device to record the latent x-ray image after the attenuated beam exits the patient. DSA instrumentation is comparatively complex, utilizing a series of sophisticated photoelectronic devices (including image intensifier (II), television (video) camera, and analog-to-digital convertor (ADC)) to sequentially detect, intensify, read, and digitally convert the signal information that ultimately contributes toward a subtraction image. These functions are represented schematically in Figure 37–9. Ideally, each of the components should be properly matched in terms of performance capabilities in order to ensure that signal information is accurately processed with minimal introduction of artifact. In this regard, the weak link in DSA imaging chain is typically the television camera. Most video cameras currently in use are not capable of faithfully recording the full range of light intensities that may be produced by the image intensifier. This limitation results in the introduction of annoying artifact known as either saturation or cutoff (at either extreme), caused by failure of the television camera to accurately discriminate excessively bright or dim light levels. The presence of this type of artifact represents one of the most frustrating problems of DSA, perhaps second only to motion artifacts. A basic understanding of the function and limitations of the television camera in DSA enables one to easily recognize saturation and cutoff artifacts, helping to avoid potentially serious diagnostic errors. Such knowledge also permits one to make quick and accurate decisions regarding relatively simple compensatory maneuvers that may eliminate the underlying problem.

Television Camera: The "Weak Link" in DSA

Saturation or cutoff video artifacts are manifest on DSA images because of normal variations in tissue density and body thickness that exist within a radiographic field. In order to more fully understand the problem at hand, it becomes necessary at this point to discuss several technical points. Let us briefly consider the transfer of signal information, beginning with pulsed radiation that has been variably attenuated by the anatomical field interposed between the x-ray tube and II. A latent image (spatially dependent variation in photon flux) representing a two-dimensional projection of the patient's body part is already contained in space. Operator-dependent choices (selection of kVp, mA, and exposure time) have already impacted on image contrast and potential for video camera artifact. As this burst of radiation strikes the input phosphor (cesium iodide) of the II, visible light is produced with intensity proportional to the number of impingent x-rays. An "intensified" visible light image (due to both acceleration and minification gain) is presented at the output phosphor of the II.

An optical coupling system with an iris diaphragm (for variable aperture settings) focuses the image from the output phosphor of the II onto the target assembly of the video camera. Contained within the target are numerous tiny deposits of photoconductive material (such as lead monoxide in plumbicon tubes) imbedded in an insulating matrix. As light impinges on the target, tiny dots (or domains) are discharged of electrical charge. The higher the light intensity, the more the domain is discharged. These domains act as tiny capacitors and in assemblage attempt to faithfully record the two-dimensional image presented by the output phosphor of the II. In order to "read" the image information recorded, a pencil-like beam of electrons is focused on the target material. The function, then, of this electron beam is to recharge the target material, and during this recharging process a small current signal is generated proportional to the amount of discharge in the target domain and hence proportional to the intensity of light that impinged on the target element.

When the intensity of visible light from the II becomes excessive, the tiny domains in the target are over-discharged. As this occurs, the electrons focally deposited in a rapid sweep of the target by the electron beam are quantitatively insufficient to completely fill in the over-saturated areas. Because a full-scale current (signal) is generated, detection of iodinated contrast material within a blood vessel lumen is reduced or lost entirely over the corresponding area on subtraction images. The role of the video camera in the production of saturation and its effect in subtraction images is illustrated diagrammatically in Figure 37–10. The effects of saturation carry over into subsequent video frames, and the artifact may bleed into an even larger area.

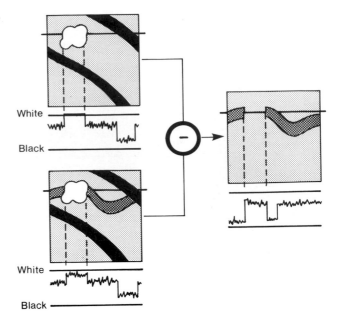

Figure 37–10. VIDEO CAMERA SATURATION ARTIFACT. In a schematic representation of the source of video camera saturation artifact, the hypothetical radiographic fields at left (mask, *top*; contrast-laden, *bottom*) depict bone as black, air as white, soft tissue as light gray, and contrast opacified blood vessel as dark gray. Locally excessive x-ray penetration through air-containing structures (such as the larynx) generates a full-scale (white) video signal even when overlapping an iodine-filled vessel lumen. At such a location, the subtraction image *(far left)* may show "subtraction" of the overlapping segment. (Courtesy P. Vonbehren, Livermore CA.)

Conversely, when the intensity of visible light emitted from portions from the II is very low, a negligible video current is generated. This phenomenon tends to occur in portions of the image which are under-penetrated (e.g., over dense cortical bone such as the petrous apices or orbital roofs) and is known as cutoff. Under such circumstances, an even lower level of x-ray penetration on a subsequent exposure due to iodinated contrast material coursing within the lumen of a blood vessel cannot be accurately recorded by the video camera. This occurs because video levels over the dense anatomy are already near zero (black) prior to the arrival of contrast material. An artifact not too dissimilar to that produced by saturation may then occur, as shown in Figure 37–11.

Video Camera Saturation ("Bright Spots")

Saturation artifact occurs most frequently on subtraction images when dealing with anatomic fields that incorporate a wide variation in tissue density, especially those including air. Hence, common sites include the paranasal sinus region, larynx, lungs, and over abdominal bowel gas. For

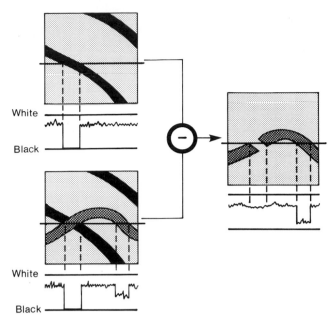

Figure 37–11. VIDEO CAMERA CUTOFF ARTI-FACT. This drawing describes schematically the source of video camera cutoff artifact (same gray scale/anatomic key as in Figure 37–10), a phenomenon that is essentially the opposite of saturation. Very low (black) video levels at sites of dense bone *(top left)* or metallic density cannot be registered below scale when iodine-filled blood vessel overlaps *(bottom left)*. Because negligible but nearly identical video levels are produced, the overlapping segment is subtracted. (Courtesy P. Vonbehren, Livermore CA.)

similar reasons, difficulty may be encountered when attempting to resolve superficial vascular anatomy such as the superior sagittal sinus (because of its proximity to air). In most cases, recognition of saturation artifact poses no special problem when large anatomic areas are involved or the configuration of homogeneously bright subtraction artifact which locally obscures blood vessels corresponds to a known anatomic structure. Selection of exposure factors in the appropriate range, guided by test exposures, coupled with adjustment of light levels by changing the iris diaphragm setting (done automatically on many systems), helps avoid gross degrees of subtraction artifact on most DSA runs.

Persistent small areas of saturation artifact may initially be difficult to recognize on DSA images, particularly by an inexperienced observer. Besides obscuration of normal and abnormal anatomy, the potential for artifactually simulated pathology, due to video camera saturation, may exist. For instance, the common carotid DSA study shown in Figure 37–12 shows what on initial inspection (in Figure 37–12A) appears to be nearly total occlusion of the proximal external carotid artery due to a thick plaque. However, examination of a later image of this same run (Figure 37–12B), after washout of contrast material, shows what is clearly recognizable as saturation artifact (over a portion of the

larynx) corresponding to the "plaque" suggested earlier in the run. Such artifact is easy to recognize because of the "bleeding" effect mentioned earlier, and its visibility is further enhanced by viewing the subtraction image at relatively narrow window settings.

The presence of saturation artifact may generate additional confusion when therapeutic procedures are performed, such as transcatheter embolizations (Figure 37–13). In such cases, it is imperative that saturation artifact, when present, be quickly recognized and accurately distinguished from cutoff artifact or embolic material lodged within a vascular channel.

It would obviously be desirable, during any DSA procedure, to prevent the occurrence of saturation artifact. However, merely reducing radiographic technique or increasing the F-stop of the iris diaphragm, although effective, is not an acceptable solution. These approaches will lead to inadequate x-ray penetration and/or low video levels, in turn leading to poor contrast resolution and cutoff artifact. Actually, the need to compensate for variations in tissue density is not unique to DSA. The use of bolus bags or simple wedge filters has been common in both conventional angiography as well as tomography for years. However, the need for a more precise and convenient method of density compensation in DSA was not accurately anticipated and planned for by the manufacturers, resulting in considerable user disappointment in the early years of DSA use.

Maneuvers that may be employed to compensate for the significant variations in tissue density include (1) increasing the kVp of the x-ray beam (with an appropriate reduction in mAs), (2) the use of added filtration positioned centrally in the x-ray beam path, and (3) attenuation devices positioned within the x-ray beam at sites corresponding to less dense anatomic regions.

Increasing the kVp of the x-ray beam may be effective up to a limit. The increased average keV of the beam reduces the relative contribution of photoelectric effect to beam attenuation (with a relative increase in Compton scatter); hence radiographic contrast (and demand for dynamic range of the DSA components) is less. Placing added filtration (typically a sheet of aluminum 2- to 4-mm thick or equivalent thickness of brass or copper) in the central path of the beam produces a similar result by absorbing predominantly low-energy photons likely to undergo photoelectric interactions. The average keV is also increased. If copper is chosen, it is advisable to use aluminum backing in order to absorb the very low energy (9 keV) characteristic x-rays, which would otherwise considerably increase patient skin dose without adding information. Relative disadvantages of these two techniques are the associated increases in radiographic technique required as well as diminished iodine resolution.

Many angiographers attempt to avoid saturation by positioning any of a variety of readily available attenuating materials within or around the field being examined. Such objects might include plastic bags filled with saline, flour, or even Vaseline. Lead apron material may be cut into strips or curves to correspond to the border of patient anatomy. Such efforts are usually followed by a series of test exposures and repeat adjustments until the desired effect is produced. These methods have several important disadvantages. First, time-con-

suming delays may jeopardize patient safety (this is particularly important with carotid or cerebral studies); second, patient radiation exposure may be unnecessarily increased, depending upon where the attenuation material is placed and how many test exposures are made; and third, devices lacking smooth transitions at their margins (beveled edges) may cause misregistration on subtraction images.

Perhaps the most attractive means of dealing

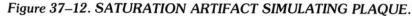

Figure 37–12. SATURATION ARTIFACT SIMULATING PLAQUE.

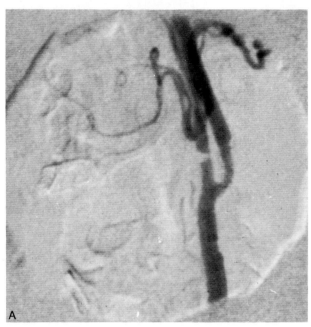

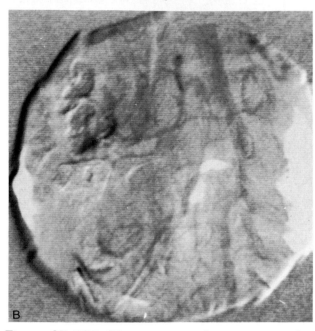

Figure 37–12A. In this common carotid IADSA, the apparent plaque causing critical stenosis of the proximal external carotid artery is not in fact present. Rather, it is simulated by saturation artifact from the overlapping air-containing larynx.

Figure 37–12B. The presence of saturation artifact *(bright spots)* is clarified on this late phase subtraction image displayed at a narrow window setting.

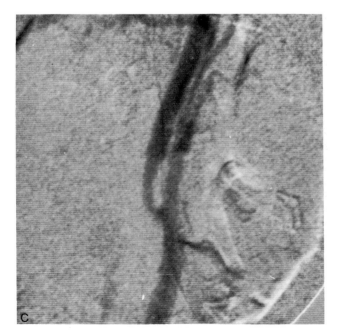

Figure 37–12C. Normal appearance of the same external carotid artery is shown on a subsequent run in the opposite projection.

Figure 37–13. SATURATION ARTIFACTS SIMULATING EMBOLI.

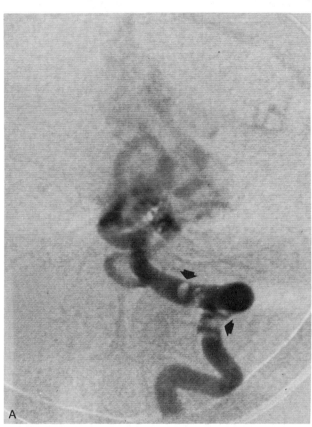

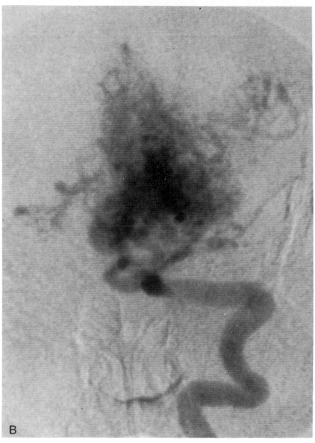

Figure 37–13A. Transfacial DSA was made immediately following embolization of a posterior fossa arteriovenous malformation. The "filling defects" (arrows) within the vertebral artery represent saturation artifacts (over-penetration through paranasal sinuses) and not embolization particles, as might have been feared.

Figure 37–13B. Repeat DSA performed immediately after the run shown in A with a beam attenuation device (dish filter) in place eliminates this potentially confusing artifact.

From: Kelly W, Brant-Zawadzki M, Norman D, Gould R. Beam attenuation devices for digital subtraction angiography. Radiology 1984; 153: 817–818. Reproduced with permission.

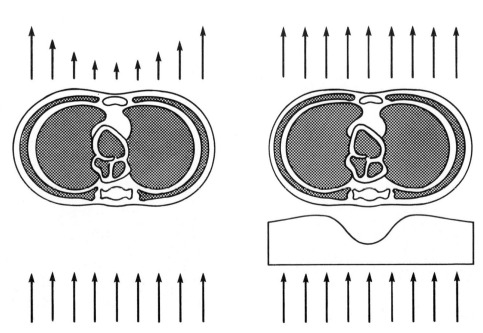

Figure 37–14. FIELD-EVEN-ING FILTERS. Beam attenuation devices, or filters, are designed to compensate for the uneven x-ray penetration that occurs because of varying tissue density and thickness. A relatively flat exit beam helps to avoid saturation artifacts.

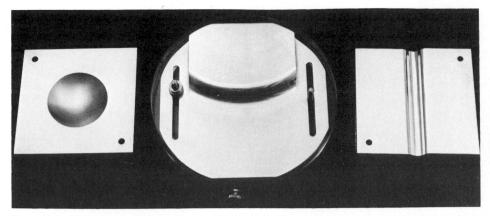

Figure 37–15. VARIABLE THICKNESS FILTERS. Variable thickness aluminum beam attenuation devices are designed for DSA. *Left,* trough filter; *center,* curved plateau filter attached to a Plexiglas mount (note the ability to adjust the position of plateau transition in the radial direction); *right,* dish filter.

From: Kelly W, Brant-Zawadzki M, Norman D, Gould R. Beam attenuation devices for digital subtraction angiography. Radiology 1984; 153: 817–818. Reproduced with permission.

Figure 37–16. EFFECT OF FILTERS ON IMAGE SIGNAL. Test exposure images were obtained before *(A)* and after *(B)* placement of the dish filter. The image and histogram shown in *A* (obtained without benefit of a filter) indicate saturation (relative over-penetration) in less dense portions of the field. Note the more uniform brightness levels and avoidance of saturation achieved with the filter in place.

From: Kelly W, Brant-Zawadzki M, Norman D, Gould R. Beam attenuation devices for digital subtraction angiography. Radiology 1984; 153: 817–818. Reproduced with permission.

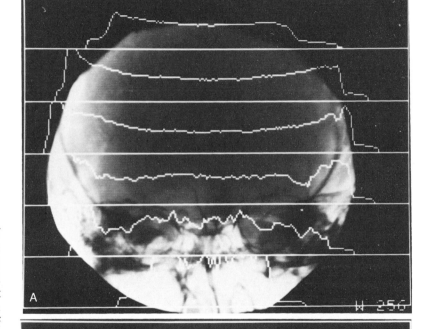

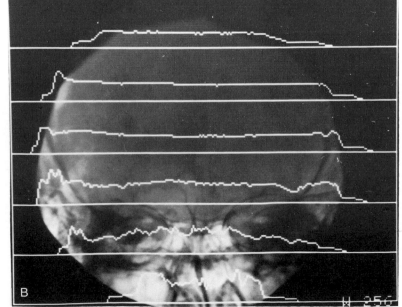

with the potential for saturation artifact is the use of an aluminum filter specifically designed and contoured to compensate for variable attenuation of the x-ray beam through a given anatomic field. For instance, a trough filter might be ideally suited for a DSA study of the aortic arch. The thin trough region of the filter, when properly aligned with the spine, would serve to normalize the exit beam before it reaches the image intensifier, a concept schematized in Figure 37–14. The clinical efficacy of a dish-type filter for eradication of saturation artifact and its value in the performance of cerebral DSA procedures are demonstrated in Figure 37–13B.

A set of several aluminum filters with beveled margins and smooth gradations in thickness can be designed and constructed to deal with a variety of angiographic fields. The three devices shown in Figure 37–15 would suffice for most commonly performed DSA procedures, and were in fact used with uniformly satisfactory results in over 200 DSA examinations.[12] Their design is simple, and their versatility is augmented by a custom Plexiglas mount that can be quickly attached to the x-ray tube housing and that allows for both rotational and radial adjustments. The additional design feature of smooth beveled edges is desirable to avoid visible misregistration of a filter if image reregistration is used in a post-processing fashion.

After selection and placement of a beam atten-uation device, a histogram of digital pixel values from an initial empirical test exposure is a useful adjunct for rapidly determining ideal exposure and/or aperture settings (Figure 37–16). This function is provided on most DSA units and consists of a bar graph display depicting the relative distribution of brightness levels (digital values) stored in the image matrix. The shape of an "ideal" histogram is not the same for different radiographic fields; however, as a general rule, one strives to adjust exposure factors and add filtration or attenuation devices so as to produce a histogram that occupies a relatively broad range of brightness levels centered near middle intensity.

Video Camera Cutoff

The test shot procedure and histogram analysis that precedes each DSA run, as described earlier, forms a basis for selection of radiographic technique and is also a useful tool in assessing the need for field compensation. Skillful use of beam attenuation devices similar to those shown in Figure 37–15 can help avoid saturation as well as cutoff. The "fine tuning" accomplished with the aid of these instruments is designed to ensure that the image intensifier sees a relatively uniform (compensated) radiographic field (Figure 37–17). At the same time, a

Figure 37–17. USE OF FILTERS FOR OPTIMAL IMAGES.

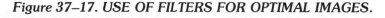

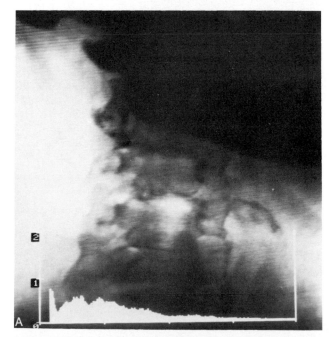

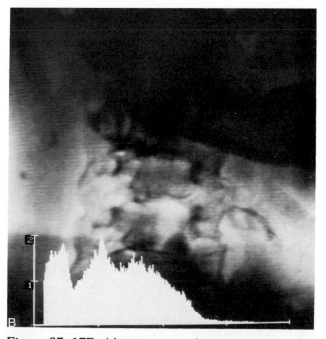

Figure 37–17A. DSA test exposure of neck was taken prior to IVDSA. As evident on the image and as depicted on the histogram, saturation is present over less dense portions, whereas the tissues over the cervical spine are underpenetrated.

Figure 37–17B. After insertion of an aluminum trough filter between the patient and x-ray tube (and after increasing exposure factors), the level and range of x-ray transmittance are optimized for this DSA study.

certain minimum level of photon flux must be maintained, typically 1 mR per image, in order to achieve satisfactory signal-to-noise levels (contrast resolution). Therefore, the iris diaphragm of the optical coupling mechanism between the image intensifier and video camera (see Figure 37–9) is adjusted so that video levels throughout each raw image are of intermediate brightness when using the target range of x-ray flux. Cutoff can result from generally inadequate x-ray flux or an excessively constricted iris diaphragm. More commonly, cutoff occurs focally within a radiographic field because of insufficient x-ray penetration through extremely dense structures that cannot be realistically compensated for using the methods described earlier. This important concept is illustrated diagrammatically in Figure 37–11. When video levels are already near zero in one portion of a mask image due to focally dense anatomy, there is little if any dynamic range remaining for faithful and proportionate de-

Figure 37–18. VIDEO CUTOFF ARTIFACT SIMULATING VASCULAR SPASM.

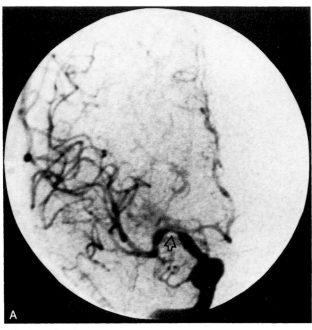

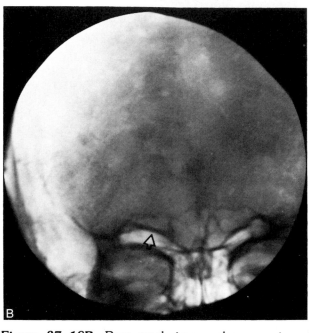

Figure 37–18A. Cerebral DSA shows segmental "narrowing" *(arrow)* of the proximal M1 segment of the middle cerebral artery, suggesting vascular spasm.

Figure 37–18B. Raw mask image shows a rim of dense cortical bone *(arrow)* (marginating aerated frontal sinus), which overlaps the segment of "spasm" in the middle cerebral artery, raising the possibility of cutoff artifact.

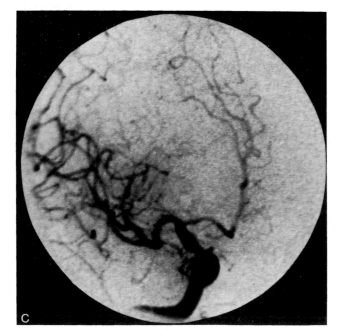

Figure 37–18C. Repeat DSA of same vessel with oblique positioning minutes later excludes spasm and supports the conclusion of focal cutoff artifact accounting for findings seen on the anteroposterior projection.

tection of even less x-ray penetration caused by an overlapping contrast opacified vessel. At such an overlapping site, video levels of the mask and contrast-laden image may be nearly identical (both close to zero), resulting in disappearance of this segment of the blood vessel when the subtraction process is performed.

Intrinsically hyperdense cortical bone within a radiographic field is usually responsible for the varying degrees of cutoff which are either too difficult or too impractical to totally eliminate with beam attenuation devices and exposure factor adjustments. The resulting subtraction artifact is depicted as a "faded," poorly seen, or "absent" segment of a blood vessel. For instance, cutoff artifact commonly limits the visibility of the intrapetrous portion of the carotid artery on cerebral DSA studies or the portion of the aortic arch superimposed over the spine on oblique thoracic aortograms. A more challenging problem is encountered when a narrow cortical margin, such as an orbital rim, only partially overlaps a blood vessel lumen. Under these conditions, recognition of cutoff artifact can be difficult,

as the subtraction image may misleadingly represent the blood vessel as focally narrowed or even simulate the appearance of spasm (Figure 37–18).

Metallic substances ranging from foreign bodies such as bullet fragments and shrapnel to iatrogenic densities, including dental amalgam, surgical clips, aneurysm clips, wires, and plates, also rank as frequent causes of cutoff artifact. It is important to fluoroscopically note the location of any such densities that may overlap blood vessels, as cutoff artifact is an inescapable result, owing to the extreme density of most metal alloys. Knowledge and anticipation of this potential problem is the key to avoiding diagnostic mistakes. Hard-copy photographs of selected raw images are also important to obtain in addition to subtraction images. Thus, one can correlate the location of any metallic density (or bony ridge) with the presence of any confusing vascular findings that may be attributable to cutoff artifact (Figure 37–19). Accurate documentation of these potential relationships (by photographing at least one raw image from each run) is especially important in DSA because, unlike screen-film an-

Figure 37–19. METALLIC ARTIFACT SIMULATING VASCULAR STENOSIS. Cutoff artifact from metallic aneurysm clip in a patient treated for anterior communicating and pericallosal aneurysms.

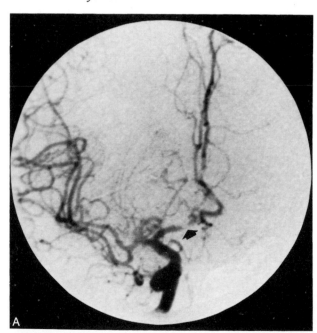 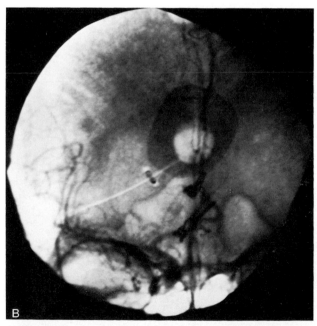

Figure 37–19A. The distal A1 segment *(arrow)* of the right anterior cerebral artery is obscured by video cutoff artifact. Although normal dynamics of blood flow into both distal anterior cerebral arteries mitigates the likelihood of stenosis, the origin of this artifact is difficult to ascertain without benefit of clinical history. The excellent subtraction of background structures (including potential sources of cutoff artifact) serves to emphasize the importance of photographing at least one raw image from each DSA run.

Figure 37–19B. Unsubtracted raw image clarifies the source of cutoff artifact (aneurysm clip).

Figure 37–20. CUTOFF ARTIFACT FROM AN ANEURYSM CLIP. This series of DSA studies illustrates cutoff artifact from an aneurysm clip that has been suboptimally placed, encroaching on the lumen of the parent vessel.

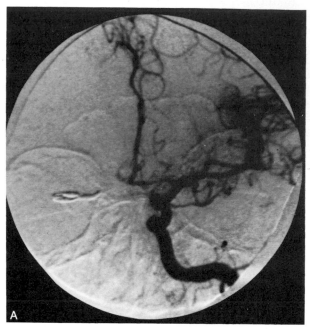

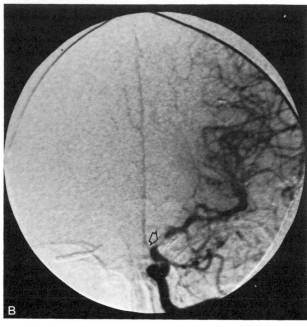

Figure 37–20A. Preoperative DSA. A right middle cerebral artery aneurysm has been previously clipped. Visualization of the metallic vascular clip is made possible due to motion artifact. The patient also has a left posterior terminal carotid aneurysm, not visible on this projection. Note the patency of the anterior cerebral artery.

Figure 37–20B. Postoperative DSA. Cutoff artifact *(arrow)* obscures the terminal carotid artery. However, occlusion of the left anterior cerebral artery (with a corresponding neurologic deficit) in conjunction with slow middle cerebral artery flow (determined from the series) indicates an excessively tight clip. The midline vessel extending superiorly is the anterior artery of the falx, originating from the ophthalmic artery.

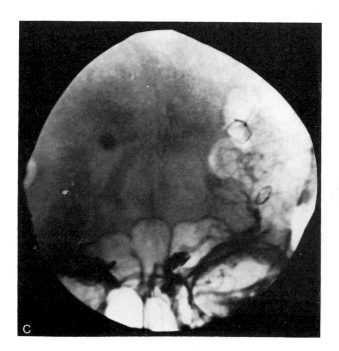

Figure 37–20C. Unsubtracted view showing position of aneurysm clip.

giography, permanent unsubtracted images are not automatically produced. Furthermore, in the absence of motion artifact, DSA obfuscates recognition of various metallic densities or anatomic interfaces because of the extremely precise subtraction process that may totally eliminate any evidence of otherwise telling contours (see Figure 37–19).

Cutoff artifact may coexist with and obscure, or even simulate, an important overlapping vascular finding that is in fact present. This confusing situation is depicted in Figure 37–20, which shows cutoff artifact from an aneurysm clip. Both the artifact and the clip encroach upon the lumen of the terminal carotid artery. That the clip has been positioned too tightly around the parent artery of the aneurysm can be deduced only by noting the altered circulatory dynamics visible distally when comparing the pre- and postoperative studies.

Acknowledgment: The author would like to thank Ms Connie Davis for her secretarial assistance and manuscript preparation.

REFERENCES

1. Chilcote WA, Modic MT, Pavlicek A, et al. Digital subtraction angiography of the carotid arteries: A comparative study in 100 patients. Radiology 1981; 139:287–295.

2. Christenson PC, Ovitt TW, Fisher HD III, et al. Intravenous angiography using digital video subtraction: Intravenous cervicocerebrovascular angiography. AJNR 1980; 1:379–386.

3. Strother CM, Sackett JF, Crummy AB, et al. Intravenous video arteriography of the intracranial vasculature: Early experience. AJNR 1981; 2:215–218.

4. Brant-Zawadzki M, Gould R, Norman D, et al. Digital subtraction cerebral angiography following intra-arterial contrast injection; comparison with conventional angiography. AJNR 1982; 3:593–599.

5. Kelly W, Brant-Zawadzki M, Pitts LH. Arterial injection–digital subtraction angiography. J Neurosurg 1983; 58:851–856.

6. Sherry RG, Anderson RE, Kruger RA, Nelson JA. Real-time digital subtraction angiography for therapeutic neuroradiologic procedures. AJNR 1983; 4:1171–1173.

7. Sider L, Mintzer RA, Deschler TW, et al. Control of swallowing by use of topical anesthesia during digital subtraction angiography. Radiology 1983; 145:563–564.

8. Seigel RS, Williams AG. Efficacy of prone positioning for intravenous digital angiography of the abdomen. Radiology 1983; 148:295.

9. Rabe FE, Yune HY, Klatte EC, Miller RE. Efficacy of glucagon for abdominal digital angiography. AJR 1982; 139:618–619.

10. Kelly WM, Gould R, Norman D, et al. ECG-synchronized DSA exposure control: Improved cervicothoracic image quality. AJNR 1984; 5:429–432.

11. Enzmann DR, Freimarck R. Head immobilization for digital subtraction angiography. Radiology 1984; 151:801.

12. Kelly WM, Brant-Zawadzki M, Norman D, Gould R. Beam attenuation devices for digital subtraction angiography. Radiology 1984; 153:817–818.

Index